Medical Radiology

Diagnostic Imaging

Series Editors

A. L. Baert, Leuven
M. F. Reiser, München
H. Hricak, New York
M. Knauth, Göttingen

Medical Radiology

Diagnostic Imaging

Emmanuel E. Coche

Benoît Ghaye

Johan de Mey

Philippe Duyck (Eds.)

Comparative Interpretation of CT and Standard Radiography of the Chest

Foreword by

A. L. Baert

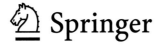 Springer

Emmanuel E. Coche
Department of Medical Imaging
Cliniques Universitaires St-Luc
Avenue Hippocrate, 10
1200 Brussels
Belgium
emmanuel.coche@uclouvain.be

Benoît Ghaye
Department of Medical Imaging
University Hospital of Liege
B35 Sart Tilman
4000 Liege
Belgium
bghaye@chu.ulg.ac.be
and
Department of Medical Imaging
Cliniques Universitaires St-Luc
Avenue Hippocrate, 10
1200 Brussels
Belgium
benoit.ghaye@uclouvain.be

Johan de Mey
Department of Radiology
AZ-VUB
Laarbeeklaan 101
1090 Brussel
Belgium
johan.demey@az.vub.ac.be

Philippe Duyck
Department of Radiology
UZ-Gent
De Pintelaan 185
9000 Gent
Belgium
philippe.duyck@uzgent.be

ISSN: 0942-5373

Additional material to this book can be downloaded from http://extra.springer.com

ISBN: 978-3-540-79941-2   e-ISBN: 978-3-540-79942-9

DOI: 10.1007/978-3-540-79942-9

Springer Heidelberg Dordrecht London New York

Library of Congress Control Number: 2010937977

Cover design: eStudio Calamar, Figueres/Berlin

Printed on acid-free paper

Springer is part of Springer Science+Business Media (www.springer.com)

Foreword

Although standard radiography of the chest has limitations, it still remains the first and basic radiological diagnostic modality, which is very frequently used in daily clinical practice.

The three-dimensional (3D) information on the organs of the chest, which became available by the introduction of CT, has revolutionized our knowledge of the anatomy and pathology of the chest and the modern management of chest diseases. But, in addition, CT, by virtue of producing cross-sectional as well as reformatted 2D and 3D images of the thoracic organs, offers an exquisite new approach to provide new insights and skills in the interpretation of standard radiography of the chest.

E. Coche and his co-authors, all internationally well-known chest radiology experts, have been very successful in producing this excellent comprehensive overview of chest radiography interpretation by means of side-by-side comparative presentation of chest standard radiographies and corresponding CT images.

The judicious selection and superb technical presentation of the numerous illustrations, as well as the accompanying well-written and easily readable text, makes this book an indispensable tool not only for all certified radiologists and radiologists in training, but also for pneumologists, intensive care and emergency specialists as well as for chest surgeons. It will assist them efficiently in solving the day-to-day problems in standard chest radiography interpretation. I can guarantee them that this book will not remain idle on their book shelves.

I am very much indebted to the editor and his co-authors for their brilliant performance and I am confident that this outstanding volume will meet a great success with the readership of our "Medical Radiology – Diagnostic Imaging" series.

Leuven   Albert L. Baert

Preface

The first chest radiography was obtained more than 100 years ago. Despite Computed Tomography (CT) revolutionizing diagnostic thoracic imaging 30 years ago, chest radiography still remains one of the most performed imaging modality in radiology worldwide, due to low costs, low radiation and wide availability. Chest radiographs are obtained for detection, diagnosis and follow-up of many forms of thoracic diseases, evaluation of chest trauma, and many other conditions including screening purposes.

Its interpretation is notoriously difficult and needs to receive a careful attention for teaching and learning. With the advent of multi-slice CT scanners (MDCT) enabling isotropic reconstructions and high-quality reformats, new tools are available for both radiologists and clinicians for re-interpreting chest radiographs in light of orthogonal views or additional planes.

The concept of this book was imagined in 2008, just after a successful symposium dedicated to a "side-by-side comparison with MDCT" that we held in Brussels. The idea was to provide a comprehensive approach of chest diseases using a direct comparison between the old two-dimensional technology and the up-to-date three-dimensional technology of MDCT. In collaboration with Belgian and international experts in chest radiology, we have elaborated the content of this book on three different parts. The first part summarizes clinical indications and technical aspects of chest radiography and CT with emphasis on reconstructions and tools for image comparison. The second part is related to the semeiology of normal variants and diseased chest using an anatomically based classification. The third part deals with some diseases presenting a peculiar aspect on chest radiography.

This book is designed for radiologists, internists, pneumologists, surgeons and acute unit physicians involved in the care of patients with chest diseases, and students who want to improve their understanding in chest radiography. At the end of this book, a link to a web site containing additional clinical cases is available for the most curious readers.

Brussels

Emmanuel E. Coche
Benoit Ghaye

Acknowledgements

We wish to thank the following individuals for their assistance in bringing this book to publication: Françoise Martin, secretary in the Department of Medical Imaging, Cliniques Universitaires St-Luc (UCL) in Brussels, Walter Rijsselaere, secretary in the Department of Radiology, Universitair Ziekenhuis (VUB) in Brussels.

Contents

Part I

Introduction

Chest Radiography Today and Its Remaining Indications

1

Emmanuel E. Coche

Contents

E.E. Coche
Department of Medical Imaging, Cliniques Universitaires
St-Luc, Avenue Hippocrate, 10, 1200, Brussels, Belgium
e-mail: emmanuel.coche@uclouvain.be

Abstract

› Today, chest radiography remains the cornerstone for the diagnosis of many pulmonary diseases but it has received less attention during the past several years due to the explosion of new imaging techniques. However, chest radiography has many advantages. It offers simplicity, low cost, low radiation, large amounts of information, and is widely available throughout the world.

› In this chapter, the remaining indications for the use of chest radiography in adults will be discussed in the context of MDCT. In pneumonia, chest radiography plays a pivotal role in the initial evaluation and follow-up of patients. In immunocompromised patients, chest radiography should be considered as a screening test and will often be followed by MDCT. In the intensive care unit (ICU), chest radiography can be easily performed to detect malposition of medical devices, but difficult cases still will be assessed by MDCT. In the emergency room, chest radiography is the recommended initial imaging study for the patient, and its results will often initiate additional imaging examinations such as MDCT. Chest radiography is also the most commonly used imaging tool for follow-up of benign conditions such as pneumothorax, pneumonia, pleural effusion. Its role in the follow-up of malignant conditions is less obvious. At the end of the chapter, the role of chest radiography in lung cancer screening, assessment of preoperative patients, and daily follow-up will be discussed.

E.E. Coche et al. (eds.), *Comparative Interpretation of CT and Standard Radiography of the Chest*,
Medical Radiology, DOI: 10.1007/978-3-540-79942-9_1, © Springer-Verlag Berlin Heidelberg 2011

1.1 Introduction

Despite continuous advances in cross-sectional imaging, chest radiography remains the cornerstone for the diagnosis of many pulmonary diseases and the most commonly performed diagnostic imaging test in western countries and probably throughout the world. This imaging modality is responsible for approximately 30–40% of all X-ray examinations performed, regardless of the level of health care delivery. International commission on radiological protection (ICRP 1993). Over the period of 1993–1999, chest radiography was the most frequently used radiologic examination in the United States (Maitino et al. 2003). In many instances, it is the first–and frequently the only–diagnostic imaging test performed in patients with a known or suspected thoracic abnormality. In various clinical situations, chest radiography will be performed first and its results will dictate complementary investigations (Figs. 1.1 and 1.2). However, some serious chest diseases can present as normal chest radiographs in the early stages, and sometimes even at more advanced stages. This point will be discussed in 'further detail in Chap. 15 (Missed Lung Lesions).

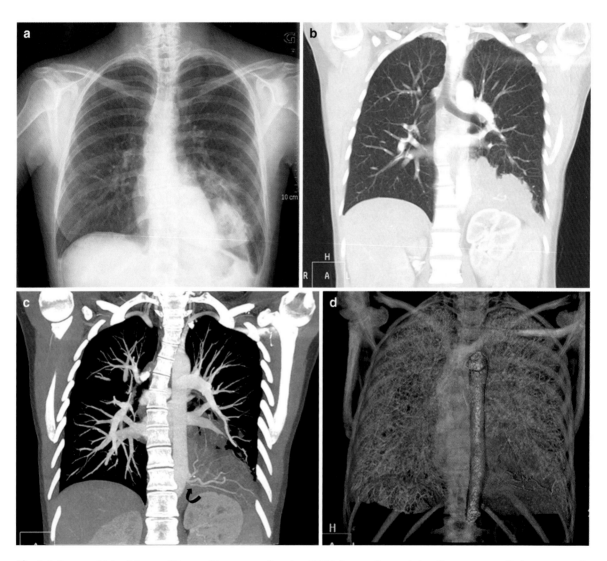

Fig. 1.1 Images obtained from a 35-year-old woman referred for chronic cough and fever. (**a**) Chest radiography demonstrates a left retrocardiac mass containing a lucent area. (**b**) Frontal reformatted CT image demonstrates, in the lung window setting, the irregular borders of the mass. (**c**) Maximal Intensity Projection (MIP) image demonstrates the presence of aberrant vessels (*curved arrow*) originating directly from the thoracic aorta and feeding the lung abnormality. (**d**) Volume rendered image highlights in *red* the aberrant vessels linked to an intralobar sequestration

In patients with respiratory complaints, CT examination should be performed promptly to avoid disease progression even when the chest radiograph is normal (Fig. 1.3).

Compared to other modalities of imaging, chest radiography has many advantages. It offers simplicity, low cost, low radiation, large amounts of information, and is widely available throughout the world,

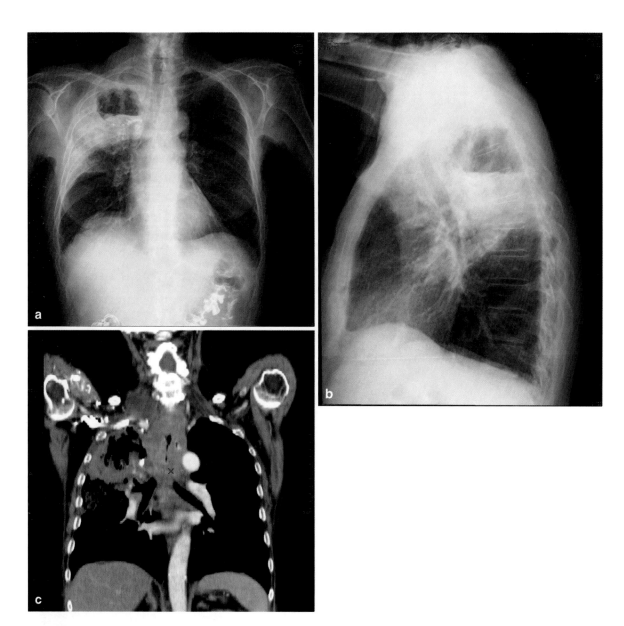

Fig. 1.2 Images obtained from a 76-year-old man with previous oropharyngeal carcinoma addressed for dysphagia and weight loss since 1 month. (**a**) Posteroanterior chest radiography reveals a large density of the right upper thorax containing a fluid level. (**b**) Lateral chest radiograph shows the posterior location of this abnormality. (**c**) Frontal reformation of spiral CT acquisition on mediastinal window setting reveals soft-tissue infiltration of the mediastinum centered on the esophagus and a large aerated cavity in the right upper lobe. (**d**) Two axial CT scans obtained at the level of the upper chest confirm the esophageal thickening. Note the right pleural effusion. (**e**) [18]Fludeoxyglucose Positron emission tomography with frontal reformation reveals intense uptake in the area of the mediastinal thickening and the right upper lobe. (**f**) Barium swallowing demonstrates a large fistula between the upper esophagus and the right lung. (**g**) Axial CT scan performed after oral opacification confirms the abnormal communication between the esophagus and the right lung. Esophageal biopsy was performed, and pathology revealed a well-differentiated squamous cell carcinoma of the esophagus

Fig. 1.2 (continued)

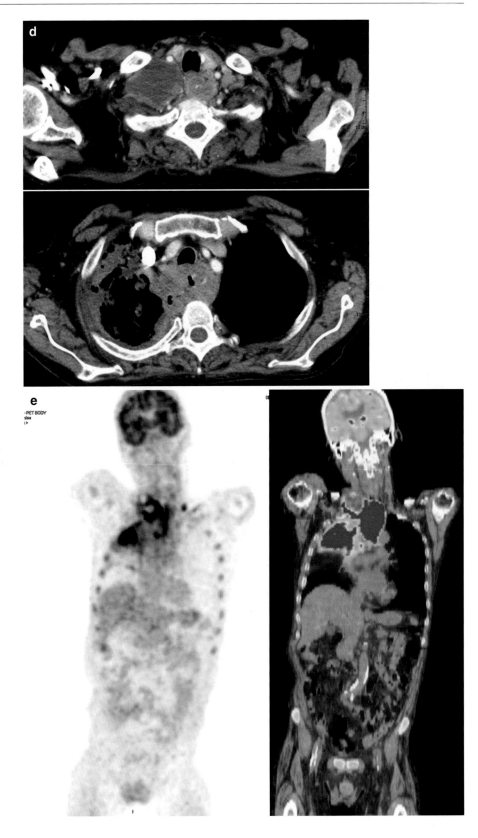

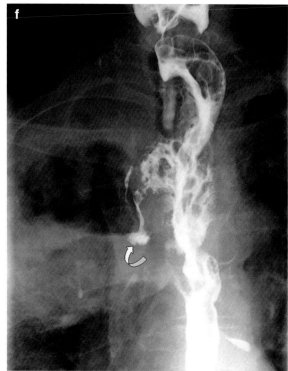

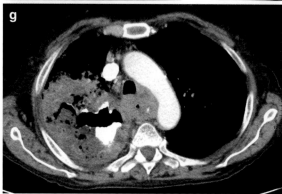

Fig. 1.2 (continued)

even in less developed countries. In addition, portable chest radiographs represent a precious tool to monitor patients with fragile conditions in the ICU and/or isolated patients. In this context, it is essential to take into account the radiation dose delivered by chest radiography because in many cases the patient may undergo repeated diagnostic radiologic examinations. Traditionally, the effective dose of chest radiography is in the order of 0.05 mSv for a posteroanterior (PA) view and 0.08–0.30 mSv for the PA and lateral views (UNSCEAR 1993). This low radiation needs to be counterbalanced by the excessive amount of radiation produced by more sophisticated techniques such as CT scanners. In a recent survey review (Stamm 2007) analyzing the delivered radiation doses for multi-detector row computed tomography (MDCT), it seems that the effective doses were in the range of 5.7–10.4 mSv, which represent at least 100- to 200-fold the radiation dose delivered by a single chest radiography.

The number of CT examinations has continuously increased in the field of thoracic medicine. In a review performed by Wittram et al. (2004) in a large academic hospital, the authors showed that there has been a significant increase in the ratio of chest CT per patient during the last years. From 1996 to 2001, there has been a 2.8-fold increase CT per admitted patient, and a 2.5-fold increase in the use of chest CT for outpatients. In the United States, CT has increasingly become the initial approach for the evaluation or detection of lung metastases, obstructive pulmonary disease, primary lung neoplasm, and others (Margulis and Sunshine 2000). The 1995–1996 workload data drawn from the ACR's survey (Sunshine et al. 1998) already showed an increase in high-technology modalities, particularly interventional radiology, CT, and MR imaging, and a decline in the percentage of use in general radiology. The drop in the share of chest radiography was approximately 17% between 1993 and 1999 (Maitino et al. 2003).

This decrease explains why residents in radiology are frequently tempted to follow educational courses in new thoracic imaging techniques, such as thoracic CT with new applications, notably coronary artery angio-CT (Miller et al. 2008; Becker 2006; Shuman et al. 2008; Roberts et al.2008), dual-energy CT techniques (Remy-Jardin and Remy 2008; Pontana et al. 2008; Boroto et al. 2008), thoracic MR (Plathow et al. 2005; Nael et al. 2005; Vogt et al. 2003), or FDG-PET (Jeong et al. 2008; Melek et al. 2008; Al-Sarraf et al.2008) rather than more traditional techniques such as thoracic radiography.

However, there has recently been a renewal of interest in the field of chest radiography thanks to several technical innovations in the fields of digital detection and post-processing (Schaefer-Prokop et al. 2008; Mc Adams et al. 2006). These technical advances, which will be further detailed in Chap. 2, have resulted in improved image quality and the reduction of radiation delivered to patients. Post-processing techniques

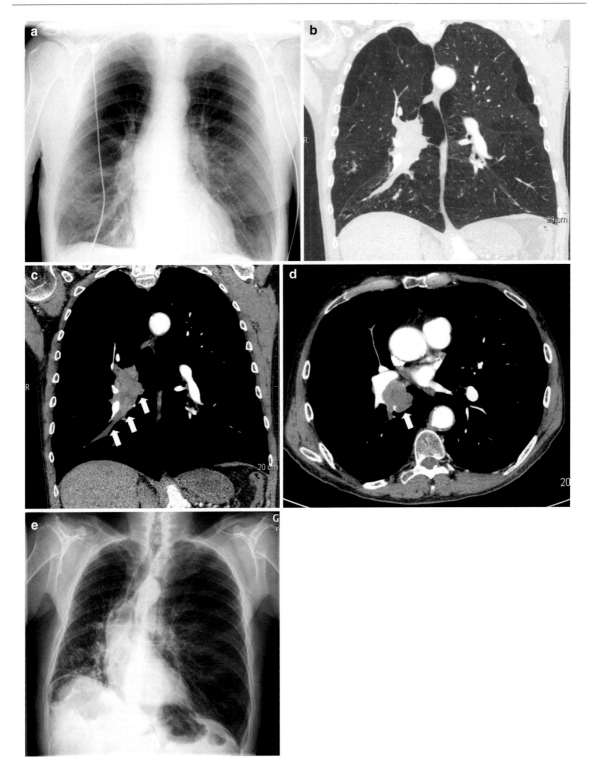

Fig. 1.3 Images obtained from a 75-year-old man with chronic obstructive pulmonary disease admitted to the emergency department for exacerbation of dyspnea. (**a**) At admission, anteroposterior chest radiograph does not show any obvious abnormality. (**b**) Enhanced spiral MDCT was performed to rule out pulmonary embolism. Frontal reformation demonstrates on the lung window setting a large right hilar mass with right lower lobe mucous plugging. Note the paraseptal emphysema in both upper lobes. (**c**) The mediastinal window setting depicts well the right hilar and bronchial abnormalities (*straight arrows*). (**d**) Axial CT at the level of the aortic root shows a large right hilar (*straight arrow*) mass in relation to a squamous cell carcinoma (proved pathologically). (**e**) Chest radiograph performed several days after admission shows a mediastinal shift to the right linked to a complete obstruction of the right inferior bronchus and lung collapse. This case illustrates the usefulness of MDCT in case of discordant results between chest radiography and the patient's complaints

in digital chest radiography, which consist of temporal subtraction, dual energy subtraction, digital tomosynthesis, and computer-aided detection (CAD) (Mc Adams et al. 2006), have ensured better lung nodule detection and characterization (KELCZ et al. 1994) and thereby enhanced small lung cancer visualization (Li et al. 2008).

The aim of the present chapter is to review the remaining indications of chest radiography in adults today in the context of MDCT. Chest radiography in the pediatric population is beyond the scope of this book and will not be discussed.

1.2 Main Indications of Chest Radiography

Periodically, scientific societies edit guidelines for the performance of chest radiography to assist practitioners in providing appropriate radiological care for patients (ACR 2006a; ACR 2006b; Speets et al. 2006; Geitung et al. 1999). Those guidelines are evidence based but differ by country according to socioeconomical factors and technical developments.

1.2.1 Pneumonia

Radiologic imaging plays a prominent role in the evaluation and treatment of patients with pneumonia. Plain chest radiography is an inexpensive test and is an important initial examination for all patients suspected to have pneumonia. MDCT is a valuable adjunct in case of negative or nondiagnostic chest radiography, unresolved pneumonia, and when complications are suspected.

1.2.1.1 Community-Acquired Pneumonia

Community-acquired pneumonia (CAP) constitutes a common and serious disease despite the availability of potent new antimicrobial agents. In the United States, pneumonia is the sixth leading cause of death and the number one cause of death from infectious diseases (Garibaldi 1985; Niederman et al. 1998).

The diagnosis of pneumonia should be considered in any patient who has recently developed respiratory symptoms such as cough, sputum production, and/or

shortness of breath, especially if accompanied by fever and clinical signs such as abnormal breath sounds and crackles at auscultation. In the immunocompromised or elderly, pneumonia may present insidiously with nonrespiratory symptoms such as confusion, worsening of an underlying chronic illness, failure to thrive, or a fall (Marrie 1994; Metaly et al. 1997).

All patients suspected of having pneumonia should have a chest X-ray to establish the diagnosis and the presence of potential complications (Fig. 1.4). It is important to note that chest radiography may be not sensitive in the case of early pneumonia and must be repeated in some circumstances 24–48 h after the onset of symptoms. One study (Syrjala et al. 1998) has shown that some of these radiographically negative patients do have lung infiltrates, if a high-resolution CT scan of the chest was performed. The radiographic appearance may be useful in differentiating pneumonia from other conditions that mimic it (Fig. 1.5). These include congestive heart failure, obstructing lung carcinoma, lymphoma and inflammatory lung diseases (bronchiolitis obliterans and organizing pneumonia, drug-induced lung diseases, eosinophilic pneumonia, sarcoidosis, acute interstitial pneumonitis, Wegener's granulomatosis, etc.). In addition, the radiographic findings may also suggest specific etiologies or conditions, such as lung abscess or tuberculosis, or identify a coexisting condition such as bronchial obstruction or pleural effusion.

Among patients who respond poorly to therapy, chest radiography should be repeated and a CT scan could be proposed to rule out complications such as empyema, abscess formation, or a pleuropulmonary fistula. If the patient has developed severe sepsis from pneumonia, the chest radiography and clinical course may deteriorate because of the presence of acute respiratory distress syndrome (ARDS) and multiple-system organ failure. A late complication of CAP, nosocomial pneumonia, can also complicate the illness and lead to an apparent nonresponse to therapy.

1.2.1.2 Pneumonia in the Immunocompromised patient

Pneumonia remains a major cause of morbidity and mortality in patients with AIDS or those treated with immunosuppressive drugs. Early diagnosis and effective curative treatment are both essential for a favorable outcome.

Standard chest radiography in immunosuppressed patients should be viewed as a screening test, and some authors (Nyamande et al. 2007; Heussel et al. 1997; Gulati et al. 2000) encourage early use of the CT scan (Fig. 1.6). In a study of 87 consecutive patients with febrile neutropenia, Heussel and colleagues 1997) noted that in 50% of subjects the CT scan revealed a pulmonary lesion that was not visible on the chest X-ray. A similar study in renal transplant recipients confirmed that chest radiography initially might be normal in immunosuppressed patients with pulmonary complaints, whereas a subsequent CT scan may

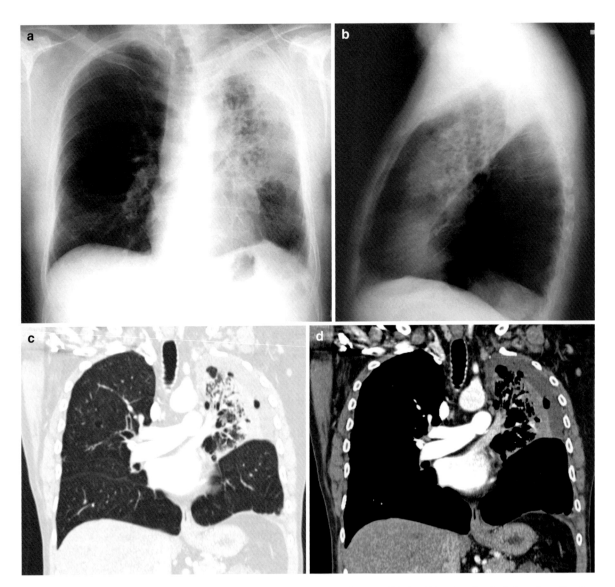

Fig. 1.4 Images obtained from a 65-year-old man who was admitted for fever and dyspnea. (**a**) Postero-anterior osteroanterior chest radiograph shows a left upper lobe consolidation with air bronchogram suggestive of lobar pneumonia. (**b**) Lateral chest radiography confirms the consolidation delimited by the great fissure posteriorly and involving the left upper lobe. Multiple small radiolucencies are observed within the consolidation area. (**c**) Frontal reformation of spiral CT acquisition on lung window setting confirms the infectious nature of the left upper lobe consolidation. Note the nice depiction of small radiolucencies linked to preexisting emphysema. (**d**) Frontal reformation of spiral CT acquisition on mediastinal window setting rules out the possibility of an obstructive lung carcinoma. (**e**) Sagittal reformation of spiral CT acquisition on lung window setting shows the nice side-by-side comparison with the corresponding chest radiography. (**f**) Sagittal reformation of spiral CT acquisition on mediastinal window setting highlights the anatomical delineation of the consolidation by the great fissure

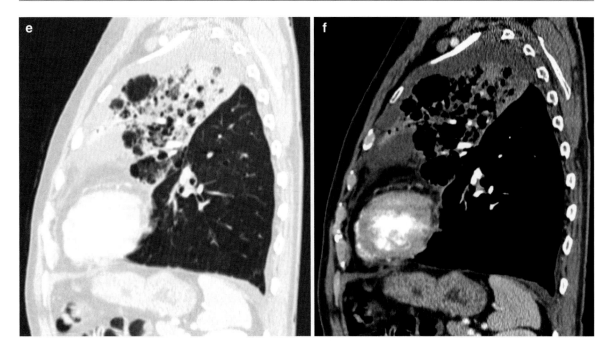

Fig. 1.4 (continued)

demonstrate multiple abnormalities (Gulati et al. 2000). In both reports, reliance on early CT scanning led to alterations in patient management. A larger, follow-up study of febrile neutropenia, examining only patients with normal chest radiographs ($n=112$), underlined the value of chest CT (Heussel et al. 1999); as it showed pneumonia in approximately 60% of them. Based on these findings, the investigators concluded that the sensitivity and specificity of CT scan were superior to the screening value of the standard chest radiograph. In addition to identifying pulmonary pathology that would otherwise be missed on plain radiographs, chest CT is used for guiding invasive diagnostic procedures, such as bronchoalveolar lavage or transbronchial biopsy.

The differential diagnosis of pulmonary lesions in this setting is broad. It is important to search for both infectious and noninfectious etiologies such as drug toxicity, pulmonary edema, alveolar proteinosis, or extrinsic allergic alveolitis. Frustratingly, many of the processes that result in pulmonary infiltrates present in a similar fashion, with nonspecific syndromes consisting of infiltrates, dyspnea, and hypoxemia. No single pattern of symptoms or radiographic findings can conclusively exclude a diagnostic possibility.

1.2.2 The Patient in Intensive Care Unit

Chest radiography is frequently performed in intensive care unit patients (ICU) (Trotman-Dickenson 2003). It is readily available and inexpensive but has technical and diagnostic limitations. Although chest radiographs have high diagnostic accuracy for detecting malposition of indwelling devices like translaryngeal tubes or central venous catheters (Henschke et al. 1996), diagnostic accuracy with respect to other abnormalities such as cardiogenic edema, pneumothorax, and pleural effusion is low (Graat et al. 2006). In this setting, MDCT certainly has an important role to play in the detection of small air collections and distinguishing pleural effusions from parenchymal processes, particularly when the patient is in the supine position. MDCT is certainly the modality of choice to detect pulmonary embolism, atelectasis, and interstitial emphysema in ICU patients as well as various complications such as pulmonary artery aneurysm following Swan-Ganz catheter placement.

Recently, portable chest radiography has benefited from the implementation of digital technology with increased diagnostic accuracy and increased confidence in interpretation. The connection to the Picture Archiving

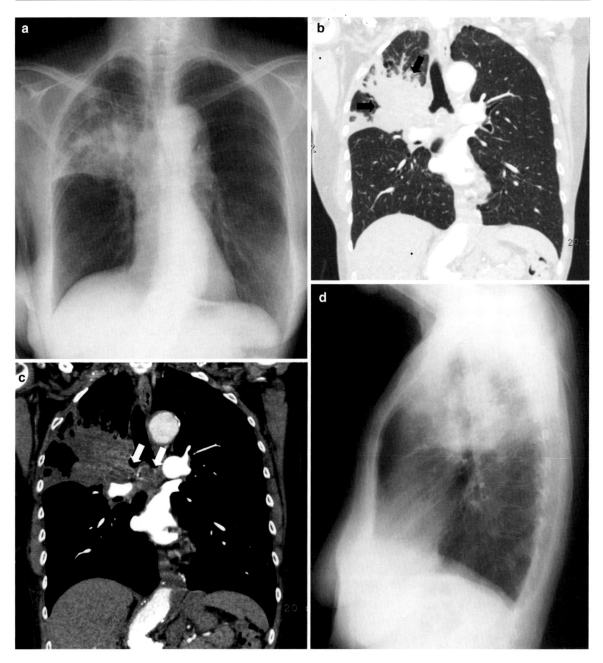

Fig. 1.5 Images obtained from a 60-year-old female smoker admitted to the emergency room because of loss of consciousness. White blood cell count was measured at 18.8 10^3/mm^3 (4–10 10^3/mm^3), C-reactive protein: 5.7 mg/dl (<1 mg/dl), carcioembryonic antigen: 3.7 ng/ml (<3 ng/ml), neuron-specific enolase: 14.4 ng/ml (<12 ng/ml). (**a**) PA chest radiography performed demonstrates a right upper lobe consolidation with air bronchogram consistent with a lobar pneumonia. (**b**) Frontal reformation of enhanced spiral CT acquisition on lung window setting reveals a suspicious mass (*straight arrows*) in the right upper lobe. (**c**) Mediastinal window setting reveals the mediastinal infiltration (*straight arrows*) by the lung mass. (**d**) Lateral chest radiography shows the lung mass in supra-hilar location. (**e**) Sagittal reformation on lung window setting confirms the suspicion of a superimposed mass within the parenchymal consolidation. (**f**) Pathology reveals neoplastic cells of a poorly differentiated lung carcinoma

Fig. 1.5 (continued)

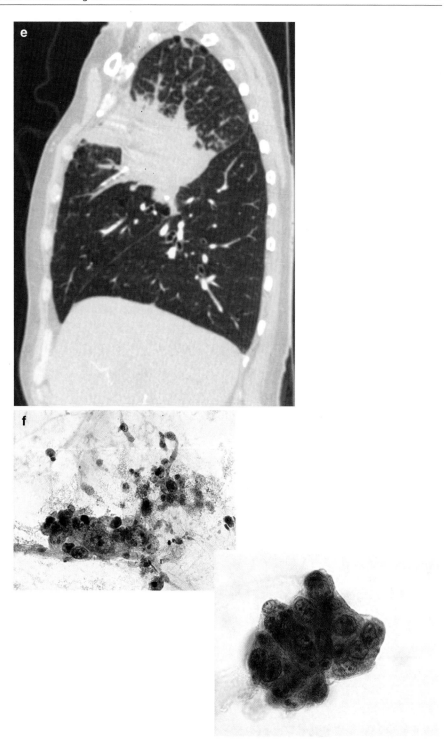

System (PACS) has also greatly facilitated the access to the thoracic images by ICU clinicians.

1.2.3 Position of Catheters and Thoracic Devices

Chest devices are encountered on a daily basis by almost all radiologists (Hunter et al. 2004). Clinical judgment does not reliably predict malpositioning after central venous catheter or the presence of postprocedural complications. For many practitioners, chest radiography after central venous catheter placement in the critically ill should remain the standard of care. However, in some instances, CT can depict more accurately the course of the catheter or the relationship of the medical devices to the anatomical structures. Unfortunately, in these situations, CT is often limited by the presence of metallic artifacts generated by the device. The position of pleural devices, endotracheal and esophageal tubes, vascular catheters, and pacemakers can be assessed accurately by chest radiography only. Mechanical valves and circulatory assist devices (Fig. 1.7) usually require additional evaluation by other imaging modalities such as ultrasonography or MDCT (Labounty et al. 2009).

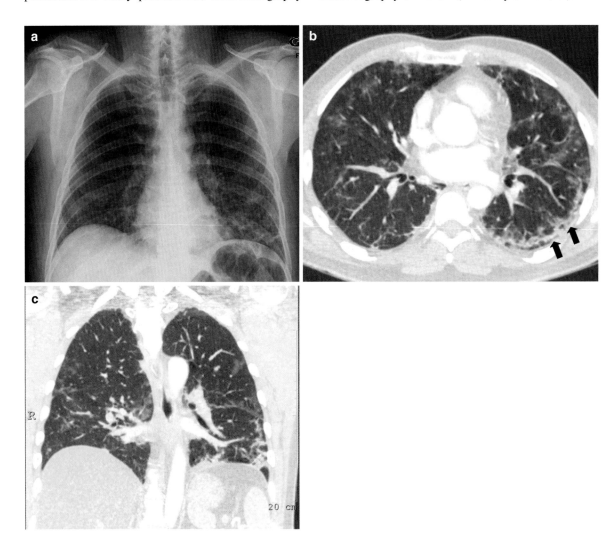

Fig. 1.6 Images obtained from a 37-year-old male HIV patient complaining of fever (38°C) for 15 days, cough, and shortness of breath. The patient has lost 20 kg in 5 months. Blood sample analysis reveals a low white blood cell count at 1.8 10^3/mm^3 (4–10 10^3/mm^3) and normal C-reactive protein: 0.9 mg/dl (<1 mg/dl). (**a**) Anteroposterior chest radiography reveals interstitial abnormalities more prominent in the left lower lobe. (**b**) Axial CT scan obtained at the level of the left atrium shows bilateral ground glass opacities and increased septal lines. Curvilinear sub-pleural bands are observed at the left lower lobe (*arrows*). (**c**) Frontal reformation of spiral CT acquisition on lung window setting depicts well the bilateral involvement of both lungs intersecting the inferior two thirds of the thorax. The CT aspect was in favor of viral or parasitic infection. (**d**) Pathology reveals cellular inclusions due to *Pneumocystis jirovecii*

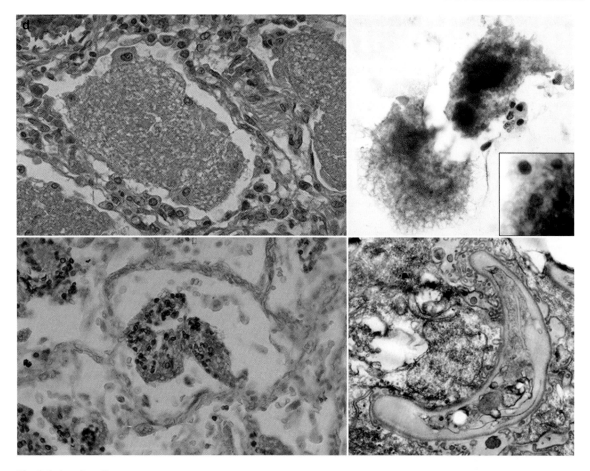

Fig. 1.6 (continued)

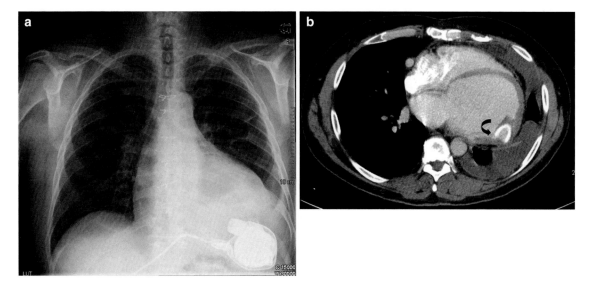

Fig. 1.7 Images obtained from a 48-year-old man referred for dysfunction of an external cardiac device. The cardiac assistance was placed 4 months previously for cardiac failure, possibly viral in origin, with normal coronary arteries. (**a**) Anteroposterior chest radiograph shows that the external device is in good position.

(**b**) Enhanced spiral CT performed at the level of the left ventricle reveals that the tube placed at the top of the left ventricle is against the posterior wall (*curved arrow*) of the left ventricle and is probably responsible for the cardiac dysfunction

1.2.4 The Patient in the Emergency Room

Chest pain represents one of the most common causes of admission to the emergency department. As proposed by ACR (Stanford et al. 2000), chest radiography is the recommended initial imaging study. This examination can diagnose various conditions such as acute and chronic infections, pneumothorax (Fig. 1.8), pleural effusions, pneumomediastinum, malignancies, and fractured ribs. Other conditions producing chest pain, such as aortic aneurysms/dissections and/or pulmonary embolism (PE), may be suspected from the chest radiograph, but the overall sensitivities are rather poor. Massive PEs may be present even with a normal chest radiograph (Fig. 1.9). The presence of a Hampton hump, Westermark sign, or pulmonary artery enlargement on chest radiograph may suggest PE (Coche et al. 2004). In this context, chest radiography also has the potential to play a role in the determination of subsequent imaging tests (i.e., scintigraphy or MDCT). It has been shown that the presence of any abnormality on the initial chest radiograph decreases the utility of scintigraphy (Forbes et al. 2001)

Although CT is not recommended for the initial evaluation of patients with chest pain, it is frequently

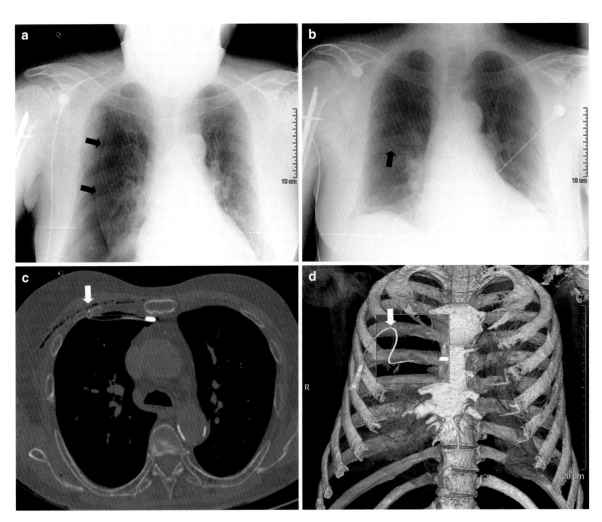

Fig. 1.8 Images obtained from a 78-year-old man admitted for dyspnea and chest pain. (**a**) Bedside chest radiography revealed a right hyperlucent lung in relationship with a pneumothorax (*straight arrows*). (**b**) A chest tube was placed, and a chest radiography was performed, confirming the good position of the chest tube (*straight arrow*). (**c**) The axial CT scan performed at the level of the upper chest reveals that the chest tube was inserted through a rib (*straight arrow*) and not through an intercostal space as usually done. (**d**) Volume rendered CT images highlight the aberrant course of the chest tube through the bony structures in the box (*straight arrow*)

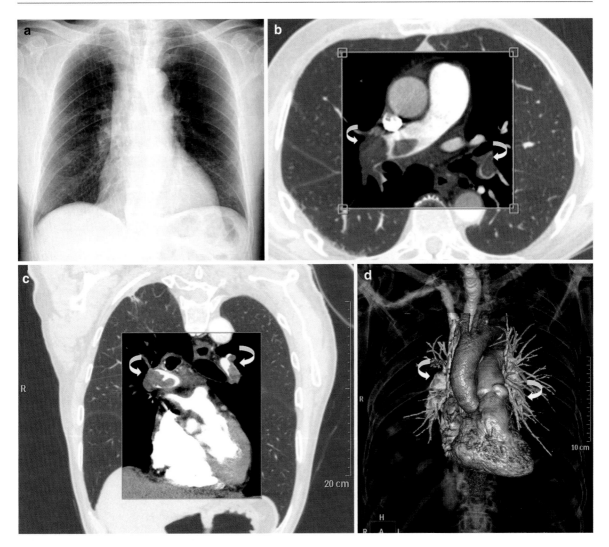

Fig. 1.9 Images obtained from a 72-year-old man treated for lymphoma and small cell carcinoma. He was admitted to the emergency room for hypoxemia. (**a**) Posteroanterior chest radiograph shows no significant abnormality. (**b**) Contrast-enhanced MDCT reveals bilateral massive pulmonary embolism (*curved arrows*) on the mediastinal window setting (in the central box) and a normal lung parenchyma on a lung window setting (outside the central box). (**c**) Frontal reformation of spiral CT acquisition on mediastinal window setting depicts well the extensive clots in the pulmonary arteries (*curved arrows*) (in the central box) with a normal lung parenchyma (outside the central box). (**d**) Volume rendered images with a transparent mode shows the bilateral clots (*curved arrows*) in the pulmonary arteries

appropriate when the results of the clinical, radiographic, and laboratory studies are either suggestive of significant disease or nondiagnostic. This strategy is still evolving; the advent of very rapid MDCT scanners allows a triple rule-out protocol (PE, aortic dissection, and coronary heart disease) for chest pain during a short breath-hold (Frauenfelder 2009; Takakuwa 2008).

Patients with dyspnea may have various conditions that may justify the realization of chest radiography (Fig. 1.10). Two studies (Butcher et al. 1993; Pratter et al. 1989) suggest that the chest radiograph adds enough additional useful information to recommend its routine use in patients with chronic and acute dyspnea. Another study (Benacerraf et al. 1981) found that acute dyspnea was a strong predictor of radiographic abnormality in patients above the age of 40 (only 14% had normal chest radiographs). Among dyspneic patients younger than 40 years of age, chest radiography was normal in 68% and revealed acute and chronic findings in 13% and 18%, respectively. Among patients with acute findings, the vast majority had either a positive physical examination or hemoptysis. The authors concluded that chest radiography was not warranted in patients under the age of 40 unless physical examination was positive or the patient had hemoptysis or limited differential diagnosis.

Among patients presenting in the emergency room with nonmassive hemoptysis (less than 1,000 ml/24 h), chest radiography should be obtained after careful history and clinical evaluation (Fig. 1.11). Hemoptysis should be differentiated from hematemesis. In the primary care setting, the most common causes of hemoptysis are acute and chronic bronchitis, pneumonia, tuberculosis, and lung cancer. If a diagnosis remains unclear, further imaging with chest CT or direct visualization by bronchoscopy is often indicated. In high-risk patients with normal chest radiographs, fiberoptic bronchoscopy should be considered to rule out malignancy.

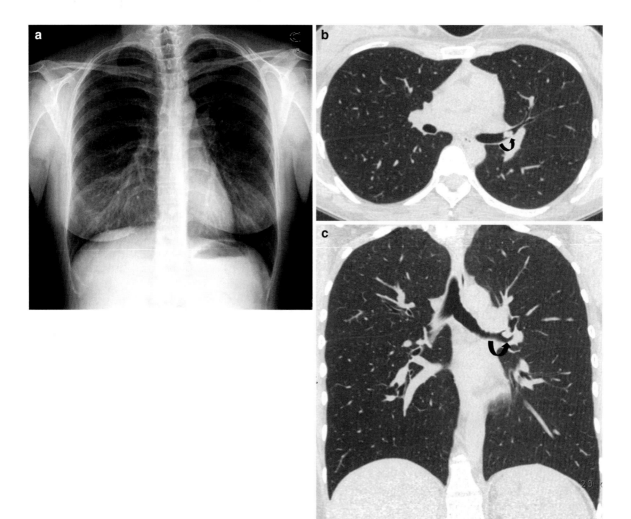

Fig. 1.10 Thirty-seven-year-old woman with previous asthma presented for acute dyspnea when laying down. (**a**) Posteroanterior chest radiograph does not show any significant abnormality. (**b**) Axial CT reveals a small endobronchial mass (*curved arrow*) located at the proximal portion of the culminal bronchus. (**c**) Reformatted frontal CT image shows a small tumor (*curved arrow*) that was not visible on frontal chest radiograph, even retrospectively. (**d**) Virtual bronchoscopy shows an endobronchial tumor (*straight arrows*). (**e**) Real bronchoscopy was performed with a perfect correlation with the CT findings (*straight arrows*). (**f**) Pathology is consistent with an endobronchial hamartoma

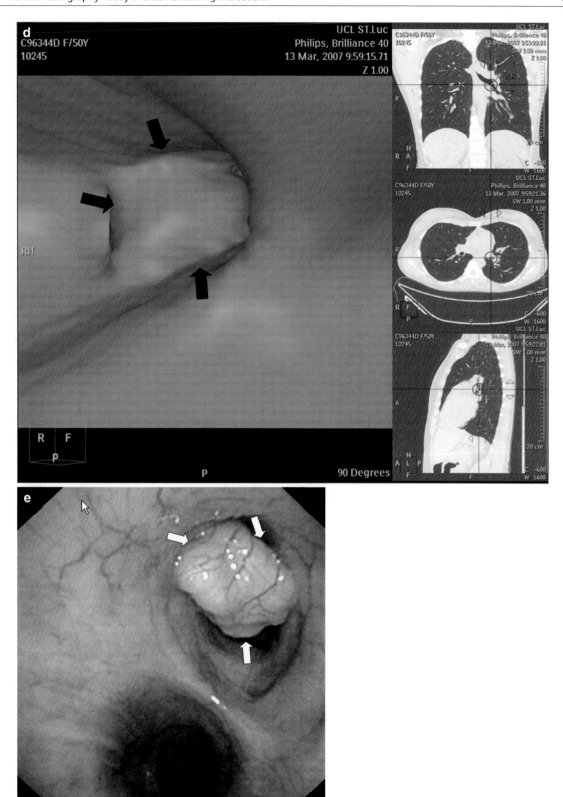

Fig. 1.10 (continued)

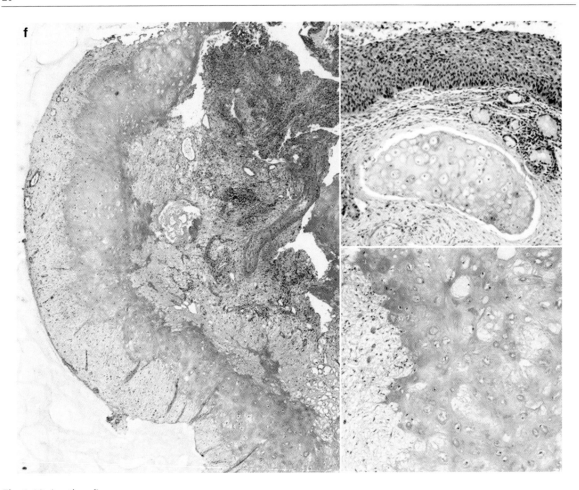

Fig. 1.10 (continued)

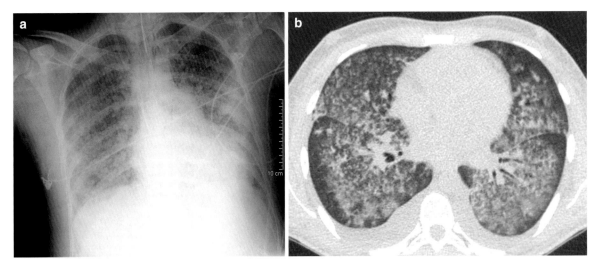

Fig. 1.11 Images obtained from a 21-year-old man with Goodpasture syndrome and massive hempotysis. (**a**) Bedside chest radiograph shows bilateral consolidation suspicious of massive hemorrhage in the clinical context. (**b**) Chest CT confirms on this axial view a bilateral alveolar syndrome respecting the sub-pleural area and consistent with pulmonary hemorrhage. (**c**) Reformatted frontal CT image shows on the right side thick reconstructed image and fuzzy densities related to the alveolar syndrome. On the *left*, in the box, the image appears thin and highlights the dark bronchus sign, as described in alveolar hemorrhage

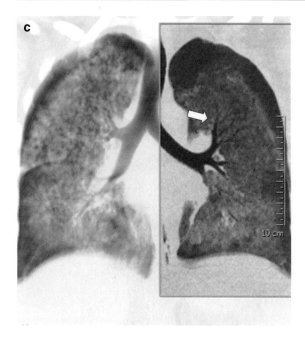

Fig. 1.11 (continued)

1.2.5 The Patient's Follow-Up

Chest radiography is less sensitive than chest CT in the detection of various disorders, but the intrinsic characteristics (low radiation dose, excellent cost benefit ratio, accessibility and speed) of chest radiography place this technique in an interesting position to follow some patients with various conditions. Chest radiography is the most commonly used imaging tool for follow-up of benign conditions such as treated pneumonia, pneumothorax after drain placement, pleural effusion, cardiac failure, and pulmonary edema after cardiac stabilization.

Some follow-up strategies for malignant conditions also use chest radiography. Some authors (Pickhardt et al. 1998) have shown that chest radiography is a simple imaging method to detect lymphoproliferative disorders in lung transplant recipients. In this context, CT is more sensitive than chest radiography for evaluating the extent of the disease, but this increased sensitivity for discovering additional lesions did not result in better prediction of survival. A survey (Beitler et al. 2000) concerning the follow-up after potentially curative resection of extremity sarcomas revealed that most examinations occurred with chest X-rays and routine office visits rather than repeated expensive CT scans. Lord et al. (Lord et al. 2006) recommend a 6-month chest radiograph follow-up in patients with high-grade sarcomas. The low cumulative dose of radiation received from chest radiography makes this a safe, simple, and appropriate first-line tool. Chest radiography may also be used in clinical routine to grossly evaluate the effect of chemotherapy on lung tumor volume reduction and detect respiratory complications (Fig. 1.12).

1.2.6 Clinical Situations in Which Chest Radiography Has Been Abandoned or Its Role Discussed

1.2.6.1 Lung Cancer Screening

The first screening test for lung cancer used to be chest radiography. In the 1960s and 1970s, there were large randomized trials conducted both in the USA and Europe in which volunteers underwent either periodic chest radiography or a simple clinical follow-up as baseline examination (Brett 1969; Fontana et al. 1986). Although these studies found a higher incidence of resectable disease in the screened population, none of them showed a lung cancer mortality reduction with screening.

During the past decades, large randomized trials have been conducted, mainly in the USA, addressing the role of chest radiography and sputum cytology examination when screening for lung cancer. The Memorial-Sloan Kettering and Johns Hopkins University studies compared lung cancer detection rates using annual chest radiography alone (control arm) and annual radiography plus sputum cytology analysis every 4 months (intervention arm) (Flehinger et al. 1984; Frost et al. 1984). The Memorial Sloan Kettering study enrolled 4,968 men to chest radiography and 5,072 to dual (chest radiography and sputum cytology) screen. There were 144 lung cancers detected in each group. The investigators found no significant difference in stage distribution, resectability, survival, or disease-specific mortality between groups and concluded that the addition of a sputum cytology examination offered no advantage over annual screening with chest radiography (Melamed et al. 1984). In the Johns Hopkins study, 5,161 men were randomized to chest radiography and 5,226 to dual screening.

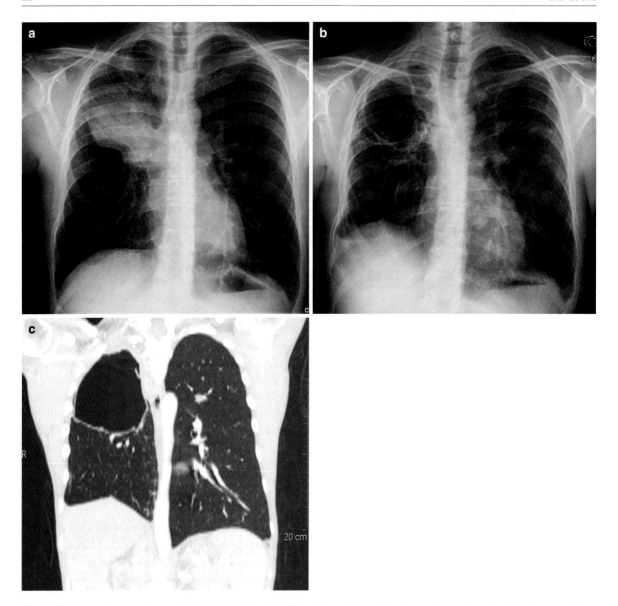

Fig. 1.12 Images from a patient with lung cancer (poorly differentiated adenocarcinoma) treated by surgery and an anti-angiogenetic agent. (**a**) At admission chest radiograph reveals a large mass located in the right upper lobe. (**b**) Posteroanterior chest radiograph performed several months after therapy with an anti-angiogenetic agent demonstrates a large radiolucency in the right upper lung zone. (**c**) Reformatted frontal CT image shows a large cavity in the right upper lobe due to tumor necrosis

Screening resulted in the detection of 202 cases of lung cancer in the chest radiography group and 194 cases in the dual screening group (Tockman 1986).

The Mayo Lung Project (Fontana et al. 1984) enrolled more than 10,900 subjects. Participants were offered chest radiography and sputum cytology at enrollment. They were then randomly assigned to a close-surveillance group, which underwent chest radiography and sputum cytology every 4 months, or to a control group, which was advised to have the standard surveillance of yearly chest radiography and sputum analysis. There were no statistically significant differences in either survival or lung cancer–related mortality between the two groups.

Since those disappointing results, lung cancer screening with chest radiography has been abandoned. The future role of low-dose MDCT in this field needs to be addressed. Some prospective randomized controlled trials comparing lung cancer mortality in a screening arm (with low-dose CT screening) and a control arm (without CT screening) have been initiated (National Lung Cancer Screening Trial, available at: http://www.cancernet.nci.nih.gov/nlst). At the end of those large studies, scientists hope to be able to answer whether low-dose CT screening can reduce lung cancer–related mortality.

1.2.6.2 Preoperative Patients

The recommendations for performing routine preoperative chest X-ray based on age cutoffs have been established in some countries and institutions. Some authors (Escolano et al. 1994) have suggested that X-rays should be recommended for patients over the age of 45 years old; those with a history of cardiovascular or lung disease, or of cancer; smokers of more than 20 cigarettes/day.

A review of the literature has shown that the prevalence of unexpected abnormalities in routine preoperative chest X-rays performed before noncardiac and nonthoracic surgery is highly variable and increases

with age. In a systematic review (Joo et al. 2005), most thoracic abnormalities reflected chronic disorders such as cardiomegaly (15–65%) and chronic obstructive diseases (COPD) (7–30%). The diagnostic yield of preoperative chest X-ray among patients under the age of 50 was low, ranging from 3% to 16%. The diagnostic yield for patients aged between 51 and 60 years ranged from less than 10% to as high as 59%. Between the ages of 61–70, the diagnostic yield was high, ranging between 13% and 58%, and for patients older than 70 years, it ranged between 47% and 61%. However, the influence of the detection of such incidental thoracic abnormalities on patient management is minimal. One study (Wiencek et al. 1987) reported canceling surgery as a result of the chest X-ray findings in 2% of patients. (Gagner and Chiasson 1990) reported delaying surgery for 1.3% of patients based on a preoperative chest X-ray depicting pneumonia. A large prospective study (Bouillot et al. 1996) reported that only 0.5% of patients had a change in anesthetic or surgical management because of the results of an abnormal chest radiograph.

For those reasons, some authors recommend performing targeted investigations as indicated by clinical findings rather than on the basis of arbitrary age cutoffs. In this context, patients referred for cardiac or thoracic surgery usually undergo chest radiography no matter their age to confirm the presence and location of the thoracic abnormality just before the surgery (Fig. 1.13).

1.2.6.3 Daily Routine Chest Radiography

According to some authors (Marik 1997), routine daily chest radiography may be justified in critically ill patients in a medical ICU because management decisions are made on the basis of the information obtained. Studies have indeed shown that up to 65% of daily radiographs in the ICU reveal significant or unsuspected abnormalities and lead to a change in the patient's management (Henschke et al. 1983, Bekemeyer et al. 1985, Strain et al. 1985).

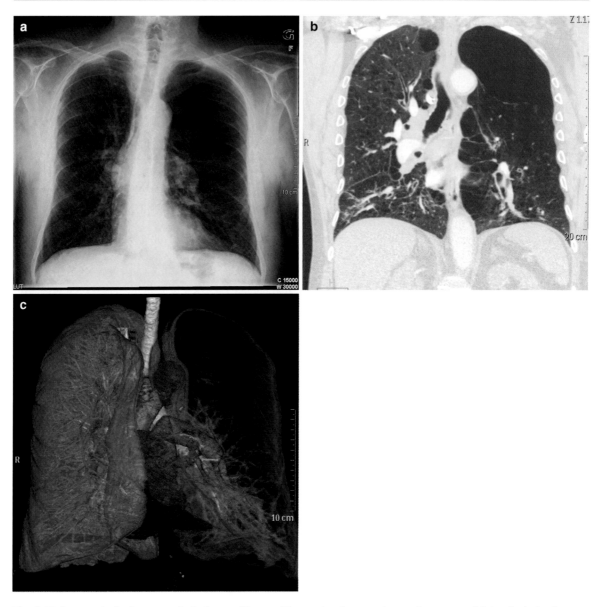

Fig. 1.13 Images obtained preoperatively from a 72-year-old man admitted for surgery related to emphysema. (**a**) Posteroanterior chest radiograph shows hyperinflatory status with reduction of pulmonary vascularity in the left upper zone. (**b**) Frontal reformatted CT image demonstrates on lung window setting the extensive emphysema, explaining the lack of vascularity in this area on the chest radiograph. (**c**) Volume rendered images in a transparent mode highlights the hypertransparency of the left lung in relationship with bullous emphysema

1.3 Conclusions

Despite spectacular advances in cross-sectional imaging techniques, chest radiography still has numerous clinical indications because of its intrinsic characteristics of simplicity, availability, low cost, and low radiation delivery. However, its interpretation is notoriously difficult and needs to receive careful attention during teaching and learning. In this context, special efforts have to be made by the academic community to maintain the standards of interpretation at a high level to continue to ensure the valuable role of chest radiography in the clinical diagnostic process.

References

ACR practice guideline for the performance of pediatric and adult chest radiography (2006a) American College of Radiology 301–306

ACR practice guideline for the performance of pediatric and adult portable (mobile unit) chest radiography (2006b) American College of Radiology 307–311

Al-Sarraf N, Gately K, Lucey J, Wilson L, McGovern E, Young V (2008) Lymph node staging by means of positron emission tomography is less accurate in non-small cell lung cancer patients with enlarged lymph nodes: analysis of 1, 145 lymph nodes. Lung Cancer 60:62–68

Becker CR (2006) Cardiac CT: a one-stop-shop procedure? Eur Radiol 16:M65–M70

Beitler AL, Virgo KS, Johnson FE, Gibbs JF, Kraybill WG (2000) Current follow-up strategies after potentially curative resection of extremity sarcomas. Results of a survey of the members of the society of surgical oncology. Cancer 88:777–785

Bekemeyer WB, Crapo RD, Calhoon S, Cannon CY, Clayton PD (1985) Efficacy of chest radiography in a respiratory intensive care unit. A prospective study. Chest 88:691–696

Benacerraf BR, McLoud TC, Rhea JT, Tritschler V, Libby P (1981) An assessment of the contribution of chest radiography in outpatients with acute chest complaints: a prospective study. Radiology 138:293–299

Boroto K, Remy-Jardin M, Flohr T, Faivre JB, Pansini V, Tacelli N, Schmidt B, Gorgos A, Remy J (2008) Thoracic applications of dual-source CT technology. Eur J Radiol 68:375–384

Bouillot LJ, Fingerhut A, Paquet JC et al (1996) Are routine preoperative chest radiographs useful in general surgery? A prospective, multicentre study in 3959 patients. Association des chirurgiens de l'Assistance Publique pour les évaluations médicales. Eur J Surg 162:597–604

Brett GZ (1969) Earlier diagnosis and survival in lung cancer. Br Med J 4:260–262

Butcher BL, Nichol KL, Parenti CM (1993) High yield of chest radiography in walk-in clinic patients with chest symptoms. J Gen Intern Med 8:115–119

Coche E, Verschuren F, Hainaut P, Goncette L (2004) Pulmonary embolism findings on chest radiographs and multislice spiral CT. Eur Radiol 14:1241–1248

Escolano F, Alonso J, Gomar C, Sierra P, Castillo J, Castaño J (1994) Usefulness of preoperative chest radiography in elective surgery. Rev Esp Anest Reanim 41:7–12

Flehinger BJ, Melamed MR, Zaman MB, Heelan RT, Perchick WB, Martini N (1984) Early lung cancer detection: results of the initial (prevalence) radiologic and cytologic screening in the Memorial Sloan-Kettering study. Am Rev Respir Dis 130:555–560

Fontana RS, Sanderson DR, Taylor WF, Woolner LB, Miller WE, Muhm JR, Uhlenhopp MA (1984) Early lung cancer detection: results of the initial (prevalence) radiologic and cytologic screening in the Mayo Clinic study. Am Rev Respir Dis 130:561–565

Fontana RS, Sanderson DR, Woolner LB, Taylor WF, Miller WE, Muhm JR (1986) Lung cancer screening: the Mayo program. J Occup Med 28:746–775

Forbes KP, Reid JH, Murchison JT (2001) Do preliminary chest X-ray findings define the optimal role of pulmonary scintigraphy in suspected pulmonary embolism. Clin Radiol 56:397–400

Frauenfelder T, Appenzeller P, Karlo C, Scheffel H, Desbiolles L, Stolzmann P, Marincek B, Alkadhi H, Schertler T (2009) Triple rule-out CT in the emergency department: protocols and spectrum of imaging findings. Eur Radiol 19:789–799

Frost JK, Ball WC Jr, Levin ML, Tockman MS, Baker RR, Carter D, Eggleston JC, Erozan YS, Gupta PK, Khouri NF (1984) Early lung cancer detection: results of the initial (prevalence) radiologic and cytologic screening in the Johns Hopkins study. Am Rev Respir Dis 130:549–554

Gagner M, Chiasson A (1990) Preoperative chest X-ray films in elective surgery: a valid screening tool. Can J Surg 33:271–274

Garibaldi RA (1985) Epidemiology of community-acquired respiratory tract infections in adults: incidence, etiology, and impact. Am J Med 78:32S–37S

Geitung JT, Skjærstad LM, Göthlin JH (1999) Clìnical utility of chest roentgenograms. Eur Radiol 9:721–723

Graat M, Wolthuis E, Choi G, Stoker J, Vroom M, Schultz M (2006) The clinical value of daily-routine chest radiographs in a mixed medical-surgical intensive care unit is low. Crit Care 10:R11

Gulati M, Kaur R, Jha V et al (2000) High-resolution CT in renal transplant patients with suspected pulmonary infections. Acta Radiol 41:237–241

Henschke CL, Pasternack GS, Schroeder S, Henschke CI, Pasternack GS, Schroeder S, Hart KK, Herman PG (1983) Bedside chest radiography: diagnostic efficacy. Radiology 149:23–26

Henschke CI, Yankelevitz DF, Wand A, Davis SD, Shiau M (1996) Accuracy and efficacy of chest radiography in the intensive care unit. Radiol Clin North Am 34:21–31

Heussel CP, Kauczor HU, Heussel G et al (1997) Early detection of pneumonia in febrile neutropenic patients: use of thin-section CT. AJR 169:1347–1353

Heussel CP, Kauczor HU, Heussel GE et al (1999) Pneumonia in febrile neutropenic patients and in bone marrow and blood stem-cell transplant recipients: use of high-resolution computed tomography. J Clin Oncol 17:796–805

Hunter TB, Taljanovic MS, Tsau PH, Berger WG, Standen JR (2004) Medical devices of the chest. Radiographics 24:1725–1746

International commission on radiological protection ICRP (2004) Managing patient dose in digital radiology. ICRP publication 93 Annals of the ICRP, Elsevier, p 21

Jeong SY, Lee KS, Shin KM, Bae YA, Kim BT, Choe BK, Kim TS, Chung MJ (2008) Efficacy of PET/CT in the characterization of solid or partly solid solitary pulmonary nodules. Lung Cancer 61:186–194

Joo HS, Wong J, Naik VN et al (2005) The value of screening preoperative chest X-rays: a systematic review. Can J Anaesth 52:568–574

Kelcz F, Zink FE, Peppler WW, Kruger DG, Ergun DL, Mistretta CA (1994) Conventional chest radiography vs dual-energy computed radiography in the detection and characterization of pulmonary nodules. AJR 162:271–278

Labounty TM, Agarwal PP, Chughtai A, Kazerooni EA, Wizauer E, Bach DS (2009) Hemodynamic and functional assessment of mechanical aortic valves using combined echocardiography and multidetector computed tomography. J Cardiovasc Comput Tomogr 3:161–167

Li F, Engelmann R, Doi K, MacMahon H (2008) Improved detection of small lung cancers with dual-energy subtraction chest radiography. AJR 190:886–891

Lord HK, Salter DM, MacDougall RH, Kerr GR (2006) Is routine chest radiography a useful test in the follow up of all adult patients with soft tissue sarcoma? Br J Radiol 79:799–800

Maitino AJ, Levin DC, Parker L, Rao VM, Sunshine JH (2003) Nationwide trends in rates of utilization of noninvasive diagnostic imaging among the Medicare population between 1993 and 1999. Radiology 227:113–117

Margulis AR, Sunshine JH (2000) Radiology at the turn of the millennium. Radiology 214:15–23

Marik PE, Janower ML (1997) The impact of routine chest radiography on ICU management decisions: an observational study. Am J Crit Care 6:95–98

Marrie TJ (1994) Community-acquired pneumonia. Clin Infect Dis 18:501–513

Mc Adams HP, Samei E, Dobbins J, Tourassi GD, Ravin CE (2006) Recent advances in chest radiography. Radiology 241:663–683

Melamed MR, Flehinger BJ, Zaman MB, Heelan RT, Perchick WA, Martini N (1984) Screening for early lung cancer. Results of the Memorial Sloan-Kettering study in New York. Chest 86:44–53

Melek H, Gunluoglu MZ, Demir A, Akin H, Olcmen A, Dincer SI (2008) Role of positron emission tomography in mediastinal lymphatic staging of non-small cell lung cancer. Eur J Cardiothorac Surg 33:294–299

Metaly JP, Schulz R, Li Y-H et al (1997) Influence of age on symptoms at presentation in patients with community-acquired pneumonia. Arch Intern Med 157:1453–1459

Miller JM, Rochitte CE, Dewey M, Arbab-Zadeh A, Niinuma H, Gottlieb I, Paul N, Clouse ME, Shapiro EP, Hoe J, Lardo AC, Bush DE, de Roos A, Cox C, Brinker J, Lima JA (2008) Diagnostic performance of coronary angiography by 64-row CT. N Engl J Med 359:2324–2336

Nael K, Laub G, Finn JP (2005) Three-dimensional contrast-enhanced MR angiography of the thoraco-abdominal vessels. Magn Reson Imaging Clin N Am 13:359–380

Niederman MS, McCombs JI, Unger AN, Kumar A, Popovian R (1998) The costs of treating community-acquired pneumonia. Clin Ther 20:820–837

Nyamande K, Lalloo UG, Vawda F (2007) Comparison of plain chest radiography and high-resolution CT in human immunodeficiency virus infected patients with community-acquired pneumonia: a sub-Saharan Africa study. Br J Radiol 80:302–306

Pickhardt PJ, Siegel MJ, Anderson DC, Hayashi R, DeBaun MR (1998) Chest radiography as a predictor of outcome in post-transplantation lymphoproliferative disorder in lung allograft recipients. AJR 171:375–382

Plathow C, Schoebinger M, Fink C, Ley S, Puderbach M, Eichinger M, Bock M, Meinzer HP, Kauczor HU (2005) Evaluation of lung volumetry using dynamic three-dimensional magnetic resonance imaging. Invest Radiol 40:173–179

Pontana F, Faivre JB, Remy-Jardin M, Flohr T, Schmidt B, Tacelli N, Pansini V, Remy J (2008) Lung perfusion with dual-energy multidetector-row CT (MDCT): feasibility for the evaluation of acute pulmonary embolism in 117 consecutive patients. Acad Radiol 5:1494–1504

Pratter MR, Curley FJ, Dubois J, Irwin RS (1989) Cause and evaluation of chronic dyspnea in a pulmonary disease clinic. Arch Intern Med 149:2277–2282

Remy-Jardin M, Remy J (2008) Vascular disease in chronic obstructive pulmonary disease. Proc Am Thorac Soc 5:891–899

Roberts WT, Bax JJ, Davies LC (2008) Cardiac CT and CT coronary angiography: technology and application. Heart 94:781–792

Schaefer-Prokop C, Neitzel U, Venema HW, Uffmann PM (2008) Digital chest radiography: an update on modern technology, dose containment and control of image quality. Eur Radiol 18:1818–1830

Shuman WP, Branch KR, May JM, Mitsumori LM, Lockhart DW, Dubinsky TJ, Warren BH, Caldwell JH (2008) Prospective versus retrospective ECG gating for 64-detector CT of the coronary arteries: comparison of image quality and patient radiation dose. Radiology 248:431–437

Speets AM, van der Graaf Y, Hoes AW et al (2006) Chest radiography in general practice: indications, diagnostic yield and consequences for patient management. Br J Gen Pract 56:574–578

Stamm G (2007) Collective radiation dose from MDCT: critical review of survey studies. In: Tack D, Gevenois PA (eds) Radiation Dose from Adult and Pediatric Multidetector Computed Tomography. Heidelberg, Springer, pp 81–97

Stanford W, Levin DC, Bettmann MA, Gomes AS, Grollman J, Henkin RE, Hessel SJ, Higgins CB, Kelley MJ, Needleman L, Polak JF, Wexler L, Abbott W, Port S (2000) Acute chest pain – no ECG evidence of myocardial ischemia/infarction. American College of Radiology. ACR Appropriateness Criteria. Radiology 215:79–84

Strain DS, Kinasewitz GT, Vereen LE, George RB (1985) Value of routine daily chest X-rays in the medical intensive care unit. Crit Care Med 13:534–536

Sunshine JH, Bushee GR, Mallick RV (1998) US radiologists' workload in 1995–1996 and trends since 1991–1992. Radiology 208:19–24

Syrjala H, Broas M, Suramo I, Ojala A, Lahde S (1998) High-resolution computed tomography for the diagnosis of community-acquired pneumonia. Clin Infect Dis 27:358–363

Takakuwa KM, Halpern EJ (2008) Evaluation of a "triple rule-out" coronary CT angiography protocol: use of 64-Section CT in low-to-moderate risk emergency department patients suspected of having acute coronary syndrome. Radiology 248:438–446

Tockman M (1986) Survival and mortality from lung cancer in a screened population: the John Hopkins study. Chest 89:325S–326S

Trotman-Dickenson B (2003) Radiology in the intensive care unit (Part I). J Intensive Care Med 18:198–210

UNSCEAR (1993) Report to the General Assembly, with Scientific Annexes. United Nations, New York

Vogt FM, Goyen M, Debatin JF (2003) MR angiography of the chest. Radiol Clin North Am 41:29–41

Wiencek RG, Weaver DW, Bouwman DL et al (1987) Usefulness of selective preoperative chest X-ray films. A prospective study. Am Surg 53:396–398

Wittram C, Meehan MJ, Halpern EF, Shepard JA, McLoud T, Thrall JH (2004) Trends in thoracic radiology over a decade at a large academic medical center. J Thorac Imaging 19:164–170

Difficulties in the Interpretation of Chest Radiography

2

Louke Delrue, Robert Gosselin, Bart Ilsen,
An Van Landeghem, Johan de Mey, and Philippe Duyck

Contents

Abstract

> Reading chest X-rays is a difficult and challenging task, and is still important despite the development of powerful imaging techniques such as computed tomography, high-resolution computed tomography, and magnetic resonance. For a correct reading and interpretation of chest X-rays, it is necessary to understand the techniques, their limitations, basic anatomy and physiology, and to have a systematic system of scrutiny. However, we have to keep in mind that interpretation is submitted to perceptual and cognitive limitations and errors. In this chapter, chest X-ray will be discussed from prescription to report in all its facets.

L. Delrue (✉), R. Gosselin, and A. Van Landeghem
Ghent University Hospital, Ghent, Belgium
e-mail: louke.delrue@uzgent.be
e-mail: robert.gosselin@uzgent.be

B. Ilsen
Department of Radiology, Universitair Ziekenhuis Brussel,
Laarbeeklaan 101, 1090, Brussel, Belgium
e-mail: bart.ilsen@uzbrussel.be

J. de Mey
Department of Radiology, AZ-VUB, Laarbeeklaan 101,
1090 Brussel, Belgium
e-mail: johan.demey@az.vub.ac.be

P. Duyck
Department of Radiology, UZ-Gent, De Pintelaan 185,
9000 Gent, Belgium
e-mail: philippe.duyck@uzgent.be

2.1 Introduction

In recent years, continuing trends in radiology have tended to diminish the importance of conventional thorax radiology. Computed tomography (CT), high-resolution CT and magnetic resonance have been applied with great success to the investigation of a range of thoracic diseases. Used separately or in sequence, they have extended our ability to evaluate many diseases. Through the use of axial imaging techniques, a lot of pulmonary images have become more understandable and interpretable for radiologists. Nowadays, the conventional chest X-ray, cheap and easily accessible but limited in scope and sensitivity, often seems irrelevant in the presence of such powerful imaging techniques. However, it would be unwise to neglect or dismiss the information conventional chest

X-rays often provide. Reading chest X-rays is still an important, difficult, and challenging task. New literature about radiological signs and symptoms mandatory for understanding chest images is scarce and sometimes inadequate, and for young radiologists basic literature is often unavailable or too concise in textbooks.

Needless to say that for a correct reading of chest X-rays, it is important to understand their limitations, basic anatomy and physiology, and to have a systematic system of scrutiny (Wright 2002). A chest radiograph is, after all, a 2-dimensional projection of a complex 3-dimensional volume in which several different tissues overlay each other.

During the last 2 decades, improvements in technique (including the use of a higher kilovoltage (kV), shorter exposure time, and the transition from conventional film to digital radiography) have had a significant impact on chest X-rays and the way radiologists and clinicians analyze thoracic images. Lots of effort has been made to facilitate the visualization of disease on chest X-rays (e.g., zooming, windowing, bone filtration). However, even when subjected to the best technical conditions, medical images are of little value unless interpreted by an expert reader; perceptual and cognitive processes directly influence the clinical utility and effectiveness of X-rays (McAdams et al. 2006). With each examination, the radiologist is still confronted with radiological findings that require interpretation in correlation with the clinical presentation and information.

2.2 Technique

For a correct interpretation of chest X-rays, proper technique is mandatory, otherwise abnormalities that should be noted may be missed.

2.2.1 Exposure

High peak kilovoltage (kVp) (e.g., 120–130 kVp) views are considered essential and the standard for most purposes; low-kV (e.g., 50–70 kVp) examinations can fail to display 30% or more of the lungs, e.g., retrocardiac, retrodiaphragmatic areas, and areas hidden by the ribs. Selection of an appropriate kV should primarily provide adequate penetration from the hila to

the periphery of the lung fields and is restricted to the patient thickness, habitus, and pathology.

A high kVp, in combination with a thick body part and a large field of view, which is the case with a chest X-ray, results in a large amount of scattered radiation, called image noise or radiographic noise (McAdams et al. 2006). Too much image noise reduces the contrast between the lung fields and the mediastinum, which results in a loss of inherent contrast. Moreover, the visualization of small low-density lesions (e.g., small noncalcified nodules, nondisplaced fractures of the ribs, foreign bodies) becomes difficult. The use of a filtering device, attached to the light-beam diaphragm of the X-ray beam, can solve this problem (Swallow et al. 1986).

However, an increase in kVp is required for penetration of the dense mediastinum and the heart to show the lung tissue behind those structures and behind the diaphragm, as well at the lung bases in a large-breasted individual.

The high kVp technique is also used to reduce obscuring effects of the ribs on underlying pulmonary pathology. The ribs cause anatomic noise and about two thirds of the lung is covered by them. Anatomic noise limits the detection of subtle abnormalities on chest X-rays, even more substantially than radiographic noise (Austin et al. 1992; Boynton and Bush 1956).

An ultrashort exposure time is necessary to obtain a high-quality chest image, preferably in the millisecond range; it reduces involuntary subject movements (Swallow et al. 1986).

Exposure factors are used correctly if the end plates of the lower thoracic vertebral bodies are visible through the cardiac shadow.

2.2.2 Positioning and Inspiration

The choice of erect or decubitus position is mainly predetermined by the condition of the patient, with the majority of X-rays taken with the patient in an erect position. Very ill patients or those who are immobile are X-rayed in decubitus or semi-recumbent position (Swallow et al. 1986).

The posteroanterior (PA) projection is generally implemented in preference to the anteroposterior (AP) projection because the arms can more easily be positioned to enable the scapulae to be projected out of the lung fields, and there is less cardiac enlargement. The mediastinal and heart shadows, however, obscure a considerable part of the lung fields, and therefore a lateral radiograph is recommended as part of an initial survey. Lesions obscured on the PA view are often clearly visible on the lateral view, such as hilar disease. In contrast, clear-cut lesions on the PA view may be difficult to identify on the lateral view because of the superposition of both lung fields. Another advantage of the lateral view is that the pleural effusion not seen on the PA projection can be identified.

2.2.2.1 Frontal View Posteroanterior Erect View

The patient is placed facing the cassette with the chin extended and centered to the middle of the top of the cassette. The feet are placed slightly apart so that the patient achieves a stable stance. The median sagittal plane is adjusted at a right angle to the middle of the cassette. The dorsal side of both hands is positioned below and behind the hips with the elbows brought forward. Alternatively, the arms encircle the cassette to allow the shoulders to rotate forward and downward and come in contact with the cassette (Swallow et al. 1986). This position avoids a superimposition of the

scapulae over the lung fields. The breasts should be compressed against the screen to prevent them from obscuring the lung bases and diaphragm.

The horizontal central X-ray is directed first at right angles to the cassette at the level of the fourth thoracic vertebra, and then angled 5° caudally to make the central ray coincide with the middle of the cassette. This results in a confining of the radiation field to the film/detector without unnecessary exposure to head and eyes (Swallow et al. 1986). Inappropriately centered X-rays may lead to hyperlucency simulating pulmonary emphysema, massive vascular embolism, or an anomaly of the soft tissues. Improper positioning (rotation) of the patient can obscure certain regions of the lung such as the hila and mediastinal lines, and borders cannot be seen anymore. It can also produce a distorted position of the trachea, which can be misinterpreted as a paratracheal mass. Exposure is made in full arrested inspiration for optimal visualization of the lung bases (the diaphragm must descend to the level of the tenth or eleventh ribs posteriorly, or to the level of the sixth ribs anteriorly). Poor inspiration may lead to under-expansion of the thoracic cage with crowding of basal vessels simulating congestion or fibrosis. Moreover, small pleural effusions will be masked (Fig. 2.1).

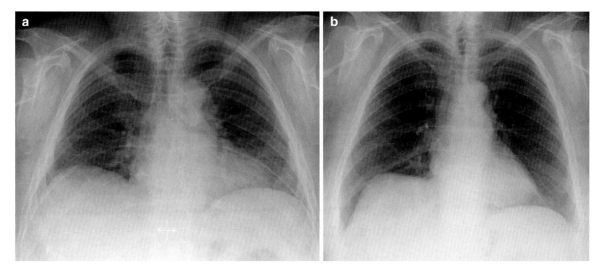

Fig. 2.1 A 60-year-old female patient was admitted to our hospital for the evaluation of persistent pain of unknown origin in the left limb. She was treated for colon carcinoma in 1993 (in remission), a transient ischemic attack in 2000, and she underwent resection of uterine polyps in 2003. A chest radiograph was performed for a general check-up. (a) Posteroanterior chest X-ray reveals decreased lucency at both lung bases suggesting consolidations. X-ray also shows accentuation of vessels and enlarged heart shadow: a sign of vascular congestion? (b) A second Posteroanterior chest X-ray of the same patient taken in deep inspiration, did not confirm any of these abnormalities: there were no consolidations and no signs of congestive heart disease. The second view only revealed an asymmetric position of the diaphragm. Poor inspiration may lead to accentuation of vessels simulating congestion, the heart shadow will be enlarged, and the visualization of consolidations can be compromised

A pattern of under-expansion is not always caused by the noncooperation of patients but may also be due to diseases that decrease lung compliance: pulmonary disease such as lung fibrosis, neurologic disorders such as multiple sclerosis, or thoracic deformity generated by kyphoscoliosis.

PA erect view is an alternative when the patient's condition makes it difficult or unsafe for the patient to stand. The patient sits (or stands) with his or her back against the cassette. Again, the shoulders are brought downward and forward, with the back of the hands below the hips and the elbows well forward. If the patient's condition does not allow proper realization of this movement, it is preferable that the arms be laterally rotated and supported with the palms of the hands facing forward. In this position the scapulae are superimposed but visibility of the upper lateral segments is easier because of the reduced absorption effects (Swallow et al. 1986). Notice the greater object–cassette distance of the heart compared to the PA view, which makes accurate measurement of the heart size difficult (overestimation).

2.2.2.2 Lateral View

The patient is turned with his or her left side against the cassette and the median sagittal plane parallel to the cassette. The arms are folded over the head or raised above the head to rest on a horizontal bar. The midaxillary line coincides with the middle of the cassette. The volume between the apices and the lower lobes to the level of the first lumbar vertebra should be covered by the cassette. The central ray is directed at right angles to the middle of the cassette in the midaxillar line (Swallow et al. 1986). Exposure is made in full arrested inspiration.

2.2.2.3 Other

Exposure made in full arrested *expiration* has the effect of increasing intrapleural pressure, in turn resulting in compression of the lung parenchyma, which makes the pneumothorax bigger and therefore, more easily visualized (Swallow et al. 1986).

In selected patients *paired inspiratory* and *expiratory PA exposures* can demonstrate air trapping. Areas of akinesis or hypokinesis of the diaphragm can be detected by *fluoroscopy*, called the sniff test: a paradoxical motion of a hemidiaphragm when a patient sniffs vigorously suggests phrenic nerve paralysis or paresis of the hemidiaphragm. Rapid upward movement of the diaphragm during brisk sniffing in the supine position is highly suggestive of paralysis of the ipsilateral diaphragm.

Other views, such as *oblique view, apical view,* and *lordotic view,* are superseded by CT.

2.2.3 Image Processing and Post-Processing

Radiological imaging is undergoing revolutionary changes and traditional film–screen imaging has been rapidly replaced by digital imaging during the past several years (Mettler et al. 2004). Variability of image quality in conventional radiography, due to the developing procedure of the X-ray film, vanished with the introduction of digital radiography (DR) (Bacher et al. 2006). Moreover, digital images are very flexible in terms of processing and archiving, thereby providing a solution to the major disadvantages of the screen–film systems. Regardless of whether digital radiography or computed radiography (CR) is used, readjustment of an analog signal to a digital signal by an analog-to-digital converter is common to both. Once the digital signal is produced, it may be displayed, processed, and manipulated to maximize visualization of anatomical structures and disorders. The image quality depends on spatial and contrast resolutions. The *spatial resolution* of a digital image is defined or limited by a matrix of pixels running in horizontal and vertical rows. More pixels generate a better spatial resolution. The matrix size of the monitors on which the image is displayed can influence the visibility of a disease. 3 K monitors (3,000 × 3,000 pixels) are a minimal requirement for chest radiography (Bacher et al. 2006). Both the pixel depth and the range of gray shades that can be assigned to the pixels are responsible for image quality. They are also referred to as the dynamic range. The dynamic range, measured in bits, influences the *contrast resolution* of a digital system. The higher the contrast resolution, the more distinct the adjacent structures of close opacity (Shephard 2003).

An important advantage of digital imaging (CR or DR) over conventional radiographic imaging is that once the digital image is created it becomes available in an electronic form that can be archived and manipulated on a diagnostic workstation by optimizing display contrast regardless of the exposure level (McAdams et al. 2006). The visibility can be optimized depending on the region of interest. Digital imaging may offer additional information, dose reduction, and fast availability of images, resulting in clinical benefits, a favorable cost-benefit ratio and increased quality and efficiency (Nitrosi et al. 2007).

The combination of storage phosphor technology and post-processing technology enables the visualization of large absorption differences in one image. Post-processing is guided by three types of algorithms: gray-scale processing, edge enhancement, and multi-frequency processing (McAdams et al. 2006). (1) Gray-scale processing involves the conversion of detector signal values to display values in such a way that digital images appear similar to conventional film images. (2) The edge enhancement algorithm aims to enhance fine image details by manipulating the high-frequency content of the image by using a variant of the unsharp masking technique (a blurred version of the image is formed and a fraction of the resulting image is subtracted from the original image). (3) In multi-frequency processing, the image is decomposed into multiple frequency components. Each of them is weighted separately and then recomposed into one image. This results in more visibility of the opaque regions—retrocardial, paramediastinal, and paradiaphragmatic—without compromise of the contrast in the lung regions (McAdams et al. 2006). The large dynamic range of the storage phosphor technology and its post-processing capabilities allow visualization of the entire lung even with a large field of view, as in chest X-rays, despite the lower spatial resolution of the digital technique compared to conventional film–screen images. Busch (1997) demonstrated that digital imaging yields additional information through its clearly higher-contrast perceptibility; particularly, the quality of visualization of the mediastinal and retrocardial structures is much higher. This advantage is even more pronounced in "bedside-image" chest radiographs. It leads to a much better localization of probes and catheters. Busch (1997) showed a decrease in the number of low-quality images from 22% to 8% and a decrease in the number of images of insufficient quality from 8% to 2% when phosphor storage technology is used instead of conventional film–screen technology in chest X-rays without exposure control.

2.3 Interpretation

Correct interpretation of plain chest X-rays will often obviate the need for more expensive and sophisticated examinations.

The main ways to minimize interpretation errors are thorough knowledge of the normal anatomy of the thorax, and the basic physiology of chest diseases; analyzing the radiograph through a fixed pattern; evaluating the evolution over time; knowledge of clinical presentation and history; and knowledge of the correlation with other diagnostic results (laboratory results [blood, sputa], electrocardiogram, respiratory function tests).

2.3.1 Knowledge of Anatomy and Physiology

Before a diagnosis can be made, any abnormalities must be distinguished from normal variations. Therefore, radiologists must have a knowledge of the pattern of linear markings throughout the normal lung (Fraser et al. 1988). Such knowledge cannot be gained through literature or didactic teaching; it requires exposure to thousands of normal chest X-rays to acquire the ability to distinguish normal from abnormal. This requires not only familiarity with the pattern and the distribution of branching of these markings, but also knowledge of normal caliber and changes that may occur in different phases of respiration and in various body positions. Normally, the distribution of the pulmonary blood flow is controlled primarily by gravitational forces. The vessels branch like a tree, gracefully and gradually from the hilum toward the periphery of the lung in the erect position. This normal flow pattern is called "caudalization" (Chen 1983). A change in caliber of the arteries and veins remains one of the most variable radiological signs of pulmonary arterial and pulmonary venous hypertension. A redistribution of vessels may constitute major evidence for pulmonary collapse or previous surgical resection. A firm understanding of anatomy and physiology is helpful in radiographic interpretation. The lungs can be likened to a mirror reflecting the underlying pathophysiology of the heart (Chen 1983). Failure of the right side of the heart will result in a scanty flow, small vessels, and unusually radiolucent lungs.

2.3.2 Basic Principles of a Chest X-Ray

2.3.2.1 Three Basic Principles

Being familiar with the *basic principles of a chest radiograph* will help the radiologist to overcome some difficulties because they indicate the fundamental nature of diseases.

A radiograph is not a shadow but a complex summation of a polychromatic beam of X-rays (Milne 1993).

Remember the following three basic principles (Squire 1970; Novelline and Squire 1997):

1. Roentgen white–gray–black values are the result of variations in the number of rays that have passed through the object of interest to expose the X-ray detector.

Therefore, they are always summation shadow grains of all the masses in the full thickness of the object that has been interposed between the beam-source and the detector.

Because it is a summation/projection of several layers, subtle lesions such as early lung cancer or focal pneumonia can be overlaid by background anatomy. Austin and colleagues (1992) concluded that confusion by background structures is the leading cause of nondetection of nodules in well-penetrated lung zones. Dual-energy radiography, which is a clinical application of digital imaging, can overcome this difficulty through the elimination of the background with the subtraction technique. Ishigaki and others (1986) described this technique in 1986 by using two storage phosphor plates separated by a filter for a single shot based on the difference in spectral absorption characteristics of bone and soft tissue. Dual-energy imaging with bone subtraction (called soft imaging) has been shown to be advantageous for

- the detection of lung nodules, even those obscured by overlaying structures
- other types of focal opacities, such as those caused by infection
- the visualization of central airways

There was, however, no advantage in the characterization of interstitial patterns when compared with conventional standard images (MacMahon et al. 2008b). The bone image can help to detect the presence of calcification in lung nodules, referring to benign etiology, and in pleural plaques. It also has been shown to be advantageous in the evaluation of coronary and cardiac calcifications and radio–opaque devices, and it helps in the detection of sclerotic skeletal metastases.

2. The margin of any shadow on the X-ray represents a tangentially seen interface between two structures of different roentgen density.

The silhouette sign is based on the premise that an intrathoracic opacity, if in anatomic contact with a border of the heart or aorta, will obscure that border (Felson 1973). The mechanism responsible for the sign is still debated. The silhouette sign can be used in two ways (Armstrong et al. 1990):

- To localize a density on a chest X-ray
- To detect lesions of low density when the shadow is less obvious than the loss of the silhouette

Most anatomic structures bordering the lung (such as the heart, aorta, and diaphragm) are not visible themselves; their recognition depends on the presence of adjacent air-filled (normal) lung tissue: loss of silhouette sign (Wright 2002). Thus, obliteration or absence of the outline of those structures indicates that airless tissue, such as fluid or a solid tumor, is adjacent to those structures. For example, collapse or consolidation of the left upper lobe will obliterate the left cardiac border, and collapse or consolidation of the right middle lobe will obliterate the right cardiac border.

Using the same principle, a well-defined mass seen above the clavicles is located posteriorly and in contact with the aerated lung parenchyma, whereas a mass located anteriorly is in contact with mediastinal soft tissues and so is poorly defined. This is also known as the *cervico-thoracic sign.*

The *hilum overlay sign* is used to distinguish a hilar mass from a nonhilar mass: When the hilar vessels can still be seen through a mass, then the mass does not arise from the hilum. Because of the geometry of the mediastinum, most of these masses will be located in the anterior mediastinum.

3. Awareness of the range of atomic numbers (roentgen densities) of objects or tissues plus the information you will deduce about their thickness,

shape and form, make it possible to identify an object by name from its radiograph. The atomic composition of objects or tissues will strongly influence the amount and the energy of the X-rays that will interact with the X-ray detector. Together with the information about their thickness, shape, and form, objects can be identified by name from a radiograph.

2.3.2.2 Threshold Visibility

The *threshold visibility* is defined at 3 mm: a structure must be at least 3 mm in thickness to be radiologically visible on a chest X-ray. The 3-mm limit of visibility can only be applied if the margins of the structure are parallel to the X-ray beam. It decreases progressively when the margins are beveled (Fraser et al. 1988). Four mm is considered to be the lower limit of visibility for noncalcified intrapulmonary densities by Westra (1990) and Brogdon et al. (1983). The threshold visibility is not only influenced by the border of the lesion shadow (sharply defined or beveled margins), but also by its location. The visibility is higher when a lesion can be projected in such a way that it is related to air-containing parenchyma without a superimposed confusion by overlying structures. This leads to relatively "blind" areas. Those areas are located in close proximity to the pleura and the rib cage, in the paramediastinal regions, and near the diaphragm (Brogdon et al. 1983; Fraser et al. 1988)

2.3.3 Analyzing the Radiograph Through a Fixed Pattern

One of the most challenging tasks when viewing chest X-rays is to visualize and depict all lesions regardless of their location, whether a lesion is primarily in the lung, the hilum, the mediastinum, the pleura, the chest wall, the diaphragm, or outside the thorax.

A chest X-ray can be inspected in two ways (Fraser et al. 1988):

- Direct search is a method whereby a specific pattern of inspection is carried out.
- Free global search, in which the X-ray is scanned without a preconceived orderly pattern.

There is subjective and objective evidence that experienced radiologists use to perceive the most important abnormalities within the first few seconds of viewing; a single display of less than 300 ms may be sufficient for the identification of major features of lesions, and this rapid identification of abnormalities increases with experience (Brogdon et al. 1983). This proposition supports the free global search and suggests that fragmentary images are filled in from the observer's memory bank (Kundel and Nodine 1983).

We believe a systematic approach to radiological interpretation is of profound importance, especially for radiologists in training. Radiologists must develop a routine when examining X-rays that ensures that all areas of the radiograph are scrutinized. It is only through this exercise during thousands of examinations that the pattern of a normal chest can be recognized. The radiologist must try to appreciate signs such as the size, number, and density of pulmonary lesions in combination with their border sharpness, homogeneity, anatomic location, and distribution as well as the presence or absence of cavitation or calcification.

A suggested scheme is as follows, examining each point in turn (Murfitt 1993):

1. Request form	Name, age, date, sex Clinical information
2. Technical	Centering, patient position Markers
3. Trachea	Position, outline
4. Heart and mediastinum	Size, shape, displacement
5. Diaphragms	Outline, shape Relative position
6. Pleura	Position of horizontal fissure Costophrenic, cardiophrenic angles
7. Lung fields	Local, generalized abnormalities Comparison of the translucency and vascular markings of the lungs
8. Hidden areas	Apices, posterior sulcus Mediastinum, bones
9. Hila	Density, position, shape
10. Below diaphragms	Gas shadows, calcifications
11. Soft tissues	Mastectomy, gas, densities, etc.
12. Bones	Destructive lesions, densities, etc.

1. *Request form:* age, sex, and clinical information can help in making the distinction between normal and abnormal structures. It is important to know that the area of the pulmonary trunk is frequently very prominent in young women. In babies and young children (more frequently in boys than girls) normal thymus tissue can be present as a triangular sail-shaped opacity with well-defined borders projecting on one or both sides of the mediastinum and causing an enlarged mediastinal appearance. Patients recovering from disease can present with an enlarged thymus (thymus rebound). In a young healthy person, a nodule present in the lung parenchyma is most probably benign (Fig. 2.2).

2. *Technique:* any adjustment of the regular procedure must be mentioned and marked clearly on the image: PA or AP, left/right label, inspiration/expiration. It is important to correctly diagnose pathologies such as Kartagener syndrome. Kartagener syndrome is defined by the combination of primary ciliary dyskinesia, an inherited disorder of special respiratory tract cells, along with positioning of the internal organs on the opposite side from normal (called situs inversus). For example, the heart is on the right side of the chest instead of the left.

3. *The trachea:* this conduit is located on the midline in its upper part and deviates slightly to the right at the level of the aortic knuckle. This deviation is more pronounced during expiration. During expiration, the trachea becomes shorter. This implies that an endotracheal tube that is situated just above the carina during inspiration can occlude the main bronchus during expiration. The translucency of the tracheal air column decreases caudally in normal conditions. Widening of the carina occurs during inspiration and the angle may measure 60–75°.

4. *The heart:* the position of the heart relative to the midline and the transverse cardiac diameter on the PA view is quite variable, even among healthy people. The average normal value of the cardiothoracic ratio is 0.45 in adults (Chen 1983). The heart shadow is enlarged without being pathological on expiration X-rays, in the supine position, in AP projection, when the diaphragm is elevated, and in patients with kyphosis or scoliosis. Measurement in an isolated event is of less value than when previous X-rays are available for comparison. For example, an increase in the transverse cardiac diameter of 1.5 cm in sequential X-rays is significant and should be investigated further (Murfitt 1993).

5. *The diaphragm:* the diaphragm is a thin musculotendinous structure, which is not or only partially visible on conventional X-rays (Bogaert and Verschakelen 1995). Nevertheless, the diaphragmatic area is noteworthy because it can provide important information. For example, the detection of a diaphragmatic defect after trauma can be life-saving. It has been shown that missing this difficult diagnosis results in higher morbidity and mortality in trauma victims (Meyers and McCabe 1993).

6. *The pleura:* the pleura consist of two thin layers covering a serous membrane lining the inside of the chest cavity and covering the lung, with a small amount of fluid in between. The pleura serves an important role in lung function; it acts as a cushion for the lungs and allows for smooth movement of the lungs within the chest cavity. It is not visible in normal conditions and barely visible in the case of ventral pleural detachment. The increase of the transparency of the lung can be very subtle or even masked by overlying tissue (Ball et al. 2005).

Pay attention to pneumothorax "*ex vacuo*"; in this condition, acute bronchial obstruction from mucous plugs, aspirated foreign bodies, or badly positioned endotracheal tubes cause acute lobar collapse and a significant increase in negative intrapleural pressure around the collapsed lobe. As a consequence, gas is attracted into the pleural space around the collapsed lobe while the seal between the visceral and parietal pleura of the adjacent lobe or lobes remains intact. The remaining pleural attachment is characteristic. Correct interpretation of this kind of pneumothorax is crucial in directing treatment, which consists of relieving the bronchial obstruction rather than inserting a chest tube into the pleural space. Once the bronchial obstruction is relieved, the lobe will re-expand and the pneumothorax will resolve spontaneously (Ashizawa et al. 2001; Florman et al. 2001) (Fig. 2.3).

Other difficulties of pleural processes include determining whether a "pleural" abnormality really originates from the pleura (Fig. 2.4) and distinguishing lung nodules from pleural irregularities (Fig. 2.5).

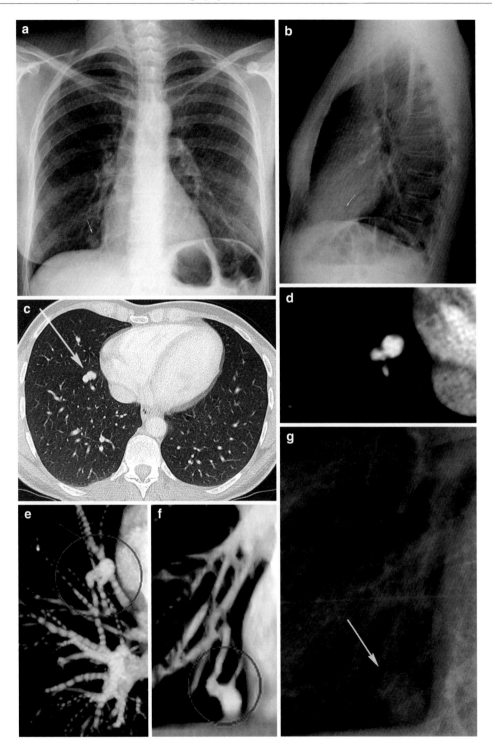

Fig. 2.2 A 40-year-old female patient with chronic headaches consulted the hospital to exclude underlying general physical causes. She smokes 12 cigarettes a day. In this setting she received a chest X-ray. (**a**, **b**) Chest X-ray reveals a well-defined nodule projected alongside the heart at the right lung base on PA view and projected on the heart shadow on lateral view. Multidetector row CT (MDCT) was performed to exclude neoplastic nodule. (**c**, **d**) MDCT demonstrates a dense lobulated nodule in the anterior right lower lung lobe. (**e**, **f**) On the 3-dimensional reconstructions, the nodule is connected to a small artery and vein. No other parenchymal abnormalities are visualized. Final diagnosis was a pulmonary arterio-vascular malformation. (**g**) A digital magnified spot view of the chest X-ray reveals the vascular malformation

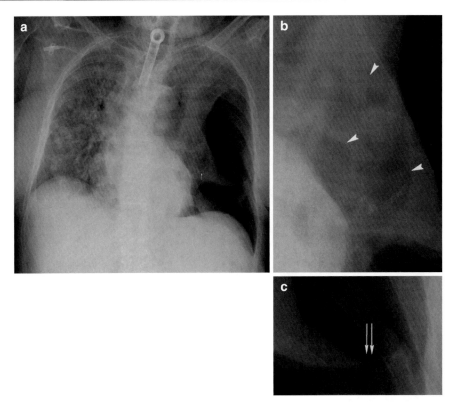

Fig. 2.3 A 63-year-old female patient was sent to the emergency radiology department for a chest X-ray to exclude aspiration pneumonia. Her clinical history reveals severe interstitial lung pathology based on chronic nephropathy, and a 3-month period of recurrent pneumonia resulting in open lung biopsy (negative culture) and in increasing respiratory insufficiency. For that reason, the patient underwent the placement of a permanent tracheostomy. At the time of presentation, the patient showed no signs of acute dyspnea, fever, or sudden chest pain. (**a**) The bedside anteroposterior X-ray confirmed severe alveolo-interstitial lung pattern of the right lung, a small shift of the cardio-mediastinum to the right, and a lobar collapse in the left hemi-thorax with hyperlucency around the collapsed lobe (notice surgical stitches projecting on the heart after open lung biopsy [*arrow*]). The X-ray also reveals (**b**) conglomerate of trapped air and irregular dense particles at the left hilum and (**c**) a seal connecting the parietal and visceral pleura of the lobe(s). The patient suffered from a pneumothorax ex vacuo caused by bronchial obstruction. Immediate relief of bronchial obstruction is crucial and lifesaving (no tube into pleural space but tracheal aspiration)

7. *The lung fields:* normal intrapulmonary airways are invisible unless they end in the X-ray beam, but air within bronchi or bronchioli, passing through airless parenchyma, may be visible as a branching linear lucency known as an "air bronchogram." An air bronchogram within an opacity means that the opacity is intrapulmonary in location (Armstrong et al. 1990). The most common causes of an air bronchogram are pneumonia or pulmonary edema. Air bronchograms can be seen in atelectatic lobes provided the airways are patent. Because of the specific growth of bronchioalveolar carcinoma, as well as lymphoma around airways without compressing them, both diseases can also be associated with an air bronchogram.

By comparing the lung fields, areas of abnormal translucency or even distribution of lung markings are more easily detected. However, confusing the interpretation of diffuse lung disease in X-rays is not surprising. Much of the confusion arises because of doubt over precisely what is seen and what can be seen on a chest X-ray. The radiologist is sometimes confronted with the problem of superimposition of many layers of opacity. As mentioned by Fraser and Paré (1998), superimposition of small nodules can cause an apparent reduction in the size of the individual nodules and in the formation of curvilinear and nodular opacities.

Another major reason for confusion during the interpretation of interstitial lung disease in X-rays is the lack of specificity of the presented radiological

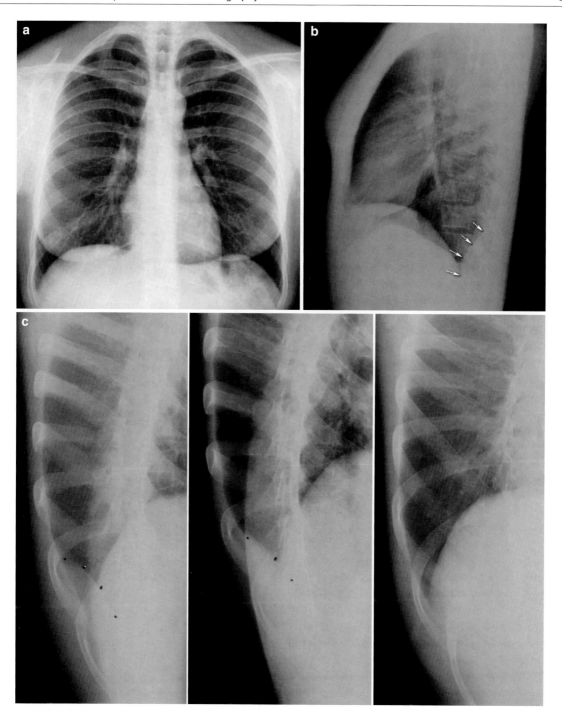

Fig. 2.4 A 37-year-old female patient was admitted to our hospital with right latero-dorsal thoracic pain without history of a traumatic event. There was no fever, weight loss, or nocturnal sweating. Clinical investigation revealed a painful hard mass at the right hemi-thorax; the lung auscultation was normal. The patient mentioned recent travel to Australia. (**a, b**) Posteroanterior and lateral X-rays of the chest show a deformation of the dorsal costo-dia-phragmatic sinus (*arrows*). (**c**) An oblique magnified view confirmed the existence of the deformation: pleural mass? soft-tissue tumor? localized pleural effusion? (**d**) Contrast-enhanced Multidetector row CT demonstrates a cystic lesion with dense rim in the right costophrenic pleura (*white arrow*) with expansion in the dorsal thoracic wall (*white arrowhead*). Final diagnosis was a hyatid cyst (positive for Echinococcus antibodies)

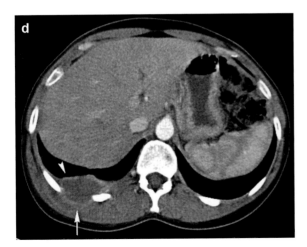

Fig. 2.4 (continued)

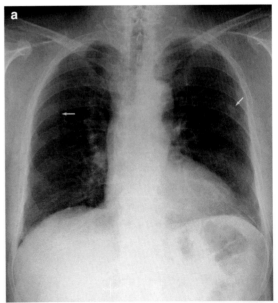

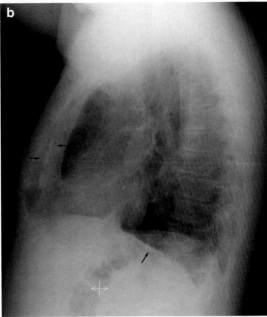

patterns. Basic radiological patterns of interstitial lung disease are reticular, nodular, reticulonodular, and linear, which are well known. However, sometimes diseases present as reticular at the beginning and evolve into a nodular or mixed reticulonodular pattern. Similarly, in a reticular network, particularly if it is coarse, many linear densities will be seen "en face" and thus appear as a reticular pattern, but many must be seen on end and thus simulate nodules (Fraser et al. 1988; Stolberg et al. 1964). Because of this obvious visual effect, it might seem logical to designate all these diseases as reticulonodular (see Chap. 8: Interstitial Lung Disease).

However, the distinction between reticular and nodular is important not only morphologically, but also in relation to the impact each may have on the pulmonary function (Fig. 2.6).

Unilateral pulmonary hyperlucency with decreased vascularity and airtrapping on expiration is signature of the Swyer-James-MacLeod syndrome (Lucaya et al. 1998) (Fig. 2.7).

8. *The hidden areas:* apices, posterior sulcus, mediastinum, hila, and bones remain a challenge on chest X-rays, even in digital imaging, multi-detector row CT can be necessary for further differentiation (Fig. 2.8).

9. *The hila:* the dimension of the normal hila, delineated mostly by the large pulmonary arteries and upper lobe pulmonary veins, varies considerably within and among individuals (left versus right). A difference in the relative density of the two hila

Fig. 2.5 A 62-year-old male patient with a persistent cough was sent by his general physician for a chest X-ray to exclude lung pathology. The patient was a smoker but had no other items in his medical history. (**a**) Posteroanterior chest X-ray revealed a non-sharply delineated nodular structure of limited density projected on the posterior part of the sixth rib in the right hemi-thorax (*arrow*). A second fanciful dense opacity projected on the posterior part of the left sixth rib (*arrow*). (**b**) Linear densities projected posterior of the sternum and above the diaphragm, best revealed on the lateral chest X-ray (*arrows*). (**c**) Multi-detector row CT shows several pleural irregularities, e.g., at the level of the sixth rib bilateral. Some of the irregularities were partially calcified, specifically those located at the diaphragm. Irregular focal thickening of the pleura can simulate a suspicious parenchymal opacity on a chest X-ray

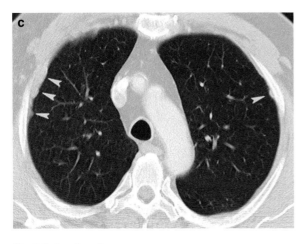

Fig. 2.5 (continued)

could imply hilar pathology and is an indication for additional CT. A lack of sharpness of the lateral hilum also requires CT examination because of the implications of the silhouette sign. The hilum overlay and hilum convergence sign are based on that principle (Felson 1973) (Fig. 2.9).

10. *Areas below the diaphragm:* a pneumoperitoneum is more easily detected on a lateral chest X-ray in erect position than on an erect abdominal view. Chilaiditi syndrome, which is the interposition of the colon between the liver and diaphragm, is very common, especially among the elderly. The haustral pattern helps to distinguish it from free intraperitoneal gas.

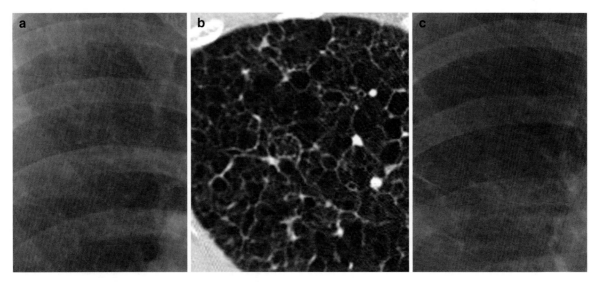

Fig. 2.6 Several cases of parenchymal lucencies associated with the presence of cysts, which are difficult to distinguish on a conventional X-ray. (**a, b**) Pulmonary Langerhans cell histiocytosis. The X-ray reveals diffuse parenchymal lucencies and reticulonodular pattern of the interstitial space. High-resolution CT (HRCT) demonstrates cystic airspaces, which are mainly less than 10 mm in diameter, with typical sparing of the costophrenic angles. The lung cysts have distinct walls ranging from thin and barely perceptible to several millimeters in thickness and have varying shapes (mostly round, some bizarre in shape). (**c, d**) Lymphangioleiomyomatosis. The X-ray again reveals diffuse small parenchymal lucencies with a reticulonodular interstitial pattern. HRCT shows numerous thin-walled lung cysts with varying diameters (ranging from 2 mm to 5 cm) and round in shape, diffusely distributed and surrounded by patchy areas of ground-glass opacity. (**e, f**) Centrilobular emphysema. Only moderate to severe emphysema can be diagnosed on plain radiographs. The X-ray can only suggest parenchymal hyperlucency; perhaps reduction in the size of pulmonary vessels or vessel tapering can be detected. On HRCT there is the presence of multiple small, round areas of abnormally low attenuation,

several millimeters in diameter. The areas of lucency are grouped near the centers of secondary pulmonary lobules, surrounding the centrilobular artery branches, and often lack distinct walls. (**g, h**) Panlobular emphysema. The X-ray reveals an increased hyperlucency with size reduction of pulmonary vessels and vessel tapering, which is not a sensitive or reliable sign of emphysema. HRCT demonstrates widespread areas of abnormally low attenuation by uniform destruction of the pulmonary lobule. The pulmonary vessels appear as fewer, smaller, and inconspicuous. Panlobular emphysema is easily distinguished from lung cysts by the lack of distinct walls. (**i, j**) Paraseptal emphysema. The X-ray shows no aberrancy in parenchymal pattern. On HRCT there are some focal hyperlucent areas in the subpleural areas (involvement of the distal part of the secondary lobule) with visible, very thin walls corresponding to the interlobular septae. (**k, l**) Fibrosis. The X-ray reveals a reticulonodular pattern *with small nodular opacities*. HRCT confirms the reticulonodular pattern caused by subpleural intralobular interstitial thickening predominantly involving the subpleural lung regions, in combination with irregular opacities, honeycombing, architectural distortion, and traction bronchiectasis

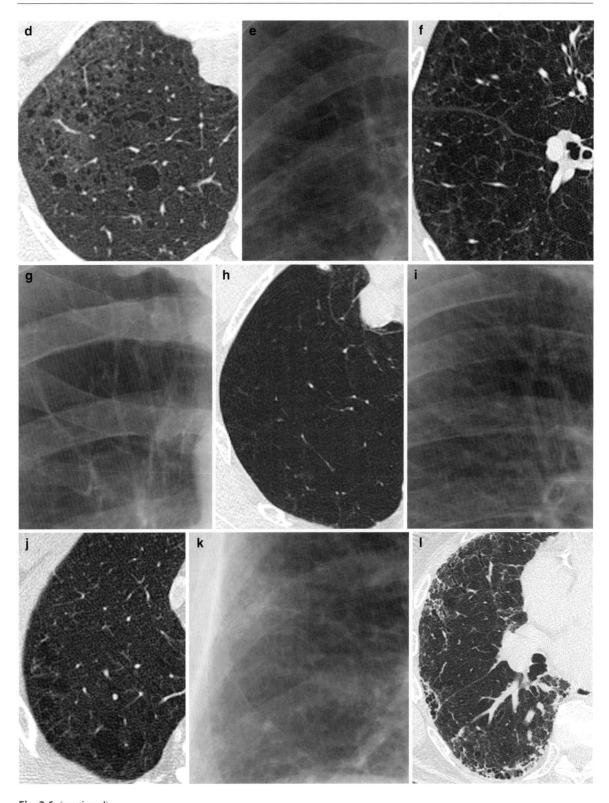

Fig. 2.6 (continued)

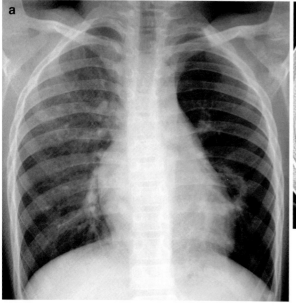

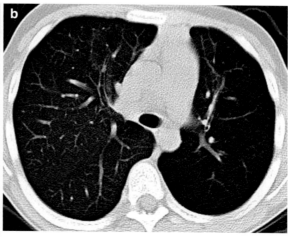

Fig. 2.7 (**a**) A chest X-ray of an 11-year-old child reveals a discrepancy in translucency between the left and the right hemithorax. Because of the asymmetric presentation of the lung fields, an overlaying interstitial or alveolar lung pathology cannot be excluded. There are no arguments for pneumothorax in the left hemithorax. Notice the tiny displacement of the mediastinum to the left side. (**b**) Multi-detector row CT shows a unilateral hyperlucent left lung with reduced lung volume in inspiration, diminuation of the vascularisation, and air-trapping. No disturbance of the interstitial or alveolar pattern can be seen. The patient suffered from Swyer-James-MacLeod syndrome, caused by incomplete development of the alveolar buds as a result of damage to the terminal and respiratory bronchioles, usually due to viral lower respiratory tract infection in infancy or early childhood

11. *Soft tissues:* the breasts may partially obscure the lung bases. Physiological breast asymmetry or previous surgery can mislead and be misinterpreted as parenchymal shadowing or hyperlucency. Identification of the nipple shadow is necessary to distinguish from neoplasm and vice versa. Repeat X-rays with nipple marking or fluoroscopy can help out if in doubt.

    The anterior axillary fold frequently causes an ill-defined shadow on the lung fields and must be differentiated from a consolidation.

    The caudal border of the opacity of the sternocleidomastoid muscles can simulate a cavity or bulla at the lung apices. Subpleural fat or prominent intercostal muscles can mimic pleural pathology.

12. *Bones:* bone alterations can be the only sign of pathology on chest X-rays; a fracture of the clavicula or fracture of the first rib can cause a pneumothorax and/or vascular rupture, both life-threatening situations. Hemi-vertebrae may be associated with neuro-enteric cysts.

As mentioned previously, more than 66% of the lung parenchyma is superimposed by bony structures, which may result in missed lung nodules. On the other hand, focal bone opacities, such as a benign bone island (enostosis), also can result in false-positive abnormal chest X-rays (Fig. 2.10).

2.3.4 Evolution Over Time

An additional source of information is the *evolution over time*. It is imperative to compare studies carried out at different dates whenever they are available (Fig. 2.11). A sudden or progressive increase in the cardio-mediastinal shadow width may be the only indicator of a mediastinal tumor. Minimal thickening of the right paratracheal stripe, which is an indirect sign of paratracheal lymphadenopathy, may be detected only when compared with a previous chest X-ray.

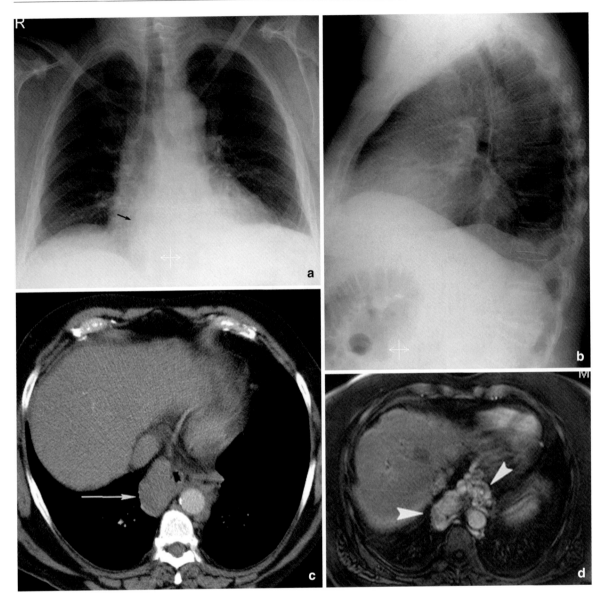

Fig. 2.8 A 66-year-old male patient with ethylic liver cirrhosis was admitted to the hospital for diminished consciousness and deterioration of his general condition. (**a**) Posteroanterior and lateral view of the chest demonstrate vascular calcifications at the descending aorta, widening of the carina, and a dense pericardial mass near the right atrial border (*arrow*). (**b**) Two vertebral collapses are also visualized on the lateral view: at the fifth dorsal and first lumbar vertebra. (**c**) Nonenhanced multi-detector row CT confirms a relatively dense paraesophageal and paraaortic soft tissue structure. (**d**) T1-weighted magnetic resonance image after Gadolinium demonstrates a knot of vessels in the middle and posterior mediastinum. The pericardial mass visualized on the chest X-ray was periesophageal varices in this patient who has liver cirrhosis

The speed of growth of a lesion over time indicates the cell replication rate within the lesion and gives information about its benign or malignant character. The rate of growth is disclosed by the doubling , or the time it takes a given tumor to double in volume, and requires sequential exposures over time (Garland et al. 1963). Tumor doubling time is an independent and significant prognostic factor for lung cancer patients (Usuda et al. 1994). Spratt et al (1963). found a mean doubling time of 3.1 months for squamous cell carcinoma, 9 months for adenocarcinomas, and 3 months for undifferentiated cancer on chest X-rays.

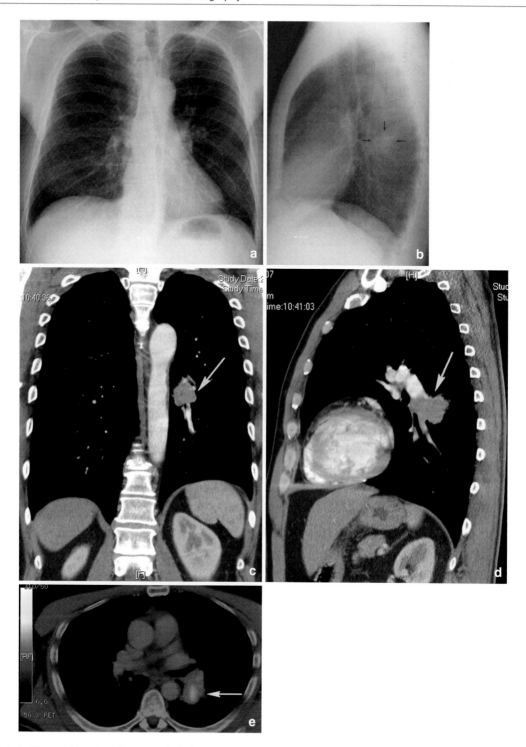

Fig. 2.9 A 56-year-old male patient consulted the hospital for persistent dry cough, dyspnea when exercising, asthenia, and weight loss despite a good appetite. History revealed nicotine abuse (25–30 pack years) and exposure to asbestos. (**a, b**) Chest X-ray suggests an additional opacity (*arrows*) at the left hilum, best visualized on the lateral view projected on the anterior border of the thoracic vertebral column. (**c, d**) Multi-detector row CT confirms a homogeneous mass at the origin of the main bronchus of the left lower lobe, as illustrated here in coronal and lateral reformatted reconstructions of the mediastinum (*arrows*). (**e**) Positron emission tomography-CT shows elevated fludeoxyglucose uptake in the mass. Bronchoscopy confirmed a suspicious mass in the ostium of the bronchus of the left lower lobe. Pathology revealed a non–small-cell lung carcinoma, spinocellular type

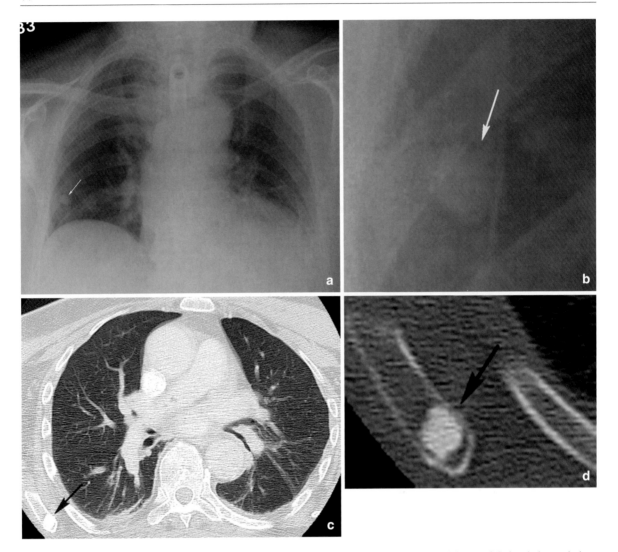

Fig. 2.10 A 64-year-old male patient was sent to the emergency radiology department with spontaneous intracranial bleeding. He received surgical cranial decompression and a tracheostomy. (**a**) A bedside chest X-ray in the intensive care ward shows a dense nodular structure in the eighth intercostal space on the right side (*arrow*). (**b**) Digital magnified spot view confirms the nodular density with nonsharp margins (*arrow*). (**c**) Mutli-detector row CT shows no parenchymal nodule on axial view in lung window. At the scapular point a nodular density is revealed (*arrow*) and confirmed on (**d**) the magnified spot reconstructed with bone window (*arrow*). This is an incidental finding of a solitary dense nodule on a chest X-ray in a patient with spontaneous intracranial bleeding. This nodule was located in the scapular point and consisted of dense osseous tissue (benign bony island)

Temporal subtraction may be the innovation that reveals a significant improvement in the accuracy of detection of nodules and hazy pulmonary opacities such as pneumonia and pneumonitis (Difazio et al. 1997; MacMahon et al. 2008b; Tsubamoto et al. 2002). This advanced image-processing technique enhances interval changes by using the previous radiographs as subtraction masks (MacMahon et al. 2008a). DiFazio and others (1997) reported not only a substantial and highly significant improvement in diagnostic accuracy when using temporal subtraction, they also stated that the chest X-ray interpretation time was reduced by 19%. One of the difficulties of this technique is its dependence on reproducible patient positioning. The

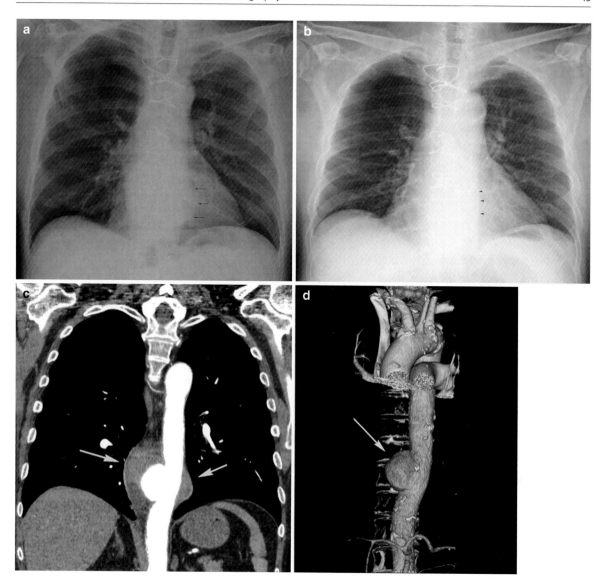

Fig. 2.11 A 64-year-old male patient known since 2001 with severe chronic obstructive pulmonary disease (III) was recently hospitalized with pneumonia, erysipelas of the right lower limb, and reflux oesophagitis grade B. Because of this medical history, he received subsequent chest X-rays for a period of 2 months. (**a**) On the anteroposterior chest radiograph of April 2008 there was an impression of a deviation of the left paravertebral line. (**b**) Looking back to previous chest radiographs, no displacement of the left paravertebral line was visualized (e.g., chest X-ray DD March 2008). This suggests a para-vertebral pathology, such as an aneurysm of the thoracic aorta. For that reason the patient underwent urgent CT examination. (**c, d**) Multi-detector row CT of the thoracic aorta confirms the presence of a para-aortic dense heterogeneous mass and reveals a saccular dilatation of the thoracic aorta, illustrated here in coronal reformatted reconstructions of the mediastinum (*arrow* in **c**) and 3-dimensional reconstructions (**d**). Final diagnosis was a leaking thoracic aortic aneurysm, for which the patient was successfully treated with an endovascular stent procedure. This case proves the importance of a good technical quality, which is obligatory for transparency of the mediastinum to detect displacement of the paravertebralline and the need for comparison with previous chest X-rays

majority of the artefacts in thoracic temporal subtraction are due to bone misregistration, which can be reduced or even eliminated in combination with dual-energy imaging (see above).

Evolution over time can also make interpretation more difficult and complex. As diseases progress, identified patterns can disappear. Several lung diseases, each with a different diagnostic pattern, may all eventually evolve into lung fibrosis; all present the same pattern of honeycomb formation.

2.3.5 Knowledge of Clinical Presentation, History, and Correlation to Other Diagnostic Results

When there is no clinical information or medical history available, the exact diagnosis of a rounded peripheral mass on plain chest X-ray can be very challenging because benign or malignant lesions, infection, rounded atelectasis (as seen in asbestosis), lung sequestration (Fig. 2.12), or congenital disorders such as broncho-genic cysts can be the responsible underlying disease.

Another example illustrating the unavoidable need for clinical information or medical history is acute lung fibrosis. Chemotherapy may induce acute lung fibrosis and can lead to respiration failure. Immediate chemotherapy interruption and oxygen support are mandatory.

Another difficulty relating to fibrosis is differentiating fibrosis from an infectious disease in a patient with chronic obstructive pulmonary disease, as described in Fig. 2.13.

The integration of information obtained from systematic interpretation of the chest X-ray and correlation with the clinical status often results in an allowable degree of diagnostic accuracy in chest diseases.

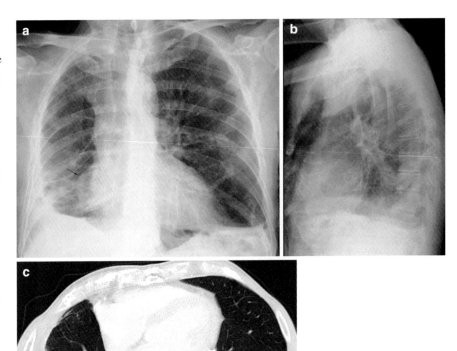

Fig. 2.12 A 63-year-old male patient with cough, fever, and dyspnea. (**a, b**) PA and lateral chest X-ray reveals a right mediastinal shift, a mass projected on the right cardiac border, posteriorly located in the right lung lower lobe and associated with pleural thickening and obliteration of the cardiophrenic sinus. The hyperlucency of the retrosternal space on the lateral view is due to an asymmetry in expansion of both lungs and causing a distortion of the sternum (**c**) CT confirmed pleural effusion and thickening, right mediastinal shift, and the mass posteriorly located in the right lower lung. This rounded dense mass is swirled by vessels and bronchi converging upon the density (comet sign). Notice the presence of calcified pleural plaques on the diaphragm and flattening of the diaphragm. This patient was exposed to asbestos and was diagnosed with a rounded atelectasis

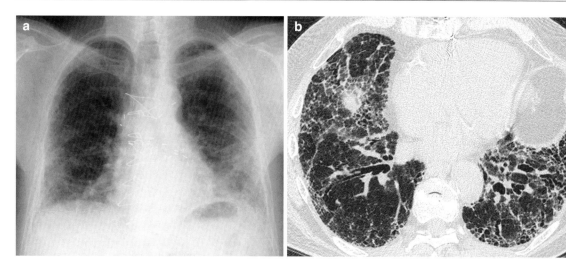

Fig. 2.13 An 84-year-old male patient, 10 years after coronary artery bypass graft, was admitted with dyspnea and cough, present during the last 2 months. (**a**) A routine PA chest X-ray revealed a reticulo-nodular pattern of the parenchyma of both lungs and enlargement of the trachea. Differential diagnosis included fibrosis, pneumonia, or co-morbidity of fibrosis and pneumonia. (**b**) High-resolution CT demonstrates massive fibrosis with dilatation of bronchi and bronchioles, accentuation of the interlobular septae, peripheral honeycombing, and ground-glass opacity as a sign of active fibrosis. There were no arguments for associated bacterial pneumonia

2.4 Errors and Perception

2.4.1 Perceptual and Cognitive

The radiological diagnosis of chest disease begins with the identification of an abnormality on a chest X-ray; in other words, that which is not seen cannot be appreciated (Fraser et al. 1988). That appreciation is submitted to the perceptual and cognitive limitations that have a direct bearing on the clinical utility and effectiveness of chest X-rays (McAdams et al. 2006).

Experience gives the radiologist the perceptual and cognitive skills to know what information to look for and how to interpret that information based on the accumulation and integration of information processed from previous encounters with the same type of images (Krupinski 2003). What makes the task difficult, is that, although the basic anatomy is essentially the same in all images, the degree of natural variation in both normal and abnormal structures is high and radiologists will never be able to see all possible variations during their career. The results of all this variation in normal and abnormal features are variation and error in interpretation. Kundel et al

(1978). found that perceptual errors can be grouped into three general categories

- Some missed lesions are never looked at.
- Some missed lesions are looked at, but not long enough to allow detection or recognition.
- Some lesions are looked at for long period of time but either are not recognized as a lesion or are actively dismissed as normal structure.

2.4.2 Observer Errors

Observer errors provoke false-negative or false-positive readings. In case of a false-positive reading, a finding without pathological significance is interpreted as a lesion; in case of a false-negative reading, a pathological finding is misinterpreted as normal. Inter-observer disagreement in some cases may reach astonishing levels (Fraser et al. 1988). Observer errors are very complex and every physician concerned with the correct reading and interpretation of a chest X-ray must also have proficient knowledge of the physical and physiological principles of perception, so errors will be diminished to a minimum. It is important to read chest X-rays from a certain distance, at least 6–8 ft, both because the slight nuances of density variation between similar zones can be better detected at a distance and because the visibility of shadows with ill-defined margins is improved with minification (Fraser et al. 1988). This was previously discussed by Tuddenham in 1963 (Tuddenham 1963). Shea and Ziskin (1972) mentioned that reading X-rays at a fixed distance increases the risk of failure of abnormality detection.

Another mechanism to reduce the frequency of misreading X-rays is double reading: dual interpretation by the same observer on two separate occasions or by two independent observers. This procedure improves the diagnostic accuracy, but is difficult to implement routinely in large radiology departments (Fraser et al. 1988). However, since double reading improves sensitivity, Stitik et al. recommend to double read a chest X-ray by removing the eyes from the image for a short period and looking at it a second time before finalizing the report (Stitik and Tockman 1978).

Psychological aspects in interpretation should also be mentioned as a source of errors when reading chest X-rays. No experienced radiologist can deny the diminution in visual and mental acuity when exposed to a heavy work load, the so called "reader fatigue." Errors owing to reader fatigue can be reduced through frequent "rest periods" away from the viewbox and a reasonable work load each day. Attention to comfort and convenience in the viewing facilities, e.g., light intensity, background illumination, and noise, reduces the risk of interpretation failure. *Intra-observer disagreements* are also bound to occur, probably ascribed to "a state of mind" that is continually fluctuating, and they represent an intangible influence on one's approach to a problem (Fraser et al. 1988). *Satisfaction of search* is also a source of errors in reading chest X-rays: underreading errors (false-negative responses) occur when lesions remain undetected after detection of an initial lesion (Berbaum et al. 1990).

2.5 Radiologic Report

The radiologic report should be built up in two parts: a descriptive part and a conclusive part (Westra 1990).

Lesions must be depicted in the descriptive part in such a way that the conclusion can be anticipated (Westra 1990). It is mandatory that, in the conclusive part, an attempt be made to answer the specific questions that were the reason for performing the examination and to guide the clinician toward possible further procedures or examinations when necessary.

Words must be carefully chosen. The Fleischner Society, whose purpose is to advance knowledge of the normal and diseased chest, proposed the "Glossary of terms of thoracic radiology" (Hansell et al. 2008; Tuddenham 1984) to standardize terms so exchange of information would be facilitated. This glossary helps to identify nuances of meaning that distinguish words of similar connotation and to reject the argument that "everyone says it that way" as a justification for a misused term. The term "infiltrate" is almost invariably used in the sense of any poorly defined opacity in the lung, and serves no useful purpose. Due to the lack of any specific connotation, it causes great confusion. It should only be used as a descriptor to distinguish processes that do not distort the lung architecture from expanding processes that do (Tuddenham 1984).

There is also considerable variation in the terms used for describing pulmonary "dense" structures.

The term "opacity" in a radiograph refers to any area that appears more opaque (or of lesser photometric density) than its surroundings. It is an essential and recommended radiologic descriptor that does not indicate the size or pathologic nature of the abnormality (Hansell et al. 2008).

The term "nodule" is any pulmonary or pleural lesion represented in a radiograph by a well or poorly defined, discrete, nearly circular opacity of 2–30 mm in diameter and is a descriptor recommended to be always qualified with respect to size, location, border characteristics, number, and opacity (Hansell et al. 2008; Tuddenham 1984). The term "micronodule" is reserved for a sharply defined, discrete, nearly circular opacity of less than 3 mm in diameter. "Mass" is used if the opacity is larger than 30 mm in diameter (Hansell et al. 2008; Tuddenham 1984).

Every radiologist must be thoughtful in his or her choice of words; not only is visualizing the disease a basic condition for medical treatment, but so is the right description of this visualization.

In conclusion, despite the long existence of conventional radiography, which is based on the inherent contrast of the connecting components in the thorax (soft tissue – bone – air – fat), and despite the development of newer and more exciting imaging techniques, chest

X-ray still remains one of the most challenging diagnostic tools due to the wide range of possible diseases, especially when performed in the approved manner with all the trimmings.

References

Armstrong P, Wilson AG, Dee P (1990) Imaging of diseases of the chest. Mosby – Year Book, London

Ashizawa K, Hayashi K, Aso N et al (2001) Lobar atelectasis: diagnostic pitfalls on chest radiography. Br J Radiol 877:89–97

Austin JHM, Romney BM, Goldsmith LS (1992) Missed Bronchogenic-Carcinoma – radiographic findings in 27 patients with a potentially resectable lesion evident in retrospect. Radiology 1:115–122

Bacher K, Smeets P, De Hauwere A et al (2006) Image quality performance of liquid crystal display systems: influence of display resolution, magnification and window settings on contrast-detail detection. Eur J Radiol 3:471–479

Ball CG, Kirkpatrick AW, Laupland KB et al (2005) Factors related to the failure of radiographic recognition of occult posttraumatic pneumothoraces. Am J Surg 5:541–546

Berbaum KS, Franken EA Jr, Dorfman DD et al (1990) Satisfaction of search in diagnostic radiology. Invest Radiol 2:133–140

Bogaert J, Verschakelen J (1995) Spiral CT of the diaphragm. J Belge Radiol 2:86–87

Boynton RM, Bush WR (1956) Recognition of forms against a complex background. J Opt Soc Am 9:758–764

Brogdon BG, Kelsey CA, Moseley RD Jr (1983) Factors affecting perception of pulmonary lesions. Radiol Clin North Am 4:633–654

Busch HP (1997) Digital radiography for clinical applications. Euro Radiol 7(suppl 3):S66–S72

Chen JT (1983) The plain radiograph in the diagnosis of cardiovascular disease. Radiol Clin North Am 4:609–621

Difazio MC, MacMahon H, Xu XW et al (1997) Digital chest radiography: effect of temporal subtraction images on detection accuracy. Radiology 2:447–452

Felson B (1973) Chest roentgenology. WB Saunders, Philadelphia

Florman S, Young B, Allmon JC et al (2001) Traumatic pneumothorax ex vacuo. J Trauma 1:147–148

Fraser RG, Paré JAP, Paré PD et al (1988) Diagnosis of diseases of the chest. WB Saunders, Philadelphia

Garland LH, Coulson W, Wollin E (1963) The rate of growth and apparent duration of untreated primary bronchial carcinoma. Cancer 16:694–707

Hansell DM, Bankier AA, MacMahon H et al (2008) Fleischner society: glossary of terms for thoracic imaging. Radiology 3:697–722

Ishigaki T, Sakuma S, Horikawa Y et al (1986) One-shot dual-energy subtraction imaging. Radiology 1:271–273

Krupinski EA (2003) The future of image perception in radiology: synergy between humans and computers. Acad Radiol 1:1–3

Kundel HL, Nodine CF (1983) A visual concept shapes image perception. Radiology 2:363–368

Kundel HL, Nodine CF, Carmody D (1978) Visual scanning, pattern recognition and decision-making in pulmonary nodule detection. Invest Radiol 3:175–181

Lucaya J, Gartner S, Garcia-Pena P et al (1998) Spectrum of manifestations of Swyer-James-MacLeod syndrome. J Comput Assist Tomogr 4:592–597

MacMahon H, Li F, Engelmann R et al (2008a) Dual energy subtraction and temporal subtraction chest radiography. J Thorac Imaging 2:77–85

MacMahon H, Li F, Engelmann R et al (2008b) Dual energy subtraction and temporal subtraction chest radiography. J Thorac Imaging 2:77–85

McAdams HP, Samei E, Dobbins J 3rd et al (2006) Recent advances in chest radiography. Radiology 3:663–683

Mettler F, Ringertz H, Vañó E (2004) Managing patient dose in digital radiology: a report of the International Commission on Radiological Protection. Ann ICRP 1:1–73

Meyers BF, McCabe CJ (1993) Traumatic diaphragmatic hernia Occult marker of serious injury. Ann Surg 6:783–790

Milne EN (1993) Reading the chest radiograph. A physiologic approach. Mosby – Year Book, St Louis

Murfitt J (1993) The normal chest: methods of investigation and differential diagnosis. Churchill Livingstone, Oxford

Nitrosi A, Borasi G, Nicoli F et al (2007) A filmless radiology department in a full digital regional hospital: Quantitative evaluation of the increased quality and efficiency. J Digit Imaging 2:140–148

Novelline RA, Squire LF (1997) Squire's fundamentals of radiology. Harvard University Press, Cambridge

Shea FJ, Ziskin MC (1972) Visual system transfer function and optimal viewing distance for radiologists. Invest Radiol 3:147–151

Shephard CT (2003) Radiographic image production and manipulation. McGraw-Hill Columbus, Ohio

Spratt JS Jr, Spjut HJ, Roper CL (1963) The frequency distribution of the rates of growth and the estimated duration of primary pulmonary carcinomas. Cancer 16:687–693

Squire LF (1970) Exercises in diagnostic radiology. WB Saunders, Philadelphia

Stitik FP, Tockman MS (1978) Radiographic screening in the early detection of lung cancer. Radiol Clin North Am 3:347–366

Stolberg HO, Patt NL, Macewen KF et al (1964) Hodgkin's disease of the lung. Roentgenologic-pathologic correlation. Am J Roentgenol Radium Ther Nucl Med 92:96–115

Swallow RA, Naylor E, Roebuck EJ et al (1986) Clark's positioning in radiography. Heinneman Medical Books, Oxford

Tsubamoto M, Johkoh T, Kozuka T et al (2002) Temporal subtraction for the detection of hazy pulmonary opacities on chest radiography. Am J Roentgenol 179(2): 467–471

Tuddenham WJ (1963) Problems of perception in chest rontgenology: facts and fallacies. Radiol Clin North Am 1:277

Tuddenham WJ (1984) Glossary of terms for thoracic radiology: recommendations of the Nomenclature Committee of the Fleischner Society. AJR Am J Roentgenol 3:509–517

Usuda K, Saito Y, Sagawa M et al (1994) Tumor doubling time and prognostic assessment of patients with primary lung cancer. Cancer 8:2239–2244

Westra D (1990) Radiologic diagnosis of chest disease. Springer, Berlin

Wright FW (2002) Radiology of the chest and related conditions. Taylor and Francis, London

Part

II

Technical and Practical Aspects for CT Reconstruction and Image Comparison

The Use of Isotropic Imaging and Computed Tomography Reconstructions

3

Alain Vlassenbroek

Contents

Abstract

> With modern multislice computed tomography (CT) scanners, which combine ultrafast acquisition with high spatial resolution, isotropic imaging of the chest can be performed during a short breathold. Adapting the slice thickness, the reconstruction increment, filter, and matrix enable an optimal isotropic visualization of each organ. The very large high-quality 3-dimensional datasets that are then generated require the use of various postprocessing techniques for an improved diagnostic. These tools have become a vital component for the visualization and the interpretation of the large volumetric data and to present the results to the clinicians. New dynamic modes of visualization have recently been introduced to reduce the storage capacity and to improve the workflow and the image quality for any organ interpreted by the user. Despite this gain in information obtained with modern multislice CT scanners, the patient's dose has not been increased. On the contrary, it has been reduced thanks to the use of automatic dose modulation which adapts the X-ray tube output to maintain adequate dose and image quality when moving to different body regions.

3.1 Introduction

One of the most significant advantages of computed tomography (CT) imaging over conventional radiology lies in the vastly improved contrast discrimination it makes possible.

A. Vlassenbroek
Philips Healthcare, Rue des Deux Gares 80,
1070 Brussels, Belgium
e-mail: alain.vlassenbroek@philips.com

E.E. Coche et al. (eds.), *Comparative Interpretation of CT and Standard Radiography of the Chest*,
Medical Radiology, DOI: 10.1007/978-3-540-79942-9_3, © Springer-Verlag Berlin Heidelberg 2011

A conventional radiograph always provides a projection image that renders the total attenuation along an X-ray path that goes from the X-ray source to each picture element. The radiograph gives the shadow pattern of the X-rays as they pass through the body. In such a projection image, only structures that exhibit very high differences in attenuation with respect to their surroundings can be recognized, and the contrast is dominated by the anatomical structures with the highest attenuation, such as bones and contrast media or by differences in object thickness. Contributions from structures with low attenuation, typically soft tissue structures, are therefore completely hidden.

Instead of superposition images of complete body sections, CT provides cross-sectional images (slices) of the body, which are reconstructed from the X-ray projection data collected from many different directions during the rotation of the X-ray tube and detectors around the patient. The exceptional contrast sensitivity in CT images is the result of the reconstruction technique that almost completely eliminates the superposition of anatomical structures, leading to an improved visualization of the soft tissue structures (Kalender 2000). This major advantage led to the immediate breakthrough of CT when it was introduced in 1972.

During the last 10 years, CT scanners have been subject to tremendous technological innovations. The most important improvement was the stepwise replacement of the one-dimensional detection system, which consisted of one single row of detectors, to two-dimensional large area detectors with a detector array consisting of more than a single row of detectors. A scanner with two rows of detectors (CT Twin, Elscint Haifa Israel) had already been on the market since 1992 when multislice CT (MSCT) scanners with four rows were introduced in 1998 by several manufacturers. The primary advantage of MSCT scanners is their acquisition speed (Pappas et al. 2000). They allow substantial reduction in examination time for standard protocols and, most importantly, substantially improved longitudinal resolution by the use of thinner slices without the drawback of extended scan times. In other words, MSCT scanners combine ultrafast acquisition with high spatial resolution.

In the early days of spiral CT, the ability to acquire volume data paved the way for the development of three-dimensional (3D) image processing techniques such as multiplanar reformation (MPR), maximum intensity projections, and volume rendering techniques (Flohr et al. 2005). These various postprocessing techniques are helpful for interpreting the large datasets and presenting them to clinicians. With the current MSCT scanners, the availability of higher resolution datasets provides MPR and 3D reconstructions of superior quality and enables a significant improvement in the diagnostic approach. These image processing tools have become a vital component of medical imaging today and are commonly available on separate 3D-workstations and/or on the main scanner console.

The current generation of MSCT acquires 256 slices simultaneously with an extremely fast gantry rotation (0.27 s) and nearly accommodates a 1,000-fold increase in speed over single-slice CT (SSCT). New clinical applications, such as perfusion studies (Youn et al. 2008) or cardiac imaging (Hoffmann et al. 2004), are currently within the reach of CT. All the traditional CT applications are also enhanced and strengthened by these remarkable improvements in scanner performance. Fast isotropic acquisitions are achieved during routine examinations and fundamentally improve the management of chest disease. The faster scanning enables volumetric high-resolution image acquisition with isotropic resolution and with reduced motion artefacts. Due to the shorter exam time with MSCT, patients tolerate it better than SSCT and are more likely to hold their breath for a full thorax coverage with submillimeter slices. The advantage of thin slice collimation is not associated with an increased radiation dose because low noise/thick sections can still be visualized in real-time and in any plane at the workstation (Galanski et al. 2002).

For pulmonary angiography, the volume of intravenous contrast material injected is also decreased due to faster scanning (Fleischmann 2002; Salgado et al. 2007). All these combined advantages result in an improved diagnosis, a faster patient throughput, and a reduced cost.

An important consideration is the minimization of radiation dose. Because the lung parenchyma has a high natural contrast, low-and even ultralow-dose scanning protocols may be used in routine practice. In all cases, a good contrast-to-noise ratio has to be maintained combined with the best possible spatial resolution, enabling all MPR and 3D reconstructions to be done. With MSCT scanners, additional dose reduction can be accomplished by using dose modulation techniques which automatically adjust the amount of radiation to the size of the patient, to the shape of the patient, and to the thickness of the body part being scanned based on attenuation measurements obtained from the scout view (McCollough et al. 2006).

3.2 MSCT Spiral Acquisition and Reconstruction

3.2.1 MSCT Spiral Acquisition

A fundamental concept in 3D imaging for any application is that the quality of the reconstructed images is ultimately limited by the quality and resolution of the dataset. The latter is affected by the performance of the CT scanner that is used to acquire the dataset. An SSCT scanner with a 1-s rotation is unable to scan the entire thorax of an adult patient with submillimeter slices during a comfortable breathhold. For a 30-cm scan length corresponding to an average chest size and with a 0.8 mm slice thickness, the scan time would be approximately 375 s (assuming a 1-s rotation and a pitch of 1). If such a large scan range has to be covered within a single breath hold, a thick collimation of minimum 10 mm must be used, which results in an acquisition time of 30 s. The consequence of this slow single-slice acquisition is a considerable mismatch between the longitudinal and the in-plane spatial resolution, which, for a high-resolution thorax, should be in the range 0.3–0.5 mm. To achieve increased coverage with an improved longitudinal resolution, more slices must be acquired simultaneously per gantry rotation and/or the gantry rotation speed should be increased (Klingenbeck-Regn et al. 1999; Hu 1999; Hu et al. 2000).

Simultaneous acquisitions of M slices result in an M-fold increase in speed if all other parameters are unchanged. Alternatively, the scan range that can be covered during a certain scan time is extended by the same factor M. The most important clinical benefit is the ability to scan a given anatomical volume within a given scan time with a reduced slice thickness, providing an increase in spatial resolution by a factor M.

Alternatively, this increase in spatial resolution could also be achieved with an M-fold increase in the gantry rotation speed ω (expressed in turns/second). The major limitations in speeding up the gantry rotation are due to the mechanical constraints associated with the increased centripetal acceleration $\omega^2 R$, which is proportional to the square of the rotation frequency ω and to the radius of rotation R. The typical centripetal acceleration of an SSCT with a 1-s rotation is around 3 g (where g is the acceleration due to gravity). The centripetal acceleration of a modern 256-slice CT scanner with the shortest gantry rotation time of 270

ms is around 40 g. To give an order of magnitude, the effective weight of the X-ray tube (~40 kg at rest) during the rotation is around 1.6 tons. Thus mechanical design has to withstand this very fast rotation and the additional forces acting on the X-ray tube.

An interesting parameter that combines both the M factor and the gantry rotation speed ω is the slice acquisition rate (SAR), given by $SAR = M\omega$ (slices/second). SAR indicates the number of slices that can be acquired per second for a given CT scanner and should be used whenever one wants to compare the acquisition speed of two different scanners. An SSCT scanner with a gantry rotation time of 1 s has an $SAR = 1$, whereas a 256-slice CT with a rotation time of 270 ms has an $SAR = 948$. In other words, modern MSCT scanners are approximately 1,000 times faster than the old SSCT scanners. As a consequence, modern MSCT scanners are now fully capable of isotropic imaging, providing a longitudinal resolution matching the in-plane resolution. They achieve this in routine practice and for all applications, including very large acquired volumes in a short scan time. A full 30-cm thorax would be scanned in less than 1 s with 0.8-mm slices compared to the 375 s needed with an SSCT of the early 1990s.

Isotropic imaging is characterized by an isotropic spatial resolution, i.e., a spatial resolution identical in the three spatial directions. The main parameters that affect the spatial resolution are the slice thickness, the reconstruction increment, and the reconstruction filter.

3.2.2 MSCT Image Reconstruction

3.2.2.1 Slice Thickness, Reconstruction Increment

On most CT scanners, different slice thicknesses can be selected, ranging from 10 to 0.5 mm. The choice of the slice thickness will have a predominant influence on the spatial resolution (Kalender 2000). As far as image sharpness is concerned, the thickness of the slice is crucial in controlling the partial volume effect, and consequently in enhancing the spatial resolution in the axial plane (characterized by coordinates XY). Figure 3.1 reveals that each pixel in the image of an object represents a volume element in the body, and it has a "depth." Perceived three-dimensionally, the pixel may be referred to as a "voxel." Within each voxel, the

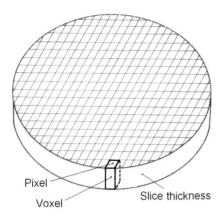

Fig. 3.1 Reconstruction of the collected data results in a numeric matrix, in which each pixel is assigned a value, or computed tomography (CT) number (expressed in Hounsfield units), related to the attenuation coefficient of the object traversed by the X-ray beam in the corresponding point. The pixel size is determined by the size of the reconstruction matrix and by the diameter of the circle of reconstruction (or, equivalently, field of view). Each pixel in the CT image actually represents a volume element in the body (a voxel) and has a depth that corresponds to the slice thickness of the reconstructed image

attenuation of the tissues is averaged. As a result of this volume averaging, the perception of structures that are included only partially into the voxel may be diminished. This is known as the partial volume effect. This effect is most damaging to the CT image when the scanned object includes many small, high-density structures, where only a portion of the structures extends into the slice thickness. Naturally, objects that extend only part of the way into the thickness of the slice will be measured by the detector as less attenuating, and hence less dense than they really are. Volume averaging can cause further damage to the CT image: soft-tissue lesions present in a voxel that contains high-attenuation bones may not be resolved at all. By definition, the partial volume effect can never be eliminated completely. However, volume averaging may be reduced by decreasing the depth of the voxel, which is the slice thickness. Thus, objects previously blurred by volume averaging will be resolved as discrete structures if scanned and/or reconstructed with narrower slices (Fig. 3.2). Consequently, thin slices should always be used to reduce partial

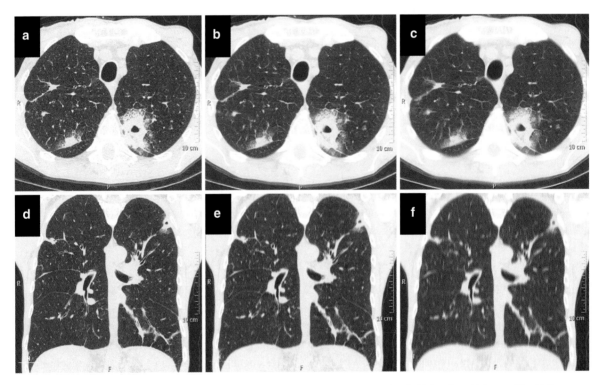

Fig. 3.2 Upper row shows axial computed tomography images reconstructed with different slice thicknesses: (**a**) 0.8 mm, (**b**) 2.5 mm, and (**c**) 5 mm. Lower row shows coronal reformatted images (**d**), (**e**), and (**f**) obtained from (**a**), (**b**), and (**c**), respectively. In each case, the reconstruction increment was chosen to be equal to half the slice thickness. The highest spatial resolution is achieved with the thinnest slices in both the axial and longitudinal directions. The blurring of small structures is progressively increased in both directions when the slice thickness is increased

volume effects and to improve the localization of small structures in the axial slices.

A disadvantage of the use of thinner slices is the effect it has on the quantum noise. Quantum noise is the noise in an image that is related to the number of X-ray photons (N) that are utilized to generate the image. It can be shown that the quantum noise is inversely proportional to the square root of N (Brooks and DiChiro 1976). By decreasing the slice thickness by a factor of 4, we also decrease the number of X-ray photons contributing to a particular voxel by a factor of 4, so that the quantum noise rises by a factor of 2. Inversely, several slices can be combined during the reconstruction process or by postprocessing to reduce the noise. This makes it possible to reconstruct images with different slice thicknesses, trading off, in this way, spatial resolution and noise.

The choice of the slice thickness also has a predominant influence on the spatial resolution in the longitudinal direction (characterized by the coordinate Z), i.e., along the axis of the body, when the stack of axial slices is used to generate MPR-reconstructed images in the sagittal or the coronal planes. This is again because an averaging of overall structures located in a slice always takes place. Multiplanar reconstructions demonstrate this in a simple way (Fig. 3.2) and show that the use of thinner slices strongly improves the sharpness of the MPR-reformatted images. While the Z-resolution depends, above all, on the slice thickness (sw), it also depends strongly on the scan or reconstruction increment (ri) between individual slice images. Because in spiral CT it is possible to freely select the number and the Z-positions of the images to be reconstructed, the availability of overlapping images in spiral CT brings a fundamental advantage with regard to spatial resolution in the Z-direction (Fig. 3.3). An image reconstruction increment equal to the slice thickness ($ri=sw$) corresponds to a sequential CT and does not utilize the special advantages of spiral CT, leading to a certain loss of resolution and small-detail contrast. Wang and Vannier (1994) showed that, for $ri<sw$, longitudinal resolution can be improved up to a limit, which depends on the pitch used during the spiral acquisition. The theoretical limit corresponds to a longitudinal resolution of approximately half the effective slice thickness and is approached when a strong overlapping is used, corresponding to three to four slices reconstructed per slice thickness (Kalender et al. 1994). As an example, in the case of

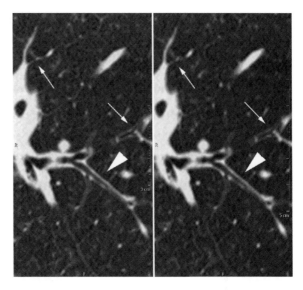

Fig. 3.3 Zoomed coronal reformatted images showing details of the lung parenchyma. The *left* image was reformatted from a stack of axial images with $sw=0.8$ mm and $ri=0.4$ mm. The *right* image was reformatted from a stack of adjacent axial images with $sw=0.8$ mm and $ri=0.8$ mm. The use of overlapping axial images clearly increases the sharpness of the resulting reformatted images (see, for example, the details pointed to by the *arrows*) and removes the stair-step artefacts that are visible on the coronal image reformatted from the nonoverlapping axial images (see *arrow heads*)

an acquisition performed with an effective slice thickness of 1.25 mm, the smallest resolvable detail in the longitudinal direction will measure approximately 0.62 mm. In practice, the authors recommend using 50% overlap ($ri=sw/2$) in clinical routine, with two images reconstructed per slice thickness, and recommend 67% overlap ($ri=sw/3$) whenever high longitudinal spatial resolution is needed and to obtain MPR and 3D-reconstructed images of excellent quality.

3.2.2.2 The Reconstruction Filter

The reconstruction technique commonly employed in current MSCT scanners is the 3D filtered back projection technique, which is a process that converts the attenuation data collected by the detectors (usually named "raw data") into the final CT numbers that make up the clinical image (Kak and Slaney 1988). Cross-sectional CT images are reconstructed from sets of attenuation projections that have to be convolved with dedicated mathematical functions; these are known as "reconstruction filters" or "convolution kernels." The choice and design of these convolution kernels offer the possibility to influence image quality (Kalender 2000). With highly resolving or high-pass reconstruction filters, spatial resolution is improved but noise is increased; the opposite happens with smoothing or low-pass filters, which reduce noise at the expense of spatial resolution (Fig. 3.4). The ultimate goal is to optimize the signal-to-noise ratio of the images. For this purpose, modern MSCT scanners offer a combination of high- and low-pass filters to suit a variety of smoothing or enhancement needs, depending on the properties of the scanned object.

One typical measure that is routinely used to assess scanner resolution in the image plane is the modulation transfer function (MTF), which describes the system's effective frequency response (Rossmann 1969) and is another way of defining the system's spatial resolution. The MTF of an ideal CT scanner would be a horizontal line; such a scanner would be able to transmit each spatial frequency with 100% efficiency. Of course, this is impossible to achieve and the MTF is always high for low spatial frequencies and decreases for increased spatial frequencies. At some point, the MTF becomes zero, which is known as the cutoff

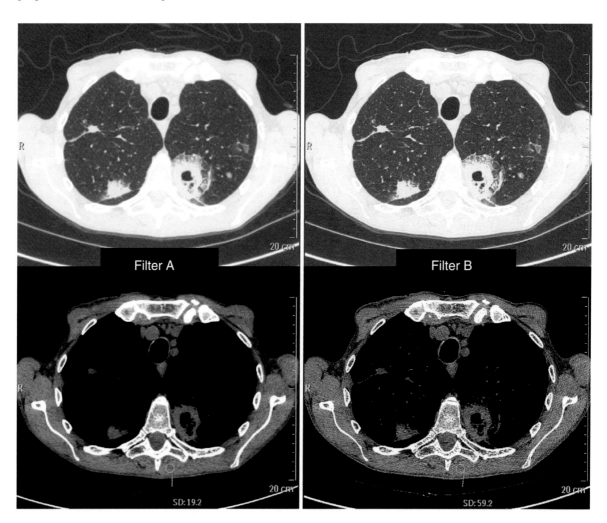

Fig. 3.4 Images on the *left* were reconstructed with a smooth reconstruction filter (filter A), optimized for the visualization of the soft tissues and characterized by a cutoff frequency of 8 Lp/cm. The standard deviation of the pixel value (noise) measured on the image is 19.2 Hounsfield units (HU). With filter A, the images are smooth and the noise is low. The lung parenchyma is not displayed optimally and appears unsharp.

Images on the *right* were reconstructed with a sharper filter (filter B), optimized to visualize the small lung details and characterized by a cutoff frequency of 12 Lp/cm. The noise measured on the image is 59.2 HU. This large increase in the noise damages the contrast resolution and therefore this filter is not adequate for an improved visualization of the soft tissues

Fig. 3.5 Modulation transfer function (MTF) curves of the two reconstruction filters (filters A and B) used to reconstruct the images of Fig. 3.4. Filters A and B are characterized by a cutoff frequency of 8 and 12 Lp/cm, respectively. As seen on the images of the high-contrast bar phantom, spatial frequencies above the cutoff do not appear in the images and are imaged as uniform gray without modulation. This phantom allows accurate measurment of the MTF of the filter used to reconstruct the computed tomography images at spatial frequencies of 1, 2 Lp/cm, etc.

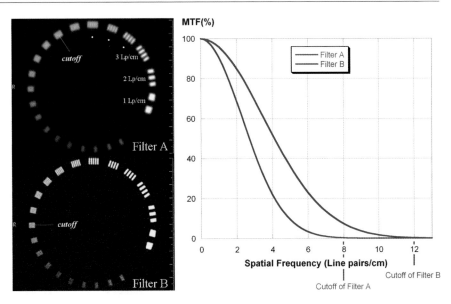

frequency (Fig. 3.5). A spatial modulation above the cutoff frequency will image as uniform gray, with no variation in contrast. Such spatial modulations with frequencies above the cutoff do not appear in the images. The MTF can be measured accurately by scanning a high-contrast bar phantom (Fig. 3.5) (Droege and Morin 1982). From such a scan, the cutoff frequency can also be easily determined. It is expressed as pairs of Lines per cm (Lp/cm) and roughly corresponds to the spatial resolution of the CT image in the axial direction. From the cutoff frequency (f_c), the smallest high-contrast detail size that can be resolved in a CT axial image can be calculated from

$$(cm) = \frac{1}{2 f_c (Lp/cm)}$$

As an example, with a cutoff frequency of 8 Lp/cm, the smallest detail that can be resolved in a CT axial image is 0.62 mm.

One of the most significant advantages of CT imaging over conventional radiology lies in the vastly improved contrast discrimination it makes possible. Contrast resolution is a function of the statistical noise in the image, which arises from the detection of a finite amount of X-ray photons. Both statistical noise and contrast resolution may be modified by the reconstruction filter. Noise may be reduced and contrast improved by smoothing, at the expense of a certain blurring of the image. It is apparent that spatial and contrast resolution are closely interrelated. To determine a scanner's overall response, both spatial and contrast resolution together

need to be taken into account. The choice and design of the reconstruction filter influences the sharpness/contrast in the axial images, and the response of each filter is characterized by its own MTF curve. When plotting a MTF curve, it is useful to think of the area under the curve as a measure of how "fuzzy" and "out of focus" an image will appear. The less area under the curve, the less sharp and less noisy an image will appear, with the highest contrast resolution. In other words, the image noise depends on the surface below the MTF curve. Figure 3.5 shows the MTF curves of two reconstruction filters: smooth filter A with a cutoff frequency of 8 Lp/cm and a sharper filter B with a cutoff frequency of 12 Lp/cm. The use of filter B (δ=0.41 mm) will enable to resolve smaller details in the images than filter A (δ=0.625 mm) but, because the area under the MTF curve of filter B is larger than the area under the MTF curve of filter A, the images with filter B will be more noisy than with filter A, and with a reduced contrast resolution (Fig. 3.4).

As discussed in Sect. 3.2.2.1, objects blurred in the axial slice by volume averaging will be resolved as discrete structures if scanned and/or reconstructed with narrower slices. In other words, an improvement of the Z-resolution will also improve the spatial resolution of the axial XY images (Fig. 3.2). Figure 3.6 shows that the opposite is also true and that an improvement of the XY-resolution will improve the spatial resolution of longitudinally reformatted images. The choice of the reconstruction kernel will thus also have an influence on the spatial resolution and image noise of MPR images.

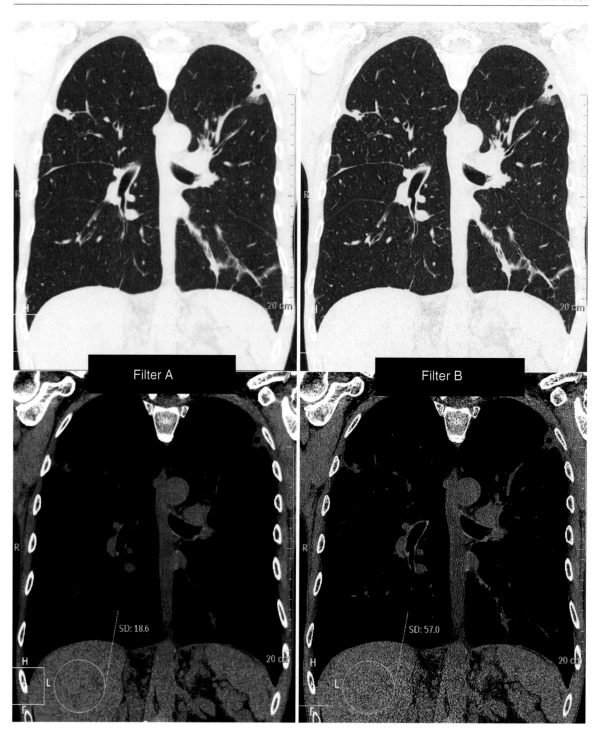

Fig. 3.6 Coronal images reformatted from a stack of axial images with sw=0.8 mm and ri=0.4 mm and reconstructed with the filters A (*left*) and B (*right*), respectively (see modulation transfer function in Fig. 3.5). The noise measured on the images is 18.6 HU (**a**) and 57 Houndsfield units (HU) (**b**). The images show that an improvement of the XY-resolution also improves the spatial resolution of longitudinal reformatted images and, hence, that the choice of the reconstruction filter influences the spatial resolution and image noise of multiplanar reformated images

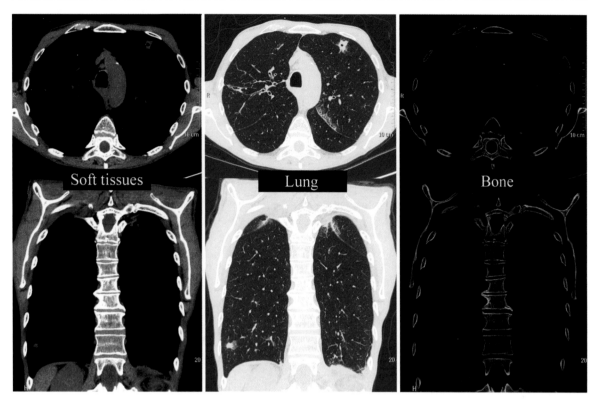

Fig. 3.7 Multidetector computed tomography imaging of the thorax might require multiple reconstructions from the same raw data, with each reconstruction being optimized for each organ. In these isotropic reconstructions, the image quality of the coronal reformations (characterized by the spatial resolution and contrast resolution) is, for each organ, identical to the one of the original axial images. *Soft tissues*: sw =1.25 mm, ri=0.62 mm, filter A (8 Lp/cm), *Lung*: sw=0.8 mm, ri=0.4 mm, filter B (12 Lp/cm), *Bone*: sw =0.62 mm, ri=0.31 mm, filter C (16 Lp/cm)

MDCT imaging of the thorax might require multiple reconstructions, with each reconstruction being optimized for each organ (Fig. 3.7). An adequate visualization of the mediastinum will be obtained with a soft tissue kernel (~8 Lp/cm) providing a good low contrast resolution between the lesion and the non-pathological surrounding tissues whereas an accurate visualization of the smaller details of the lung parenchyma will require the use of a sharper reconstruction filter (~12 Lp/cm). The increased noise level will not be problematic because of the high natural contrast of the lung parenchyma. A third reconstruction filter could be needed to optimize the visualization of the bone structure with a very sharp filter (>16 Lp/cm).

The properties of reconstruction filters are not subject to standardization. Therefore, kernels of equal or similar designation may vary considerably from one scanner to the next. Equally, reconstruction filters used for head or body scans carrying the same name are by no means identical. Labels such as "smooth" or "sharp"

can be used only as coarse indicators of the balance between spatial resolution and image noise (Galanski et al. 2002).

3.2.2.3 Isotropic Imaging

3D and MPR reconstructions should always be performed on an isotropic dataset, i.e., on an axial dataset reconstructed with a reconstruction filter and a slice thickness/increment that are such that the spatial resolution will be identical in the three spatial directions X, Y, and Z. As explained in Sects. 3.2.2.1 and 3.2.2.2, this isotropic condition will be fulfilled if

$$sw(cm)/2 = \quad (cm) = \frac{1}{2f_c(Lp/cm)} \Rightarrow sw = \frac{1}{f_c} = 2 \quad ,$$

or in other words, if the smallest detail that can be resolved in the axial plane is equal to half the slice thickness, which is the maximum longitudinal resolution and is approached when strong overlapping is used. As an example, a dataset reconstructed with a filter characterized by a cutoff frequency of 8 Lp/cm should use a slice thickness of 1.25 mm and a reconstruction overlap of at least 67% ($ri < sw/3$). In this case, the smallest high-contrast detail that will be resolved in any axial, sagittal, or coronal plane will measure 0.62 mm. In practice, we usually limit the reconstruction increment to $ri = sw/2$ to limit the number of reconstructed slices.

In summary, an isotropic thorax examination, with an optimized image quality for 3D visualization of every organ, requires three typical reconstructions:

1. *Soft tissue*: Soft reconstruction filter (~8 Lp/cm)
   Isotropic: $sw = 1.25$ mm, $ri \leq 0.62$ mm (≥ 480 slices for a 30 cm scan length)
2. *Lung parenchyma*: Sharp reconstruction filter (~12 Lp/cm)
   Isotropic: $sw = 0.80$ mm, $ri \leq 0.40$ mm (≥ 750 slices for a 30-cm scan length)
3. *Bone*: Very Sharp reconstruction filter (~16 Lp/cm)
   Isotropic: $sw = 0.62$ mm, $ri \leq 0.31$ mm (≥ 960 slices for a 30-cm scan length)

An example of such an isotropic acquisition with three reconstructed datasets optimized for the soft tissue, lung, and bone visualization, respectively, is shown in Fig. 3.7. This figure shows that the image quality of coronal reconstructions performed on an isotropic dataset is identical to the one of the original axial images.

With an average scan length of 30 cm, this requires a minimum of 2,200 slices for an adequate thorax visualization and full diagnostic capability. This is a huge amount of images to reconstruct that requires time and storage capacity. An alternative solution that is used in many institutions is to use only one single reconstruction (for example, the soft tissue reconstruction, which provides the less noisy dataset) and to require additional reconstructions only when suspicious lesions are detected in the lung parenchyma or in the bone. The major penalty is that the optimal image quality is not obtained right away. A simplified solution that could improve the workflow considerably while maintaining the full image quality obtained immediately will be described in Sect. 3.4.

It is often erroneously stated that an isotropic dataset is a dataset characterized by an isotropic voxel, i.e., with a pixel size equal to the slice thickness (*sw*) (Fig. 3.1). This is wrong because the spatial resolution in the axial plane is limited by the cutoff frequency of the reconstruction filter and should not be limited by the pixel size. In other words, the reconstruction matrix should always be chosen such that the corresponding pixel size does not reduce the spatial resolution in the images. With this condition, the spatial resolution will be limited by the reconstruction filter only and will not depend on the reconstructed field of view *FOV* and matrix. This condition will introduce the concept of ideal reconstruction matrix (Kalender 2000) and is discussed in the next section.

3.2.2.4 The Reconstruction Matrix

The ideal reconstruction matrix size (m_{ideal}) is the one providing a pixel size equal to the smallest resolvable detail (δ) in the reconstructed image and that is determined by the cutoff frequency of the reconstruction filter. From this,

$$\text{pixel size } (cm) = \frac{FOV(\text{cm})}{m_{ideal}} = \delta = \frac{1}{2 f_c (\text{Lp/cm})}$$

$$\Rightarrow m_{ideal} = 2 FOV(\text{cm}) f_c (\text{Lp/cm})$$

where *FOV* is the reconstructed field of view expressed in cm. As an example, a high-resolution thorax reconstructed with an *FOV* of 32 cm and a reconstruction filter of 12 Lp/cm will require $m_{ideal} = 768$ ($\delta = 0.042$ cm). If the pixel size is larger than δ (or equivalently $m < m_{ideal}$), then the spatial resolution will be reduced due to spatial averaging over the larger pixel. At the same time, image noise will be decreased as a consequence of this spatial averaging. On the other hand, a matrix size larger than m_{ideal} would not result in an improved image quality compared with an image reconstructed with m_{ideal}. In that case, the spatial resolution of the image is not affected by the pixel size but by the reconstruction filter only (Fig. 3.8). The use of a matrix above m_{ideal} only brings the penalty of increasing the storage size and the loading/processing/transfer time of the images. In the previous example, if a maximum matrix size of 512 is available for the reconstruction (and not larger matrices), then the smallest resolvable detail size in the image would measure $\delta = 32/512 = 0.062$ cm for a full *FOV* visualization of 32 cm. This corresponds to a spatial resolution of 8 Lp/cm. To achieve the full 12 Lp/cm of the reconstruction

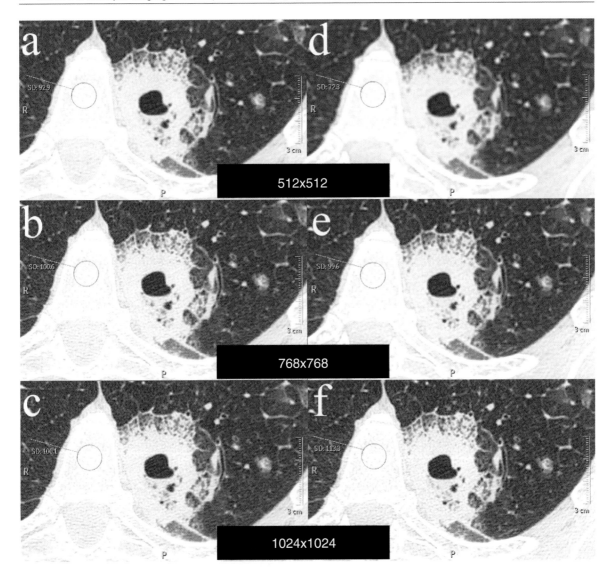

Fig. 3.8 Images (**a**), (**b**), and (**c**) were reconstructed with a field of view (FOV) equal to 32 cm and increasing matrix sizes of 512, 768, and 1,024, respectively. With a reconstruction filter having a cutoff of 12 Lp/cm, the ideal matrix is 768. The noise measured in the images is 92.9, 100.6, and 100.1 Houndsfield units (HU), respectively. Spatial resolution is improved when increasing the matrix size from image (**a**) to image (**b**), with a resulting increased noise. In image (**a**), the reconstruction matrix is below the ideal matrix and the spatial resolution is limited by the pixel size. However, no change in image quality is noticed when going from image (**b**) to image (**c**), because the recon-struction matrix is then above the ideal matrix. In that case, the spatial resolution is not affected by the pixel size but by the reconstruction filter only. Another example is given with images (**d**), (**e**), and (**f**), which were reconstructed with a $FOV=40$ cm and the same increasing matrix sizes. With this filter, the cutoff is 16 Lp/cm and the ideal matrix is 1,280. The noise measured in the images is 72.3, 99.6 and 113.3 HU, respectively. Spatial resolution is improved from image (**d**) to image (**e**) and again from image (**e**) to image (**f**) with increasing noise. In all three cases, the reconstruction matrix is below the ideal matrix and the spatial resolution is determined by the pixel size

filter, an alternative solution would be to decrease the reconstructed *FOV* to 21.3 cm. In this case, two recon-structions would be needed for a high-resolution visu-alization of the complete thorax: one for the right and one for the left lung.

Finally, let us also stress the fact that the adequate matrix size also depends on the viewing conditions and that an improvement in spatial resolution resulting from large matrix sizes can only be used when the size of the display is sufficiently large.

3.2.3 Postprocessing

The goal of postprocessing is to obtain additional information through improved image analysis tools. In fact, all the information is contained in the axial slices but is sometimes difficult to perceive. To reach the maximum quality, volume datasets should always be acquired isotropically since this forms the basis for image display in arbitrarily oriented imaging planes. Several image postprocessing tools are available to allow clinically useful information to be extracted from several hundreds of individual axial images generated during a chest MSCT examination. The evaluation often begins with scrolling through the volumetric dataset in a slab mode using a *slab viewer*. One important advantage is being able to interactively change the thickness of the reconstructed slab with a minimal value that corresponds to the voxel size. Thick reconstructed slabs in the sagittal and coronal planes mimic the superposition image of conventional

radiographs obtained after anteroposterior and lateral exposures (Fig. 3.9). Contrary to radiographs, however, the slab thickness and position can be adapted to better visualize an organ or a volume of interest, which can be chosen arbitrarily (Fig. 3.10).

A reconstructed image with a slab thickness corresponding to the minimal value would be more adequate when visualizing nonsuperposed small high-contrast structures, but might be too noisy when visualizing larger lower-contrast lesions. The latter could be better recognized after a small increase of the slab thickness, which can improve substantially the signal-to-noise ratio (Fig. 3.11).

Both the axial and the longitudinal planes should be reviewed because typical findings are sometimes more easily recognized in longitudinal planes whereas they would be very difficult or impossible to assess in the axial plane (Beigelman-Aubry 2007). Curved MPR reconstructions can also help in the evaluation of

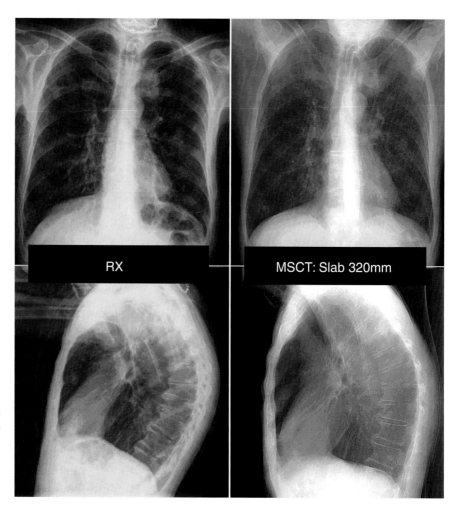

Fig. 3.9 Thick reconstructed slab in the coronal and sagittal planes from multislice computed tomography images mimic the superposition image of conventional radiographs obtained after anteroposterior and lateral exposures

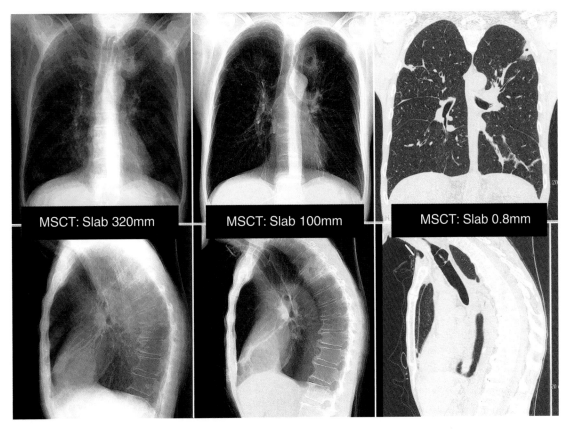

Fig. 3.10 The advantage of multislice computed tomography (MSCT) over the radiograph is that the slab thickness and its position can be adapted to better visualize an organ or a volume of interest, which can be chosen arbitrarily

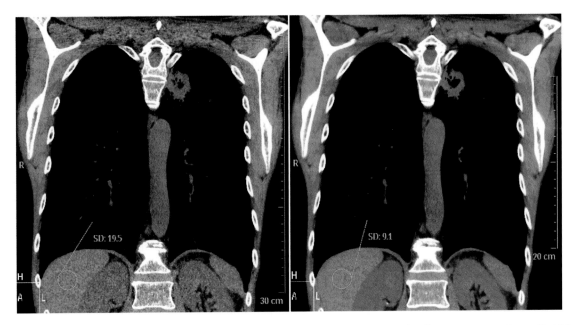

Fig. 3.11 A change in the slab thickness of the reformatted images substantially changes the signal-to-noise ratio of the corresponding images. In the example shown, the slab thickness of the *left image* is 0.8 mm (noise = 19.5 Houndsfield units [HU]) and of the *right image* is 3.0 mm (noise = 9.1 HU). A thin slab is more adequate to visualize nonsuperposed, small, high-contrast structures but might be too noisy to visualize larger lower-contrast lesions. The latter could be better recognized after a small thickening of the slab thickness, which reduces the noise and improves the contrast resolution substantially

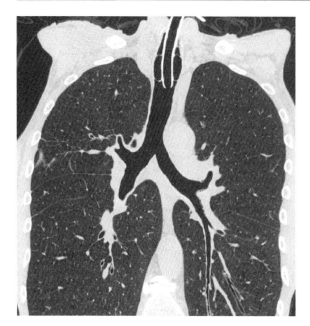

Fig. 3.12 Curved multiplanar reformat along the left main bronchus enables a complete visualization in a single reconstructed image

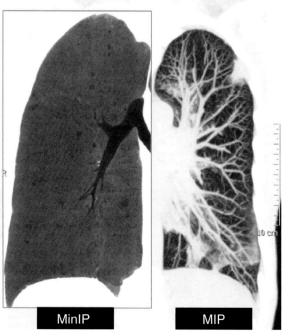

Fig. 3.13 *Left*: Slab minimum intensity projection (MinIP) is useful to display the airways and to characterize the abnormalities of the bronchial tree and of the lung parenchyma. Emphysema bubbles are nicely visualized. *Right*: Slab maximum intensity projection (MIP) provides an excellent assessment of pulmonary arteries and veins and is an excellent tool to analyze the lung parenchyma and to improve the detection of lung nodules

curved structures since they enable a complete visualization of the structure in a single reconstructed image (Fig. 3.12). MPR reformations, such as along the bronchi, have been used to demonstrate stenosis of major airways and can help a bronchoscopist to appreciate the lengths of structures, in particular those beyond a stenosis that cannot be passed by the bronchoscope (Quint et al. 1995; Lacrosse et al. 1995)

Another major tool for thoracic imaging is *maximum intensity projection* (MIP). With MIP, the voxel with the highest density along the direction from the observer's eye to the image plane is determined and this maximum value is displayed in the image. In other words, this reconstruction technique represents the most dense voxels in each projection axis. MIP is the basic postprocessing tool for the study of blood vessels. In the case of pulmonary angiography, the use of slab MIP of variable thickness provides an excellent assessment of pulmonary arteries and veins. Slab MIP is also an excellent tool to analyze the lung parenchyma (Beigelman-Aubry 2007) and to improve the detection of high-contrast lung nodules, which, in contrast to projection X-ray, cannot be hidden by ribs or other overlying structures (Fig. 3.13).

As an alternative to the voxels with the highest intensity, projection images that display the lowest

intensities can also be generated. This tool, named *minimum intensity projection* (MinIP), can be useful to display the airways and to characterize the abnormalities of the bronchial tree and lung parenchyma (Fig. 3.13).

With the *3D volume rendering* technique, for each direction from the observer's eye to the resulting image pixel, all voxels contribute to the resulting image (and not only the voxel with the maximum density as in MIP), using a weighting function that assigns a different opacity, brightness and color to each CT value (Fig. 3.14). Volume rendering is considered the method of choice for 3D display because of its great variability of display possibilities and the attractive images, close to the macroscopical pathological view that it generates (Fig. 3.15).

Virtual endoscopy is precisely what it says. It is a software tool that generates perspective views of the environment of the virtual endoscope's tip. It is a dedicated form of the volume rendering technique described above, where the opacity and color functions are selected in such a way as to present the transition from

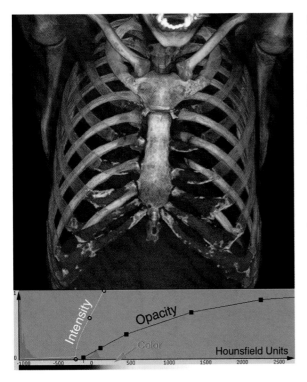

the organ wall to the surrounding tissues (Kalender 2000). "Fly through" through the volume can be generated, which provides the impression of a virtual flight through the selected body region. Virtual endoscopy can be used to complete the evaluation of the airways (Fig. 3.16) and a precise assessment of endoluminal anomalies (Richenberg and Hansell 1998).

3.3 Dosimetric Aspects of MSCT

3.3.1 Chest CT: A High-Dose Examination?

During the last 10 years, radiation exposure to the patient during MSCT has gained considerable attention in the radiological community. The problem is that, although MSCT represents only a small percentage of all the radiological procedures, it contributes largely to the population dose arising from medical procedures (Bernhardt et al. 1995). Despite its undisputed clinical benefits, MSCT scanning is often considered to be a "high-dose" technique. Contrary to the general expectation that, with the advent of magnetic resonance imaging, the usefulness of X-ray would quickly decline, CT continues to gain in importance. The introduction of MSCT has drastically

Fig. 3.14 With three-dimensional volume rendering, all voxels contribute to the image using a weighting function that assigns a different opacity, intensity, and color to each CT value. A histogram of the CT values within the volume of interest is displayed with the functions describing how the opacity, intensity, and color is assigned to each computed tomography (CT) value. In this example, opacity increases with the CT# and bones can be visualized through the more transparent soft tissues

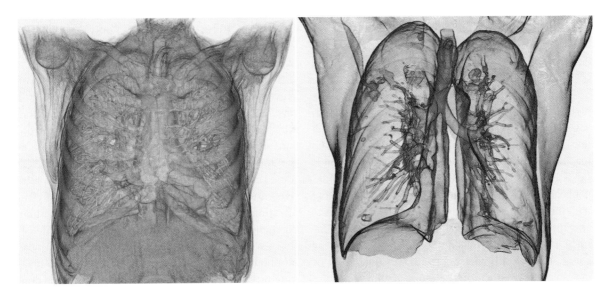

Fig. 3.15 Three-dimensional volume-rendered images obtained with two different weighting functions

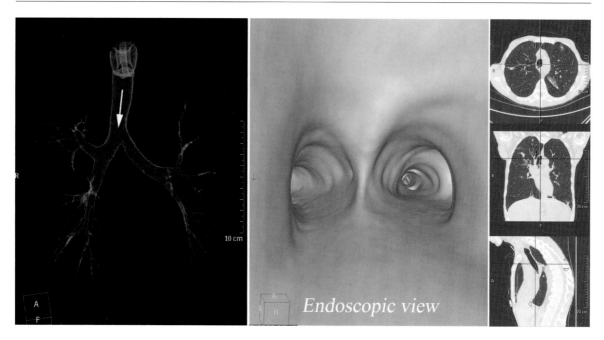

Fig. 3.16 Virtual endoscopy of the trachea. The volume-rendered image of the trachea and the multiplanar reformatted images can be used as a guide for the virtual navigation. The endoscopic view, which shows the bifurcation between the right and left bronchi, is a perspective view, which represents the environment of the virtual endoscope's tip and can be used to assess the airways

increased the performance capability and simplified the CT examinations. The range of CT applications has been extended with, for example, the introduction of cardiac CT (Hoffmann et al. 2004) or, more recently, large-coverage perfusion CT enabled by the introduction of large-area detectors (Youn et al. 2008). The relative contribution of CT to the dose delivered by all radiological examinations is of course increasing proportionally. For this reason, there are demands to limit or reduce the dose delivered during CT examinations.

In addition, the average dose level with MSCT is higher than for SSCT (Brix et al. 2003). The main reason is the preference to go to isotropic imaging with thin slices, generating noisier images and often causing the user to apply increased milliampere-seconds (mAs) settings. This is a bad reaction and there should not be a need to increase the dose when reconstructing with thin slices. The reduction in partial volume gives an improved contrast of small details that increases linearly when the slice thickness is decreased, whereas quantum noise only increases with the square root of the slice-thickness ratio. Therefore, if thin slices are used, the visibility of small details improves despite the increased noise (Galanski et al. 2002). In addition,

the use of a slab viewing software enables low noise/thick sections to be visualized in real time and in any plane at the workstation (Fig. 3.11). In other words, the trend should be to reconstruct thin and noisy datasets and to visualize thicker, lower noise sections of high quality in any 3D plane.

Typical value for the effective dose to the patient for a chest CT is in the range of 5–7 mSv (McCollough 2003), a value that must be compared with the annual average natural background radiation, which is 2–5 mSv. In other words, chest CT is not a high-dose procedure. With regard to X-ray, the chest is a low attenuating organ because of its composition, which is mainly air. This means that a low dose exposure still results in a large detector signal because of the low attenuation and, hence, low mAs factors (dose) can be used and still provide images with relatively low noise. In addition, when only a good visualization of high-contrast lesions of the lung parenchyma (airways anomalies, lung nodule detection, etc.) is of importance, good image quality can be obtained with low-and even ultralow-dose scanning protocols (<1 mSv) due to the high natural contrast of the lung parenchyma (Fig. 3.17) (Ley-Zaporozhan et al. 2008). The increased noise

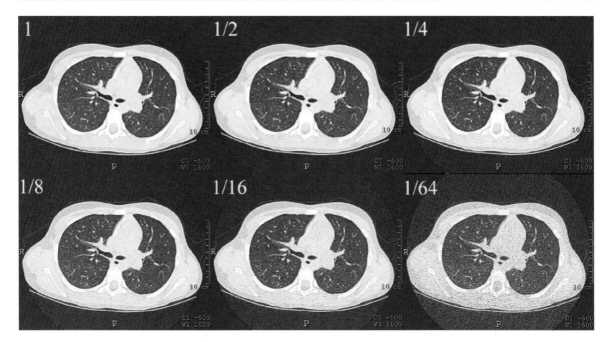

Fig. 3.17 Simulated low-dose images (Amir et al. 2003) at 1/2, 1/4, 1/8, 1/16, and 1/64 of the maximum dose of the original image, located in the upper left corner, and which was acquired at 120 kV and 100 mAs. Simulated low-dose scans show that the noise at an extremely low dose does not jeopardize the visualization of high-contrast structures

level due to the low dose scanning does not jeopardize the diagnostic quality because of the high intrinsic contrast. For example, low-dose chest CT allows detection of lung nodules that are usually too small to be seen on chest X-ray.

In summary, chest CT is a naturally low-dose technique. As we shall see in the next section, additional dose savings can still be achieved using dose modulation.

3.3.2 Dose Modulation

The most important factor for reducing radiation exposure is the adaptation of the patient dose to the patient's size. As a general rule, the dose necessary to maintain constant image noise has to be doubled if the patient diameter is increased by 4 cm. Inversely, for a patient diameter that is 4 cm smaller than average, half the standard dose is sufficient to maintain adequate image quality (Fig. 3.18). This is of particular importance in pediatric imaging, where considerable dose saving can be achieved because of the small patient size among this population (Morgan

and Braunstein 2001; Morgan 2002; Boone et al. 2003). In more sophisticated approaches, tube output is modified according to the patient geometry not only during each rotation but also in the longitudinal direction to maintain an adequate dose when moving to different body regions (McCollough et al. 2006). Figure 3.19 shows the typical variation of the mAs for a CT scan of the chest–abdomen–pelvis of an average sized adult patient.

3.4 Future Perspectives

As discussed in Sect. 3.2.2.2, MSCT imaging of the thorax might require multiple reconstructions, with each reconstruction being optimized for each organ. It would seem advantageous for most applications to modify the sharpness-noise tradeoff of a stack of images in real time without having to go back to several reconstructions with different reconstruction filters. In other words, the proposed idea is to use a single default reconstruction providing the highest in-plane resolution that is needed for the particular application and to smooth in real time the sharp reconstructed images when contrast resolution is needed, instead of performing a new

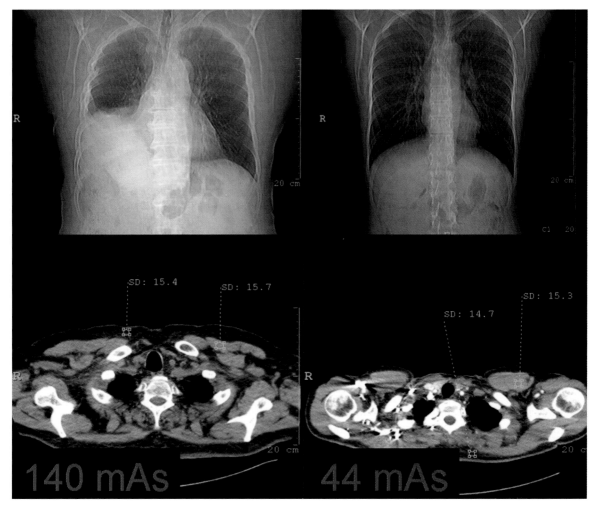

Fig. 3.18 Two different scans performed with a dose adapted to the patient's size show that the image quality can be maintained with considerable dose savings for small patients. In the exam- ple shown, the dose is reduced by a factor 3.2 and the noise measured in the images is similar

reconstruction of the entire axial stack with a smoother reconstruction kernel (Schaller et al. 2003). With this simplification, the image quality is very similar to the one obtained with a smoother reconstruction filter (Fig. 3.20). Preliminary tests (Poty et al. 2008) show that the accuracy is still sufficient for practical purposes and the image quality of the resulting smoother images does not jeopardize the diagnostic efficiency. One of the main advantages of this image filtration technique is that it can be applied to provide an adequate visualization of the soft tissues in any MPR image from an isotropic sharp dataset in a few milliseconds (Fig. 3.21),

and it has the potential to replace the lengthy operation, which consists of reconstructing the entire axial stack of images with a smoother reconstruction filter before the MPR reconstruction can be applied (see, for example, Fig. 3.6) (Feldman et al. 2008).

In conclusion, this approach significantly simplifies the workflow by requiring only one set of images reconstructed with one reconstruction kernel. This means there is only one reconstruction, one set of images archived, one set of images loaded to the slab viewer, and a very high image quality for any window displayed by the user.

Fig. 3.19 Typical variation of the dose needed to achieve a constant image quality for a chest–abdomen–pelvis examination when taking into account the variation of the body size along the longitudinal direction. For such an examination, a typical dose savings of 50% can be achieved compared with a scan that would be performed with the fixed maximum value of the dose. Note that the minimum value of the dose is needed in the thorax because of its low X-ray attenuation

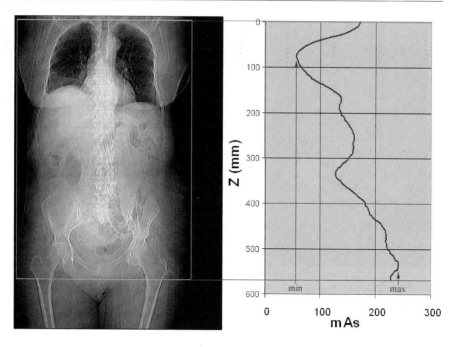

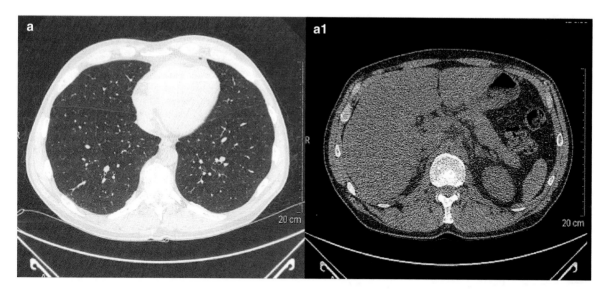

Fig. 3.20 Images (**a**) and (**b**) are reconstructed with a lung filter (sharp) and an abdominal filter (smooth), respectively. Image (**a1**) displays image (**a**) with an abdominal window. Note that the noise is too high with this window setting because of the use of a sharp reconstruction filter optimized for the visualization of the lung. Gaussian filtration (smoothing) of image (**a1**) gives image (**a2**), which has an image quality very close to image (**b**)

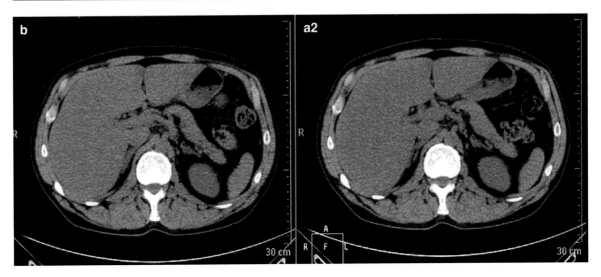

Fig. 3.20 (continued)

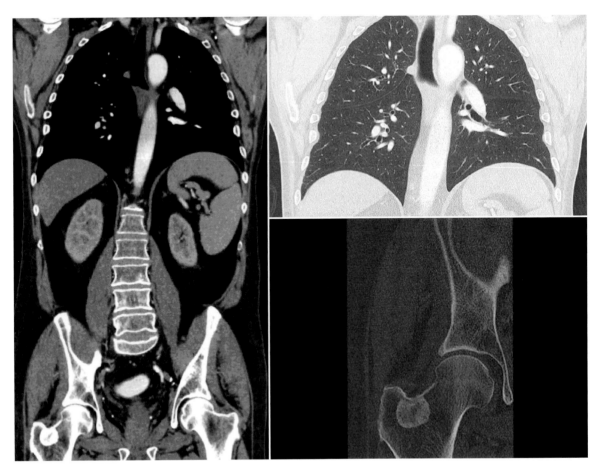

Fig. 3.21 Various amount of Gaussian filtration and slice thickening can be applied online to the multiplanar-reconstructed images according to the window width, which is chosen to improve the visualization of all organs. The image quality obtained is then very high for any window displayed by the user, with only one reconstructed "sharp and thin" dataset

References

Amir O, Braunstein D, Altman A (2003) Dose optimization tool. Proc SPIE Conf 5029:815–821

Beigelman-Aubry C (2007) Post-processing and display in multislice CT of the chest. JBR–BTR 90:85–88

Bernhardt J, Veit R, Bauer B (1995) Erhebung zur Strahlenexposition der Patienten bei der Rontgendiagnostik. Med Phys 5:33–39

Boone JM, Geraghty EM, Seibert JA, Wootton-Gorges SL (2003) Dose reduction in pediatric CT: a rational approach. Radiology 228:352–360

Brix G, Nagel HD, Stamm G et al (2003) Radiation exposure in multi-slice versus single-slice spiral CT: results of a nationwide survey. Eur Radiol 13(8):1979–1991

Brooks RA, DiChiro G (1976) Statistical limitations in x-ray reconstructive tomography. Med Phys 3:237–240

Droege RT, Morin RL (1982) A practical method to measure the MTF of CT scanner. Med Phys 9(5):758–760

Feldman A, Rabotnikov M, Nae Y, Vlassenbroek A (2008) A new concept for acquisition and image reconstruction in ct, aimed to significantly boost the workflow and to improve the image quality. RSNA 2008 abstract SSA21–01

Fleischmann D (2002) Present and future trends in multiple detector-row CT applications: CT angiography. Eur Radiol 12(Suppl 2):11–15

Flohr T, Schaller S, Stierstorfer K, Bruder H, Ohnesorge B, Schoepf UJ (2005) Multi-detector row CT systems and image-reconstruction techniques. Radiology 235(3):756–773

Galanski M, Hidajat N, Maier W, Nagel HD, Schmidt T (2002) Radiation exposure in computed tomography, 4th edn. CTB, Hamburg

Hoffmann M, Heshui S, Schmid F et al (2004) Noninvasive coronary imaging with MDCT in comparison to invasive conventional coronary angiography: a fast-developing technology. AJR Am J Roentgenol 182(3):601–608

Hu H (1999) Multi-slice helical CT: scan and reconstruction. Med Phys 26(1):5–18

Hu H, He HD, Foley WD, Fox SH (2000) Four multidetector-row helical CT: "Image quality and volume coverage speed." Radiology 215:55–62

Kak AC, Slaney M (1988) Principles of computerized tomographic imaging. IEEE, New York

Kalender WA (2000) Computed tomography: fundamentals, system technology, image quality, applications. Publicis MCD Verlag, Munich

Kalender WA, Polacin A, Suss C (1994) A comparison of conventional and spiral CT: an experimental study on the detection of spherical lesions. J Comput Assist 18(2):167–176

Klingenbeck-Regn K, Schaller S, Flohr T, Ohnesorge B, Kopp AF, Baum U (1999) Subsecond multi-slice computed tomography: basics and applications. Eur J Radiol 31(2):110–124

Lacrosse M, Trigaux JP, Van Beers BE, Weynants P (1995) 3D spiral CT of the tracheobronchial tree. J Comput Assist Tomogr 19(3):341–347

Ley-Zaporozhan J, Ley S, Krummenauer F et al. (2010) Low dose multi-detector CT of the chest (iLEAD Study): Visual ranking of different simulated mAs levels. Eur. J. Radiol. February 2010:73(2):428-33.

McCollough CH (2003) Patient dose in cardiac computed tomography. Herz 28:1–6

McCollough CH, Bruesewitz MR, Kofler JM (2006) CT dose reduction and management tools: overview of available options. Radiographics 26:503–512

Morgan H (2002) Dose reduction for CT pediatric imaging. Pediatr Radiol 32:724–728

Morgan H, Braunstein D (2001) A computed tomography dose index for infants and young children. Med Phys 28:1818

Pappas JN, Donnelly LF, Frush DP (2000) Reduced frequency of sedation of young children with multisection helical CT. Radiology 215:897–899

Poty V, Ferain J, Vlassenbroek A, Defrize L, Coche E (2008) Apport de la filtration dynamique des images dans le suivi oncologique thoraco-abdominal au scanner. J Radiol 89: 1493–1494

Quint LE et al (1995) Stenosis of the central airways: evaluation by using helical CT with multiplanar reconstructions. Radiology 194:871–877

Richenberg JL, Hansell DM (1998) Image processing and spiral CT of the thorax. Br J Radiol 71:708–716

Rossmann K (1969) Point spread function, line-spread function and modulation transfer function: tools for the study of imaging systems. Radiology 93:257–272

Salgado RA, Spinhoven M, De Jongh K, Op de Beeck B, Corthouts B, Parizel PM (2007) Chest MSCT acquisition and injection protocols. JBR–BTR 90:97–99

Schaller S, Wildberger JE, Raupach R, Niethammer M, Kingenbeck-Regn K, Flohr T (2003) Spatial domain filtering for fast modification of the tradeoff between image sharpness and pixel noise in CT. IEEE Trans Med Imaging 22(7):846–853

Wang G, Vannier MW (1994) Longitudinal resolution in volumetric x-ray CT – analytic comparison between conventional and helical CT. Med Phys 21:429–433

Youn SW, Kim JH, Weon YC et al (2008) Perfusion CT of the brain using 40-mm-wide detector and toggling table technique for initial imaging of acute stroke. AJR Am J Roentgenol 191:120–126

PACS – Tips and Tricks for Imaging Comparison

Roger Eibel, Sven Thieme, and Peter Herzog

4

Contents

Abstract

> The advent of multislice computed tomography (CT), which makes a lung examination with more than 1,000 axial slices in few seconds possible, and the progressive improvements in CT technology have dramatically changed our daily practice. Picture Archiving and Communication Systems (PACS) and especially the introduction and widespread availability of viewing and diagnostic workstations become essential to handle the data and work load. The fundamental meaning of image postprocessing is the application of imaging techniques to original axial images to derive additional information or hide unwanted information that distracts from the clinical findings. The aim of image manipulation is to improve the diagnostic quality, but it is important to keep in mind that the axial source images contain the basic information of a CT scan and have to be first. In this chapter, some basic principles of PACS workstations and postprocessing techniques are mentioned. The cases illustrate the different methods for imaging manipulation and give some insights for imaging comparison.

R. Eibel (✉)
Department of Radiology and Neuroradiology, HELIOS Clinics Schwerin, Teaching Hospital of the University of Rostock, Wismarsche Str, 393,19049, Schwerin, Germany
e-mail: roger.eibel@helios-kliniken.de

S. Thieme and P. Herzog
Department of Clinical Radiology, University Hospitals-Grosshadern, Ludwig Maximilians University of Munich, Marchioninistr. 15, 81377, Munich, Germany
e-mail: sven.thieme@med.uni-muenchen.de
e-mail: peter.herzog@med.uni-muenchen.de

4.1 Introduction

Never change a winning team. Sounds like a good idea, in sports for example. But is this wise statement valid in the world of radiology? For almost 100 years radiology has been based on viewing photographic images on transparent plastic polymer sheets. And

E.E. Coche et al. (eds.), *Comparative Interpretation of CT and Standard Radiography of the Chest*,
Medical Radiology, DOI: 10.1007/978-3-540-79942-9_4, © Springer-Verlag Berlin Heidelberg 2011

during this time the winning team has not changed fundamentally. X-rays were transmitted through a body and the attenuated radiation at the opposite side exposed a film in inverse proportion to its absorption. After conversion processes this latent image could be stored, viewed, distributed, and archived (Carter 2008). Only one important modification has to be mentioned. As described, the film was exposed only by the X-radiation. With the advent of intensifying screens, the radiation dose could be dramatically reduced because of an amplification of the number of photons used to expose the film by light emitted as the screens fluoresced in response to X-rays (Fauber 2009). But with the significant reduction in radiation dose the spatial resolution of the radiograph was considerably reduced. However, the dose aspect clearly outweighed the lower resolution, which partially is compensated for by using grids.

For decades, there was no need to change this winning team. The only imaging modality available in the daily medical practice was projection radiography. And For the radiologist this meant interpreting a few studies in the morning, going home for lunch, and interpreting a few more in the afternoon, as Colonel Thompson outlined in his diary at Walter Reed in 1956 (Dreyer et al. 2006). Perhaps at this moment the reader is thinking about or remembering the good old times. Gone are the days when a radiologist interpreted single-or two-view studies with dictated and manually transcribed reports. But also gone are the days when the film was not in the film jacket and when the surgeon gets his outcome in the film reading room while the patient is already under general anesthesia in the operation theater. Gone are the days when it takes minutes or hours to receive previous images from a dusty archive. Gone are the days when the radiologist carries 30 or more film jackets into the demonstration room then finds they are not the most important for the clinician's purpose. This list can be continued.

Who or what has made these "good old days" a thing of the past? The answer is computers, computed tomography (CT), magnetic resonance imaging (MRI), and the demands of managing a practice and providing modern clinical care. The earliest CT unit built by Hounsfield took several hours to acquire a single slice of information. The machine then took a few days to reconstruct the raw data into a recognizable image. In 1998 one of the first four-row CT scanners was installed and it was the first time that we felt

unable to handle the amount of images using film printouts. In 2009, 64-row scanners are widely distributed and a radiology department that wants to differ from others now is installing 256-row, dual source CT, 640-row, or even more sophisticated machines. Whether they are necessary or not, more than 1,000 images commonly are generated for every CT examination in many institutions. This amount of images is far beyond film's capacity and this image explosion made the transition to filmless interpretation mandatory. In MRI the development is comparable when thinking about MR angiography and functional imaging. The second was the demand of modern clinical care. It is far beyond the scope of this chapter to discuss the pros and cons of modern clinical care. But five needs should be taken into account: accessibility (access to the images independent of location), urgency (instantaneous access to imaging data and interpretation), security (on a need-to-know basis), simplification (use of multimedia reports), and service (improve the ability to and ease of scheduling exams) (Dreyer et al. 2006).

In summary, because of technical and health care developments, a change in the performance of radiology and the organization of a radiology department was necessary. The "good old days" are gone, and after almost 100 years the wind of change reached even film–screen radiology.

4.2 RIS and PACS

As previously mentioned, demands from the referring clinician, market competition, and the need to become more efficient to balance the losses from the steady decline in reimbursement rates make it necessary to organize and perform radiology as effectively as possible. Being effective in a patient setting means to handle more and more patients (with many more images) in shorter times with fewer staff. Enhancement of the productivity and efficiency investments in technology are necessary. This increase in quality and clinical effectiveness, and meeting the pressure of market competition, never could be provided in the analog world (Dreyer et al. 2006). This chapter deals with the three most important systems in the radiologic world of today and the near future.

4.2.1 RIS

The Radiology Information System (RIS) is designed to support both the administrative and clinical operations of a radiology department. It manages general radiology patient demographics and billing information, procedure descriptions and scheduling, diagnostic reports, patient arrival scheduling, film location, and examination room scheduling. Realistically, "only" a computer system with peripheral devices (workstations, normally without images display, printers, and possibly bar code readers) are necessary. The "only" is justified because in daily practice a network, server, and clients that work well are sometimes more a dream than reality. So, the RIS is the nervous system of the digital department (Dreyer et al. 2006). However, this system is more effective when it is integrated in to the Hospital Information System (HIS) and in the Picture Archiving and Communication System (PACS). The HIS is a computerized management system for handling three categories of tasks in a healthcare environment: support for the clinical and medical patient care activities in the hospital, administration of the hospital's daily business transactions, and evaluation of hospital performance and costs.

4.2.2 PACS

Speaking and writing about PACS can be very time consuming and complex. In the scope of this chapter we want to give a short summary about the fundamentals of the functions and the basic technology of PACS and then focus on workstations and features necessary in daily practice.

To begin, PACS is a computer system designed for digital imaging that can capture, store, distribute, and display digital images. A network system links multiple computers so that images, patient data, and interpretations can be viewed simultaneously by people at different workstations and desktops at multiple locations in the hospital. PACS was developed in the late 1980s, serving small modules of the total operation of a radiology department. By adding more and more of these modules the system failed because of a lack of connectivity and cooperation between the modules. Today the performance of PACS is strictly linked to connectivity. PACS now is a general multimedia data management system that must be easily expandable, flexible, and versatile in its operation and calls for both top-down management to integrate various hospital information systems and a bottom-up engineering approach to build a foundation (i.e., PACS infrastructure).

4.2.2.1 Basic Elements of PACS

The basic skeleton of PACS infrastructure consists of hard- and software components:

- Image device interface
- Storage devices
- Host computers
- Communication networks
- Display systems
- Software for communication, database management, storage management, job scheduling, interprocessor communication, error handling, and network monitoring (Dreyer et al. 2006)

To bring such a system into life, image acquisition is the major task for three reasons. First, the imaging modality is not under the auspices of the PACS. Many vendors supply various imaging modalities, each of which has its own DICOM-compliant statement. As a consequence the images cannot be administered or handled by PACS. Second, image acquisition is a slower operation than other PACS functions. It takes time for the imaging modality to acquire the necessary data for image reconstruction. Third, images and patient data generated by the modality sometimes may contain information in a format that is not accepted by the PACS operation. So The major functions of a PACS controller and archive server are summarized in Table 4.1.

One important benefit of PACS is the abovementioned automatic retrieval of comparison images, called prefetching. Most prefetching is initiated as soon as the archive server detects the arrival of a patient via a message from the HIS. The prefetching algorithm is based on predefined parameters such as examination type, disease category, radiologist, referring physician, location of the workstation, and the number and age of the patient's archived images (Huang 2004), but it can be modified. In the authors' hospital, prefetching includes the entire previous examinations of the patients. But this works only because the hospital is filmless and has been for a few years. Soon the workload for the network and the computer systems will be probably so high that a more subtle prefetching algorithm will be necessary, if storage capacity is limited. It is absolutely essential to have all the examinations in digital form and stored in the PACS for such a system to work properly. It is time consuming and cumbersome to make reports comparing examinations on a workstation in one case and on a film–screen in another. It is not necessary and no one will recommend digitizing an old film archive and importing it into the new PACS. But in a filmless hospital, scanning of recent hardcopies from an outpatient facility would be very helpful.

The second important task is image routing. Exams are immediately and automatically sent to the archive server and the archive server automatically distributes the PACS exams to the workstations on the referring wards or even makes them available on all workstations in the hospital (i.e., intensive care unit, operation theater) (Huang 2004).

Table 4.1 Major functions of a PACS controller and archive server (Huang 2004)

Receive images from examination via acquisition gateway computers
Extract text information describing the received exam
Update a network-accessible database management system
Determine the destination workstations to which newly generated exams are to be forwarded
Automatically retrieve necessary comparison images from a distributed cache storage or long-term library archive system
Automatically correct the orientation of computed radiography images
Determine optimal contrast and brightness parameters for image display
Perform image data compression if necessary
Perform data integrity check if necessary
Archive new exams into long-term archive library
Delete images that have been archived from acquisition gateway computers
Service query/retrieve requests from workstations and other PACS controllers in the enterprise PACS
Interface with PACS application servers

4.3 Workstations

A workstation includes communication network connection, local database, display, resource management, and processing software. The major functions of a PACS workstation are summarized in Table 4.2.

There are two general types of workstations: diagnostic and review. The characteristics that distinguish between them are resolution and functionality. The diagnostic workstation is used by the radiologist to perform primary interpretation of the exams. It depends not least on the financials whether this is basically only a computer with a high-enough monitor resolution or a fully equipped workstation. The resolution of a display monitor is most commonly specified in terms of the number of lines. For example, the 1 K monitor has 1,024 lines; the 2 K monitor 2,048 lines. As a rule of thumb, when making reports of ultrasound, CT, and MRI, multiple 1 K monitors are sufficient. For conventional lung and skeletal exams at least 2 K monitors are necessary. For digital mammograms 5 K monitors should be used (Carter and Vealé 2008). Review workstations are not as powerful as the diagnostic types. The difference can be in hardware (resolution), available software functionality, or both. The most important features of a diagnostic workstation are briefly listened and explained in the next section.

Table 4.2 Major functions of a PACS workstation (Huang 2004)

Function	Description
Case preparation	Accumulation of all relevant images and information belonging to a patient examination
Case selection	Selection of cases for a given subpopulation
Image arrangement	Tools for arranging and grouping images for easy review
Interpretation	Measurement tools for facilitating the diagnosis
Documentation	Tools for imaging annotation, text, and voice reports
Case presentation	Tools for comprehensive case presentation
Image reconstruction	Tools for various types of image reconstruction for proper display

4.3.1 Fundamental Functions

In this context three major groups must be mentioned: navigation, image manipulation, and image management.

4.3.1.1 Navigation and Image Manipulation

Navigation functions are used to move through images, series, studies, and patients. Moving the grab bars by using the mouse conforms to the well-known look and feel of Windows® (Microsoft, Redmond, WA, USA). Hanging protocols means the way a set of images will be displayed on the monitor. For example, for chest X-ray images there would be one exam on each monitor; for CT images there would be perhaps four on one monitor; It depends on the preferences of the radiologist. Navigation through a study brings two new terms: frame mode and stack mode. Frame mode is an example of a static mode in which images are displayed in a matrix similar to that typically printed to film. Stack mode displays images sequentially in a single window in a movie like format. Here the images can be quickly moved through manually using the mouse, and most vendors have an additional automatic setting that runs through the images at a preset pace.

The most commonly used functions for imaging manipulation include:

- Window/level to change brightness and contrast
- Annotations, i.e., allows the circling of a special pathology for the attention of the referring physician
- Flip and rotate to orientate the image in the anatomical position desired
- Pan and zoom to increase the size of the region of interest for better outlining of the pathology
- Measurements to depict the size of a lesion or using a region of interest to determine the pixel intensity of a certain area (Dreyer et al. 2006, Carter and Vealé 2008)

Image management functions are necessary when, for example, patients' demographics need to be corrected after the transmission of the images into the PACS archive. Of course even switching of examinations from one folder to the other must be possible. But it is easy to understand why only very few persons in a hospital are allowed to have access to and to manipulate this critical data base.

4.3.2 Advanced Functions

These functions are definitely beyond the scope of review workstations but are absolutely necessary in the world of multislice CT and high-end MR scanners. The isotropic data set obtained by modern CT scanners consists of more than 500 axial slices of the lung, acquired in less than 10 s. This amount of images cannot be handled by film and the interpretation of those 0.6-mm thick axial slices with a reviewing workstation is time consuming; most of the time it is not the best way to detect and interpret pathologies. A lot of different techniques and algorithms have been applied to handle this large data set and to enhance a special kind of anatomy and pathology, called postprocessing (Neri et al. 2008). It is beyond the scope of this chapter to discuss the different techniques in detail. First of all, the radiologist must know that postprocessing starts with the reconstruction of axial slices from the raw data. Both lung and soft-tissue reconstructions should be performed for chest CT to improve detectability of the various structures. These primary overlapping axial reconstructions with a very thin slice thickness are called the secondary raw data set and are the basis for further postprocessing.

Because of the lower signal-to-noise ratio and the large amount of images, making a report of these images is not recommended. For routine evaluation, it is generally sufficient to reconstruct 5-mm thick slices with 4 mm increments, resulting in 20% overlap (Eibel et al. 2001b). Of course the raw data set also allows a high-resolution reconstruction and with comparable image quality, similar to that of sequential high-resolution CT. As mentioned above, axial slices are not sufficient for many diagnostic purposes, because of the orientation of the anatomical structures or diseases. Sometimes reconstructions in a sagittal or coronal plane enhance the visualization. Because such reconstructions are possible in every orientation they are termed multiplanar reformations (MPRs). The fundamentals for all of the following reconstruction techniques are the entire or a partial selection of the secondary axial raw data set. Because these images are commonly achieved by overlapping reconstructions (increment < 1), this data set is also called the 3-dimensional (3D) volume.

4.3.2.1 MPR

In MPR, a plane is defined by the technician or the radiologist inside the 3D volume and only the data in this plane are displayed. An MPR can be performed by using either straight planes or curved planes (Dalrymple et al. 2005). When performing an MPR with straight planes, the thickness of the selection is the same slice thickness as the voxel and is set as the default. When a greater thickness is selected, a slab MPR is created (Lee et al. 2008). To reduce the number of images, a coronal or sagittal MPR thickness of 5 mm is generally sufficient (Eibel et al. 2001b). Advantages of MPR are the ease of use and speed of the MPR algorithm. Furthermore, MPR provides images containing all available information (all Hounsfield unit values are retained). A major disadvantage of the MPR method is the high dependence on the manual orientation of the planes. Interactive viewing of this type of image from multiple viewing angles is easily possible with workstations.

MPRs can be used as a fundamental tool for direct comparison of plain film and CT. It is daily practice that a lung nodule on a plain film must be further investigated with chest CT. But it can be difficult to decide if the lesions are identical. It is possible that the lesion in the plain film corresponds to a summarization of vessels and/or bony structures or even belongs to a skin alteration and the corresponding CT shows another lesion. To resolve this problem, thick MPRs containing the whole data sets in a coronal direction are reconstructed similar to the chest X-ray. After identification of the lesion, the thickness of the MPRs is reduced step by step, with great attention paid so that the nodule at the thinner MPR is not lost. At the end of the reconstruction the nodule is clearly visible. While reconstructing perpendicular directions to the coronal image the lesion can be displayed in axial or sagittal view. Perhaps more in an academic setting the other direction is also possible. After identifying a nodule on an axial CT slice, a coronal reformation can be performed, centered to the lesion. Then the thickness of the MPR can be increased step by step until the MPR contains the whole data sets. Now an easy correlation is possible with the chest X-ray.

4.3.2.2 MIP

With maximum intensity projections (MIPs), only the highest-attenuation voxels are preserved. This algorithm casts a ray through the 3D data for each pixel in the resulting image, and only the highest-attenuation voxels found on each ray are preserved (Dalrymple et al. 2005). Disadvantages of MIP result from this because only a fraction of the available data is used. Furthermore, many artifacts are known to exist in MIP images and no 3D depth is obtained. To preserve the depth information in MIP, two principle advantages had been developed. In the rotating MIP, the radiologist has to define a center, the direction of rotation (left/right, or top/bottom), and the degree of the angles (i.e., 10°). Another technique is the sliding thin-slab MIP (STS-MIP). To obtain this MIP format, a thin-slab MPR is selected, from which an MIP image is reconstructed. This slab is moved through the volume, with the distance of slab movement smaller than the slab thickness, and at each step an MIP is created (Remy-Jardin et al. 1996). In this particular case the information of depth is preserved because the different MIP slices can be clearly localized within the volume (Eibel et al. 1999; Fishman et al. 2006). But, to mention again, the highlighting of only the highest-attenuation voxels can be either good or bad (Parrish 2007). MIP reformations on the basis of multidetector CT data sets are superior in the depiction and diagnosis of pulmonary nodules as compared with axial standard reconstructions and MPR (Eibel et al. 2001; Remy et al. 1998; Ueno et al. 2004; Dreyer et al. 2006). However, small lung emboli can be overlooked using only MIP images when the thrombus does not entirely occlude the vessel and little amounts of contrast medium flow between the thrombus and the vessel wall.

4.3.2.3 MinIP

Minimum intensity projection (MinIP) consists of projecting the voxel with the lowest attenuation value on every view throughout the volume onto a 2-dimensional image (Remy-Jardin et al. 1996; Dalrymple et al. 2005). This technique displays only 10% of the data set. The subtle difference in density between the endobronchial (pure) air and the lung parenchyma, corresponding to a difference in attenuation of 50–150 HU, permits visualization of the bronchi below the subsegmental level (Lawler and Fishman 2001). MinIP is the optimal tool for the detection, localization, and quantification of ground-glass attenuation patterns and pulmonary emphysema (Remy et al. 1998; Satoh et al. 2008). Similar to MIP, the MinIP can also be achieved as STS-MinIP to preserve information of depth within the lung volume.

4.3.2.4 Averaging

In multiplanar averaging, the mean attenuation value of the voxels on every view throughout the volume is projected onto a 2-dimensional image. This technique allows concomitant evaluation of the tracheobronchial tree in the setting of diffuse lung disease. Figure 4.1 briefly illustrates the different reformation and projection techniques.

The above-mentioned techniques use the whole data set and display the data in an alternative direction or by focusing on the highest or lowest pixels/voxels. Segmentation, on the other hand, extracts or classifies a specific region or volume of interest. Image segmentation provides quantitative data about relevant anatomy and it also enables an accurate 3D visualization of a particular structure. There is no single approach that can generally solve the problem of segmentation, and different methods will be more effective depending on the image modality being processed. Pham et al. (2000) and Preim and Bartz (2007) provide detailed reviews of the classic segmentation algorithms, many of which are now implemented within the radiological software supplied by the scanner manufacturers.

4.3.2.5 SSD

A relatively simple form of segmentation is the shaded surface display (SSD). The main landmark of this surface-rendering technique is the thresholding segmentation, which results in a binary classification of the voxels (Remy 1998). Everything below the threshold will be removed, and everything above will be assigned a color and shown as a 3D object. It is important to keep in mind that voxels belonging to the structure of interest may be misclassified because of partial volume averaging. Consequently, they will be eliminated from the final 3D image. The SSD technique requires minimal computing power and is not time consuming. Another advantage is that the depth impression is optimally rendered. Disadvantages of this method are pitfalls related to the thresholding range and pitfalls related to the slice thickness; either can be responsible for partial volume artefacts or stair-step artefacts. Pitfalls may be caused by motion during data acquisition (Magnusson et al. 1991).

4.3.2.6 VRT

One of the most complex forms of reformat is volume rendering techniques (VRTs) beyond the above mentioned SSD. Volume rendering involves applications of opacity maps based on the image histogram values, as well as different grayscale and/or color lookup maps, such that voxels may be displayed with a variable opacity as well as variable intensity/color depending on the voxel values that are displayed in a continuous range (Cody 2002; Dalrymple et al. 2005; Lee et al. 2008).

Surface rendering and VR are useful when viewing bony anatomy, organ surfaces, and blood vessels

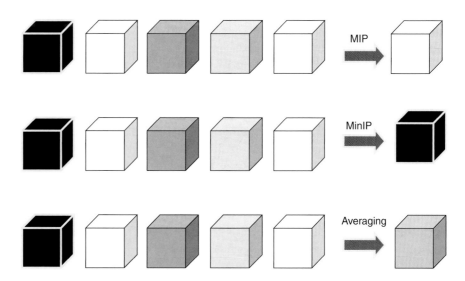

Fig. 4.1 The principles of MIP, MinIP, and averaging

(Cody 2002; Fishman et al. 2006). Volume rendering also allows variable viewing of different tissues. The specific type of image reconstruction depends on the anatomy, the purpose, and the customer's needs. VRTs are time consuming and require a maximum computing power (Remy 1998). Of course, there are presumably a lot of indications for VR, especially when bringing up special information in a very instructive and easy-to-understand way for the referring clinician. The clinical value of VR is usually limited and it is not a method used to make a diagnosis, only to present it.

4.3.2.7 VE

A further development of VR and SSD is virtual endoscopy (VE), also referred to as "fly through" (Ueno et al. 2004). Because of the high intrinsic contrast between the air-filled lumen of the trachea and bronchi and their walls, good endoluminal views are possible. The advantage of VE is that the radiologist can move interactively in the tracheobronchial tree and that the data set will be available without additional scanning of the patient. Furthermore, the radiologist can call up the corresponding cross-sectional images for localization of the special lesion (Neri et al. 2008; Remy et al. 1998). However, it is necessary to take into account that the color of the tracheal wall is artificial and that subtle details of surface morphology are lost.

4.3.2.8 CAD

The last technique that has to be mentioned briefly in this short list is computer-aided detection (CAD) (Ravenel et al. 2001). CAD doesnot stand for computer-aided diagnosis! CAD means that computer algorithms analyze special information in the images and compare it with huge imaging databases. They assist the radiologist in the recognition and classification of disease (Dreyer et al. 2006). But the final judgment and, as a consequence, the diagnosis will remain with the radiologist. In the chest, the focus is on the automated detection of nodules in the multi-slice CT data set, the detection of pulmonary emboli, and the textural analysis by classification of pixels, e.g., for the quantification of the extent of sarcoidosis or emphysema (Parrish 2007). Other CAD applications include calcium scoring, polyp detection in virtual colonography, and detection of breast masses.

4.3.3 Applications (MPR, MIP, MinIP, VRT, and Averaging)

This section gives some examples and fundamentals important for application of reformations. The fundamental necessity of all reformations is a data set consisting of the thinnest slice thickness the CT machine is able to offer. Of course, the examination time must be one during which the patient can stop breathing during the scan period. Breathing and motion artefacts can substantially degrade the image quality. Although the axial slices are relatively robust for these kinds of artefacts, coronal and sagittal reformations and especially VR can be severely influenced.

The type of reformation to use is determined by the underlying pathology and the anatomic structure to be displayed. In general, for an evaluation of the trachea, bronchi, and pulmonary parenchymal diseases it is helpful to start with MPRs or averaging. A slice thickness of 3–5 mm is a good compromise between the number of images and z-resolution (Eibel et al. 2001b). The differentiation between vessels and small lung nodules can be problematic and time consuming, especially when using thin axial slices. In this particular case, the coronal or sagittal reformation can provide only a little more confidence. The 5-mm STS-MIP reconstruction, on the other hand, allows a significantly higher detection rate. However, thicker reconstructions can make the vessels so prominent that smaller lung nodules can be overlooked. For evaluation of pulmonary embolism, MIP can be positive or negative. The higher detectability of vessels is accompanied by the drawback that the peripheral flow around a central embolus can mimic the visualization of the embolus. Lung parenchymal diseases and especially the distribution can be delineated nicely with MPRs. For the detection of emphysema and tiny ground-glass opacities the minIP should be applied.

In *case 1* (Fig. 4.2a–j), an overview is given with regard to the different types of reformations. The thorax of 48-year-old male smoker was investigated using a 64-row scanner to exclude lung cancer. The secondary raw data set consists of 0.6-mm thick axial slices, which results in a nearly isotropic data volume.

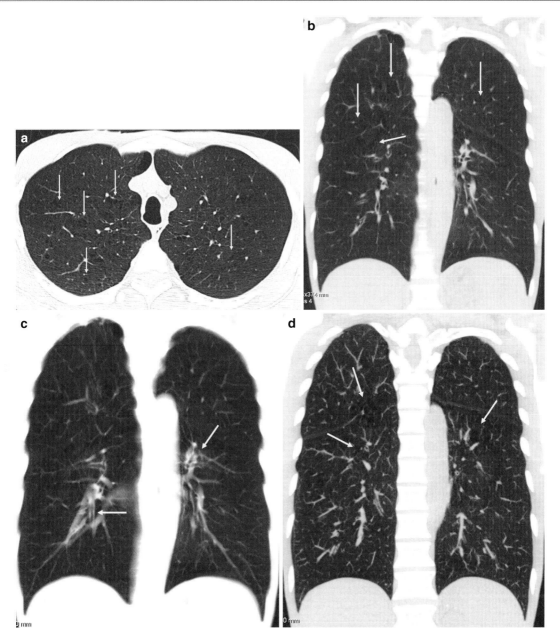

Fig. 4.2 (**a**) Axial MPR, 2.5-mm slice thickness. Centrilobular emphysema in both upper lobes (*arrows*). (**b**) Coronal MPR, 4 mm. The coronal plane nicely demonstrates the upper lobe predominance of the emphysema (*arrows*) and the concomitant rarefaction of pulmonary vasculature. (**c**) Coronal MPR, 10 mm. The images looks smoother and vascular structures are easy to delineate. The drawback is the loss of detailed resolution; for example, the deterioration in the visualization of bronchi (*arrows*). The signs of emphysema have nearly gone. (**d**) Coronal MIP, 3 mm. The advantage of MIP is the delineation of vascular structures. In 3-mm thickslices, some areas of emphysema are still detectable (*arrows*). (**e**) Coronal MIP, 10 mm. The vasculature is so prominent that the bronchi and areas of emphysema could no longer be detected. (**f**) Coronal minIP, 3 mm. The value of this technique is the visualization of emphysematous lung areas, now even detectable in the lower lobes (*arrows*). On the other hand, this technique comes with a loss of further anatomic information. (**g**) Coronal minIP, 3 mm, inversion. The areas of emphysema are now displayed brightly (*black arrows*). The darker zones adjacent to the diaphragm correlate with normal lung parenchyma. (**h**) VR, coronal view. Using presets for bone imaging, nice overviews of the skeleton and the rib cartilage (*blue color*) can be obtained. (**i**) VR, coronal view. Using presets for air and lung surface, a totally different aspect of the data set is highlighted. (**j**) VR, endoscopic view. The carina is seen from the trachea. Please note the steep right and the more horizontal left main stem bronchus. The flat fibromuscular membrane of the trachea is shown at the bottom of the image (*arrow*)

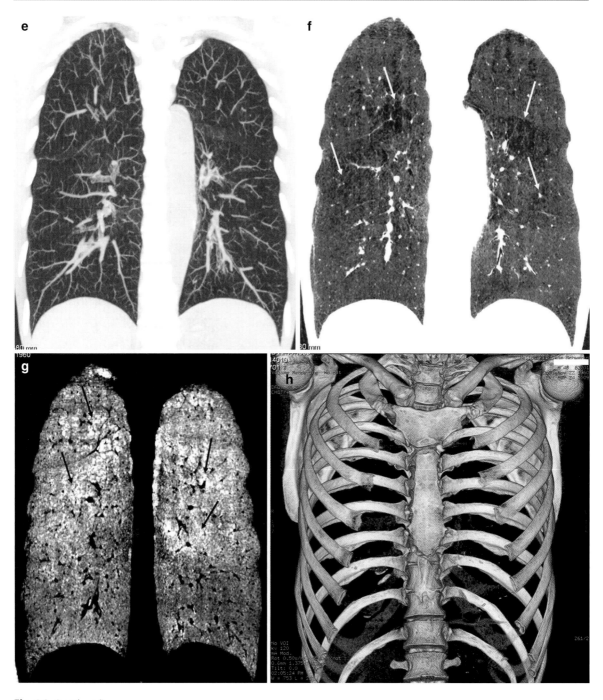

Fig. 4.2 (continued)

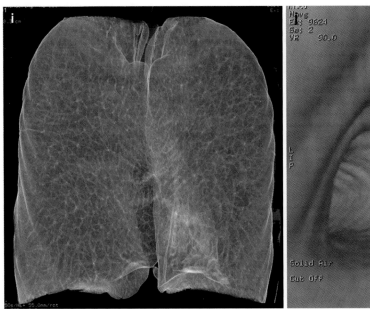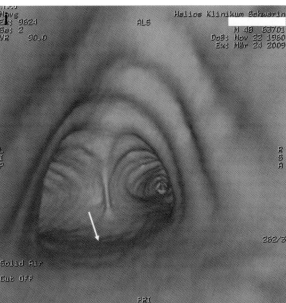

Fig. 4.2 (continued)

Case 2 (Fig. 4.3a–i) refers to a 57-year-old male with lung cancer in the right upper lobe and a left hilar metastasis. The chest X-ray shows a small lung nodule on the right side below the horizontal fissure. On the lateral view the small lung lesion is masked. The presented images show a nice reconstruction technique of the secondary raw data set of the CT, which confirms that the small lesion on plain film definitely correlates with the nodule on axial slices. The principle is to start with a thick average of MPR, including the entire thickness of the thorax. This initial reconstruction looks similar to the plain films. Now it possible to either rotate the images or reduce the slice thickness step by step, until a thin slice with high resolution remains. During the reduction of the slice thickness it is important that the lesion of interest remains in the reconstruction area.

Another tool for lung nodule detection is MIP. Again, it can help to start with thicker collimation and become thinner, centering on a specific lesion (Fig. 4.3j–l).

In *case 3* (Fig. 4.4a, b) MIP is demonstrated not to be the best reformat for investigation of pulmonary embolism, although this reconstruction technique superiorly delineates the pulmonary vessels. A shortcoming of MIP views is that objects within a high-signal object may be obstructed from view because only the brightest pixel along a ray is displayed. This may be the case when the vessel is not entirely occluded and contrast material is flowing around a central embolus. In this particular case, the embolus is masked by the high density of the adjacent contrast material.

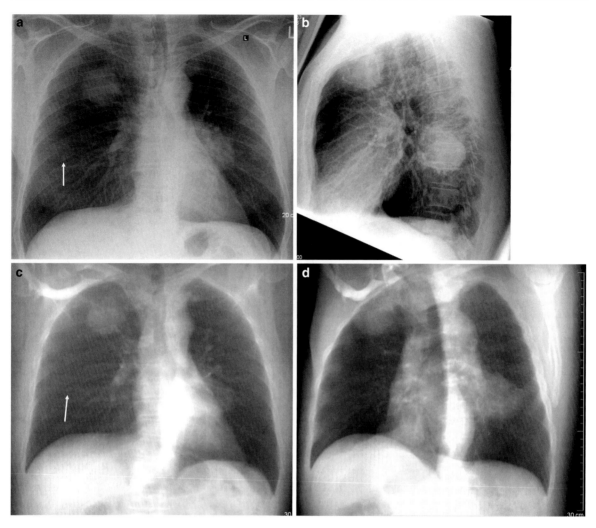

Fig. 4.3 (a) Chest X-ray, posteroanterior (PA) view. Apart from the two large masses in the right upper lobe and the left perihilar region, a small lung nodule below the horizontal fissure is detectable (*arrow*). (b) Same patient. Plain film in lateral view. The small lung nodule is masked. (c) Average coronal reconstruction of the entire 0.6-mm thick secondary raw data set, resembling a PA view of the plain film. Slice thickness, 400-mm. The small nodule is visible (*arrow*). (d) Average coronal reconstruction, 400-mm slice thickness, 20° rotation. The nodule is no longer detectable. (e) Average coronal reconstruction, 400-mm slice thickness, 50° rotation. (f) Average coronal reconstruction. 400-mm slice thickness, 90° rotation (lateral view). The lung nodule is again masked. (g) Average coronal reconstruction in PA view. 200-mm slice thickness. The small nodule can be detected (*arrow*). (h) Average coronal reconstruction in PA view. 100-mm slice thickness. (i) Average coronal reconstruction in PA view. 50-mm slice thickness. (j) Average coronal reconstruction in PA view. 5-mm slice thickness. Now the lesion is clearly visible (*arrow*). (k) MIP in coronal reconstruction. 50-mm slice thickness. Two additional lung nodules on the right side are detectable (*arrows*). (l) MIP in coronal reconstruction focusing on known lung nodule. 25-mm slice thickness. The smaller lesion above the known lung nodule is still visible (*arrows*). The smallest lesion above the right diaphragm is no longer included in the selected slice. (m) MIP in coronal reconstruction. 5-mm slice thickness. The amount of superimposing vessels is reduced; the two lesions are further visible (*arrows*). (n) VR in coronal view, 100-mm slice thickness. The small lung nodule is detectable, as is the large right upper lobe mass. However, the medical advantage of this technique falls far short of the benefit of the other techniques

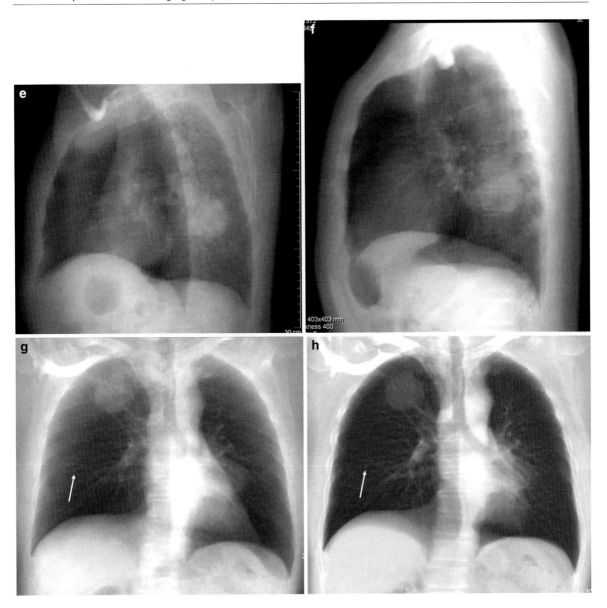

Fig. 4.3 (continued)

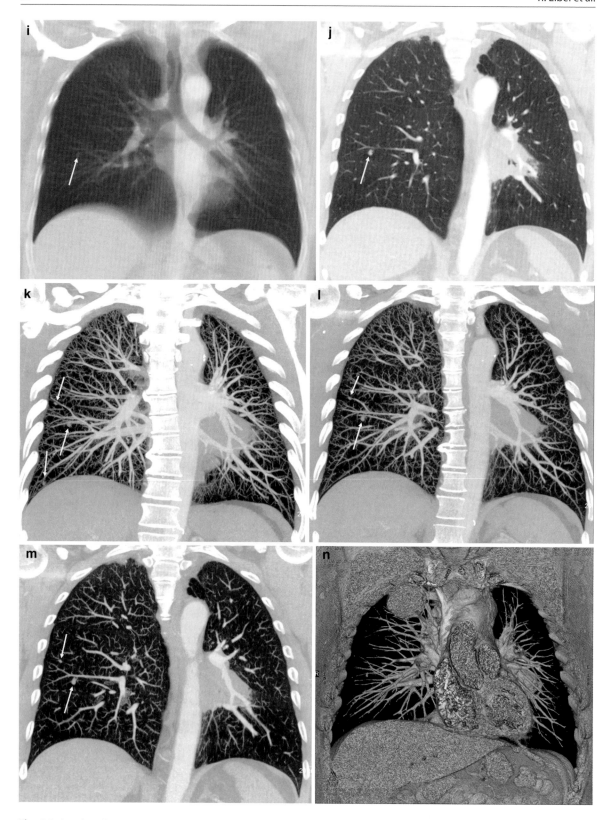

Fig. 4.3 (continued)

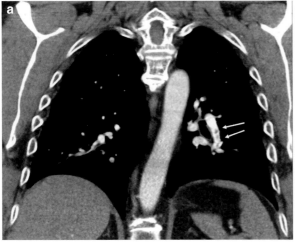
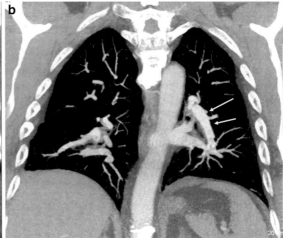

Fig. 4.4 (a) 53-year-old male with shortness of breath and deep venous thrombosis. The coronal MPR shows a filling defect in a left lower lobe pulmonary artery and corresponds with the diagnosis of acute pulmonary embolism (*arrows*). **(b)** In the MIP reconstruction, the filling defect is masked due to the fact that the brightest pixels result from the intravenously applied contrast material (*arrows*)

References

Armato SG 3rd, Li F et al (2002) Lung cancer: performance of automated lung nodule detection applied to cancers missed in a CT screening program. Radiology 225:685–692

Baldwin DR, Eaton T et al (2002) Management of solitary pulmonary nodules: how do thoracic computed tomography and guided fine needle biopsy influence clinical decisions? Thorax 57:817–822

Carter CE, Vealé BL (2008) Digital radiography and PACS. Elsevier, Mosby

Cody DD (2002) AAPM/RSNA physics tutorial for residents: topics in CT. Image processing in CT. Radiographics 22:1255–1268

Cooper JD (2002) Management of the solitary pulmonary nodule: directed resection. Semin Thorac Cardiovasc Surg 14:286–291

Dalrymple NC, Prasad SR, Freckleton MW, Chintapalli KN (2005) Informatics in radiology (infoRAD): introduction to the language of three-dimensional imaging with multidetector CT. Radiographics 25:1409–1428

Decamp MM Jr (2002) The solitary pulmonary nodule: aggressive excisional strategy. Semin Thorac Cardiovasc Surg 14:292–296

Diederich S, Wormanns D et al (2003) Lung cancer screening with low-dose CT. Eur J Radiol 45:2–7

Dreyer KJ, Hirschhorn DS, Thrall JH, PACS MA (2006) A guide to the digital revolution, 2nd edn. Springer, New York

Efilm User's Guide 3.0 (2007) Merge Heathcare

Eibel R, Bruening R, Schoepf UJ, Leimeister P, Stadie A, Reiser MF (1999) Image analysis in multiplanar spiral CT of the lung with MPR and MIP reconstructions. Radiologe 39:952–957

Eibel R, Tuerk TR, Kulinna C, Herrmann K, Reiser MF (2001a) Multidetector-row CT of the lungs: Multiplanar reconstructions and maximum intensity projections for the detection of pulmonary nodules. Fortschr Rontgenstr 173:815–821

Eibel R, Tuerk TR, Kulinna C, Schoepf UJ, Bruening R, Reiser MF (2001b) Value of multiplanar reformations (MPR) in multislice spiral CT. Fortschr Rontgenstr 173:57–64

Fauber TL (2009) Radiographic imaging and exposure, 3rd edn. Elsevier, Mosby

Ferretti G, Félix L, Serra-Tosio G, Brambilla C, Moro-Sibilot D, Brichon PY, Coulomb M, Lantuejoul S (2007) Non-solid and part-solid pulmonary nodules on CT scanning. Rev Mal Respir 24:1265–1276

Fishman EK, Ney DR, Heath DG, Corl FM, Horton KM, Johnson PT (2006) Volume rendering versus maximum intensity projection in CT angiography: what works best, when, and why. Radiographics 26:905–922

Fletcher JW (2002) PET scanning and the solitary pulmonary nodule. Semin Thorac Cardiovasc Surg 14:268–274

Garg K, Keith RL et al (2002) Randomized controlled trial with low-dose spiral CT for lung cancer screening: feasibility study and preliminary results. Radiology 225:506–510

Hartman TE (2002) Radiologic evaluation of the solitary pulmonary nodule. Semin Thorac Cardiovasc Surg 14:261–267

Hasegawa M, Sone S, Takashima S, Li F, Yang ZG, Maruyama Y, Watanabe T (2000) Growth rate of small lung cancers detected on mass CT screening. Br J Radiol 73:1252–1259

Huang HK (2004) PACS and imaging informatics. Basic principles and applications. Wiley-Liss, Hoboken

Kido S, Kuriyama K et al (2002) Fractal analysis of small peripheral pulmonary nodules in thin-section CT: evaluation of the lung-nodule interfaces. J Comput Assist Tomogr 26:573–578

Kishi K, Gurney JW et al (2002) The correlation of emphysema or airway obstruction with the risk of lung cancer: a matched case-controlled study. Eur Respir J 19:1093–1098

Lawler LP, Fishman EK (2001) Multi-detector row CT of thoracic disease with emphasis on 3D volume rendering and CT angiography. Radiographics 21:1257–1273

Lee EY, Boiselle PM, Cleveland RH (2008) Multidetector CT evaluation of congenital lung anomalies. Radiology 247:632–648

Magnusson M, Lenz R, Danielsson PE (1991) Evaluation of methods for shaded surface display of CT volumes. Comput Med Imaging Graph 15:247–256

Mazzone PJ, Stoller JK (2002) The pulmonologist's perspective regarding the solitary pulmonary nodule. Semin Thorac Cardiovasc Surg 14:250–260

Miller DL (2002) Management of the subcentimeter pulmonary nodule. Semin Thorac Cardiovasc Surg 14:281–285

Neri E, Caramella D, Bartolozzi C (2008) Image processing in radiology. Current applications. Springer, New York

Parrish FJ (2007) Volume CT: state-of-the-art reporting. AJR Am J Roentgenol 189:528–534

Pham DL, Xu C, Prince JL (2000) Current methods in medical image segmentation. Ann Rev Biomed Eng 2:315–337

Preim B, Bartz D (2007) Visualization in medicine: theory, algorithms, and applications. Morgan-Kaufmann, San Francisco

Ravenel JG, McAdams HP, Remy-Jardin M, Remy J (2001) Multidimensional imaging of the thorax: practical applications. J Thorac Imaging 16:269–281

Remy J, Remy-Jardin M, Artaud D, Fribourg M (1998) Multiplanar and three-dimensional reconstruction techniques in CT: impact on chest diseases. Eur Radiol 8:335–351

Remy-Jardin M, Remy J, Gosselin B, Copin MC, Wurtz A, Duhamel A (1996) Sliding thin slab, minimum intensity projection technique in the diagnosis of emphysema: histopathologic-CT correlation. Radiology 200: 665–671

Revel MP, Merlin A, Peyrard S, Triki R, Couchon S, Chatellier G, Frija G (2006) Software volumetric evaluation of doubling times for differentiating benign versus malignant pulmonary nodules. AJR Am J Roentgenol 187:135–142

Satoh S, Kitazume Y, Taura S, Kimula Y, Shirai T, Ohdama S (2008) Pulmonary emphysema: histopathologic correlation with minimum intensity projection imaging, high-resolution computed tomography, and pulmonary function test results. J Comput Assist Tomogr 32:576–582

Schafer JF, Vollmar J et al (2002) Imaging diagnosis of solitary pulmonary nodules on an open low-field MRI system–comparison of two MR sequences with spiral CT. Fortschr Rontgenstr 174:1107–1114

Schoepf UJ, Bruening R et al (1999) Imaging of the thorax with multislice spiral CT. Radiologe 39:943–951

Schultz EM, Silvestri GA, Gould MK (2008) Variation in experts' beliefs about lung cancer growth, progression, and prognosis. Thorac Oncol 3:422–426

Suzuki K, Asamura H et al (2002) Early peripheral lung cancer: prognostic significance of ground glass opacity on thin-section computed tomographic scan. Ann Thorac Surg 74:1635–1639

Swensen SJ (2002) CT screening for lung cancer. AJR Am J Roentgenol 179:833–836

Swensen SJ, Jett JR et al (2002) Screening for lung cancer with low-dose spiral computed tomography. Am J Respir Crit Care Med 165:508–513

Sykes AM, Swensen SJ et al (2002) Computed tomography of benign intrapulmonary lymph nodes: retrospective comparison with sarcoma metastases. Mayo Clin Proc 77: 329–333

Ueno J, Murase T, Yoneda K, Tsujikawa T, Sakiyama S, Kondoh K (2004) Three-dimensional imaging of thoracic diseases with multi-detector row CT. J Med Invest 51:163–170

Valencia R, Denecke T, Lehmkuhl L, Fischbach F, Felix R, Knollmann F (2006) Value of axial and coronal maximum intensity projection (MIP) images in the detection of pulmonary nodules by multislice spiral CT: comparison with axial 1-mm and 5-mm slices. Eur Radiol 16:325–332

Wallace MJ, Krishnamurthy S et al (2002) CT-guided percutaneous fine-needle aspiration biopsy of small (< or =1-cm) pulmonary lesions. Radiology 225:823–828

Xu DM, van der Zaag-Loonen HJ, Oudkerk M, Wang Y, Vliegenthart R, Scholten ET, Verschakelen J, Prokop M, de Koning HJ, van Klaveren RJ (2009) Smooth or attached solid indeterminate nodules detected at baseline CT screening in the NELSON study: cancer risk during 1 year of follow-up. Radiology 250:264–272

Yankelevitz DF, Reeves AP, Kostis WJ, Zhao B, Henschke CI (2000) Small pulmonary nodules: volumetrically determined growth rates based on CT evaluation. Radiology 217: 251–256

Yoon YC, Lee KS et al (2002) Benign bronchopulmonary tumors: radiologic and pathologic findings. J Comput Assist Tomogr 26:784–796

Yuan Y, Matsumoto T et al (2002) Role of high-resolution CT in the diagnosis of small pulmonary nodules coexisting with potentially operable lung cancer. Radiat Med 20:237–245

Zhang L, Wang M et al (2002) Clinico-pathological study of 98 patients with pulmonary solitary nodule. Zhonghua Zhong Liu Za Zhi 24:491–493

Semeiology of Normal Variants and Diseased Chest

Semeiology of the Mediastinum

Robert Gosselin, Louke Delrue, Bart Ilsen,
Catherine Heysse, Johan de Mey, and Philippe Duyck

5

Contents

R. Gosselin (✉), C. Heysse, and P. Duyck
Department of Radiology, UZ Gent, De Pintelaan 185,
9000 Ghent, Belgium
e-mail: robert.gosselin@uzgent.be; philippe.duyck@uzgent.be

L. Delrue
Ghent University Hospital, Ghent, Belgium
e-mail: louke.delrue@uzgent.be

B. Ilsen
Department of Radiology, Universitair Ziekenhuis Brussel,
Laarbeeklaan 101, 1090, Brussel, Belgium
e-mail: bart.ilsen@uzbrussel.be

J. de Mey
Department of Radiology, AZ-VUB, Laarbeeklaan 101,
1090 Brussel, Belgium
e-mail: johan.demey@az.vub.ac.be

Abstract

> In the past, the mediastinum has been considered as the so-called "black-box" of thoracic radiology.

> Nowadays, CT and MRI nicely depict and explain "the who's and the why's" of the mediastinal lines in physiological as well in pathological conditions. The aim of this chapter is to emphasize on the important role of basic radiological findings in standard diagnostic chest XR interpretation and to correlate the radiological anatomy with cross-sectional imaging.

> The mediastinal lines can be defined as linear structures (reflections) visible on the conventional X-ray, formed by points of contact of the mediastinal soft tissues and the adjacent aerated lung or contact of pulmonary tissue by intervening soft tissue.

> Normal anatomic structures of the mediastinum may be altered by mediastinal disease.

> This alteration of normal anatomy and the accompanying displacement of the mediastinal lines and spaces may alert the radiologist to the presence of a mediastinal mass.

> Thus, familiarity with the appearance of normal mediastinal structures on chest radiography is the first crucial part in locating and identifying an abnormality.

> These elements will further on permit to narrow the differential diagnosis and possibly influence the choice of modality for further diagnostic imaging.

E.E. Coche et al. (eds.), *Comparative Interpretation of CT and Standard Radiography of the Chest*,
Medical Radiology, DOI: 10.1007/978-3-540-79942-9_5, © Springer-Verlag Berlin Heidelberg 2011

5.1 Introduction

Currently, chest radiography is the most common and most frequently performed radiological examination because of its low cost, easy accessibility, and low irradiation.

Standard radiography can by itself provide a large amount of useful information to obtain a differential diagnosis before proceeding to cross-sectional imaging.

This information is derived from the configuration and interrelationship of the anatomical structures of the lung, mediastinum, and pleura, and forms the basis of the "mediastinal lines approach," which we shall discuss in this chapter (Gibbs et al. 2007; Whitten et al. 2007).

Before the advent of cross-sectional imaging, the mediastinum has been considered the so-called "black-box" of thoracic radiology; now computed tomography (CT) and magnetic resonance imaging (MRI) nicely depict and explain "the who's and the why's" of the mediastinal lines in physiologic as well as in pathologic conditions. The aim of this chapter is to emphasize the important role of basic radiologic findings and, more precisely, the mediastinal lines. Those anatomic structures remain important in standard diagnostic chest radiographic interpretation.

The mediastinal lines can be defined as linear structures (reflections) visible on the conventional radiograph, formed by points of contact of the mediastinal soft tissues and the adjacent aerated lung or contact of pulmonary tissue with intervening soft tissue (Gibbs et al. 2007; Neufang and Beyer 1980; Divano et al. 1983).

- Lines are very thin structures less than 1 mm in width. They are formed by air outlining thin intervening tissue on both sides, e.g., the anterior and posterior junction lines.
- Stripes are thicker structures formed by air outlining thicker slabs of intervening soft tissue, e.g., the left and right paratracheal and retrotracheal stripes.
- The edge, or interface, represents the third linear structure that we can identify on conventional radiographs and is formed when layers of different densities come in close contact with each other, e.g., the paravertebral and para-aortic lines.

Normal mediastinal lines and spaces can be altered by mediastinal disease.

This alteration of normal anatomy may alert the radiologist to the presence of a mediastinal mass. Thus, familiarity with the appearance of normal mediastinal structures on chest radiography is the first crucial part in identifying an abnormality. It is important that the lung–mediastinal interfaces (lines, stripes, edges, and spaces) are evaluated in every chest radiograph during routine work.

Identifying the exact location of a mass will narrow the differential diagnosis and possibly influence the choice of modality for further diagnostic imaging.

Whenever a mass is depicted on a chest radiograph and is possibly located within the mediastinum, the following three basic points should be determined:

- Is it a mediastinal mass?

  The following features indicate that a lesion truly originates within the mediastinum:
  - Unlike some lung lesions, a mediastinal mass will not contain air bronchograms.
  - The margins with the lung will be obtuse. A mediastinal mass lies under the pleural surface, creating obtuse angles with the lung, whereas a lung mass abuts the mediastinal surface and creates acute angles with the lung.
  - Mediastinal lines (azygoesophageal recess, anterior and posterior junction lines) will be disrupted. Some spinal, costal, or sternal abnormalities can also be associated.
- Is it located in the anterior, middle, or posterior mediastinum?
- Is it possible to further characterize the lesion by determining whether it has any fatty, fluid, or calcified components?

Traditionally, the mediastinum was subdivided into anterior, medial, posterior, and superior parts.

Felson used the findings on the lateral chest radiograph and, more specifically, the posterior heart border and the anterior tracheal wall to differentiate the anterior from the middle mediastinum; he used an imaginary line 1 cm posterior from the anterior vertebral wall to differentiate the middle and the posterior mediastinum; finally, a second imaginary line above the aortic arch was used to achieve the differentiation with the superior mediastinum (Felson 1969; Fraser et al. 1999).

A popular variation of the Felson method does not recognize a separate superior compartment.

The more complex Heitzman method divided the mediastinum into the following anatomic regions: the thoracic inlet, the anterior mediastinum, the supra-aortic area, the infra-aortic area, the supra-azygos area, and finally, the infra-azygos area (Heitzman 1997).

However, in clinical practice, a pathologic process is not necessarily primarily limited to one compartment (Fig. 5.1); for example, infection, hemorrhage,

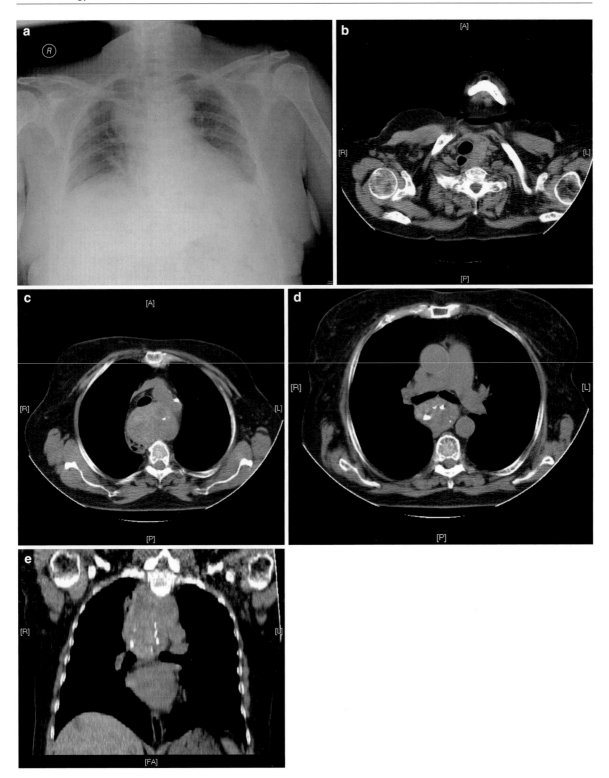

Fig. 5.1 Frontal chest radiograph (**a**), MDCT with axial (**b**, **c**, **d**) and coronal (**e**) reformats. Mediastinal lesions are not necessarily bound to one single compartment. A huge goiter, initially located in the lower neck and the superior middle mediastinum, and tracheal and oesophageal compression and deviation, extending inferiorly behind the trachea and the carina. The mass is quite heterogeneous and calcified in its lower portion

and neoplasia can secondarily spread from one compartment to another because there are no true physical boundaries between the different mediastinal compartments. Each subdivision of the mediastinum is therefore rather theoretical than physical (Whitten et al. 2007; Fraser et al. 1999; Zylak et al. 1982; Armstrong et al. 2000).

Basically for this reason, the subdivision of each mediastinal compartment (anterior, medial, and posterior) used in this chapter to explain the anatomy, the formation, and the identification of mediastinal lines, stripes, and spaces is based on a modified anatomical method, conceiving the mediastinum to be composed of three uninterrupted longitudinal compartments extending from the thoracic inlet to the diaphragm without a separate superior compartment (Whitten et al. 2007; Fraser et al. 1999).

The main goal of this modified classification is to be as precise as possible in the nonequivocal location of the abnormality in an effort to be efficient by taking into account that a pathology causing the disruption of one (or more) specific mediastinal line(s) should be associated with a specific mediastinal compartment.

However, one should always keep in mind that every classification has its practical limitations and is not necessarily totally related to a physical, anatomical, and anatomopathological reality!

Once again, it needs to be emphasized that, in contradistinction to the traditional Felson method, according to this modified classification, the heart and the great vessels are part of the middle mediastinum.

5.2 Mediastinal Compartments and Contents

5.2.1 Anterior Mediastinum

The anterior mediastinum is limited anteriorly by the sternum; posteriorly by the pericardium, the aorta, and the brachiocephalic vessels; superiorly by the thoracic inlet; and inferiorly by the diaphragm.

The following organs and tissues are included in the anterior mediastinum: thymus, lymph nodes, fat, internal mammary arteries and veins, and the thyroid when it extends into the mediastinum.

The anterior mediastinum can thus be regarded as the "prevascular space."

We shall subsequently discuss the anterior junction line and the retrosternal line and space in the anterior mediastinal compartment.

5.2.2 Middle Mediastinum

The middle mediastinum is limited anteriorly and posteriorly by the pericardium and more superiorly by the posterior tracheal wall; the superior and inferior limits are the same as for the anterior mediastinum.

The middle mediastinum includes the heart with the pericardium, the ascending aorta and the aortic arch, the superior and inferior vena cava, the brachiocephalic vessels, the pulmonary vessels, the trachea and the main bronchi, lymph nodes, vagus and recurrent nerves, and fat.

The middle mediastinum can thus be regarded as essentially a "vascular and tracheal" space.

We shall subsequently discuss the aortopulmonary stripe and window on frontal and lateral films, the right and left paratracheal line or stripe, the retrotracheal stripe, and the posterior wall of the bronchus intermedius on lateral films in the middle mediastinal compartment.

5.2.3 Posterior Mediastinum

The posterior mediastinum is limited anteriorly by the posterior tracheal wall and pericardium and posteriorly by the spine; the superior and inferior borders are the thoracic inlet and the diaphragm.

The posterior mediastinum contains the esophagus, the descending aorta, the azygos and hemiazygos veins, the thoracic duct, the vagus and splanchnic nerves, lymph nodes, and fat.

The posterior mediastinum can thus be regarded as the "postvascular" space and continues into the neck in the plane of the retropharyngeal space (Zylak et al. 1982).

We shall subsequently discuss the posterior junction line, the azygoesophageal line and recess, the para- and preaortic lines, and the paraspinal lines in the posterior mediastinal compartment.

5.3 The Anterior Mediastinal Compartment

5.3.1 Anterior Junction Line

The anterior junction line is formed by the anterior apposition of the two lungs together with their respective pleural coverings and a thin, variable layer of mediastinal tissue posterior to the sternum; the line is visible in up to 25% of chest radiographs (Fig. 5.2) (Gibbs et al. 2007; Whitten et al. 2007; Webb and Higgins 2005).

It courses retrosternally, anterior to the ascending aorta, and runs downward over a variable distance, usually obliquely to the left (Proto 1987; Proto et al. 1987).

The superior limit is formed by its superior recess behind the inferior portion of the manubrium sterni, not extending above the level of the superior sternal notch, and presents an inverted triangular morphology with concave sides (sometimes called "the anterior mediastinal triangle") (Gibbs et al. 2007; Proto 1987; Proto et al. 1987; Webb and Higgins 2005; Wright 2002).

The inferior limit is formed by the inferior recess. At this location there is considerably less tissue than at the level of the superior recess; thus, it can virtually be restricted to a thin membrane.

The anterior junction line should be considered in relation to the retrosternal line and space, the latter being essentially the lateral projection of the same structures (Wright 2002).

Absence of the anterior junction line occurs physiologically in children due to the presence of an enlarged thymus (Wright 2002). Widening of the anterior junction line is seen in cases of mediastinal fat proliferation or any anterior mediastinal mass. The most frequently seen masses are goiters, thymic tumors, germ cell tumors, lymphoma or enlarged internal mammary lymph nodes, vascular masses, and pericardial cysts (Fig. 5.3).

Obliteration or opacification on one side is noted with a tumor mass in the anterior mediastinum; adjacent lung consolidation or atelectasis with the latter is associated with volume loss of the corresponding lobe, and in the case of significant adjacent pleural effusion.

Accentuation of the anterior junction line is noted in patients who have emphysema in relation to hyperinflation and in patients who have pneumothorax.

Displacement of the anterior junction line occurs with lung or lobar collapse (Gibbs et al. 2007; Wright 2002).

In this context, we have to consider anterior lung herniation, seen with collapse or reduced volume of the lung or upper lobe or after pneumonectomy (Fig. 5.4), and also in cases of lung and pulmonary artery hypoplasia. It is due to compensatory overexpansion of the contralateral upper lobe moving the anterior junction line, the displaced line being formed by the interface between consolidated, atelectatic lung and the hyperinflated contralateral lung (Webb and Higgins 2005; Wright 2002).

The superior recess may be displaced laterally by thyroid masses or dilation of the innominate veins.

As mentioned above, anterior mediastinal masses in the prevascular space can obliterate the anterior junction line, although it is usually the preservation of more posterior lines that suggest the location of the lesion (Whitten et al. 2007). Three classical semiological signs are of great use in this particular situation: the hilum overlay sign, the cervicothoracic sign, and the silhouette sign.

The *hilum overlay sign* stipulates that if the hilar vessels are seen through the mass, it does not arise from the hilum and, due to the mediastinal geometry, the mass will likely be located in the anterior mediastinum (Fig. 5.5) (Whitten et al. 2007; Felson 1969; Fraser et al. 1999; Matsushima et al. 2007; Satoru et al. 1999). Most commonly this will be a mass of thymic or lymphatic origin (lymphoma).

The *cervicothoracic sign* is based on the fact that the anterior mediastinum ends at the level of the superior aspect of the clavicles. Therefore, when a mass extends above the superior aspect of the clavicles, it is located either in the neck or in the posterior mediastinum.

Posterior mediastinal masses situated above the level of the clavicles have an interface with the lung because lung tissue inserts between the mass and the neck; thus, the mass will be sharply demarcated (Figs. 5.6 and 5.7). In contradistinction, anterior mediastinal masses extending into the neck do not have an interface with the lung and their borders will appear blurred (Whitten et al. 2007; Fraser et al. 1999).

The difficulty of limiting the differential diagnosis to a single compartment is typically illustrated by thyroid disease: the thyroid gland is conventionally linked to the anterior mediastinum but is intimately related to the trachea, which explains why retrosternal goiter can

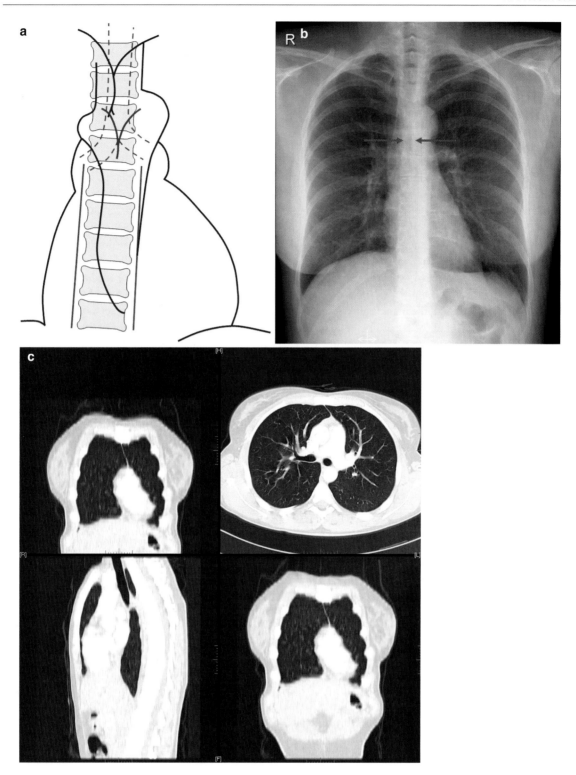

Fig. 5.2 Anterior junction line (AJL) formed by the anterior apposition of the two lungs together with their respective pleural coverings and a thin layer of mediastinal tissue. The superior limit is formed by its superior recess behind the manubrium sterni, not extending above the level of the superior sternal notch. The AJL should be considered in relation to the retrosternal line and space, the latter being essentially the lateral projection of the same structures. AJL lines (**a**, in *red*), on frontal chest radiograph (**b**, *red arrows*), clearly seen on axial and coronal reformatted MDCT images (**c**)

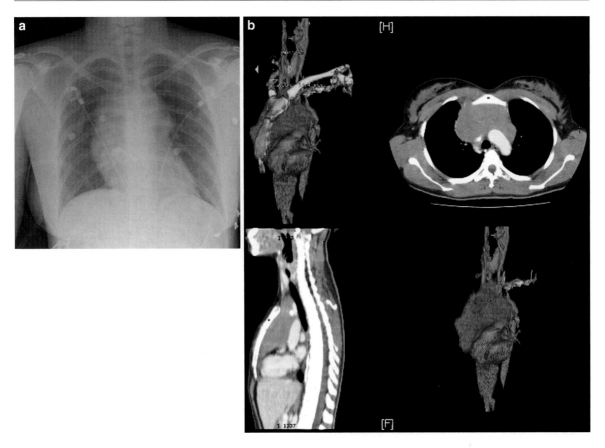

Fig. 5.3 Thymoma in a young adult. Frontal chest radiograph (**a**), MDCT with axial, sagittal and 3D volumetric reformats (**b**)

extend along the course of the trachea to all mediastinal compartments. According to the cervicothoracic sign, only the part situated in the posterior mediastinum will be clearly demarcated from the clavicles with sharply defined borders.

The classic *silhouette sign* stipulates that masses of equal density in contact with each other will be radiologically indistinguishable because of the lack of sharply demarcated borders (Figs. 5.7 and 5.8). According to this sign, anterior mediastinal masses in contact with the cardiac border or the diaphragm will have blurred borders, e.g., epicardial fat pads, pericardial cysts, and Morgagni hernias (Felson and Felson 1950).

5.3.2 Retrosternal Line or Stripe and Space

The retrosternal line or stripe is the soft tissue component situated immediately posterior to the sternum and limited to the back by the parietal pleura; it is a band-like structure of usually 2–4.5 mm thick and, in any case, less than 7 mm thick. It is located in close relationship to the retrosternal fat pad and space (Webb and Higgins 2005; Wright 2002; Whalen et al. 1973; Proto and Speckman 1979).

The retrosternal space is the radiolucent area between the sternum anteriorly and the middle mediastinum, mainly the heart and the great vessels, posteriorly. Its radiologic density is comparable to the retrocardiac space (Fraser et al. 1999).

Its anterior border, the retrosternal stripe, anatomically contains fat, internal mammary arteries, veins and lymph nodes, intercostal nerves, and innominate arteries and veins in the most superior part (Fraser et al. 1999; Williams et al. 1989). It is limited posteriorly by the pericardium and the major vascular structures of the middle mediastinum.

Both the retrosternal stripe and space are very commonly seen on chest radiographs (Webb and Higgins 2005).

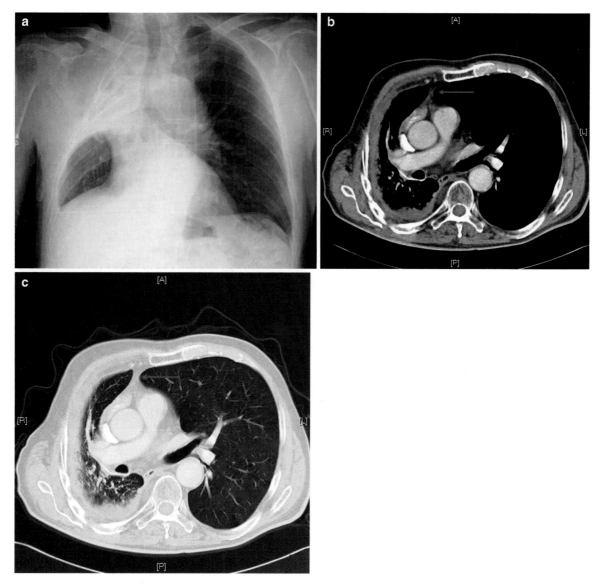

Fig. 5.4 Frontal chest radiograph (**a**), MDCT with axial reformats in mediastinal and parenchymal windowsettings (**b**, **c**) Right lobectomy with compensatory hyperinflation of the left lung, lung herniation, and displacement of the anterior junction line to the right (*red arrows*)

Enlargement of the retrosternal space may be of postural origin or due to hyperkyphosis (Dowager chest deformity) or hyperinflation and emphysema (Fraser et al. 1999; Webb and Higgins 2005; Wright 2002).

Reduction of the retrosternal space potentially has numerous origins (Fraser et al. 1999; Webb and Higgins 2005; Wright 2002):

• Postural origin (radiographs taken slightly "off lateral," rotated with projection of the retrosternal fat partially "en face." In this case, the projection of the anterior chest wall posterior to the sternum may mimic increased thickness of the retrosternal stripe; a wavy contour of the stripe in relation to the ribs may be indicative of this condition)
• Deformity and reduction in volume of one hemithorax
• Pectus excavatus
• Hypertrophic costochondral junctions and osteophytes of the manubiosternal junction
• Obesity, mediastinal lipomatosis

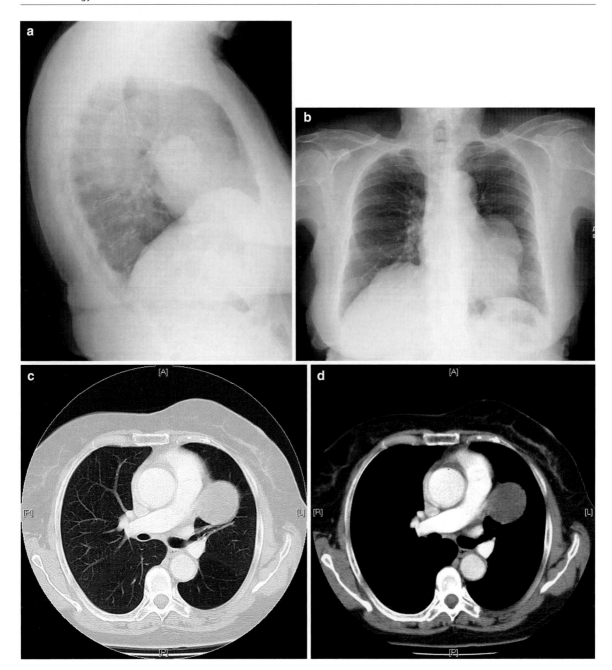

Fig. 5.5 Routine chest radiograph. The frontal film (**b**) shows a left paracardial rounded mass with the left hilar vessels clearly visible through the mass (hilum overlay sign); the lateral film (**a**) shows the central localization of the mass. MDCT with axial reformats in parenchymal (**c**) and mediastinal (**d**) window settings confirms its cystic nature, independent of the hilum. Final diagnosis: pericardial cyst

- Other fatty masses (lipoma, liposarcoma, brown fat tumors)
- Sternal tumors
- Vascular mass or dilatation (aortic aneurysm, coarctation)
- Right ventricular hypertrophy

- Main pulmonary artery hypertrophy
- Hematoma secondary to sternal fracture or surgery (Fig. 5.9)
- Lymph node enlargement (Hodgkin's disease, breast carcinoma) (Fig. 5.10)
- Any anterior mediastinal tumor (Fig. 5.11)

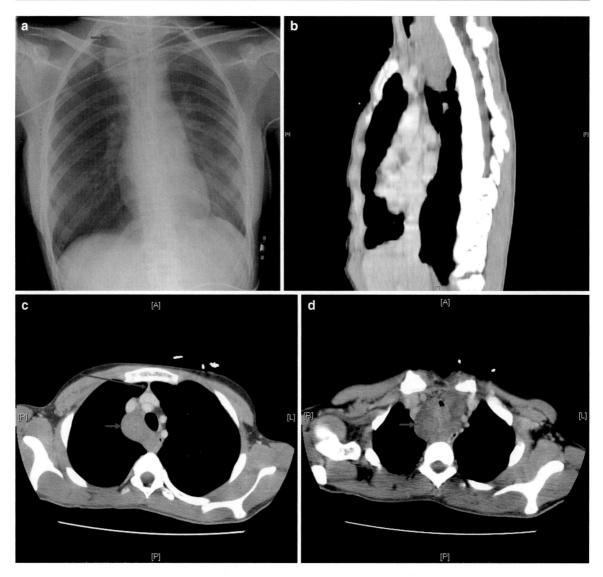

Fig. 5.6 Young female patient with dysphagia and dyspnea. Frontal chest radiograph (**a**) and MDCT with axial (**c, d**) and sagittal (**b**) reformats shows a right paratracheal mass sharply demarcated from the clavicle (*small red arrows*); note that the anterior junction line (*large red arrow*) is not displaced. Final diagnosis: cervicothoracic sign in a patient with Schwannoma. When we can depict a mass extending above the level of the clavicle with a sharp demarcation between the mass and the clavicle, there must be lung tissue in front of it (cervicothoracic sign); this mass must necessarily be located in the posterior mediastinum

5.4 The Middle Mediastinal Compartment

5.4.1 Aortopulmonary Window on Frontal Films, the Aortopulmonary Stripe

On anteroposterior films, the edge (aortopulmonary stripe) with the left lung, between the aorta and the main pulmonary artery, is almost always visible; it arises superomedially, crosses the projection of the aortic arch obliquely downward to the left, and merges inferiorly with the pulmonary artery and/or left cardiac border (Proto 1987; Webb and Higgins 2005; Blank an Castellino 1972).

It is a mediastinal interface formed by the pleura of the anterior left lung contacting and reflecting tangentially over the mediastinal fat anterolateral to the left pulmonary artery and the aortic arch.

It should have a concave or straight border toward the left lung; a convex border is considered abnormal in most cases. Examples of pathology include lymphadenopathy, masses in the anterior mediastinum moving the anterior

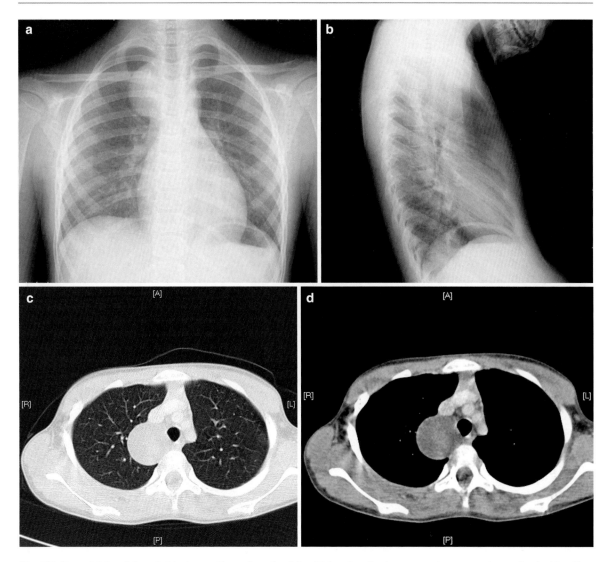

Fig. 5.7 Frontal (**a**) and lateral (**b**) chest radiograph and axial CT in parenchymal (**c**) and mediastinal (**d**) window settings. Young girl with a clinical history of mild chronic coughing. The frontal radiograph shows a well-circumscribed mass abutting the mediastinum on the right, without sharp demarcation (+ silhouette sign). On the lateral radiograph, the mass projects over the higher dorsal spine, suggesting a posterior mediastinal localization. Computed tomography shows a sharply demarcated cystic mass on the junction of the middle and the posterior mediastinum without any evident relationship with the spine. Final diagnosis: bronchogenic cyst

pleural reflection (Fig. 5.11), aortic aneurysm or dilation of the left pulmonary artery and pneumomediastinum (Gibbs et al. 2007; Whitten et al. 2007; Proto 1987; Webb and Higgins 2005; McComb 2001; Keats 1972).

5.4.2 Aortopulmonary Window on Lateral Films

The aortopulmonary window consists of the virtual space between the aortic arch and the left pulmonary artery (Fig. 5.12) and corresponds to the formal location of the ductus arteriosus of Botal. It is limited medially by the trachea and the esophagus and laterally by the left lung.

In physiologic conditions it contains fat and small lymph nodes; the left recurrent nerve branches from the vagus nerve immediately inferior to the aortic arch and its branch, the recurrent laryngeal nerve, ascends through this space to the lower neck (Gibbs et al. 2007; Whitten et al. 2007; Fraser et al. 1999; Williams et al. 1989). Therefore, paralysis of the left vocal cord

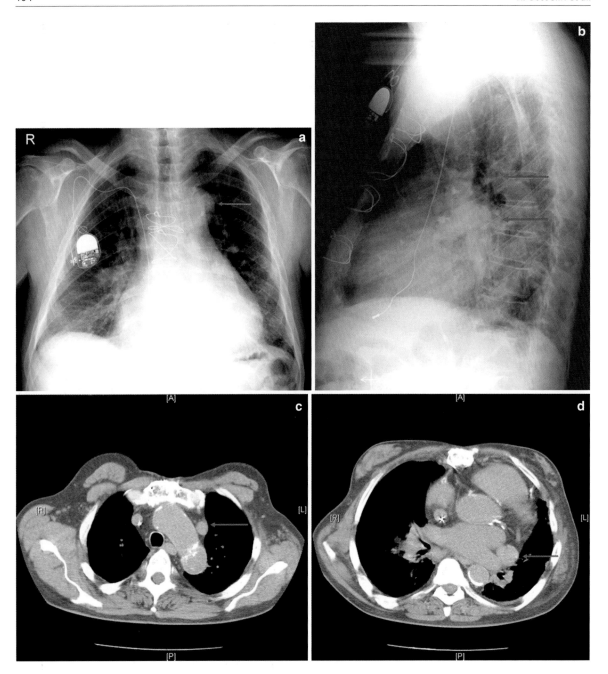

Fig. 5.8 A middle-aged patient with a long-standing history of congestive cardiopathy. Frontal chest radiograph (**a**) shows a well-defined nodular opacity immediately adjacent to the aortic arch with a+silhouette sign (*red arrow*); the lateral film (**b**) shows multiple rounded opacities of the same caliber approximately above and below the level of the left hilum (*short red arrows*). Multidetector computed tomography (**c**, **d**, **e**, **f**) in mediastinal window settings reveals a tubular structure heading along the left middle mediastinum toward the posterior aspect of the base of the right atrium (*red arrows*): left vena cava superior

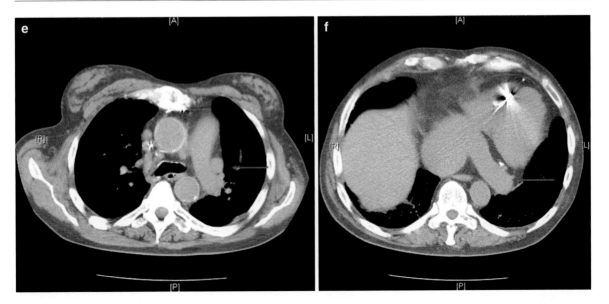

Fig. 5.8 (continued)

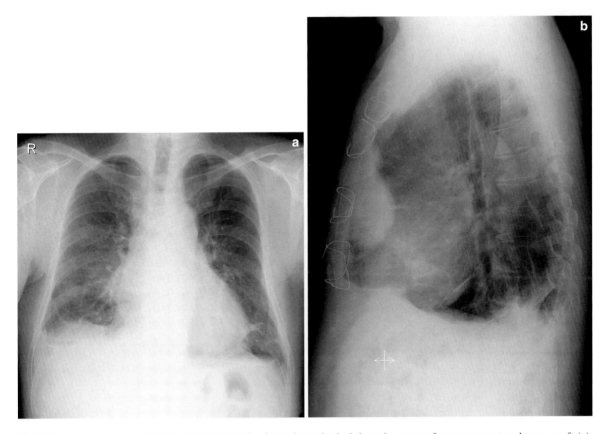

Fig. 5.9 Postoperative surveillance chest radiograph of a patient who had thoracic surgery for coronary artery bypass graft (**a**). Lobulated opacity is seen obliterating the retrosternal space on the lateral film (**b**). Diagnosis: retrosternal hematoma

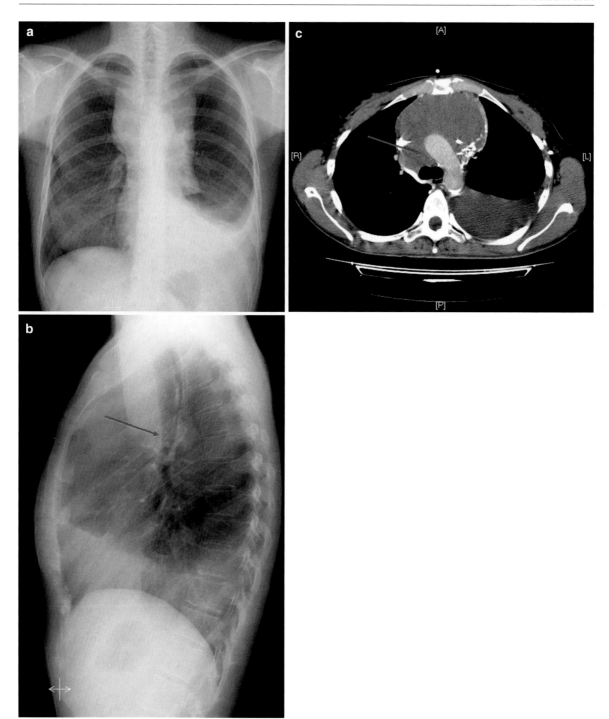

Fig. 5.10 An 18-year-old woman with B-symptoms (slight fever, night sweats, weight loss). The frontal chest radiograph (**a**) shows a huge mediastinal mass with bilateral mediastinal widening. The lateral film (**b**) and MDCT with axial (**c**) and coronal (**d**, **e**) reformats shows complete obliteration of the retrosternal space as well of the aortopulmonary window (*red arrows*), indicating the presence of the mass in the anterior as well in the middle mediastinum. Multidetector computed tomography also shows encasement of the great vessels by homogeneous hypodense tumor with vena cava superior syndrome and collateral vessels of the azygos and hemiazygos system. Final diagnosis: G-cell B-cell non-Hodgkin's lymphoma

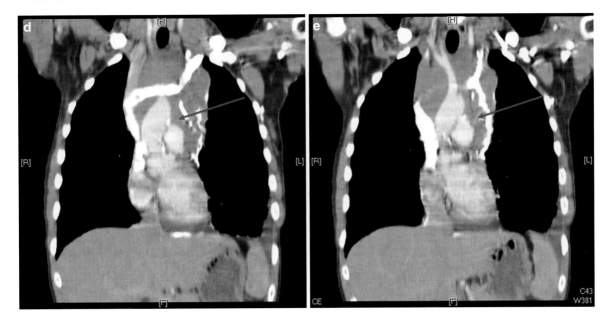

Fig. 5.10 (continued)

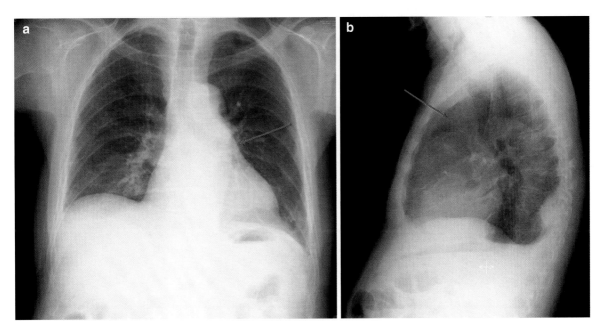

Fig. 5.11 Routine chest radiograph of a patient who had no medical history. Elevation/displacement of the aortopulmonary stripe on the frontal chest radiograph (**a**, *red arrow*). Obliteration of the retrosternal space is seen on the lateral chest radiograph (**b**, *red arrow*). These findings indicate the location of the mass in the anterior mediastinum. The multidetector computed tomography with axial (**c,d**) and sagittal (**e**) reformats shows a lobulated, slightly irregular, and heterogeneous mass in the retrosternal space without evidence of invasion of the mediastinal structures. Final diagnosis: malignant thymoma

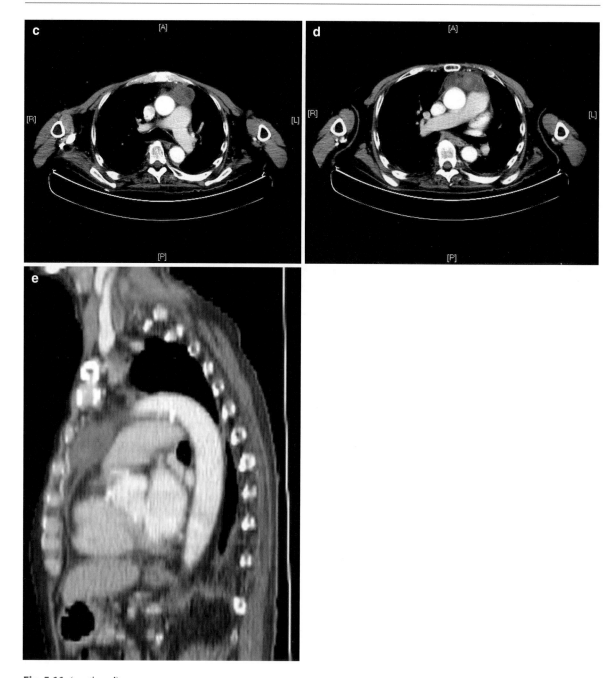

Fig. 5.11 (continued)

should induce a search for disease in the anteroposterior window (Gibbs et al. 2007; Proto 1987; Giron et al.1998; McComb 2001).

The remnant of the ductus arteriosus of Botal may calcify and cause a curvilinear calcification visible on chest CT, which often is confused with atheromatous calcification of the adjacent aorta (Armstrong et al. 2000).

The posterior turn of the azygos arch may project as a nodular opacity overlying the lower part of the aortic arch just behind the trachea; this should be distinguished from enlarged azygos lymph nodes situated more anteriorly with respect to the tracheal lucency (Wright 2002).

Masses in the anteroposterior window are common and mostly due to enlarged lymph nodes in association

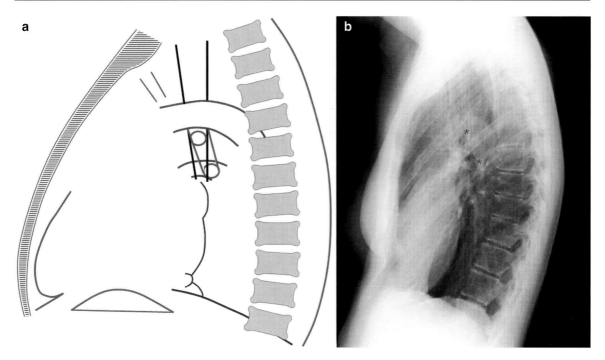

Fig. 5.12 Aortopulmonary window on lateral films. The virtual space (**b**, *asterisks*) between the aortic arch (**a**, in *red*) and the left main pulmonary artery is seen (**a**, in *red*)

with primary lung tumors or lymphoma (Fig. 5.10), with other tumors, for example, neurofibromas, being more rare.

5.4.3 Right Paratracheal Line or Stripe

The right paratracheal line is formed by the tracheal wall, mediastinal tissue, and the adjacent pleura (Fig. 5.13). Its visibility is due to the presence of air on both sides of the right tracheal wall.

Its thickness ranges from 1 to 4 mm, uniformly from top to bottom, with more than 5 mm being considered as pathological (Whitten et al. 2007).

It extends from the thoracic inlet downward to the right tracheobronchial angle where the azygos arch is located.

Most authors consider 10 mm to be the upper physiological limit for the size of the azygos vein (Whitten et al. 2007; Fraser et al. 1999; Fleischner and Udis 1952; Keats et al. 1968).

The right paratracheal line is a major landmark that should be systematically studied on all frontal chest radiographs; it is one of the most commonly seen mediastinal lines or stripes, reported in up to 97% of posteroanterior (PA) chest radiographs (Gibbs et al. 2007; Giron et al. 1998; Webb and Higgins 2005; Satoru et al. 1999; Neufang and Bülo 1981).

Thickening occurs in case of mediastinal fat proliferation and adjacent hemorrhage.

It is a very valuable sign of trauma because in most cases a normal paratracheal line permits the exclusion of adjacent hematoma and serious vascular injury (Wright 2002).

Obliteration occurs by interruption of the air–soft-tissue interface between the trachea and the right lung and is indicative of right paratracheal lymphadenopathy or local pleural, mediastinal, or tracheal masses (Figs. 5.14 and 5.15) (Gibbs et al. 2007; Whitten et al. 2007; Fraser et al. 1999; Webb and Higgins 2005; Wright 2002). Complete loss of the line occurs in consolidation or atelectasis of the right upper lobe or in the presence of adjacent pleural fluid (Wright 2002).

5.4.4 Left Paratracheal Line

In some normal subjects, the left lung lies adjacent to the left tracheal wall, medial to the left subclavian

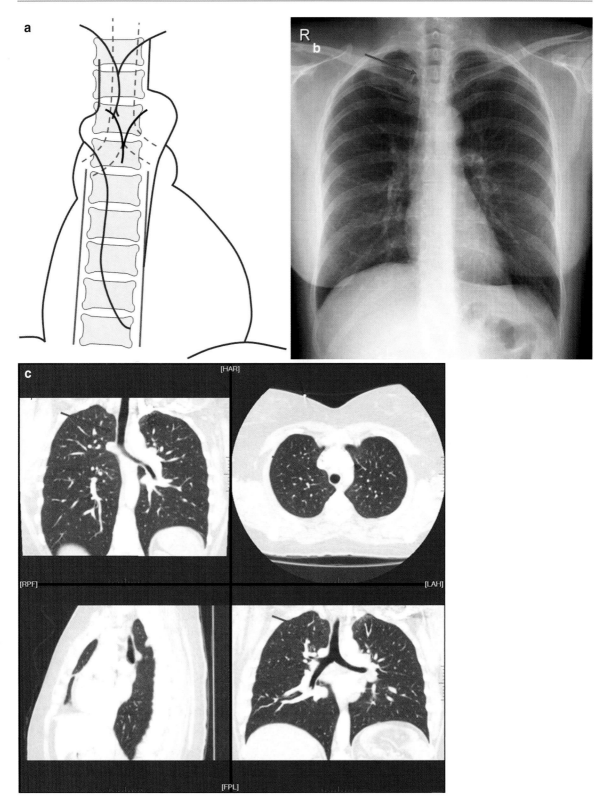

Fig. 5.13 Right paratracheal line or stripe (**a**, in *red*). Physiologically 1–4 mm thick. It extends from the thoracic inlet to the right tracheo-bronchial angle. It is formed by the tracheal wall, the mediastinal tissue and the adjacent pleura (**c**, MDCT with triplanar reformats, *red arrows*). This is a major landmark that should be checked systematically on frontal chest radiographs (**b**, *red arrows*)

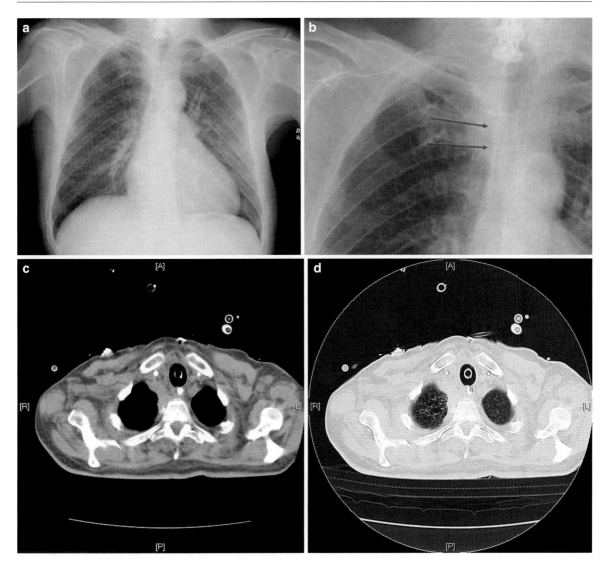

Fig. 5.14 This 55-year-old smoker has a peculiar history of chronical right cervicobrachialgia for which he had cervical spine surgery (vertebroplasty). The frontal chest radiograph (**a**) shows a discrete widening of the superior part of the right paratracheal line (**b**, magnification view, *red arrows*). Axial Multidetector computed tomography reformats in mediastinal (**c**) and parenchymal (**d**) windowsettings confirms an infiltrative tumor at the level of the thoracic outlet in a paratracheal and paravertebral location; the mass has speculated margins toward the adjacent lung. Final diagnosis: "Pancoast" tumor; the patient developed Claude-Bernard-Horner Syndrome

artery, producing a similar stripe to the more common right paratracheal line.

The line extends from the reflection of the left subclavian artery downward to the aortic arch and is visible on a maximum of 31% of PA chest radiographs. Its significantly less frequent visibility compared with the right paratracheal line can be attributed to the contact between the left lung and either the left common carotid artery anteriorly or the left subclavian artery posteriorly with respect to the higher course of the line

(Gibbs et al. 2007; Giron et al. 1998; Webb and Higgins 2005; Proto et al. 1989).

5.4.5 Retrotracheal Line or Stripe

The retrotracheal line forms the anterior border of the retrotracheal space or retrotracheal triangle of Raider, with the other borders of this space being the dorsal

Fig. 5.15 Retrotracheal Stripe (**a**, in *red*). It forms the anterior border of the retrotracheal space or retrotracheal Triangle of Raider (lateral chest radiograph, (**d**), *asterisks*); the other borders of this space are the dorsal spine posteriorly, the aortic arch inferiorly, and the thoracic inlet superiorly. It's a vertical stripe formed by air in the trachea and the right lung outlining the posterior tracheal wall and adjacent soft tissues (axial and sagittal MDCT reformats, (**b**) and lateral chest radiograph, (**c**), *red arrows*)

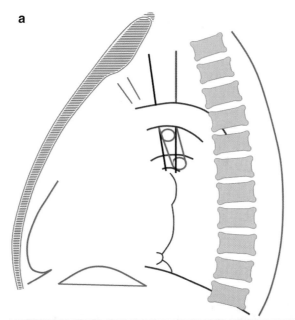

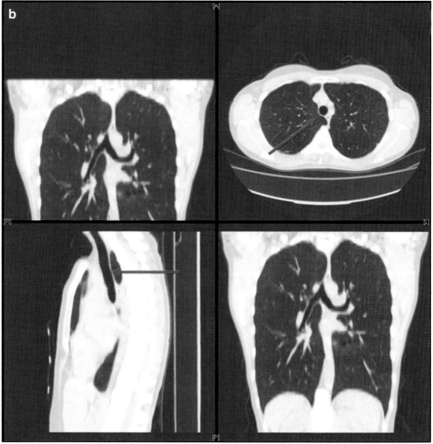

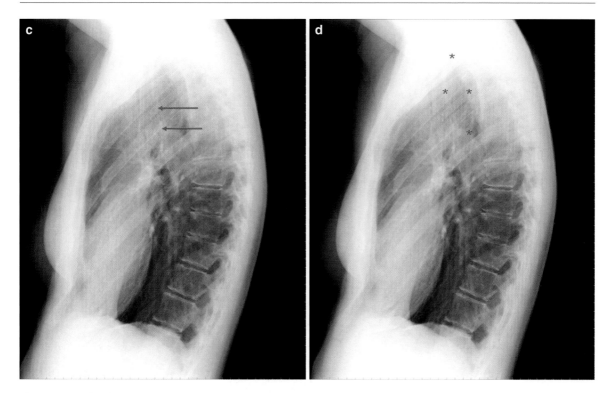

Fig. 5.15 (continued)

spine posteriorly, the aortic arch inferiorly, and the thoracic inlet at its top (Fig. 5.15).

It is a vertical line seen on lateral films in 50% to 90% of healthy adults (Neufang and Bülo 1981) and is formed by air in the trachea and the right lung outlining the posterior tracheal wall and adjacent soft tissues.

It runs from the thoracic inlet to the tracheal bifurcation and normally measures up to 2.5 mm in thickness (Gibbs et al. 2007; Wright 2002; Franquet et al. 2002).

The posterior tracheal wall, the intervening soft tissues, and the anterior esophageal wall or collapsed esophagus can combine to form the thicker tracheo-esophageal stripe, which may measure up to 5.5 mm (Gibbs et al. 2007; Fraser et al. 1999; Armstrong et al. 2000; Webb and Higgins 2005; Wright 2002; Franquet et al. 2002; Chasen et al. 1984).

Abnormal thickening of the posterior tracheal stripe can be attributed to acquired vascular anomalies, post-traumatic hematomas, esophageal masses, mediastinitis, lymphadenopathy, and neoplastic invasions (Gibbs et al. 2007; Webb and Higgins 2005).

Abnormal tissue density within the retrotracheal space consists of congenital or acquired anomalies of the aortic arch and its branches, esophageal lesions,

enlarged lymph nodes, thyroid masses, lung carcinoma, and bronchogenic cysts.

Very large masses will completely obliterate the retrotracheal space and the stripe will be completely lost because there is no more air-filled lung behind the trachea (Fig. 5.16) (Wright 2002).

5.4.6 Posterior Wall of the Bronchus Intermedius

The posterior wall of the bronchus intermedius appears as a line or stripe on the lateral chest radiograph in up to 95% of normal subjects (Fig. 5.17). Therefore, it is an important landmark in the evaluation of mediastinal disease (Gibbs et al. 2007).

It descends vertically or slightly obliquely from the origin of the right upper lobe bronchus for 3–4 cm and is formed by lung within the azygoesophageal recess, outlining the posterior wall of the bronchus intermedius projecting through the radiolucency created by the course of the left upper lobe bronchus (Wright 2002).

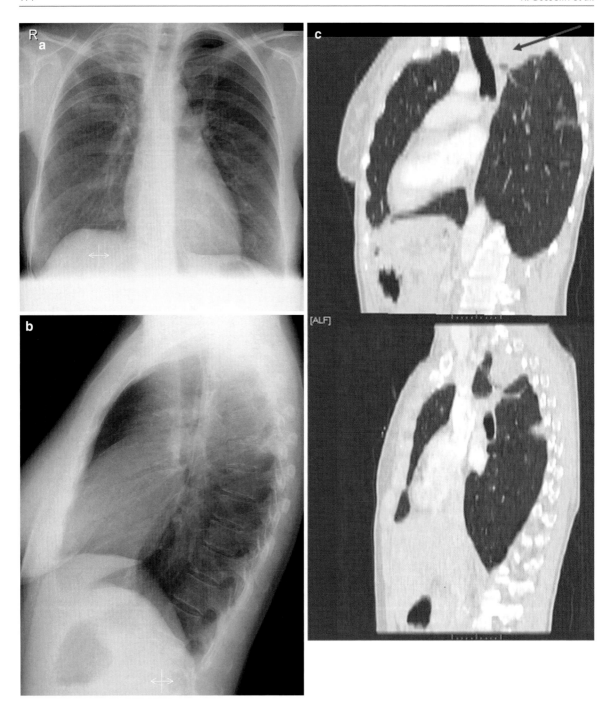

Fig. 5.16 Middle-aged woman with a long history of smoking. The frontal chest radiograph (**a**) shows retro-obstructive pulmonary condensation in the upper lobe, volume loss with elevation/retraction of the hilum, and diaphragmatic elevation; the lateral film (**b**) shows complete obliteration of the retrotracheal triangle of Raider by a mass, indicating its location in the posteriorpart of the upper middle mediastinum. The sagittal multidetector computed tomography reformats (**c,d**, *oblique arrows*) confirm the tumor mass in the right upper lobe. Final diagnosis: bronchial carcinoma with partial right upper lobe atelectasis and retro-obstructive pneumonia

Fig. 5.17 Posterior wall of the bronchus intermedius (**a**, in *red*). It appears as a line or stripe on the lateral chest radiograph (**c**, *red arrow*) and is an important landmark for the evaluation of mediastinal disease. It descends vertically or slightly obliquely from the takeoff of the right upper lobe bronchus for 3–4 cm and is formed by lung within the azygoesophageal recess (**b**, MDCT with triplanar reformats, axial and sagittal images, red arrows), outlining the posterior wall of the bronchus intermedius projecting through the radiolucency created by the course of the left upper lobe bronchus

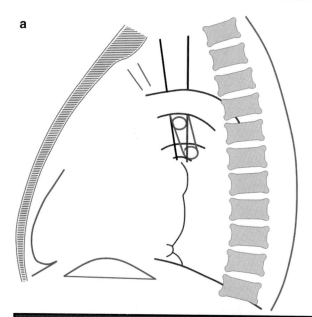

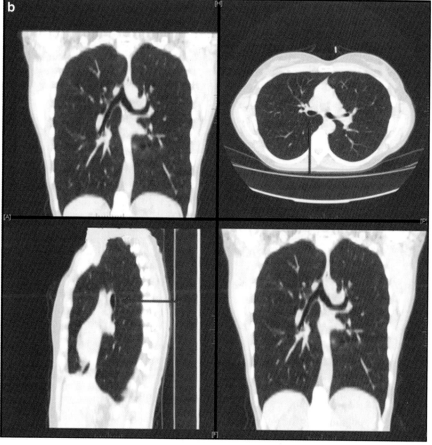

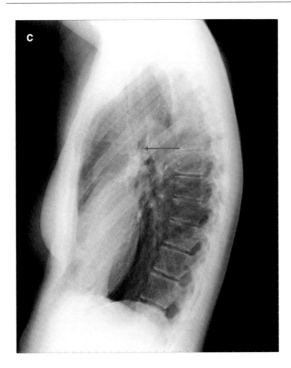

Fig. 5.17 (continued)

The posterior wall of the trachea, right main bronchus, and bronchus intermedius can sometimes merge and be seen as one continuous thin band. Normally, its thickness measures up to 3 mm.

Band-like thickening by edema is observed in congestive heart failure; irregular nodular thickening is indicative of neoplastic invasion by lung carcinoma or lymphadenopathy from lymphoma, metastatic disease, tuberculosis, and sarcoidosis (Gibbs et al. 2007; Proto and Speckman 1979; Schnur et al. 1981).

5.5 The Posterior Mediastinal Compartment

5.5.1 Azygoesophageal Line

The azygoesophageal or paraesophageal line is situated behind the heart and the mediastinum and is formed by the interface between the air-filled right lung and the posterior mediastinal tissue situated immediately laterally from the mid and lower third of the esophagus (Fig. 5.18). It curves upward with a shallow reverse-C or -S contour from the supradiaphragmatic region and laterally to the right behind the trachea to join the azygos arch and the paratracheal line above the azygoesophageal recess (Whitten et al. 2007; Armstrong et al. 2000; Proto 1987; Webb and Higgins 2005; Wright 2002; Ravenel and Erasmus 2002). It is almost always visible on correctly exposed radiographs (Webb and Higgins 2005).

It is a major landmark for the localization and the detection of pathology in this mediastinal compartment and should always be routinely evaluated on PA chest radiographs; a normally defined and situated azygoesophageal line gives a good indication of the absence of pathology in this mediastinal space.

If the esophagus is airless it is seen as a single line; however, if the esophagus contains a sufficient quantity of air, the right esophageal wall may be outlined on both sides and the azygoesophageal line may be seen as a stripe (Armstrong et al. 2000; Webb and Higgins 2005; Chasen et al. 1984).

Displacement of the azygoesophageal line is seen in the case of lung volume loss with partial or complete collapse of a lower lobe, esophageal dilation, or mass; an abscess of the posterior mediastinum; or any large posterior mediastinal mass, e.g., a neural tumor.

Indeed, the azygoesophageal recess (cfr. infra) also has an interface with the middle mediastinum; thus, the resulting line can be disrupted by both middle and posterior mediastinal pathology (Fig. 5.19). For example, large subcarinal lymph nodes may obliterate the superior aspect of the line because of the close relationship between the subcarinal space and the azygoesophageal recess (Whitten et al. 2007; Webb and Higgins 2005; Wright 2002).

Total obliteration or loss of the azygoesophageal line occurs with massive consolidation or atelectasis of the right lower lobe, right posterior pleural effusion, and ruptured aortic aneurysm with mediastinal hemorrhage and hematoma.

5.5.2 Azygoesophageal Recess

Anatomically, there are two parts in the azygoesophageal recess: one situated above and one below the level of the azygos arch. They represent a space formed by the lung lying lateral or posterior to the esophagus and anterior to the spine (Zylak et al. 1982; Armstrong et al. 2000; Wright 2002).

Fig. 5.18 Azygo-esophageal line (**a**, in *red*). Situated behind the heart and the mediastinum and formed by the interface between the air-filled right lower lobe and the posterior mediastinal tissue laterally from the mid and lower third of the esophagus (MDCT with triplanar reformats, coronal images, **b**, *long red arrows*). It describes an "inverted S" curve and joins the azygos arch and the right paratracheal lines above the azygoesophageal recess (MDCT with triplanar reformats, axial image top right, **b**, fat red arrow). It is a major landmark for the localization and the detection of pathology in this mediastinal compartment (frontal chest radiograph, **c**, *red arrows*). A normal line gives a good indication of absence of pathology in this mediastinal space

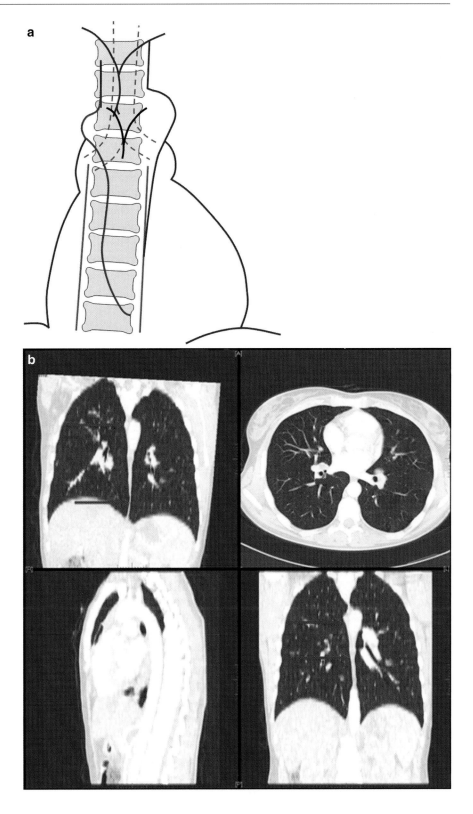

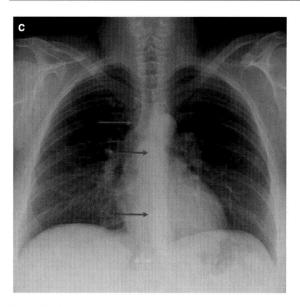

Fig. 5.18 (continued)

The upper part is less developed and plays no major role in the depiction of pathology.

The lower azygoesophageal recess is much more developed and is addressed as "the" azygoesophageal recess; it is usually well seen in conditions shown by correct X-ray exposure (Fig. 5.18) (Armstrong et al. 2000). It is filled by the apex of the right lower lobe and its medial boundary is seen as a smooth dextroconvex interface extending below the azygos arch: the azygo-esophageal line (cfr. supra).

It is accentuated by deep inspiration; hyperinflation, e.g., asthma or emphysema; left lower lobe collapse, left pneumonectomy (eventually with herniation of the right lung); hyperkyphosis; and senescent conditions.

In the case of large pleural effusions, fluid may distend and lead to left-sided herniation of the recess, which can appears as a medially situated mass (Wright 2002).

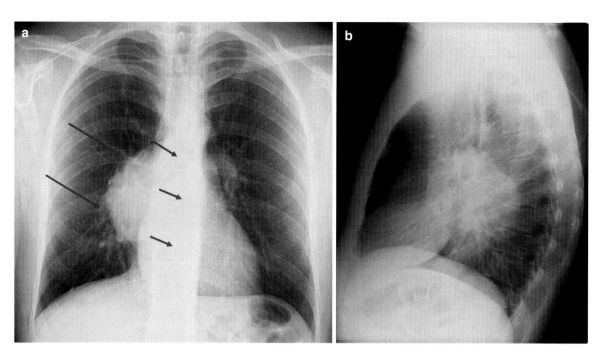

Fig. 5.19 Emergency chest radiograph and computed tomography of a 33-year-old man with no personal medical history. His younger brother had Hodgkin's lymphoma at the age of 12. He complains of having gradually worsening dyspnea for 1 week. For 3 days he has had transfixiating chest pain, nausea, and vomiting, which were unsuccessfully treated with medication. The chest radiograph and the MDCT show a huge mass projecting over the right hilar region; the hilar vessels and the main right bronchus are displaced laterally and cranially (**a**, **c**, *long* *red arrows*) and the azygoesophageal line is completely vanished (**a**, **d**, *short red arrows*). These findings indicate the central mediastinal location of the mass. Contrast-enhanced Multidetector computed tomography with axial (**e**, **f**) and coronal (**c**, **d**, **g**, **h**) reformats confirms the central mediastinal location of a huge cystic, nonenhancing mass with compression of the right main bronchus and the esophagus. Final diagnosis: huge bronchogenic cyst (Courtesy Dr. J. Lemaitre, CHU Ambroise Paré Mons)

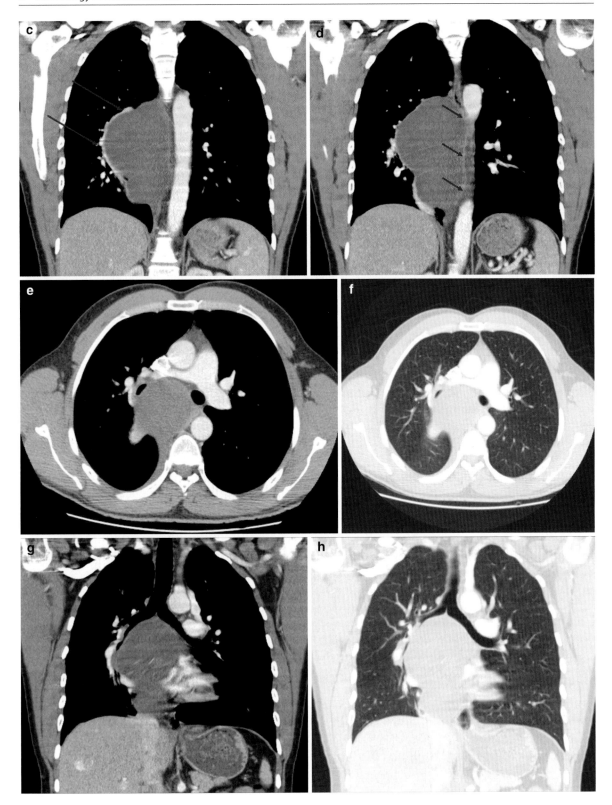

Fig. 5.19 (continued)

Hydropneumothorax may produce an air–fluid level within the recess and drainage tubes may pass to the left of the midline within the recess (Wright 2002).

Displacement of the azygoesophageal recess may occur in the case of esophageal masses or dilation; for example, achalasia may displace the recess to the right (Ravenel and Erasmus 2002). In achalasia, ballooning out of the dilated esophagus may occur both above and/or below the level of the azygos arch.

Obliteration of the azygoesophageal recess happens in two scenarios: (1) anteriorly and medially by right paratracheal and/or subcarinal lymph node enlargement, subcarinal bronchogenic cyst, left atrial hypertrophy, and a large hiatal hernia; or (2) posteriorly by esophageal dilatation, (e.g., achalasia), esophageal cancer, hiatal hernia, enlarged paraesophageal lymph nodes, and para- or prevertebral masses (Gibbs et al. 2007; Proto 1987; Wright 2002; Ravenel and Erasmus 2002).

On the lateral chest radiograph, the lung in the azygoesophageal recess outlines the posterior wall of the right main and intermediate bronchi, forming the intermediate bronchus stripe (cfr. 5.4.6.); this stripe may be thickened or obliterated by various diseases, e.g., enlarged lymph nodes, tumors, lung consolidation, and congestive heart failure.

5.5.3 Posterior Junction Line or Stripe

Similar to the anterior junction anatomy, the posterior junction anatomy includes the posterior junction line (PJL) together with its superior and inferior recesses.

The left and right lungs may be in contact with each other, giving a sagittal–pleural interface consisting of the four pleural layers anterior to the upper dorsal spine and posterior to the esophagus, thus forming the PJL (Fig. 5.20) (Gibbs et al. 2007; Proto 1987; Giron et al. 1998; Webb and Higgins 2005; Proto et al. 1983).

Compared with to the anterior junction line, the PJL extends cranially above the sternoclavicular notch toward the root of the neck (Gibbs et al. 2007; Whitten et al. 2007; Proto 1987; Wright 2002). It sweeps down from the apices toward the midline behind the tracheal air shadow at the level of D3–D5 either vertically or very slightly obliquely to the left until it splits and is reflected over the posterior aortic arch on the left and over the azygos vein on the right. It has been reported on approximately 30–40% of PA chest radiographs (Giron et al. 1998; Webb and Higgins 2005). The position of the line with respect to the midline is variable.

The superior recess is formed by the two lungs approaching the mediastinum in front of the vertebral bodies D1 and D2.

The inferior recess is formed by the lungs diverging from the midline and may present asymmetrically; the right inferior recess is usually situated lower than the left.

The thickness of the PJL varies from paper thin to a maximum of about 2 mm (Webb and Higgins 2005). The line itself may appear as a stripe up to 1 cm thick when widened by fat or when the esophagus is situated within the stripe (Gibbs et al. 2007; Webb and Higgins 2005; Wright 2002).

When the esophagus is situated at the anterior part of the line, the PJL can as such be regarded as the "mesentery" of the upper esophagus (Fig. 5.21) (Armstrong et al. 2000; Wright 2002).

The stripe can be physiologically spread by a fluid- or air-filled esophagus when it is situated within the stripe.

When air is present in the esophageal lumen, two stripes representing the air-outlined esophageal walls may be visible; these are referred to as the right and left (pleuro)esophageal stripes (Webb and Higgins 2005).

Thickening can be the only manifestation of pleural involvement in individuals who have been exposed to dust (Wright 2002). Progressive thickening is a positive indicator of active pleural disease (Wright 2002). Grossly pathological thickening can be due to mediastinal abscess or hematoma.

Pathological bulging of both the V-shaped superior and inferior recesses can be caused by overlying (supra)aortic mediastinal masses, e.g., lymphadenopathy, aneurysms, and neurogenic tumors (Gibbs et al. 2007).

Esophageal pathology also evidently affects the presentation of the stripe, but because of the variable presentation of the stripe, it remains of limited diagnostic utility and caution is needed in its interpretation (Webb and Higgins 2005).

Fig. 5.20 Posterior junction line, (**a**, in *red*). It is formed by the contact of the posterior aspects of the left and right lungs behind the esophagus creating a sagittal pleural interface (MDCT with triplanar reformats, axial and coronal images top and bottom right, **b**, *red arrows*). Contrary to the anterior junction line, it extends cranially above the sterno-clavicular notch (Frontal chest radiograph, **c**, *red arrows*). The position of the line with respect to the midline is variable

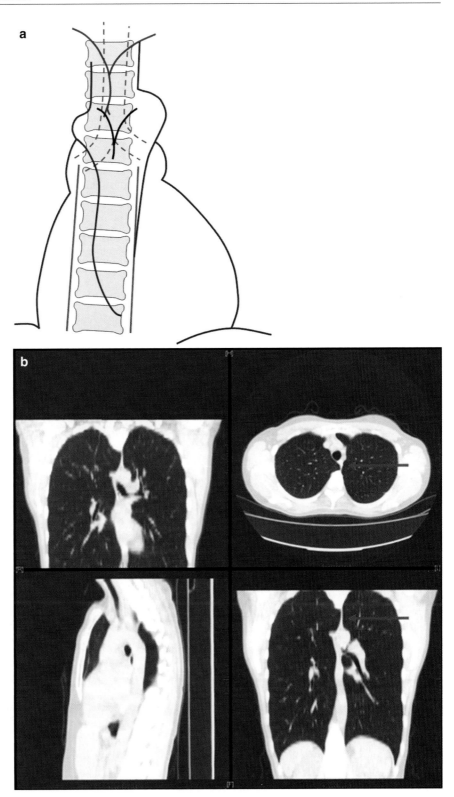

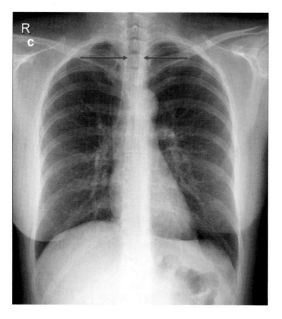

Fig. 5.20 (continued)

5.5.4 Para-aortic Line

The para-aortic line follows the descending aorta on the left side. It is formed by the interface with the aerated left lower lobe and is seen below the aortic arch, roughly parallel to the paravertebral line, extending down to the diaphragm (Fig. 5.22) (Webb and Higgins 2005). Like the paraesophageal and right paratracheal line, it constitutes a major anatomical landmark in the mediastinal anatomy and is seen on most chest radiographs (Webb and Higgins 2005).

The para-aortic line is accentuated in cases of dorsal hyperkyphosis, tortuosity of the aorta, and emphysema.

Displacement of the para-aortic line occurs in case of aortic aneurysm and para-aortic hematoma (Fig. 5.23), (para)spinal masses, significant lymph node enlargement, and neurogenic tumors, e.g., sympathetic chain neurinoma (Wright 2002).

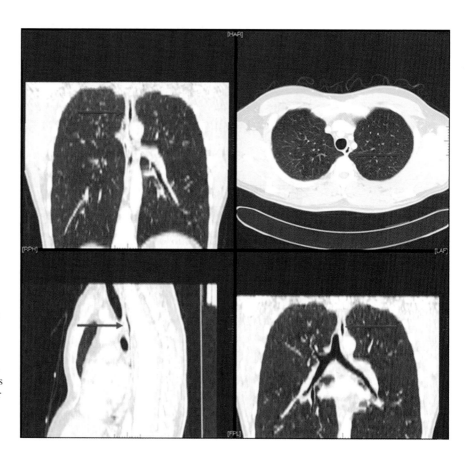

Fig. 5.21 Posterior junction line. The line itself may appear as a stripe when widened by fat or the esophagus. The anterior end of the line can be regarded as the "mesentery" of the upper esophagus (MDCT with triplanar reformats, *red arrows*)

Fig. 5.22 Para-aortic line. The para-aortic line (**a**, in *red*) follows the descending aorta on the left side. It is formed by the interface with the aerated lower left lobe (MDCT with triplanar reformats, **b**, *red arrows*). Like the paraesophageal line, it constitutes a major anatomical landmark that should be systematically checked on every frontal chest radiograph (**c**)

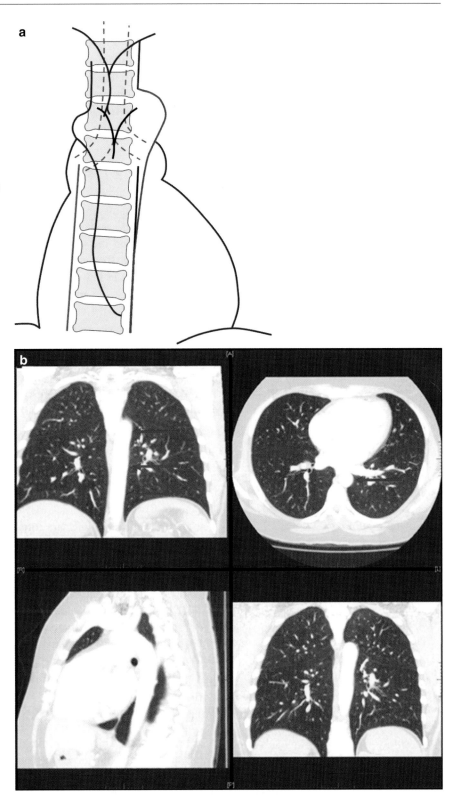

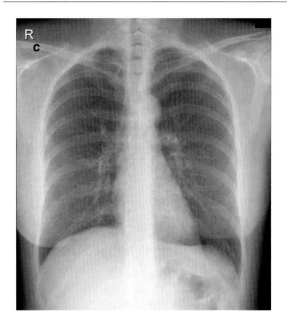

Fig. 5.22 (continued)

hypertension, or congenital anomalies of the caval, azygos, or hemiazygos circulation (Fig. 5.8).

Enlargment may also, occur with increased venous resistance, as in congestive heart failure, Budd Chiari syndrome, vena cava obstructions, or obstruction of the left brachiocephalic vein (Fig. 5.24).

5.5.5 Preaortic Line and Recess

In many subjects, the left lower lobe extends in front of the descending aorta into the aortopulmonary window behind the left lower lobe bronchus and behind the heart, forming a recess and a straight line extending down as low as D10 (Wright 2002).

It is the analog of the azygoesophageal recess and line on the right side but is usually thinner and less well seen (Webb and Higgins 2005). It can be useful in the diagnosis of esophageal and aortic lesions; a convex deviation of the inferior portion of this line can indicate the presence of a hiatal hernia or aneurysm.

The preaortic recess is accentuated in emphysema with tortuosity of the aorta and by dorsal hyperkyphosis (Wright 2002).

Loss of the para-aortic line is usually due to consolidation or atelectasis of the left lower lobe and posterior pleural effusion or abscess in the posterior left lower lobe (Wright 2002).

Lesser or invisible para-aortic line is also noted in cases of pectus excavatum and in thin patients who have a narrow anteroposterior diameter of the chest in whom the aorta tends to be "buried" deep in the mediastinum (Wright 2002).

Sometimes a small nodular opacity is visible at the margin of the aortic arch on frontal chest radiographs, called the *aortic nipple*. It is the radiological representation of the left superior intercostal vein as it runs anteriorly around the aortic arch before joining the left brachiocephalic vein.

The aortic nipple is usually found in normal, healthy patients (from 1.4% to 9.5%) (Worrell et al. 1992; McDonald et al. 1970; Hatfield et al. 1987) and is of limited clinical significance when it appears as a normal variant. CT scans show the left superior intercostal vein connecting with the accessory hemiazygous vein.

In certain conditions, the aortic nipple can become enlarged as a result of collateral flow and can mimic lymphadenopathy or aortic aneurysm (Worrell et al. 1992; Carter et al. 1985; Hatfield et al. 1987). It may be enlarged with an increase in venous flow, such as when maintaining a recumbent position, portal venous

5.5.6 Paraspinal Lines

Paraspinal lines are formed on both sides by the tangential contact of the lungs and the pleura with the posterior paravertebral soft tissues (Fig. 5.25) (Gibbs et al. 2007).

The right paraspinal line appears straight and runs vertically from the lower dorsal spine at the level of the 8th to the 12th thoracic vertebra and merges with the shadow of the diaphragmatic crus (the diaphragmatic crura blend with the anterior longitudinal ligament of the spine) (Wright 2002).

The left paraspinal line also extends vertically from the aortic arch to the diaphragm, merging with the crus. It usually lies medially to the lateral wall of the aorta, which forms the para-aortic line, but depending on the amount of mediastinal fat it can sometimes be located more laterally along the lower intrathoracic course of the aorta. It is also closely related to the hemiazygos vein (Webb and Higgins 2005).

Because of the presence of the descending aorta, the left paraspinal line is seen approximately twice as

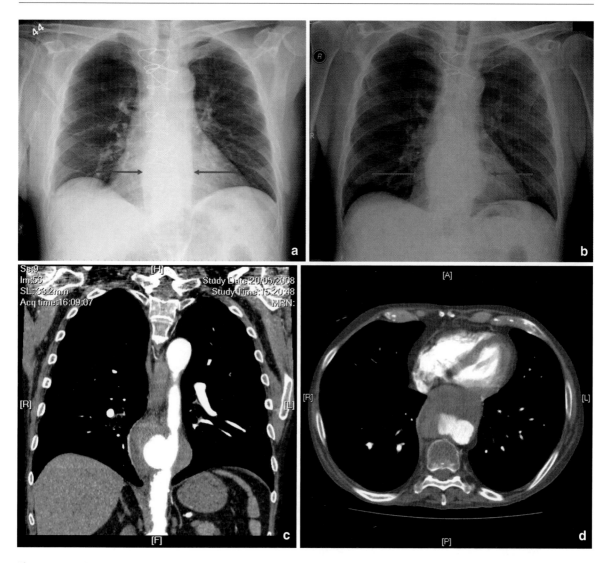

Fig. 5.23 Routine chest radiograph of a 57-year-old male patient with a long clinical history of atheromatous vascular disease. Follow-up frontal chest radiographs show a progressive widening/displacement of the lower third of both para-aortic lines (**a**, **b** *red arrows*). Multidetector computed tomography with coronal (**c**) and axial (**d**) reformats shows a saccular aneurysm of the lower thoracic aorta

often as the right (40% vs. 20%) (Gibbs et al. 2007; Whitten et al. 2007; Armstrong et al. 2000; Webb and Higgins 2005; Satoru et al. 1999).

The left paraspinal line and the para-aortic line should be clearly distinguished from each other; a paraspinal mass could obliterate the paraspinal line while the interface with the aorta and the left lower lobe is still visible (Gibbs et al. 2007).

Abnormal contours or displacement can be caused by benign entities like osteophytes and proliferation of mediastinal fat. This can also be caused by aortic tortuosity or aneurysm, hemiazygos vein enlargement,

posterior mediastinal mass, hematoma, extramedullary hematopoiesis, or esophagogastric lesions and abscesses (Fig. 5.26) (Gibbs et al. 2007; Proto 1987; Giron et al. 1998; Webb and Higgins 2005; Proto et al. 1983).

It should be noted that the paraspinal lines also continue their course inferior to the diaphragm.

The *thoracoabdominal* or *iceberg sign* is present when a lower mediastinal paravertebral thoracic mass extending inferiorly in the abdomen moves away from the spine, with its lower border no longer clearly delineated from the soft tissue shadow below the diaphragm. This means that the lesion is definitely thoracoabdominal.

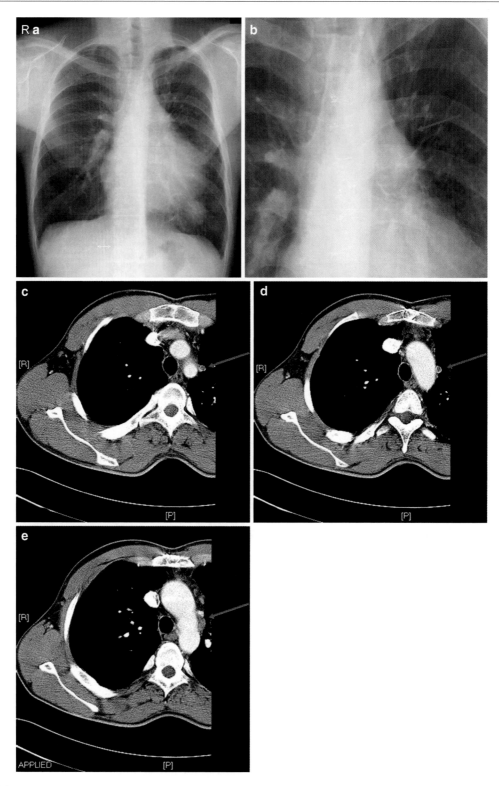

Fig. 5.24 Patient with known metastatic malignancy who had radiotherapy of the chest. Follow-up chest radiograph (**a**) with magnification view (**b**, *red arrow*) suggested a small nodular opacity projecting along the lateral border of the aortic arch, "aortic nipple." It represents the left superior intercostal vein as it runs around the aortic arch before joining the left brachiocephalic vein. Axial computed tomography scans(**c**, **d**, **e**, *red arrows*) show the left superior intercostal vein (with intraluminal thrombus, probably after radiotherapy) connecting with the accessory hemiazygous vein

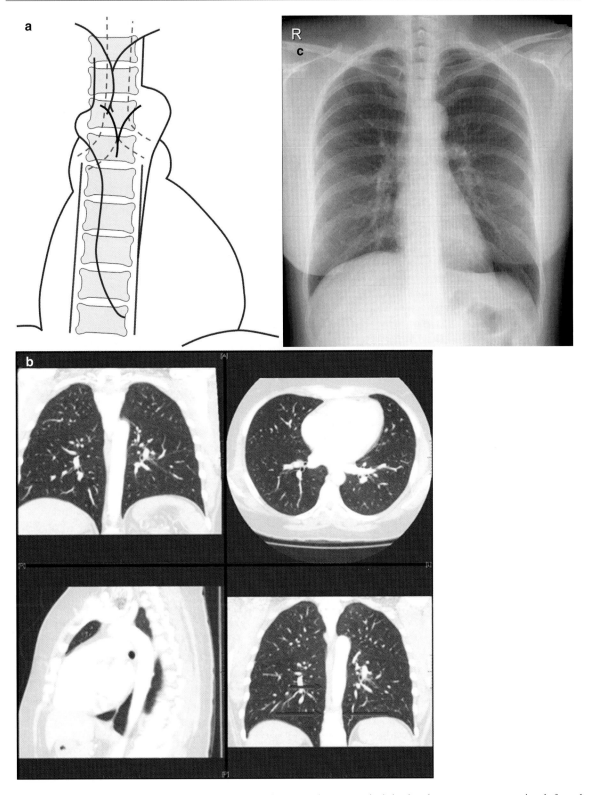

Fig. 5.25 Paraspinal lines (**a**, in *red*) are formed on both sides by the tangential contact of the lungs and the pleura with the posterior paravertebral soft tissues (MDCT with triplanar reformats, coronal image bottom right, *red arrows*) (**b**). They are major anatomical landmarks on every conventional frontal radiograph (**c**); abnormal contours or displacement can be caused by varied benign or malignant entities

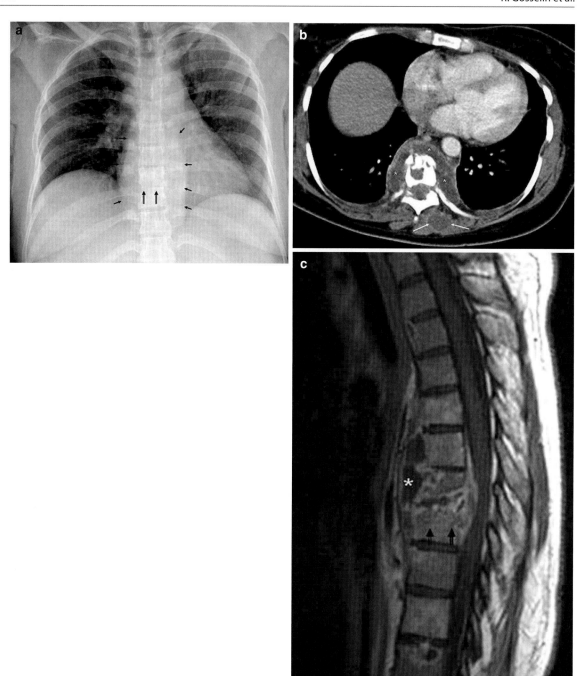

Fig. 5.26 Routine chest radiograph of a young patient with medical history of tuberculosis and recent back pain. Frontal chest radiograph shows bilateral widening/displacement of both paraspinal lines (**a**, *small black arrows*) Contrast enhanced axial computed tomography (**b**) and sagittal magnetic resonance imaging+Gd (**c**) show extensive vertebral damage (*large black arrows*) and paraspinal soft tissue component and abcess (black asterisks). Final diagnosis: cervicothoracic or iceberg sign in a patient with Pott's disease. If a mass with thoracoabdominal extension is sharply demarcated from the diaphragm and the abdominal soft tissues, it must have a mediastinal origin (cervicothoracic or iceberg sign); in the reverse situation (+ silhouette sign with the diaphragm and abdominal soft tissues), it is an abdominal mass extending cranially

Conversely, a lower mediastinal mass with a similar topography but with an inferoexernal contour rejoining the spine is entirely intrathoracic – supradiaphragmatic (Fig. 5.26) (Felson 1973; Remy et al. 1981).

References

Armstrong P, Wilson A, Dee P (2000) Imaging of disease of the chest, 3rd edn. Mosby, London, pp 47–62

Blank N, Castellino RA (1972) Patterns of pleural reflections of the left superior mediastinum: normal anatomy and distortions produced by adenopathy. Radiology 102:585–589

Carter M, Tarr R, Mazer M (1985) The "aortic nipple" as a sign of impending superior vena caval syndrome. Chest 87(6):775–777

Chasen MH, Rugh KS, Shelton DK (1984) Mediastinal impressions on the dilated esophagus. Radiol Clin North Am 22:591–605

Divano L, Osteaux M, Peetrons P (1983) Correlation between standard radiology and computed tomography in the demonstration of mediastinal lines. J Radiol 64(2):79–89

Felson B (1969) The mediastinum. Semin Roentgenol 4:41–58

Felson B (1973) Chest roentgenology. Saunders, Philadelphia

Felson B, Felson H (1950) Localisation of intrathoracic lesions by means of the postero-anterior roentgenogram: the silhouette sign. Radiology 55:363–374

Fleischner FG, Udis SW (1952) Dilatation of the azygos vein; a roentgen sign of venous engorgement. Am J Roentgenol Radium Ther Nucl Med 67:569–575

Franquet T, Erasmus JJ, Gimenez A (2002) The retrotracheal space: normal anatomic and pathological appearances. Radiographics 22:S231–S246

Fraser RS, Muller NL, Colman N, Paré PD (1999) Diagnosis and disease of the chest, 4th edn. Saunders, Philadelphia, pp 196–234

Gibbs J, Chandrasekhar C, Ferguson E (2007) Lines and stripes: where did they go? – from conventional radiography to CT. Radiographics 27:33–48

Giron J, Fajadet P, Sans N (1998) Diagnostic approaches to mediastinal masses. Eur J Radiol 27:21–42

Hatfield M, Vyborny C, MacMahon H (1987) Congenital absence of the azygos vein: a cause for "Aortic Nipple" enlargement. AJR Am J Roentgenol 149(2):273–274

Heitzman ER (1997) The mediastinum: radiologic correlations with anatomy and pathology. Mosby, St Louis, pp 216–334

Keats TE (1972) The aortic-pulmonary mediastinal stripe. Am J Roentgenol Radium Ther Nucl Med 116:107–109

Keats TE, Lipscombe GE, Betts CS (1968) Mesuration of the arch of the azygos vein and its applications to the study of cardiopulmonary disease. Radiology 90(5):990–994

Matsushima T, Eguchi K, Kuwabara M. (2007) Diseases of the chest diseases of the chest. Imaging Diagnosis Based on Pattern Classification. Thieme 149–160, chapters 4–14

McComb MH (2001) Reflecting upon the superior mediastinum. J Thoracic Imaging 16:56–64

McDonald C, Castellino R, Blank N (1970) The aortic "nipple." The left superior intercostal vein. Radiology 96: 533–536

Neufang KF, Beyer D (1980) Diagnostic value of pleuro-mediastinal lines and stripes for the radiological analysis of the mediastinum. Rontgenblatter 33(6):257–266

Neufang KF, Bülo W (1981) Frequencies of pleuro-mediastinal lines in healthy subjects: a contribution to the knowledge of the normal roentgen anatomy of the mediastinum. Rofo 135(6):673–681

Proto AV (1987) Mediastinal anatomy: emphasis on conventional images with anatomic and computed tomographic correlations. J Thoracic Imaging 2(1):1–48

Proto AV, Speckman JM (1979) The left lateral radiograph of the chest. Med Radiogr Photogr 55:29–74

Proto AV, Simmons JD, Zylak CJ (1983) The posterior junction anatomy. Crit Rev Diagn Imaging 20:121–173

Proto AV, Simmons JD, Zylak CJ (1987) The anterior junction anatomy. Crit Rev Diagn Imaging 2:1–48

Proto AV, Corcoran HL, Ball JB (1989) The left paratracheal reflection. Radiology 171:625–628

Ravenel JG, Erasmus JJ (2002) Azygoesophageal recess. J Thoracic Imaging 17(3):219–226

Remy J, Capdeville R, Coussement A (1981) Le poumon pathologique, 2nd edn. Nice

Satoru O, Tsuyoshi O, Hiroyuki O (1999) Lung-mediastinal lines and its applications. J JASTRO 11(3):141–155

Schnur MJ, Winkler B, Austin JH (1981) Thickening of the posterior wall of the bronchus intermedius. Radiology 139: 551–559

Webb R, Higgins Ch (2005) Thoracic imaging. Lippincott, Philadelphia, pp 175–211

Whalen J, Meyers M, Oliphant M (1973) The retrosternal line. AJR Am J Roentgenol 117:861–872

Whitten R, Khan S, Munneke GA (2007) Diagnostic approach to mediastinal abnormalities. Radiographics 27:657–671

Williams Pl, Warwick R, Dyson M (1989) Splanchnology. Gray's anatomy, 37th edn. Churchill Livingstone, New York, pp 1245–1475

Worrell J, O'Donnell D, Carroll F (1992) Chest case of the day. AJR Am J Roentgenol 158:1356–1362

Wright F (2002) Radiology of the chest and related conditions. Taylor and Francis, London, pp 1.02–1.60

Zylak C, Pallie W, Jackson R (1982) Correlative anatomy and computed tomography: a module on the mediastinum. Radiographics 2(4):555–592

Correlation of Chest Radiograph and CT of the Heart

6

Rodrigo A. Salgado

Contents

Abstract

> Routinely visible imaging features of the heart are many times underappreciated by general radiologists, often due to a lack of specific radiological training. Nevertheless, the increasing use of CT for evaluation of the heart and coronary arteries offers a unique opportunity to revisit the imaging findings of this organ, correlating CT and conventional radiograph imaging findings. As such, common semiologic findings can be reevaluated, with the combination of imaging modalities providing a better understanding of important pathophysiological processes. Eventually, this can lead to a better and more complete radiological report, enhancing the role of the general radiologist in the detection and management of cardiac diseases.

> Therefore, it is the aim of this chapter to provide the reader a better understanding on how the heart shadow on conventional radiographs is actually composed, and to provide a overview of the most encountered normal and abnormal findings when studying the heart using CT and conventional radiographs.

6.1 Introduction

Ever since Röntgen X-rays began being used for diagnostic purposes, radiologists have been looking at images of the heart, either intentionally or during review of a conventional chest radiograph. A chest radiograph is nearly always one of the first imaging

R.A. Salgado
Department of Radiology, Antwerp University Hospital,
Wilrijkstraat 10, 2650, Edegem, Belgium
e-mail: rodrigo.salgado@uza.be

E.E. Coche et al. (eds.), *Comparative Interpretation of CT and Standard Radiography of the Chest*,
Medical Radiology, DOI: 10.1007/978-3-540-79942-9_6, © Springer-Verlag Berlin Heidelberg 2011

modalities performed in the evaluation of suspected heart disease. Nevertheless, on many occasions the cardiac findings are not systematically reviewed by many radiologists; only a vague assessment of cardiac size (the so-called "cardiothoracic ratio") is given in the final report.

Many excellent textbooks and review articles exist about the semiology of the heart and great vessels on standard chest radiographs, both in the normal and cardiac patient (Boxt 1999; Boxt et al. 1994; Higgins 1992). Furthermore, there have also been some reviews correlating plain film chest radiographs and cardiac magnetic resonance imaging (MRI) (Baron 2001; Duerinckx 2004).

In recent years there has been an enormous interest in the noninvasive evaluation of the coronary arteries using 16- and now up to 320-slice computed tomography (CT). This also means that many general radiologists are now becoming involved in routine imaging of the heart in mainstream practices, outside specialized academic centers. Though most of the attention has focused on the evaluation and validation of computed tomography angiography (CTA) of the coronary arteries, general heart morphology is rarely systematically reviewed. Nevertheless, normal variants and pathologic morphological findings are frequently encountered during a CTA of the coronary arteries, as well as during CT of the chest that may be performed for unrelated reasons.

Therefore, the current state of noninvasive cardiac imaging offers a unique opportunity to review cardiac pathology using both conventional radiographs and multislice CT (MSCT) imaging. Furthermore, it helps to increase the knowledge of pathophysiological mechanisms involved in commonly encountered cardiac diseases, therefore increasing detection and eventually the value of the radiology report.

6.2 Anatomy Revisited

6.2.1 Review of Basic Anatomy Radiographs/CT Correlation

Multiple textbooks and dedicated reviews exist about the anatomy of the heart and great vessels on conventional chest radiographs (Boxt 1999; Boxt et al. 1994; Lipton and Boxt 2004; Higgins and Webb 2005). However, some anatomic issues can be better understood when comparing the chest radiograph findings with a multiplanar imaging modality like CT or MRI (Duerinckx 2004; Baron 2001).

Different anatomic structures contribute to the contours of the cardiac silhouette on a frontal and lateral projection (Table 6.1). When comparing a routinely acquired frontal posteroanterior chest radiograph with a coronal reformatted CT image, some key anatomic issues become apparent. First, the left border of the cardiac radiograph shadow is mainly formed by the

Table 6.1 Anatomic outline of the heart on chest radiographs

Most prominent anatomic structures contributing to the heart shadow contour	Frontal projection	Lateral projection
Left border	Distal portion of the aortic arch Main pulmonary artery Left atrial appendage Lateral wall of the left ventricle	
Right border	Superior vena cava Lateral wall of the right atrium Inferior vena cava Pars ascending aorta (when dilated)	
Anterior border		Right ventricle Main pulmonary artery Ascending aorta
Posterior border		Superimposing pulmonary veins Left atrium Left ventricle Inferior vena cava

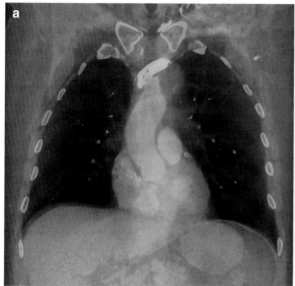
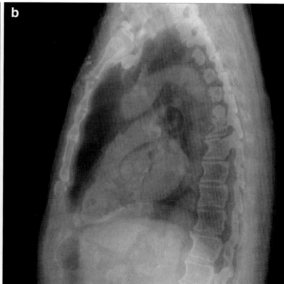

Fig. 6.1 Composite image of a conventional frontal (**a**) and lateral (**b**) chest radiograph and an multidetector computed tomography of the same patient. The contribution of the heart chambers to the cardiac contours in the frontal and lateral view is much better illustrated

slightly convex lateral wall of the left ventricle, with contributing shadows from the distal portion of the aortic arch, the main pulmonary artery, and the left atrial appendage. The right border is mainly composed by the convex lateral wall of the right atrium and the contour of the superior vena cava (Fig. 6.1a).

This implies that the frontal cardiac shadow does not usually reflect the (size of the) left atrium and right ventricle. It also means that the cardiothoracic ratio, initially developed to evaluate left ventricular dilatation, has its limitations as an initial indicator of overall heart size because it does not take all chambers' sizes into account. Furthermore, Rose et al. stated that an increase in volume of up to 66 % of the left ventricle is needed for the cardiothoracic ratio to reliably detect left ventricular enlargement (Rose and Stolberg 1982) Therefore, it is best suited for follow-up of known heart disease because a normal cardiothoracic ratio does not exclude heart chamber dilatation.

The lateral chest radiograph mostly reflects the contours of the right ventricle anteriorly and the left atrium posteriorly (Fig. 6.1b). Opposite of what is seen on the frontal chest view, the left ventricle and the right atrium occupy a more central position in the cardiac shadow, and therefore do not routinely contribute to the global heart shadow contour. Normally, the retrosternal space

remains free of any structures but becomes opacified as the right ventricle significantly dilates.

Evaluation of heart chambers on axial CT images is less straightforward than it may seem because the true axis of the heart is somewhat oblique and varies among patients. When evaluating chamber dimensions on plain axial images, cardiac chambers and structures may appear distorted and wrong assumption of size may result. Therefore, when evaluating heart morphology it is almost mandatory to be familiar with the common imaging planes of the heart which are used in MRI and echocardiography. These views provide a structural way to assess global heart morphology and atrioventricular relations and facilitate comparison of the CT imaging findings with other imaging modalities. The most commonly used imaging planes in a practical matter are the two-chamber view (both long and short axis) and the four chamber view (Fig. 6.2).

The coronary arteries are, under normal circumstances, not visible on conventional chest radiographs. Their location can become apparent when extensive coronary calcification or a coronary stent is present. Nevertheless, even calcified coronary arteries can be very difficult to visualize (Mahnken et al. 2007; Souza et al. 1978). Today, both electron-beam and conventional MSCT are far better suited to both detect and quantify coronary artery calcifications (Becker et al. 1999) (Fig. 6.3).

Like the coronary arteries, the different heart valves are normally not visible on a conventional chest radiograph. Their position can be assessed when extensive calcification is present or when the patient has one or more prosthetic valves (Fig. 6.4). The most easily detected calcified valvular structure on plain chest film is the annulus of the mitral valve (Fig. 6.5). Due to the restrosternal location of the aortic valve, calcifications are very difficult to assess on chest radiographs, but easy to evaluate with MSCT (Fig. 6.6).

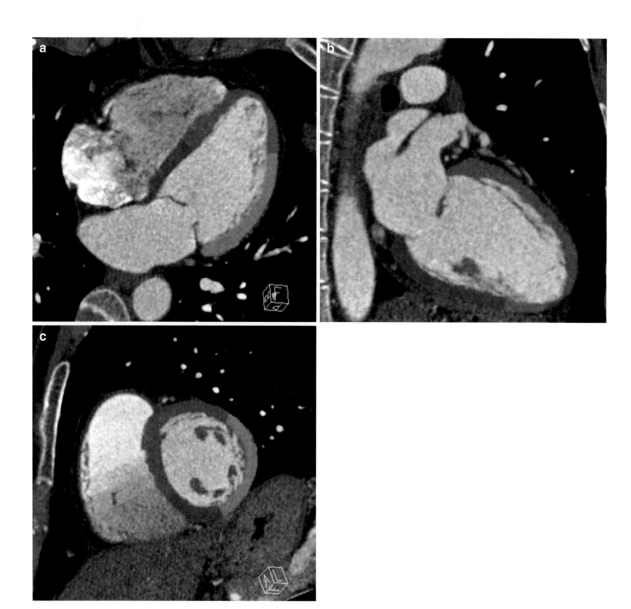

Fig. 6.2 Contrast-enhanced multidetector computed tomography images. Standardized views to look at the heart are illustrated. (**a**) Four-chamber view. (**b**) Two-chamber view long axis. (**c**) Two-chamber view short axis. These images are oriented along the actual long and short axis of the heart, and as such are better suited to evaluate heart morphology. The colors indicate the different irrigation areas of the coronary arteries: Left anterior descending (LAD) (*blue*), LAD-left circumflex (LCX) (*green*), LCX (*yellow*), and right coronary artery (*red*)

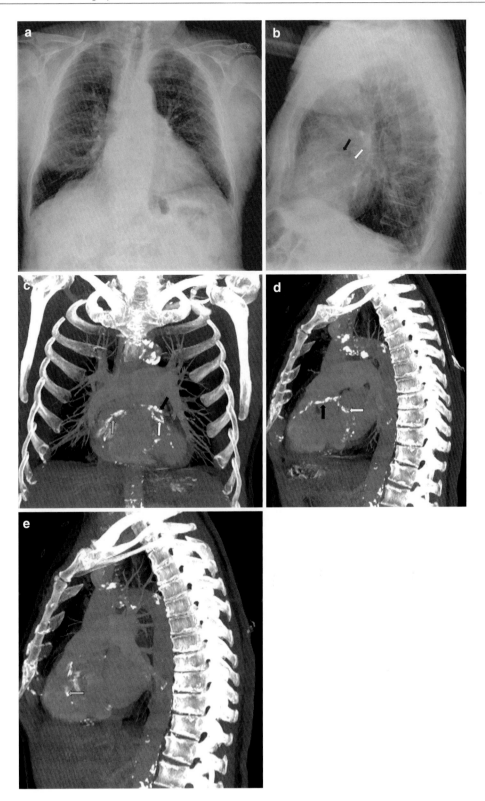

Fig. 6.3 Coronary artery calcifications. (**a** and **b**) frontal and lateral chest radiographs. (**c–e**) Coronal and sagittal maximum intensity projection computed tomography (CT) images. Even extensive coronary calcifications can be difficult to see on chest radiographs (**a** and **b**). These calcifications are nevertheless easily seen on CT images, where left anterior descending (*black arrow*), left circumflex (*open arrow*), and right coronary artery calcifications (*gray arrow*) can be identified

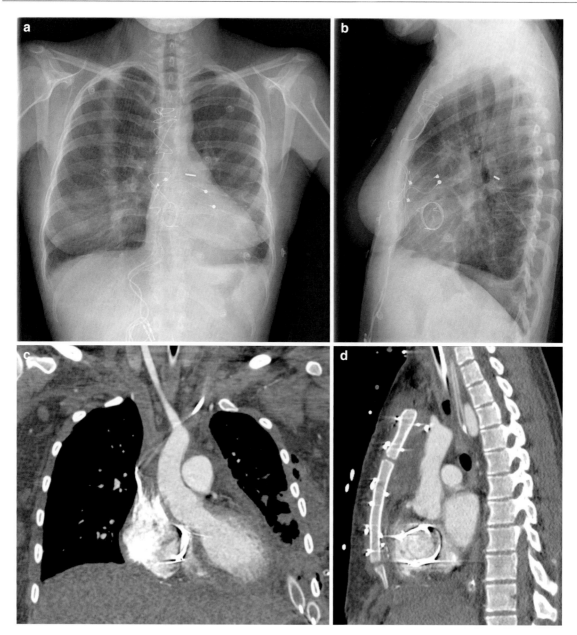

Fig. 6.4 Tricuspid valve prosthesis in a young woman. (**a** and **b**) Frontal and lateral chest radiographs. (**c** and **d**) Coronal and sagittal reformatted computed tomography images. The position of the tricuspid valve can best be evaluated when it is replaced by a prosthesis, as in this case, where valve replacement was indicated after valve destruction due to infectious endocarditis

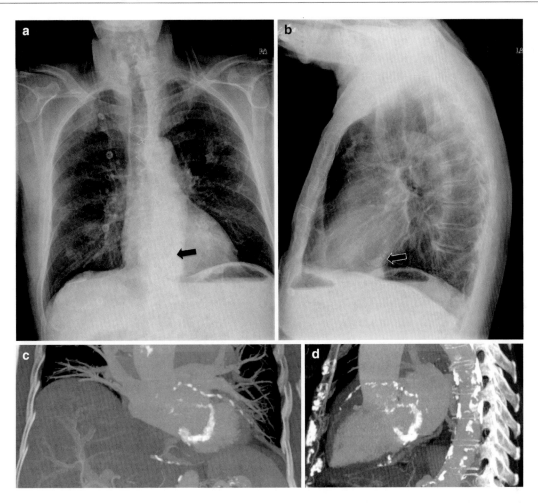

Fig. 6.5 Extensive annular mitral valve calcification in a 52-year-old man. (**a** and **b**) Frontal and lateral chest radiographs. (**c** and **d**) Coronal and sagittal reformatted computed tomography images. Extensive calcifications along the fibrous annulus of the mitral valve can be seen (*arrow*)

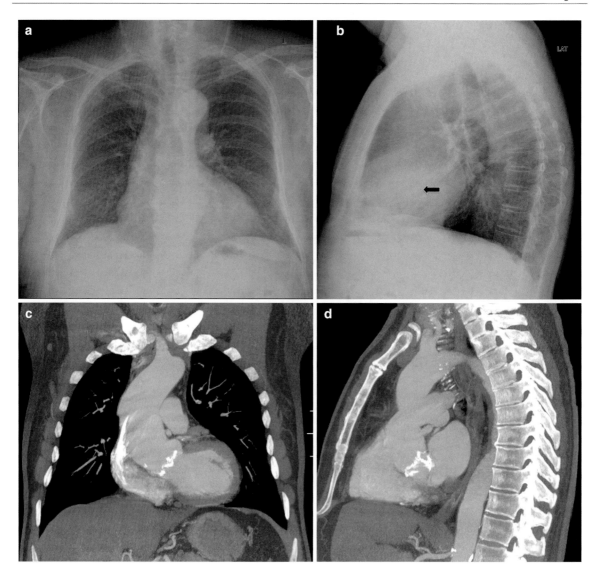

Fig. 6.6 A 63-year-old man with extensive aortic valve degeneration. (**a** and **b**) Frontal and lateral chest radiographs. (**c** and **d**) Coronal and sagittal reformatted computed tomography (CT) images. The CT images reveal extensive clunky calcifications in the aortic valve leaflets (**c** and **d**). Nevertheless, these calcifications remain difficult to see on the conventional radiographs (**a** and **b**, *arrow*)

6.2.2 Imaging Anatomy of the Left Ventricle

When describing specific portions of the heart and left ventricle, several anatomic reference terms are used that are often unfamiliar to many radiologists who are not involved in cardiac imaging. The left ventricle is subdivided in to three main segments: the apical, middle, and basal segments (Fig. 6.7). The basal and middle segments are further subdivided into anterior, anterolateral, posterolateral, posterior, posteroseptal, and anteroseptal subsegments. The apical segment is divided into anterior, lateral, inferior, and septal subsegments. This standardized and widely used segmentation of the left ventricle in 17 myocardial segments (16 + apex) has been introduced by the American Heart Association (Cerqueira et al. 2002). These different anatomic landmarks also partially reflect the distribution of irrigation of the myocardium by the coronary arteries and are applied in for example, the further specification of myocardium infarcts. As such, when speaking, for example, about a so-called "anterior infarct," it is meant that the infarct occurred in the anterior wall of the left ventricle, often indicating a significant lesion in the left anterior descending artery.

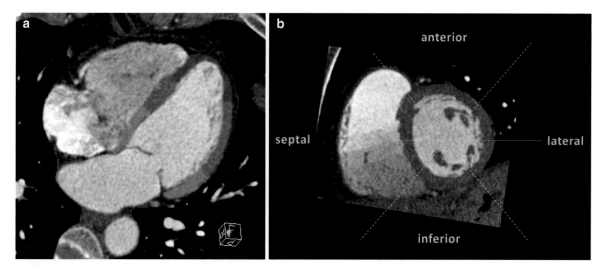

Fig. 6.7 Contrast-enhanced multidetector computed tomography anatomy of the left ventricle. (**a**) Four-chamber view. (**b**) Two-chamber view short axis. The different anatomic segments of the left ventricle are reviewed. The four-chamber view shows the apical (*red*), middle (*blue*), and basal (*green*) segments. The anatomic orientation on the two-chamber short axis view is further illustrated on the two-chamber view

6.3 Heart Chamber Evaluation

6.3.1 General Characteristics

Chamber dilatation can be difficult to assess on conventional chest radiographs. An initial evaluation could be initially directed to signs of left atrial dilatation, followed by ventricular assessment (Higgins and Webb 2005). Nevertheless, it can be very difficult to impossible to correctly identify the type of ventricular enlargement on radiographs alone (Higgins and Webb 2005).

As previously stated, chamber dilatation can occur even in patients who have a normal cardiothoracic ratio. Nevertheless, this measurement can be used in the initial heart size evaluation to make a first distinction between "small" heart and "big" heart disease (Higgins and Webb 2005). "Small" heart disease (normal cardiothoracic ratio) is mostly associated with pressure overload and reduced ventricular compliance; "big" heart disease usually has an underlying pathophysiology of volume overload or myocardial failure (Higgins and Webb 2005). Pericardial effusion can also be encountered in this group.

Other patient-related factors such as sex, age, and especially body height of the individual can also have a slight influence on atrioventricular dimensions (Vasan et al. 1997). Though there are no multiple studies with large series measuring the dimensions of the different cardiac chambers and myocardial wall on CT, a study has appeared that derived mean values for cardiac dimensions, volumes, function, and mass using CT in a normotensive, nonobese population free of cardiovascular disease (Lin et al. 2008).

Besides its contour, the myocardial wall is not directly visible on a chest radiograph unless calcifications are present (e.g., old myocardial infarction). The thickness of the myocardium varies with the heart cycle, reaching its minimum thickness at the end of the diastolic phase and its maximum during systolic phase. The myocardium thickness is commonly measured at the interventricular septum in the end-diastolic phase. As a general rule, the average thickness must not exceed 10 mm, but nevertheless can be considered as being between normal limits up to 11 mm in large individuals. Every measurement of 12 mm or higher is considered abnormal.

Although CT is better suited and more sensitive in the evaluation of chamber size because of its intrinsic slice-based imaging nature, CT images must be interpreted with caution in non-electrocardiogram (ECG) gated acquisitions. The lack of ECG-gating may result in portions of the scan being acquired, for example, in the systolic phase of the heart cycle. As such, the left ventricular myocardium may appear thicker, thereby mimicking hypertrophic changes.

6.3.2 Evaluation of Pathology with Normal Chamber Dimensions

Some heart conditions have no or only minimal impact on overall chamber size because of the nature of the underlying pathophysiological process or the presence of only minimal changes during the initial stage of disease.

Given the projection nature of conventional radiographs, they do not directly provide information about the thickness of the myocardium. Therefore, the heart shadow in conventional chest radiographs is often normal in conditions of slight or moderate myocardium thickening without obvious chamber dilatation. This can be the case in, for example, left ventricular hypertrophy (Fig. 6.8), an often-encountered heart condition

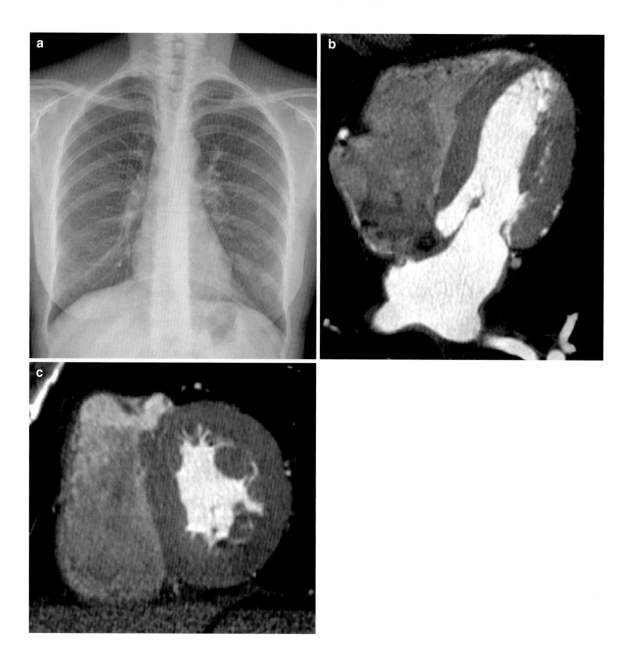

Fig. 6.8 A 52-year-old man with known arterial hypertension. (**a**) Conventional chest radiograph. (**b** and **c**) Contrast-enhanced multidetector computed tomography (MDCT) with four- and two-chamber views. The frontal chest radiograph (**a**) shows no abnormalities. The MDCT images (**b** and **c**) clearly show a uniformly thickened hypertrophic left ventricular wall, as seen in concentric left ventricular hypertrophy

with global, often concentric increase of the left ventricular mass most commonly due to arterial hypertension or valvular stenosis-regurgitation. On the other hand, CT is very well-suited to depict the concentric hypertrophic thickening of the left ventricle.

6.3.3 Left Heart Imaging

As previously discussed, the left atrium is often best appreciated on the lateral chest radiograph, but important clues of atrial enlargement can often be seen on the frontal view. In this projection, the left atrium is, under normal conditions, not very clearly visible because it occupies a rather central position and is therefore often obscured by other overlying cardiac structures and the spine. When atrial dilation occurs, known signs can be seen on conventional chest radiographs. These signs are better understood when the position of the left atrium is correlated with the surrounding structures using the better spatial relationship possibilities of MSCT.

The left atrium is only going to contribute to the frontal heart shadow projection when it is significantly increased in size. When the left atrium is significantly dilated, it will mainly extend in a laterolateral fashion, with a more prominent shadow of the left atrial appendage on the frontal projection. This leads to an additional bulge of the left heart contour, just under the level of the main pulmonary artery (Fig. 6.9). Further atrial enlargement can also lead to a "double density" on the right and/or left cardiac border as it extends into the adjacent lung.

Splaying of the carina is explained because the left atrium lies below this anatomic structure. When extensive atrial dilation occurs, it compresses the carina from the inferior, increasing the angle between the main bronchi (Fig. 6.10). This can be appreciated on coronal CT views but can be less evident on chest radiographs when left atrial dilation is not extensive.

The left border of the cardiac shadow is mainly composed of the left ventricle. When this ventricle increases in size, it will do so by extending the apical shadow in a (left) lateral, inferior, and posterior way. Furthermore, the apex will acquire a more rounded morphology. These signs are more prominent as the left ventricle increasingly dilates.

The left ventricle can globally increase in size due to increased volume or pressure, or as a result of an underlying cardiomyopathy. However, it can also dilate as a consequence of changed wall kinetics after a myocardial infarction. In such a case, the dilation can be regional according to the affected area of diminished perfusion. This can lead to a dilation of the apex of the left ventricle after an anterior infarction (Fig. 6.11).

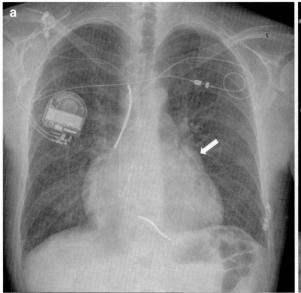
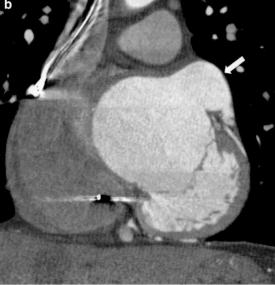

Fig. 6.9 A 63-year-old man with left atrial dilation. (**a**) Frontal conventional chest radiograph. (**b**) Coronal reformatted contrast-enhanced multidetector computed tomography. The frontal chest radiograph reveals an additional bulge on the left heart contour (**a**, *arrow*), corresponding to an enlarged left atrial appendage in left atrial dilatation (**b**, *arrow*)

The apex can also calcify and become easily detectable on chest radiographs as these calcifications become more extensive (Fig. 6.12).

One of the drawbacks of conventional chest radiographs is that it mainly depicts the contours of cardiac structures. As such, it does not provide sometimes vital diagnostic information (Fig. 6.13). In contrast, CT is very well-suited to evaluate the thickness, structure, and contrast enhancement of the ventricular wall.

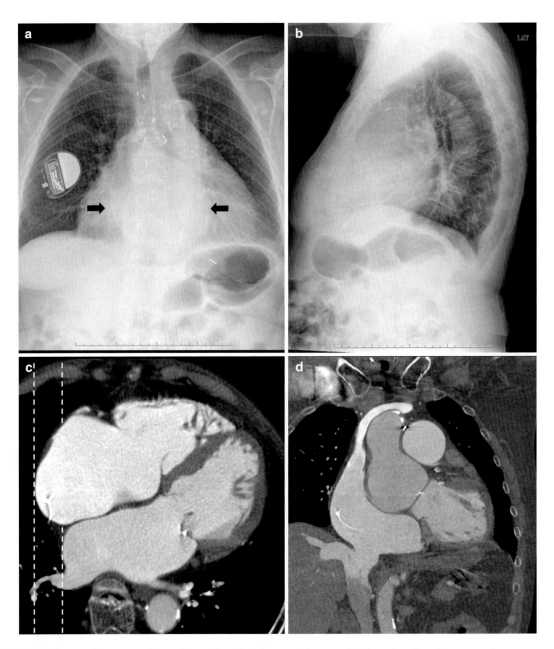

Fig. 6.10 A 71-year-old woman with cardiomegaly and right heart failure. (**a** and **b**) Conventional chest radiograph. (**c–f**) Contrast-enhanced multidetector computed tomography (MDCT). The conventional chest X-ray shows a clear dilation of the whole heart, with a double contour on the right cardiac shadow produced by an enlarged left atrium (*arrows indicate left atrial contour*). Note also the almost complete retrosternal opacification on the lateral chest view, compatible with right heart (ventricular) dilatation. The MDCT images confirm among others a prominent biatrial dilation (**c–f**), which contributes to the prominent right heart border and produces the double contour (*dashed lines*)

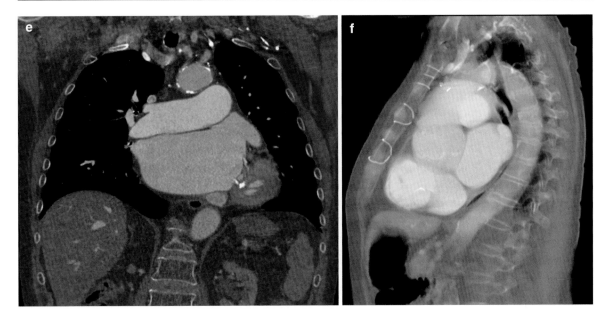

Fig. 6.10 (continued)

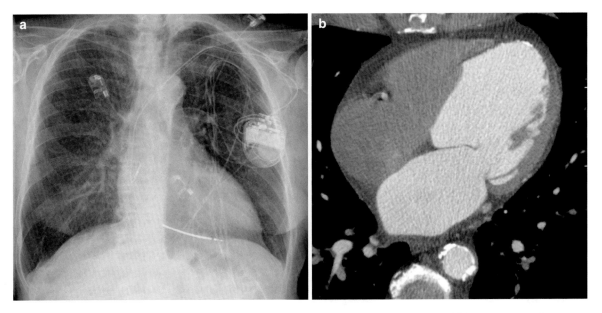

Fig. 6.11 A 54-year-old man with left ventricular dilalation secondary to an old anterior myocardial infarct. The images show leftward extension of the cardiac shadow (**a**), with left ventricular dilatation on the multidetector computed tomography image (**b**), corresponding to extensive wall thinning and apical dilatation after myocardial infarction

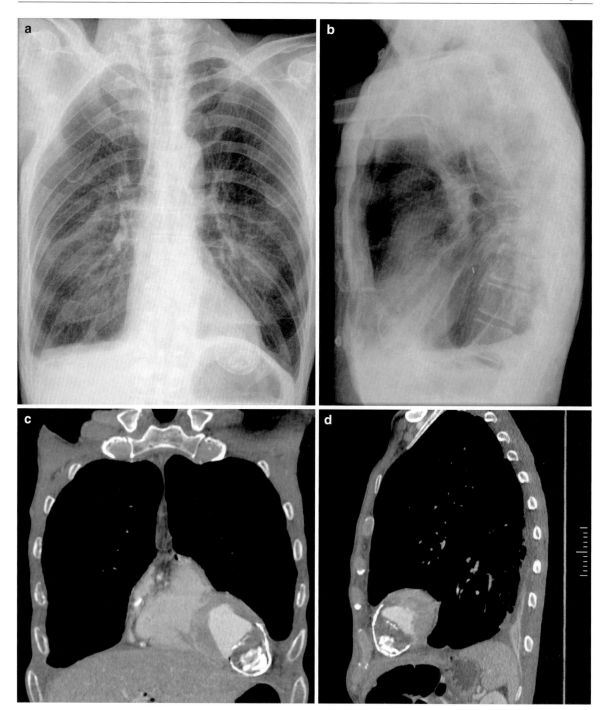

Fig. 6.12 A 63-year-old man with an old apical infarction. (**a** and **b**) Conventional chest radiograph. (**c**) Contrast-enhanced multidetector computed tomography (MDCT) image. The conventional chest radiographs reveal a semicircular calcification at the level of the left ventricular apex (**a** and **b**). The MDCT images show an old calcified apical infarction with extensive wall thinning and prominent mural thrombus due to severely diminished wall motion (**c** and **d**)

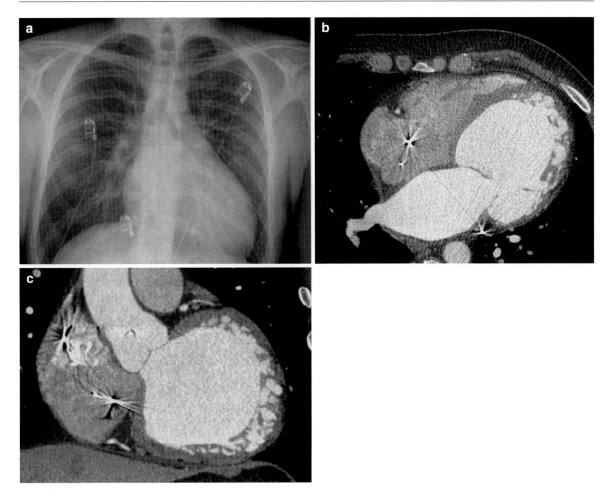

Fig. 6.13 (**a**) Conventional frontal chest radiograph and (**b** and **c**) contrast-enhanced multidetector computed tomography (MDCT) in a 24-year-old man with a nonspecific dilatation of the left ventricle (**a**). MDCT confirms the left ventricular dilation, but also shows the enlarged myocardium with a prominent trabecular morphology (**b** and **c**), compatible with a noncompaction cardiomyopathy

6.3.4 Right Heart Imaging

Analysis of right ventricular volume and function is an essential part of the detection and management of both congenital and acquired heart disease. It reflects changes in abnormal pressure or volume encountered in conditions like right ventricular outflow obstruction or intracardiac shunts, and in pulmonary pathology like pulmonary hypertension and vascular abnormalities (Greil et al. 2008). Though echocardiography and MRI are also widely used in the evaluation of the right heart, there is still an important role for conventional chest radiographs in the follow-up of right heart pathology. Furthermore, visible abnormal findings in the right heart often go undetected and underreported on chest and cardiac CT due to lack of knowledge.

As previously stated, the right border of the cardiac contour on a frontal chest radiograph is mainly formed by the right atrium. Under normal conditions, the right ventricle does not contribute to this image unless it is significantly dilated. When the right border of the cardiac silhouette enlarges, one must first consider right atrial enlargement, especially when the right border is more than 5 cm from the midline on a frontal chest radiograph (Chen 1997). One must, however, keep in mind that both left and right atrial dilation often coexist. In analogy with the left heart, a double contour formed by the left and the dilated right atrium can sometimes be appreciated on the frontal chest radiograph (Fig. 6.10).

When right heart dilation is present, it is usually be more evident on the lateral chest view because the right ventricle enlarges superiorly and anteriorly, obscuring the retrosternal space (Fig. 6.10). Other signs on the frontal projection include dilation of the pulmonary trunk, increased convexity of the left upper cardiac contour, and elevation of the cardiac apex (Cook et al. 2007; Chen 1997).

Because the myocardial wall of the right ventricle is not visible on conventional chest radiographs, CT is much better suited than conventional radiographs to detecting initial changes of increased wall thickness. Therefore, though the signs of, for example, pulmonary arterial hypertension are already visible on a chest radiograph, CT will additionally detect the hypertrophic changes of the myocardium (Fig. 6.14).

The right heart can reflect abnormalities in the pulmonary vasculature. This can be acquired conditions

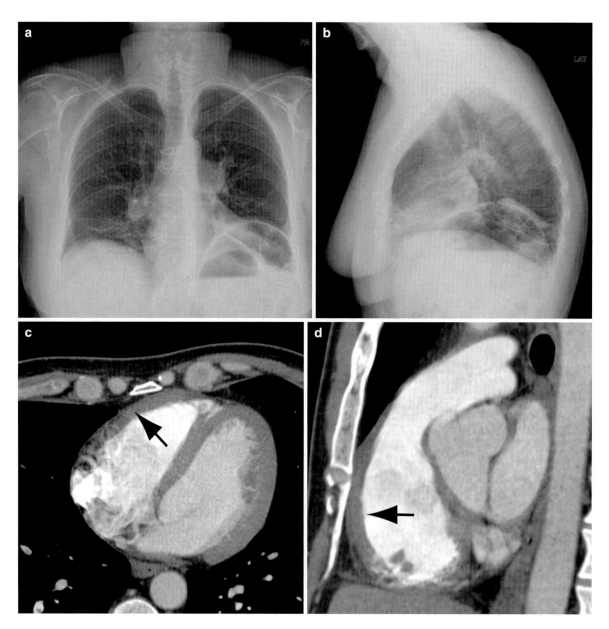

Fig. 6.14 A 65-year-old woman with pulmonary hypertension. (**a** and **b**) Conventional chest radiograph. (**c** and **d**) Contrast-enhanced multidetector computed tomography (MDCT). The conventional chest radiograph (**a** and **b**) shows prominent dilation of the pulmonary arteries but no obvious sign of right heart dilation. The MDCT images additionally reveal a thickened wall of the right ventricle (**c** and **d**, *arrow*) without concomitant dilation

like pulmonary embolism with subsequent acute or chronic right heart failure, but it can also have a congenital vascular etiology like a partially anomalous pulmonary venous connection. In such conditions, findings on chest radiographs are fairly nonspecific, but CT is excellent at showing both the vascular abnormalities and the morphological effect on the right heart chambers. Finally, a dilated pars ascending aorta can also contribute to an outward bulge of the right upper heart contour, a sign suggestive of underlying degenerative or congenital aortic valve disease (Fig. 6.15).

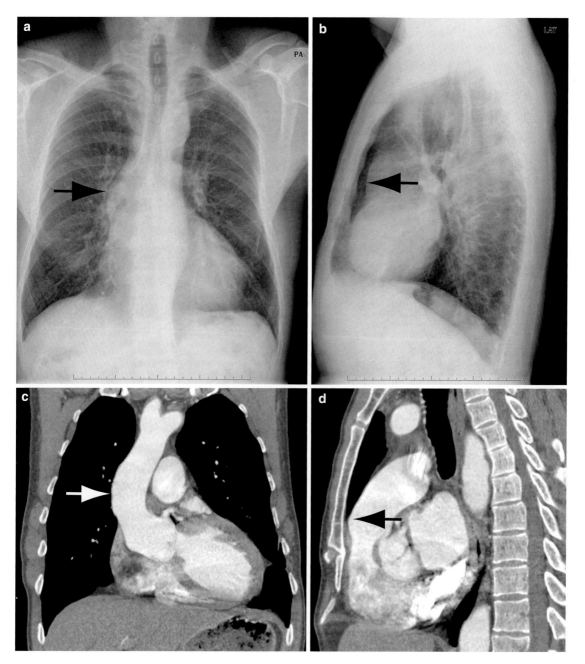

Fig. 6.15 A 32-year old man with a bicuspid aortic valve. (**a** and **b**) Conventional chest radiograph. (**c** and **d**) Contrast-enhanced multidetector computed tomography (MDCT) images. The frontal chest radiograph (**a**) reveals an outward bulge of the right upper heart contour (*arrow*). The MDCT images (**c** and **d**) clearly show a dilated ascending aorta, which causes this additional shadow (*arrow*)

6.4 Other Pathology

6.4.1 Calcifications

Cardiac calcifications are often helpful in assessing cardiac disease because they help to localize and identify anatomic structures like valves and the pericardium, and they can be a marker for specific diseases. Most visible calcifications are of a dystrophic nature, secondary to a previous inflammatory process like rheumatic mitral stenosis or as a result of myocardial infarction and scar formation. They can also appear as a sign of degeneration secondary to the wear and tear of a (congenitally) malformed structure like a bicuspid aortic valve. The shape or character of the calcifications can be helpful in determining its origin.

The visibility of calcifications on plain film depends on many factors, both technique related and patient related (Gowda and Boxt 2004). Plain films of the chest are primarily designed for visualization of the lung parenchyma and provide less detail of bone and calcium compared with a dedicated examination. In this respect, fluoroscopy is better in visualizing calcifications, with better dynamic imaging possibilities. The technical quality of the conventional chest radiograph and the circumstances in which it was acquired are also relevant; for example inadequately penetrated films or bedside taken chest films in the intensive care unit are less suitable to detect small calcifications, for obvious reasons. Finally, the calcifications have to be large enough and/or present in sufficient quantities and in a convenient location to be reliably detected during a routine chest plain film examination.

Valvular calcifications can be detected on chest radiographs but are more easily visualized with CT. The most commonly encountered calcifications are found in the aortic valve leaflets and the annulus of the mitral valve (Table 6.2). Calcifications of the fibrous mitral valve annulus are one of the most commonly visualized valve calcifications because the mitral valve is not extensively overshadowed by projection of other large adjacent anatomic structures (Fig. 6.5). Furthermore, annular calcifications are generally thick and coarse, as opposed to mitral leaflet calcifications, which have a more delicate appearance and are therefore almost never reliably visualized on chest radiographs. Annular mitral valve calcifications

Table 6.2 Differentiation between annular mitral valve and aortic valve calcifications

	Mitral valve	Aortic valve
Involved structure	Annulus	Annulus and leaflets
	Leaflets (rare)	
Etiology	chronic degeneration	<4th decade: congenital (bicuspid valve)
	accelerated by hypertension, diabetes mellitus, hyperlipidemia	>6th decade: acquired valve degeneration (tricuspid valve)
Character	Dense, ring-like clumps (annulus)	Thick, heavy calcifications (leaflets)
Function	Usually normal function	Stenosis
	Mostly insufficiency when present	

are mostly of a chronic degenerative nature, but can also be associated with end-stage renal disease.

Calcifications of the aortic valve are commonly seen in older individuals on a degenerative basis (Fig. 6.6), but can also be the result of wear and tear of a congenital bicuspid valve. Degenerative aortic leaflet calcifications are, just as annular mitral calcifications, generally dense and heavy. Because of the retrosternal position of the aortic valve and overshadowing structures like pulmonary vessels, they are not easily visualized on chest radiographs. They are nevertheless routinely seen on CT examination, which can further assess possible associated thickening of the leaflets. Finally, tricuspid and pulmonary valve calcifications are extremely rare.

Myocardial calcifications are most commonly encountered after a myocardial infarct, subsequent to necrosis, hemorrhage, or fibrosis of myocardial tissue (Gowda and Boxt 2004). Its nature is therefore dystrophic, with a location closely related to specific terminal irrigation areas of the coronary arteries. Myocardial calcifications are found in 8% of infarcts that are a minimum of 8 years old, and are mostly located in the anterior wall and in the apex of the left ventricle (Freundlich and Lind 1975; Gowda and Boxt 2004). They usually appear as dense, curvilinear calcifications in an often dilated segment of the left ventricular apex. On chest radiographs, they can be found left of the midline on a frontal projection, and anterior on a lateral projection, adjacent to the pleural lining (Fig. 6.12). Note that, because of dilatation and remodeling after an infarct, the left ventricle will regionally expand as the affected wall segment weakens, producing a more prominent convex contour of the left heart shadow. CT can additionally reveal the extensive wall thinning and the effects of changed wall kinetics, like the presence of mural thrombus (Fig. 6.12c,d). Furthermore, one must always take into account that the calcified myocardial tissue represents an underestimation of the infarct size.

Occasionally, calcifications can be encountered in the left atrium. One specific location is the left atrial wall near the appendage. The exact etiology of calcifications in this location remains not fully understood, but it is highly correlated with long-standing rheumatic disease (Salgado et al. 2008). These calcifications have a thick, coarse appearance comparable to annular mitral valve calcifications. They are located left of the midline on a frontal chest radiograph, near the vicinity of the left atrial appendage (Fig. 6.16). They may have

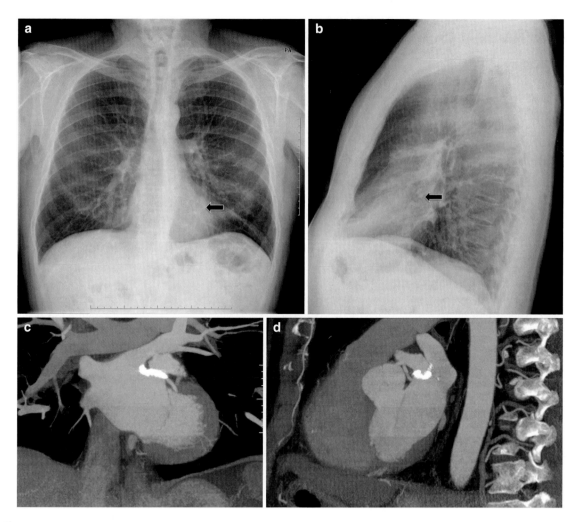

Fig. 6.16 A 57-year-old man with long-standing rheumatic disease. (**a** and **b**) Conventional chest radiographs. (**c** and **d**) Contrast-enhanced maximum intensity projection multidetector computed tomography (MDCT) images. (**e**) Volume-rendered MDCT image. The conventional chest radiographs show amorphous calcifications projecting at the level of the left atrial appendage (**a** and **b**, *arrow*). The MDCT images further reveal that these calcifications are along the orifice and proximal wall of the left atrial appendage (**c–e**, *arrow*)

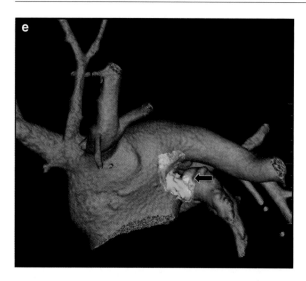

Fig. 6.16 (continued)

a semicircular appearance because they tend to appear around the orifice of the atrial appendage (Salgado et al. 2008).

Pericardial calcifications can result from an underlying infection, trauma, hemorrhage, and radiotherapy (Gowda and Boxt 2004). Although pericardial calcifications are often associated with pericarditis caused by an underlying chronic infectious or inflammatory disease, this is not always the case. In most cases, the etiology of pericarditis remains unknown. A thickened, less elastic, and more fibrotic pericardium can lead to decreased (right) heart function in constrictive pericarditis. Almost half of the cases of constrictive pericarditis seem to be idiopathic, whereas the other two main known reasons are iatrogenic: previous pericardiotomy and mediastinal radiotherapy. Other etiologies include uremia and infections, as tuberculosis continues to remain an important cause of constrictive pericarditis in the Third World (Fig. 6.17). Common imaging features of pericarditis are the presence of a thickened and enhanced pericardium, often associated with a pericardial effusion. These findings can be seen on a standard chest CT but are not depicted on a chest radiographs. Gross calcifications, which can be seen on a chest radiographs, are only seen in 28% of the cases. Nevertheless, the presence of pericardial calcification must always raise the suspicion of constrictive pericarditis.

Pericardial calcifications may appear as focal plaques and/or as a curvilinear, dense line along the pericardium (Fig. 6.18). They can be coarse and thick in long-standing disease like tuberculosis (Fig. 6.17). They always follow the contour of the heart on both frontal and lateral projections, and are usually located along the atrioventricular grooves and lower diaphragmatic portions of the pericardium. Other distinguishing features from myocardial calcifications are given in Table 6.3.

Coronary artery calcifications can occasionally be detected on conventional chest radiographs, especially when the reader is familiar with the locations of the coronary arteries (Souza et al. 1978). Coronary artery calcification may be identified on a frontal chest film in the triangular region defined by the left heart border, the spine, and the top of the left ventricle, and in the lateral view over the interventricular septum or anterior atrioventricular ring (Souza et al. 1978; Gowda and Boxt 2004). They generally appear as (curvi)linear or tram-track densities along the course of a coronary artery.

Despite the available literature about detecting coronary artery calcifications on plain chest films, this modality has little value in daily practice for this indication. During the last decade it has been clearly established that coronary artery calcifications are far better detected, evaluated, and quantified using spiral and electron-beam CT compared with a conventional chest radiograph (Fig. 6.3) (Budoff et al. 1996; Becker et al. 1999). Even when the existence of coronary calcifications is known, they still can be difficult to assess on a chest radiograph and are therefore inconsistently detected (Mahnken et al. 2007). Therefore it is better if conventional chest radiographs are not used as a replacement for a CT calcium scoring examination (Mahnken et al. 2007).

6.4.2 Pericardial Effusion and Pneumopericardium

Pericardial effusion can have many etiologies and can be serous, chylous, or hemorrhagic depending on the cause. Despite many described signs, the appearance on chest radiographs is, in practice, often nonspecific despite the cause and often reveals cardiomegaly without any further possible specification (Fig. 6.19) (Higgins and Webb 2005). Even the so-called "water-bottle appearance" is nonspecific and subject to interpretation

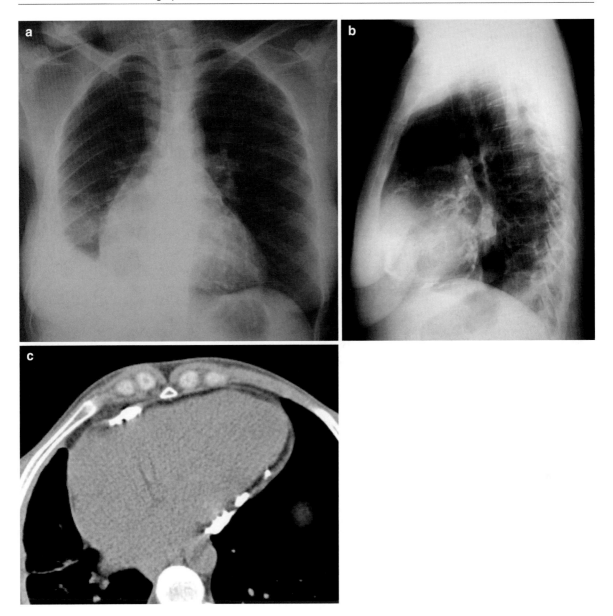

Fig. 6.17 A 30-year-old woman with known tuberculosis. (**a** and **b**) Conventional chest radiograph. (**c**) Non-enhanced multidetector computed tomography (MDCT). Coarse calcifications can be detected on the conventional chest radiographs along the lining of the left ventricle (**a** and **b**). The MDCT images confirm the presence of these calcification along a thickened pericardium (**c**). These imaging findings, together with the clinical history, are compatible with (long-standing) tuberculous pericarditis

(Higgins and Webb 2005). Furthermore, a small amount of blood in the pericardial sac can cause an acute cardiac tamponade without significantly affecting the size of the cardiac shadow on conventional radiographs. CT can easily depict pericardial effusion (Fig. 6.19b–d), but because of the widespread use of echocardiography it is almost never used solely for this indication. It is an excellent tool to assess the size and location of pericardial effusion, but it tends to overestimate the amount of fluid compared with echocardiography (Maisch et al. 2004). The density of pericardial effusion is generally between 10 and 40 HU, and as such is hypodense compared with the adjacent myocardium (Maksimovic et al. 2006). This density depends on relative amounts of the

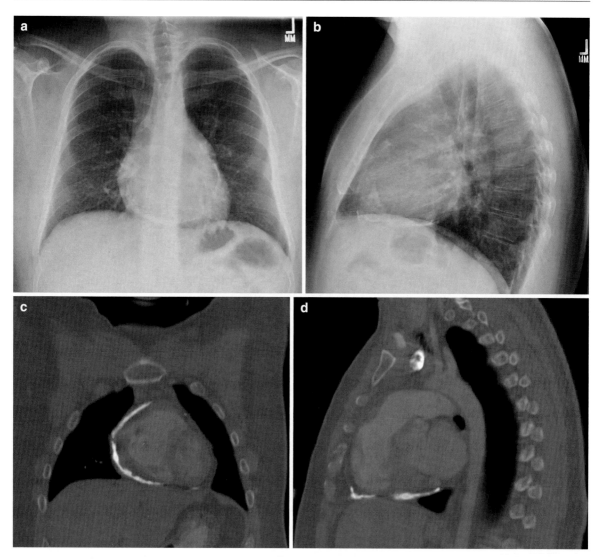

Fig. 6.18 A 56-year-old man with pericardial calcification. (**a** and **b**) Conventional chest radiograph. (**c** and **d**) Contrast-enhanced multidetector computed tomography (MDCT). There is evident calcification along the pericardial lining of the left ventricle on the conventional images (**a** and **b**). On MDCT, these calcifications are shown to a better extent (**c** and **d**) (Images courtesy of Dr. N. Goyal and Dr. S. Abbara, Massachusetts General Hospital, Boston, MA, USA)

protein (fibrin) and possible hemorrhagic content component (Maksimovic et al. 2006).

On the other hand, CT is far better suited than conventional radiographs to detect air in the pericardial sac (pneumopericardium). Pneumopericardium is far less common than pneumomediastinum and will most commonly be found after penetrating trauma and (cardiac) surgery (Fig. 6.20). These kinds of patients will nowadays nearly always be investigated with CT, which is the modality of choice to visualize gas or air in the pericardial sac. Though a pneumocardium can be detected on conventional chest radiographs as a lucency confined to the pericardial sac, this can often be obscured by superimposing structures like lung consolidations and large pleural effusions. On occasion it can be difficult to distinguish between a pneumopericardium, a pneumomediastinum, and even a pneumothorax on chest radiographs, especially in suboptimal imaging conditions like in intensive care units. Furthermore, although rare, these entities are not mutually exclusive. Sound knowledge of the involved anatomy and the properties of the involved spaces can

Table 6.3 Differentiation between myocardial and pericardial calcifications

	Myocardium	Pericardium
Etiology	Ischemic (most common)	Infection, trauma, hemorrhage, radiation
Most common location	Left ventricle (apex, anterior wall)	Atrioventricular grooves
		Lower/diaphragmatic portions of the pericardium
Distribution	Localized	Diffuse
Character	Fine, curvilinear	Small or thick (long-standing disease) clunky calcifications

nevertheless be problem-solving on many occasions (Table 6.4, adapted from Bejvan and Godwin [1996]). When doubts persist, CT has proven an excellent tool in both the detection of the abnormal air and the evaluation of its extent and possible etiology.

6.4.3 Tumors of the Heart and Pericardium

The most commonly encountered pericardial mass is the pericardial cyst. These well-defined lesions are a not uncommon finding encountered during routine chest CT that has been performed for other

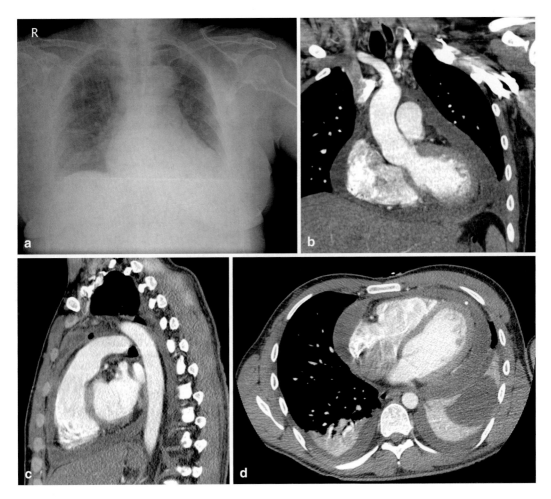

Fig. 6.19 A 72-year-old woman with infectious pericarditis and pericardial effusion. (**a**) Conventional chest radiograph. (**b–d**) Contrast-enhanced multidetector computed tomography (MDCT) images. The conventional chest radiograph reveals an enlarged heart shadow (**a**), but no further specification is possible. The MDCT images (**b–d**) show a substantial pericardial effusion due to infectious pericarditis, leading to the mentioned cardiomegaly

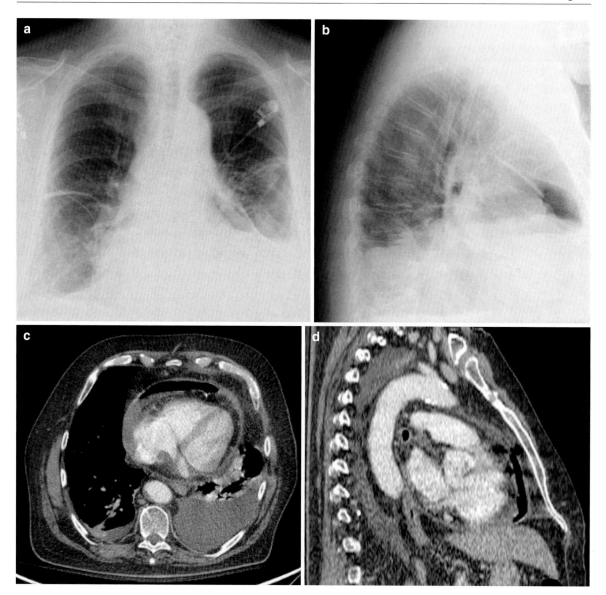

Fig. 6.20 A 72-year-old man with postoperative dyspnea after surgical abdominal aneurysm repair. (**a** and **b**) Conventional chest radiograph. (**c** and **d**) Contrast-enhanced axial and sagittal reformatted multidetector computed tomography (MDCT) images. The images show an evident pneumopericardium that developed after pericardiocentesis for drainage of a significant postoperative pericardial effusion. Though the air in the pericardial sac can be seen on the conventional chest X-ray images, it is at least partially obscured by the concomitant large pleural effusion. However, the diagnosis is straightforward on the MDCT images (Images courtesy of Prof. Dr. E. Coche, UCL, Brussels, Belgium)

reasons. They represent an embryogenic defect and are mostly asymptomatic without further clinical relevance. Though they may occur anywhere in the pericardium, the vast majority makes contact with the diaphragm and are mostly located at the right cardiophrenic angle (Fig. 6.21). Most pericardial cysts are not usually seen on conventional chest radiographs because of their size and location, but their plain film characteristics have been described (Rozenshtein and Boxt 1999). When large, they are smoothly marginated without any calcifications. CT further confirms the sharp delineation and additionally reveals the low-attenuation content. Higher density cysts can be found occasionally.

Cardiac masses can arise from different origins. They may be vegetations or thrombi secondary to infection,

Table 6.4 Differentiation between pneumopericardium, pneumomediastinum, and pneumothorax

	Pneumopericardium	Pneumomediastinum	Pneumothorax
Relative frequency	Rare	Occasionally	Frequent
Configuration of gas	Broad band surrounding heart	Multiple thin, lucent streaks of air	Apical lucency (upright), medial basal lucency (supine), deep sulcus sign (supine)
Distribution	Limited to pericardium, as such outlines ascending aorta and main pulmonary artery but does not extend to aortic arch, along trachea or bronchi, or into the neck	Outlines mediastinal structures (aorta, airway, esophagus, pulmonary artery). Commonly extends into the neck	Less likely to outline mediastinal structures. Anteromedial (supine), apical (upright)
Position variable with patient position?	Yes	No	Yes
Associated findings	Thickening of pericardium Hydropneumopericardium		

mitral valve disease, myocardial infarction, or a hyper-coagulable state caused by an underlying condition. Cardiomyopathies can also present with a more prominent focal component in the myocardium, as such mimicking a primary cardiac mass. True neoplastic processes arising from the heart are rare and can be both benign and malign. Metastatic processes to the heart and pericardium are nevertheless 20–40 times more frequent than primary heart tumors (Miller et al. 2009).

Different imaging modalities today exist to visualize a mass in the heart and pericardium. On many occasions, a conventional chest radiograph will be one of the first examinations performed. Though this exam does not have the cross-sectional capabilities of more advanced techniques like CT and MRI, it can provide an initial assessment of the location of the mass and of its hemodynamic effects on the heart (Fig. 6.22a,b). Although it is beyond the scope of this chapter to give a detailed overview of the different cardiac and pericardiac masses, there are nevertheless some imaging signs suggestive of a cardiac mass (Table 6.5, adapted from Miller et al. [2009]). CT, MRI, and other modalities like ultrasound can be further used to differentiate between a primary

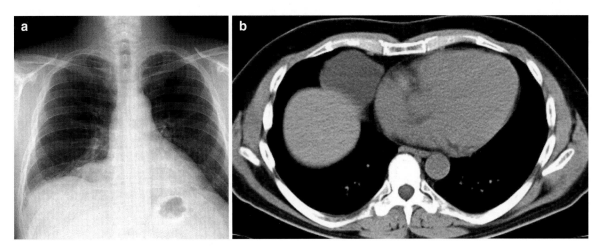

Fig. 6.21 An incidental finding in a 26-year-old man. (**a**) Conventional chest radiograph. (**b**) Non-enhanced multide-tector computed tomography (MDCT). There is an additional shadow in the right paracardial region (**a**), which on MDCT corresponds with a cystic structure located in the right paracar-dial fat. These findings are consistent with a pericardial cyst (Images courtesy of Dr. Philip Chappel, Jan Palfijn Ziekenhuis, Merksem, Belgium)

mass of the heart and an adjacent mediastinal process, and to evaluate its effect on the surrounding tissues (Fig. 6.22c,d). Though CT provides excellent anatomic detail of the investigated region, MRI has the additional benefit of providing both better tissue characterization and functional information.

6.5 The Postoperative Heart

Few organs have seen such an intensive and successful research in the development and implementation of innovative surgical techniques and various medical devices as the heart. Procedures like coronary artery

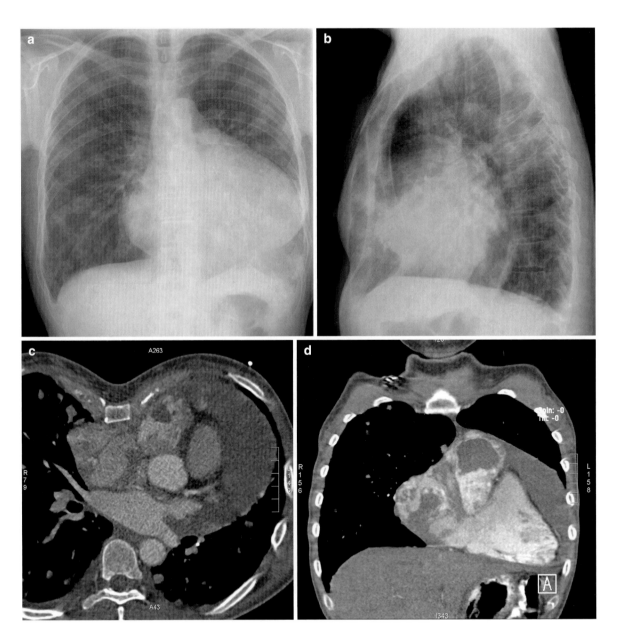

Fig. 6.22 A 56-year-old woman with an angiosarcoma of the heart. (**a** and **b**) Conventional chest radiograph. (**c** and **d**) Contrast-enhanced multidetector computed tomography (MDCT) images. An additional shadow is seen at the left heart border on conventional chest radiographs (**a** and **b**). Small nodular opacities can also be discerned in the lung parenchyma. Further investigation with contrast-enhanced MDCT (**c** and **d**) revealed an invasive angiosarcoma primary along the left heart border with lung metastasis (Images courtesy of Prof. Dr. J. Bogaert, UZ Gasthuisberg, Leuven, Belgium)

Table 6.5 Signs suggestive of a cardiac mass

Abnormal focal bulge of the heart contour
Apparent extrinsic displacement of the heart and great vessels
Pericardial effusion and/or pericardial thickening
Functional abnormalities
Intracavitary masses/filling defects
Asymmetric pulmonary edema due to pulmonary vein obstruction

bypass grafts (CABG), valve repair techniques using different kinds of valve prostheses, and the use numerous cardiac pacemakers and defibrillators are routinely encountered in almost any modern hospital. Furthermore, many devices such as left ventricular assist devices and intra-aortic balloon pumps are also increasingly being used for circulatory assistance. Therefore, it is imperative for a radiologist to become acquainted with the normal and abnormal findings after such interventions (Cascade et al. 1997; Hunter et al. 2004).

6.5.1 Cardiac Pacemakers and Implantable Cardioverter Defibrillators

There are a large number of medical electronic devices that assist with maintaining or improving heart function, as in controlling heart rhythm in patients who are at risk for rapid ventricular arrhythmias.

Both pacemakers and implantable cardioverter defibrillator (ICD) devices are permanently implanted devices consisting of a battery-operated electronic device with pacing wires or leads placed into the heart to generate electric impulses. Though pacemakers are usually used to regulate cardiac rate, ICDs are indicated for monitoring and therapy in patients who are at risk for sudden death resulting from ventricular fibrillation or tachycardia.

There are many varieties of pacemakers and ICDs and many ways of positioning the leads depending on the specific device and its intended function. Therefore, it is in many instances practically impossible for a radiologist who is unaware of the patient's specific condition to correctly establish the proper positioning of the leads (Hunter et al. 2004).

Chest radiographs are the most commonly used imaging method to visualize the position of the leads.

They can also demonstrate tip dislodgement, lead fractures, and device migration. Chest radiographs and fluoroscopy are still applied to look for pacemaker lead fractures, although nowadays this can also be achieved by electronic lead testing.

Although chest radiographs remain an important imaging tool in the evaluation of the correct positioning of pacemakers and ICDs, they lack the cross-sectional and three-dimensional capabilities of MSCT, for example for the evaluation of cardiac perforation or coronary sinus transection (Fig. 6.23a,b). However, MSCT has the significant disadvantage of beam-hardening artifacts at the electrode tip, which can complicate a correct evaluation of tip position (Fig. 6.23c,d).

6.5.2 Devices for Cardiopulmonary Support

Many devices for cardiopulmonary support are being used in mainstream and dedicated contemporary cardiovascular surgical centers, reflecting the pace of continuing innovation in this field during recent years. Most of these devices are used as a temporary device for circulatory assistance, like roller and centrifugal pumps during open heart surgery or afterwards as a short-term left ventricular assist device (Noon et al. 1995). As with pacemakers and ICDs, these devices are initially evaluated using conventional chest radiographs. Nevertheless, because they are normally applied in patients who are receiving acute clinical care, often only a portable chest radiograph taken in the intensive care unit is available. When complications are suspected, CT is often a problem-solving technique that can provide relevant answers in a single examination (Fig. 6.24a–f).

6.5.3 Coronary Artery Bypass Grafts

Conventional chest radiographs are always used in the follow-up of patients who have undergone CABG as an important parameter in the monitoring of the cardiovascular and pulmonary status. Though the findings on chest radiographs during the postoperative period have been well-documented by several authors (Narayan et al. 2005), this imaging modality is traditionally never used to asses the coronary bypass grafts. Conventional

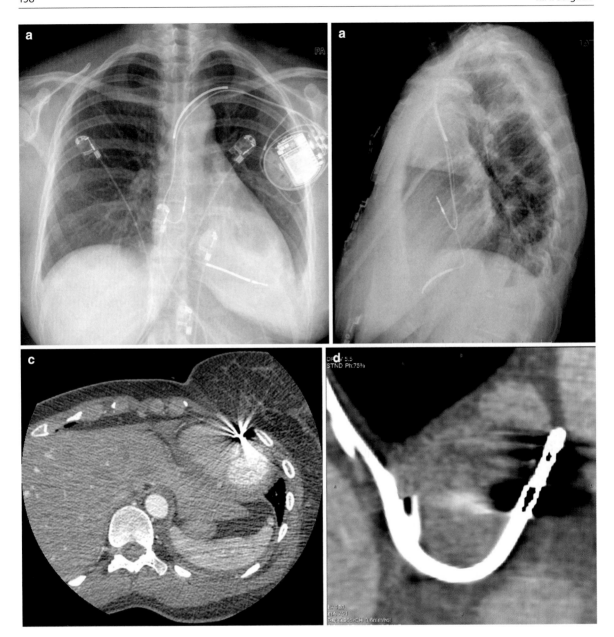

Fig. 6.23 A young woman with suspected pacemaker lead perforation. (**a** and **b**) Conventional chest radiograph. (**c** and **d**) Contrast-enhanced multidetector computed tomography (MDCT). The conventional radiographs reveal no clue regarding possible perforation with the pacemaker leads. On MDCT, the pacemaker tip at the apex of the right ventricle cannot be assessed correctly because of extensive artefacts (**c**). However, the lead at the right atrium can be better visualized, and it reveals a perforation of the right atrial wall (**d**)

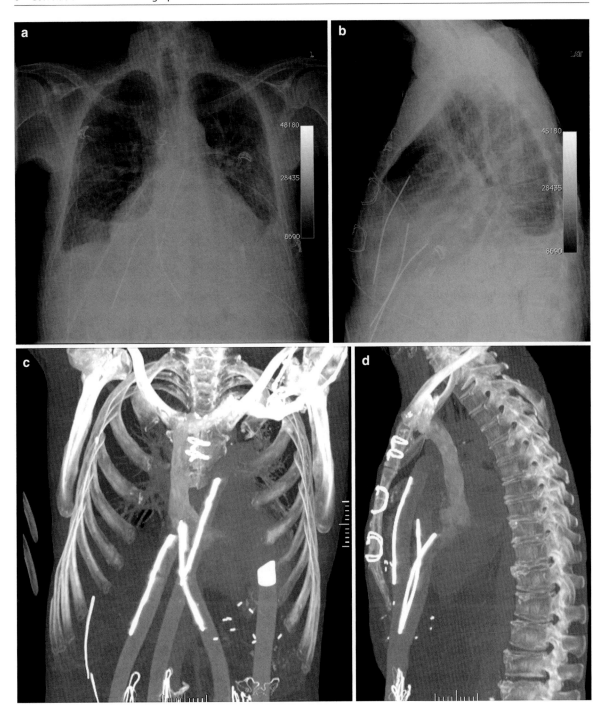

Fig. 6.24 A 68-year-old man with a left-ventricular assist device. (**a** and **b**) Conventional chest radiographs. (**c–f**) Contrast-enhanced multidetector computed tomography (MDCT) images. The chest radiographs show several bypasses from the left-ventricular assist device to the various cardiac chambers (**a** and **b**). The correct position of the bypasses is better assessed with MDCT (**c–e**), which further reveals an arterial leak adjacent to one of the bypasses (**f**, *arrow*) with subsequent development of a large hematoma

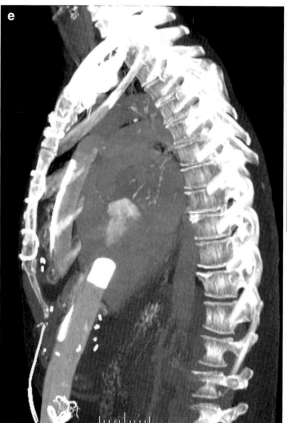

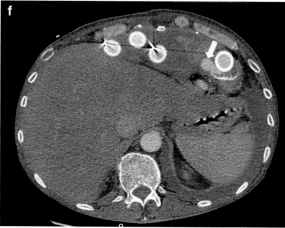

Fig. 6.24 (continued)

angiography used to be the only way to directly visualize the different arterial and venous coronary bypass grafts, but several authors have reported promising results using it to assess graft patency and dysfunction (Hamon et al. 2008). A comparison of chest radiographs and MSCT of CABG patients can provide a refreshing anatomic review of the most commonly used bypass techniques, which can help the radiologist correctly interpret the postoperative radiograph. Though the bypass grafts cannot be directly visualized on a chest radiograph, the position of the applied surgical clips can often indicate which coronary arteries have been bypassed and if an arterial and/or venous graft

was used (Fig. 6.25). Furthermore, conventional chest radiographs are often the first imaging modality to indicate a possible complication after surgery, prompting further investigation with MSCT (Fig. 6.26).

6.6 Conclusion

It has become evident that because of rapid changes in the noninvasive evaluation of the heart and coronary arteries with CT, many radiologists are becoming increasingly involved in the routine evaluation of this

Fig. 6.25 A 63-year old man with a coronary artery bypass graft. (**a** and **b**) Conventional chest radiographs. (**c–e**) Contrast-enhanced multidetector computed tomography (MDCT) images. The conventional chest images show multiple surgical clips along the course of the left internal mammary artery (LIMA)-left anterior descending (LAD) artery (*black arrow*) and venous-marginal bypass (*white arrow*). The course of the venous bypass

over the right coronary artery (RCA) is less obvious. The subsequent contrast-enhanced MDCT examination confirms the presence of an arterial LIMA-LAD bypass and a venous bypass to a marginal branch, both bypasses still patent. However, only the surgical clips along the course of the venous RCA bypass can be seen (*gray arrow*), with no opacification of the bridging vein indicating occlusion

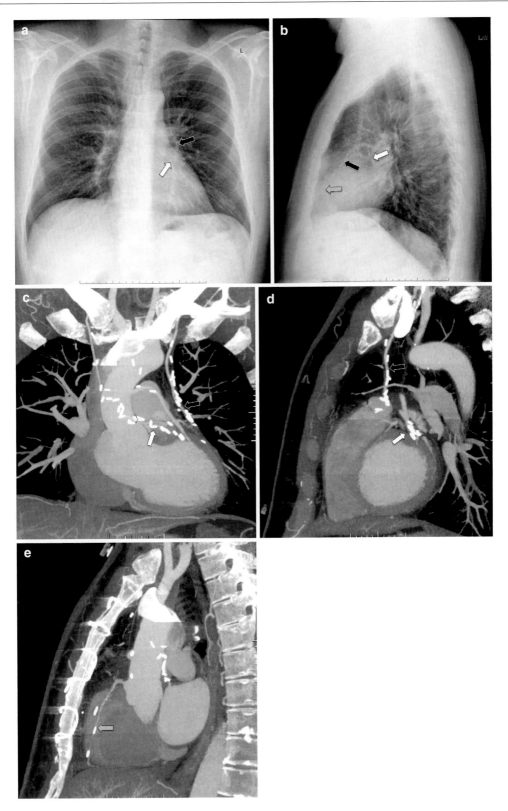

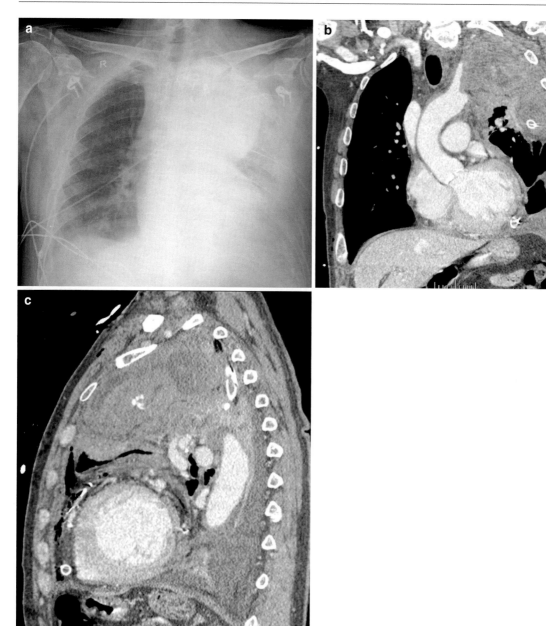

Fig. 6.26 A 65-year-old man with a sudden development of a mass in the left lung apex. (**a**) Conventional chest radiograph. (**b** and **c**) Contrast-enhanced multidetector computed tomography (MDCT) images. Two days after coronary artery bypass graft a rapidly evolving opacification was seen on a frontal chest radiograph (**a**). The suspected diagnosis at that time was an acute dissection of the aorta with subsequent rapid dilatation. However, MDCT clearly showed a postoperative hematoma with no aortic injury (**b** and **c**)

previously often neglected anatomic structure. However, it also represents a unique opportunity to refresh basic anatomic and pathophysiologic concepts of the heart, with subsequent better detection and understanding of normal and abnormal findings. The correlation of chest radiographs with CT is something that, with current picture archiving and communication systems, is increasingly available, and it provides an opportunity to become a more active player in the evaluation and management of a patient with cardiac disease.

References

Baron MG (2001) Correlation of plain films and MR of the heart. Int J Cardiovasc Imaging 17:453–456

Becker CR, Knez A, Jakobs TF et al (1999) Detection and quantification of coronary artery calcification with electron-beam and conventional CT. Eur Radiol 9:620–624

Bejvan SM, Godwin JD (1996) Pneumomediastinum: old signs and new signs. AJR Am J Roentgenol 166:1041–1048

Boxt LM (1999) Plain-film examination of the normal heart. Semin Roentgenol 34:169–180

Boxt LM, Reagan K, Katz J (1994) Normal plain film examination of the heart and great arteries in the adult. J Thorac Imaging 9:208–218

Budoff MJ, Georgiou D, Brody A et al (1996) Ultrafast computed tomography as a diagnostic modality in the detection of coronary artery disease: a multicenter study. Circulation 93:898–904

Cascade PN, Meaney JF, Jamadar DA (1997) Methods of cardiopulmonary support: a review for radiologists. Radiographics 17:1141–1155

Cerqueira MD, Weissman NJ, Dilsizian V et al (2002) Standardized myocardial segmentation and nomenclature for tomographic imaging of the heart: a statement for healthcare professionals from the Cardiac Imaging Committee of the Council on Clinical Cardiology of the American Heart Association. Circulation 105:539–542

Chen JT (1997) Radiographic anatomy. Essentials of cardiac imaging. Lippincott-Raven, Philadelphia

Cook AL, Hurwitz LM, Valente AM et al (2007) Right heart dilatation in adults: congenital causes. AJR Am J Roentgenol 189:592–601

Duerinckx AJ (2004) Plain film/MR imaging correlation in heart disease. Radiol Clin North Am 42:515–541, v–vi

Freundlich IM, Lind TA (1975) Calcification of the heart and great vessels. CRC Crit Rev Clin Radiol Nucl Med 6:171–216

Gowda RM, Boxt LM (2004) Calcifications of the heart. Radiol Clin North Am 42:603–617, vi–vii

Greil GF, Beerbaum P, Razavi R et al (2008) Imaging the right ventricle: non-invasive imaging. Heart 94:803–808

Hamon M, Lepage O, Malagutti P et al (2008) Diagnostic performance of 16- and 64-section spiral CT for coronary artery bypass graft assessment: meta-analysis. Radiology 247:679–686

Higgins C (1992) Essentials of cardiac radiology and imaging. JB Lippincott, Philadelphia

Higgins CB, Webb WR (2005) Thoracic imaging: pulmonary and cardiovascular radiology. Lippincott Williams and Wilkins, Philadelphia

Hunter TB, Taljanovic MS, Tsau PH et al (2004) Medical devices of the chest. Radiographics 24:1725–1746

JTT C (1997) Radiographic anatomy. essentials of cardiac imaging. Lippincott-Raven, Philadelphia

Lin FY, Devereux RB, Roman MJ et al (2008) Cardiac chamber volumes, function, and mass as determined by 64-multidetector row computed tomography: mean values among healthy adults free of hypertension and obesity. JACC Cardiovasc Imaging 1:782–786

Lipton MJ, Boxt LM (2004) How to approach cardiac diagnosis from the chest radiograph. Radiol Clin North Am 42:487–495, v

Mahnken AH, Wein BB, Sinha AM et al. (2009) Value of conventional chest radiography for the detection of coronary calcifications: Comparison with MSCT. Eur J Radiol 69:510–519

Maisch B, Seferovic PM, Ristic AD et al (2004) Guidelines on the diagnosis and management of pericardial diseases executive summary; The Task force on the diagnosis and management of pericardial diseases of the European society of cardiology. Eur Heart J 25:587–610

Maksimovic R, Seferovic PM, Ristic AD et al (2006) Cardiac imaging in rheumatic diseases. Rheumatology (Oxford) 45(Suppl 4):iv26–31

Miller SW, Boxt LM, Abbara S (2009) Cardiac imaging: the requisites, 3rd edn. Mosby/Elsevier, Philadelphia

Narayan P, Caputo M, Jones J et al (2005) Postoperative chest radiographic changes after on- and off-pump coronary surgery. Clin Radiol 60:693–699

Noon GP, Ball JW Jr, Papaconstantinou HT (1995) Clinical experience with BioMedicus centrifugal ventricular support in 172 patients. Artif Organs 19:756–760

Rose CP, Stolberg HO (1982) The limited utility of the plain chest film in the assessment of left ventricular structure and function. Invest Radiol 17:139–144

Rozenshtein A, Boxt LM (1999) Plain-film diagnosis of pericardial disease. Semin Roentgenol 34:195–204

Salgado RA, Shivalkar B, Parizel PM et al (2008) Left atrial calcifications: computed tomographic imaging findings of an unusual sign of rheumatic heart disease. J Comput Assist Tomogr 32:710–711

Souza AS, Bream PR, Elliott LP (1978) Chest film detection of coronary artery calcification. The value of the CAC triangle. Radiology 129:7–10

Vasan RS, Larson MG, Levy D et al (1997) Distribution and categorization of echocardiographic measurements in relation to reference limits: the Framingham Heart Study: formulation of a height- and sex-specific classification and its prospective validation. Circulation 96:1863–1873

Imaging of Hila and Pulmonary Vessels

7

Benoît Ghaye

Contents

Abstract

> Chest X-ray remains important to depict lesions located in hilar and pulmonary vessels, despite the variable accuracy of the technique. Whereas large hilar masses are easily identified, small lesions may be more difficult to detect. Knowledge and careful evaluation of hilar anatomy, however, yield significant information. There is a large variety of congenital and acquired diseases affecting the pulmonary vessels, which can be detected on chest X-ray. When the presence of a pulmonary vascular abnormality is suspected, computed tomography is invaluable because it allow analysis of the pulmonary vessels, the lung parenchyma, the heart, the pleura, the mediastinum, and the thoracic wall in a single examination.

7.1 Introduction

Although computed tomography (CT) plays a major role in the diagnostic workup of hilar and pulmonary vessels abnormalities, chest X-ray is important to depict lesions located in this area. The hila are often wrongly called abnormal when normal, and vice versa, due to the rather large variations in their normal aspect. Though large masses are easily identified, small lesions may be more difficult to detect. Knowledge and careful evaluation of hilar anatomy, however, yield significant information. Abnormalities of hilar anatomy can also be the

B. Ghaye
Department of Medical Imaging,
University Hospital of Liege, B35 Sart Tilman,
B–4000 Liege, Belgium
e-mail: bghaye@chu.ulg.ac.be

E.E. Coche et al. (eds.), *Comparative Interpretation of CT and Standard Radiography of the Chest*,
Medical Radiology, DOI: 10.1007/978-3-540-79942-9_7, © Springer-Verlag Berlin Heidelberg 2011

indirect indicator of a pathological process located elsewhere in the lung, such as an atelectasis. When the presence of a pulmonary vascular abnormality is detected on chest X-ray, CT is invaluable because it allows analysis of the pulmonary vessels, the lung parenchyma, the heart, the pleura, the mediastinum, and the thoracic wall at the same time.

7.2 Normal Anatomy

7.2.1 The Hila

The shadows of the hila on chest X-ray are mainly formed by the pulmonary arteries (PAs) and some of their main branches and the upper pulmonary veins (PVs). The wall of the bronchi accounts for little of the hilar opacity and the inferior PVs are usually too inferior to contribute to the hilar shadow. The hila are not symmetrical but contain the same basic structures on each side. In normal patients, lymph nodes, bronchial vessels, and nerves are too small, and fat and connective tissue are of insufficient quantity to contribute to the bulk of the hila (Felson 1973).

7.2.1.1 Frontal View

The main PA lies and bifurcates within the pericardial sac. It measures 4–5 cm in length and has a diameter of 3 cm. It is responsible for the middle arc on the left side of the mediastinum (sometimes together with the left PA).

Right Hilum

The right PA has a horizontal course to the right and divides within the mediastinum in two branches (Fig. 7.1). The upper branch (mediastinal PA of the right upper lobe [RUL] or truncus anterior) is directed obliquely and superiorly toward the RUL and supplies most of the pulmonary vasculature of this lobe. The mediastinal PA of the RUL contributes little to the opacity of the upper part of the right hilum because it arises inside the mediastinum. Nevertheless its recognition is important because its absence may suggest a right lobar atelectasis (Don and Hammond 1985).

The lower branch (right interlobar PA, also named intermediate arterial trunk or right descending PA) continues horizontally for 5–20 mm in the axis of the right PA, and then descends obliquely along the lateral

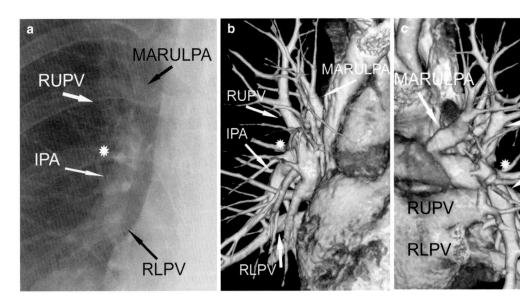

Fig. 7.1 Anatomy of the right hilum, frontal view. (**a**) Close-up view of the right hilum on a frontal chest X-ray. Correlation with computed tomography volume-rendering reformat, (**b**) anterior view, and (**c**) posterior view. *MARULPA*, main or mediastinal pulmonary artery (PA) of the right upper lobe; *IPA*, intermediate pulmonary artery; *RUPV*, right upper PV; *RLPV*, right lower PV (cutted in **c**). The *star* indicates the hilar angle

side of the bronchus intermedius. The right interlobar PA accounts for most of the right hilum shadow. The interlobar PA tapers as it branches inferiorly into the middle lobe (ML) and right lower lobe (RLL) PAs. Some branches (called ascending or fissural PA of the RUL) directed to the RUL may originate from the angle between the horizontal and descending part of the right interlobar PA (Yamashita 1978). Although those branches contribute to the arterial supply of the RUL in 90% of individuals, they may be difficult to recognize on chest X-ray due to their small size.

The right upper PV is located anteriorly to the hilar PAs and will superimpose on them. It forms the lateral margin of the right upper hilum. A shallow external angle ("hilar angle") is formed at the point where the right upper PV crosses the interlobar PA (Fig. 7.1). Its absence should raise the suspicion of a pathological process, either a lobar atelectasis or a hilar lesion (Don and Hammond 1985). The medial portion of the horizontal fissure often terminates at this angle.

Left Hilum

Contrary to the right side, the left PA arches over the left main bronchus and gives off usually two or three small PAs to the culmen of the left upper lobe (LUL) (Fig. 7.2). Thereafter it is called the left interlobar PA and descends posterolaterally to the left lower lobe (LLL) bronchus. This vessel tapers and branches as it extents inferiorly, but is less clearly seen compared with the right side, due in part to the superimposition of the heart shadow. Similar to the right side, the left upper PV is located anteriorly to the hilar PAs and will superimpose on them.

Tips and Tricks

Position: On frontal view, the right hilum cannot be located higher than the left. Indeed the left hilum is higher than the right in 97% of individuals and at the same level in the reminder (Fig. 7.3) (Felson 1973). A higher right hilum suggests a pathological process, i.e., atelectasis of the RUL or LLL.

Measurements: Measurements of hila are of uncertain usefulness because of large variations in the population. In roughly 84% both hila are equal in size, whereas the right can be larger than the left in 8%, and the left can be larger than the left in 8%. When needed, measurements may be obtained with reasonable accuracy at the level of the RLL PA. Its widest diameter should normally be 10–16 mm in men and 9–15 mm in women (Felson 1973).

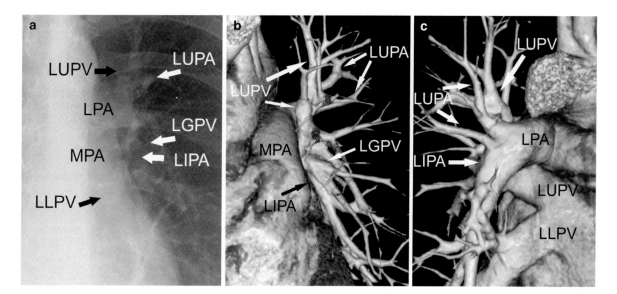

Fig. 7.2 Anatomy of the left hilum, frontal view. (**a**) Close-up view of the left hilum on a frontal chest X-ray. Correlation with computed tomography volume-rendering reformat, (**b**) anterior view, and (**c**) posterior view. *MPA*, main pulmonary artery (PA);

LUPA, left upper lobe PA; *LGPV*, lingular pulmonary vein (PV) (branch of left upper PV); *LIPA*, left intermediate PA; *LPA*, left PA; *LUPV*, left upper PV; *LLPV*, left lower PV

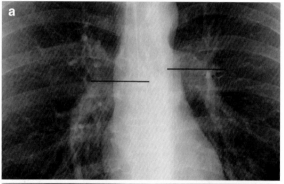

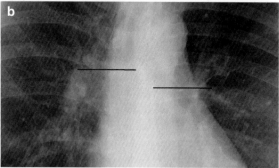

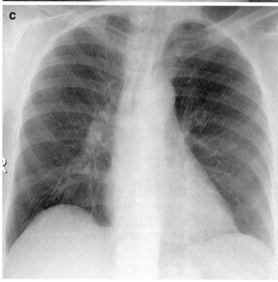

Fig. 7.3 Position of hila. (**a**) Normal position of both hila, the right being at a lower level than the left. (**b** and **c**) Abnormal position of the right hilum at a higher level than the left, in a patient with a history of radiation pneumonitis at the right lung apex caused by breast cancer treatment

Radiopacity: Opacity of both hila is similar in 91% of patients, whereas the right is more opaque in 6% and the left in 3%. All asymmetry of opacity should

raise the suspicion of a pathological process, i.e., a lesion located in or projecting on the more opaque hilum (Felson 1973).

Shape: Occasionally, the lower part of the right interlobar PA may appear rounded, mimicking a mass or enlarged lymph nodes. This is most commonly seen when lung volumes are low (Fig. 7.4).

The hilum convergence sign and hilum overlay sign are described in chapters 2 and 5.

7.2.1.2 Lateral View

Both hilar shadows are globally superimposed on the lateral chest X-ray, but specific parts of each hilum can be demonstrated around tracheal and bronchial radiolucencies. The tracheal air column ends caudally in a rounded lucency that represents the distal left main bronchus or the LUL bronchus. The RUL bronchus can be identified approximately 1–2 cm above the latter. Between the RUL and LUL bronchi that are seen end-on is a thin, vertical, white line that represents the posterior wall of the bronchus intermedius.

Right Hilum

The right PA and its central branches are located anteriorly to the major bronchi (Fig. 7.5). The right PA usually does not contribute to the hilar shadow because it is surrounded by mediastinal fat. Therefore most of the right hilum shadow on the lateral view is formed by the right interlobar PA, the mediastinal PA of the RUL, and the right upper PV, which form a large opacity that should not be confused with a mass (the left upper PV is also superimposed on the right hilum shadow) (Genereux 1983). This oval-shaped opacity is in contact with the intermediate bronchus posteriorly and the ML bronchus inferiorly.

Left Hilum

The left PA forms a comma-shaped opacity above and posterior to the lucency of the left main or LUL bronchus, parallel to but at distance below the aortic arch (Fig. 7.5).

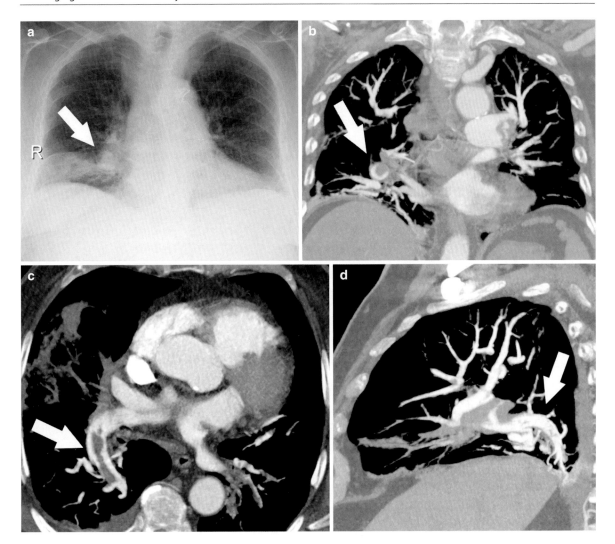

Fig. 7.4 Nodular pattern of pulmonary arteries on frontal view. (**a–d**) A 27-mm nodule (*arrows*) is depicted in the right infrahilar area on the frontal view. (**a**) Such a finding may be due to a lower lobe pulmonary artery presenting with horizontal course when a patient presents with severe hypoventilation or ascension of a hemidiaphragm. In the present case, acute pulmonary embolism is responsible for further dilation of the corresponding pulmonary artery (**b–d**)

Right and left interlobar PAs may be superimposed or not, based on the degree of inflation of lower lobes.

Inferior Hilar Window

Right and left hila form an inverted horseshoe–shaped shadow around central bronchi that is interrupted in its lower part by an area called the *inferior hilar window*. The inferior hilar window area corresponds to the area delineated by the projection of angles between the ML and the RLL bronchi on the right side, and the LUL and LLL bronchi on the left (Fig. 7.5). Normally there should be no large vessels traversing this triangular area. Therefore any opacity of more than 1 cm projecting over this zone is likely to be a mass or lymphadenopathy, with accuracy around 90% (Park et al. 1991). Such pathological processes may result in the appearance of a complete circular shadow around the central bronchi, which has been termed the "doughnut sign" (Andronikou and Wieselthaler 2004; Marshall et al. 2006) (Fig. 7.6). The side of the

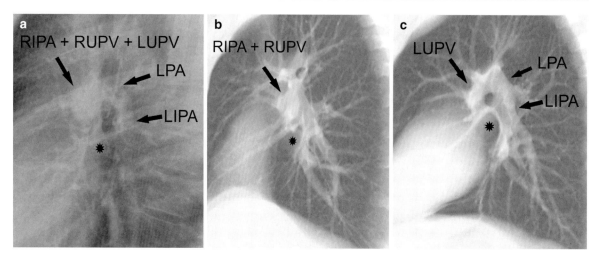

Fig. 7.5 Anatomy of the hila on lateral view, (**a**) Correlation with computed tomography MPR reformat, (**b**) on right hilum, and (**c**) MPR on left hilum. The *star* indicates the inferior hilar window. *LIPA,* left intermediate pulmonary artery (PA); *LPA* left PA; *LUPV,* left upper pulmonary vein (PV); *RIPA,* right intermediate PA; *RUPV,* right upper PV

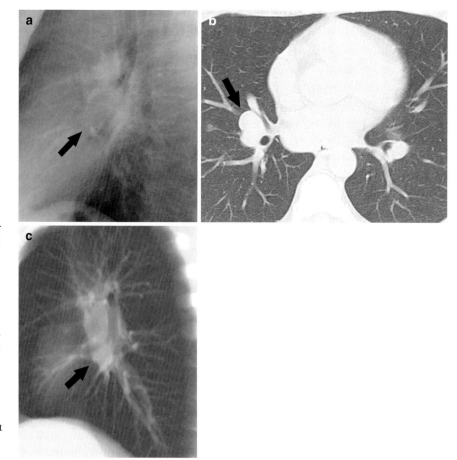

Fig. 7.6 Doughnut sign. Disappearance of the inferior hilar window on lateral chest X-ray (**a**), resulting in a complete circular shadow around the central bronchi ("Doughnut sign"). Computed tomography (**b**) confirmed that this was the result of a 13-mm lymphadenopathy located lateral to the middle lobe bronchus (*arrows*). Lateral view thick multiplanar reformat (**c**) shows filling of the space below the middle lobe bronchus and in front of right lower bronchus, namely the infrahilar window

anomaly may, however, be difficult to determine on the lateral view, but if the anterior wall of a lower lobe bronchus is visible as a linear shadow, the mass must be on the opposite side. Also, a frontal chest X-ray may help.

7.2.2 Pulmonary Veins

As previously mentioned, the upper PVs are superimposed on the hilar PA shadows on the frontal view and on the right PAs on the lateral view (Figs. 7.1–7.3). On frontal view, the right lower PV is depicted as a horizontal, slightly oblique vascular shadow crossing the PAs of the RLL and the shadow of the right atrium. The left lower PV presents with the same pattern and topography but is more difficult to demonstrate because of superimposition of the heart shadow. It may be slightly higher and posterior than the right, or it may join the left upper PV to form a common confluent (Genereux 1983; Ghaye et al. 2003).

Two particular patterns are noteworthy. On the frontal view, confluence of the PVs may occasionally be prominent and present as a convex paramediastinal opacity. This pattern is seen more frequently but not exclusively on the right in 5–27% of individuals and should not be confused with a mediastinal mass (Felson 1973; Genereux 1983) (Fig. 7.7). On the lateral view, confluence of inferior PVs may simulate a mass inferiorly to the inferior hilar window (Fig. 7.7).

7.2.3 Intrapulmonary Vessels

Pulmonary blood vessels are responsible for linear branching markings within the lungs. There are wide differences in the appearance of the pulmonary vasculature between individuals and depend on age, body habitus, and technical parameters (Felson 1973). Contrary to CT, PAs are not easily differentiated from PVs on chest X-rays. It is usually not possible to distinguish both types of vessels in the outer two thirds of the lungs. Some findings, however, may help.

Orientation: Centrally, in the lower lung zones, the orientation of PVs is more horizontal and PAs more vertical. In the upper zones, PAs and PVs show both a similar gentle curve to the hilum, although PVs may show a wider arc to the hilum.

Relation with bronchi: PAs are in close contact with their accompanying bronchi, whereas PVs are intersegmental and therefore not in contact with bronchi. As shown on CT, in the RUL and culmen PAs are internal to their bronchi; they are external in the lingula, ML, and lower lobes. PVs are external to bronchoarterial bundles in upper lobes and internal in other lobes. The relationship between PAs and bronchi can only be shown on chest X-ray when both structures are seen end-on, resulting in the "double circles" (one white and one black) pattern. Unfortunately, the anterior or posterior segmental PAs and bronchi of upper lobes are the more frequently depicted but are seen only in 50% of individuals (Fig. 7.8). Peripheral PAs (segmental, subsegmental) should have a diameter similar to that of their accompanying bronchus.

Pattern of bifurcation: PVs may show a pattern of bifurcation that may be slightly different from PAs. PA divisions are considered to be more regularly dichotomous and proportional and have a more acute angle than PVs. As a result, the size of PVs may be larger compared with PAs in the lung periphery. However, those findings should be used cautiously because of inconstancies.

7.3 Pulmonary Vascular Diseases

This chapter will review the main pulmonary vascular diseases affecting the "macroscopic" pulmonary vessels. Some "microscopic" pulmonary vascular diseases are presented in Chap. 8. All pathologies would benefit from a complete workup with CT or magnetic resonance imaging (MRI) but most are readily detectable on chest X-ray.

7.3.1 Congenital Diseases

Congenital diseases affecting the PVs are more frequent than those affecting the PAs. Although variations of the number of PVs are frequent, there is invariably one PA per side in normal individuals.

7.3.1.1 Absence of a Pulmonary Artery

Unilateral "absence" of a PA is better termed "interruption" of a PA because branches of the "absent" PA are

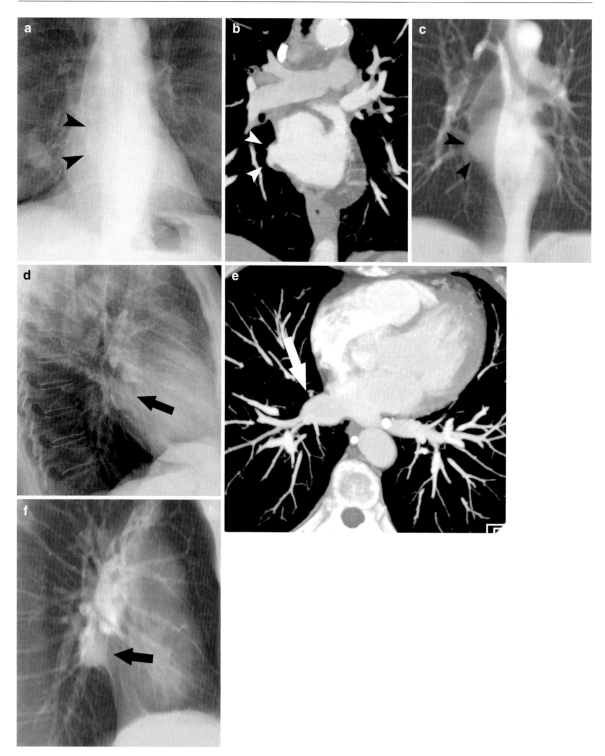

Fig. 7.7 Particular patterns of pulmonary veins (**a–c**). On the frontal view (**a**), confluence of pulmonary veins on the right side may present as a convex paramediastinal and retrocardiac opacity (*arrowheads*). Thin (**b**) and thick (**c**) multiplanar reformats (MPRs) confirm the venous origin of this finding, which should not be confused with a mediastinal mass. On the lateral view (**d**), confluence of pulmonary veins may simulate a mass inferiorly to the inferior hilar window, as confirmed on axial computed tomography section (**e**) and thick MPR (**f**) (*arrows*)

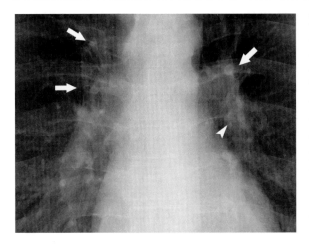

Fig. 7.8 Relation between pulmonary arteries and bronchi. Pulmonary arteries are always in close contact with their accompanying bronchi. In the right upper lobe and culmen, pulmonary arteries are internal to their bronchi (*arrows*), whereas they are external in the remaining lobes, here the superior segment of the left lower lobe (*arrowhead*). The relationship between pulmonary arteries and bronchi can only be seen on chest X-ray when both structures are viewed end-on, resulting in the "double circles" (*one white* and *one black*) pattern

present in the hilum distally to the short proximal atresia (Morgan et al. 1991). It is a rare disease more frequently found on the right side, and is found as an isolated finding in most instances. When occurring on the left side, it may be associated with various cardiovascular abnormalities as a right-sided aortic arch and tetralogy of Fallot (Ten Harkel et al. 2002). The involved lung is frequently hypoplastic but lobation, number of segments, and bronchial anatomy are normal. Collateral systemic arterial supply develops from birth to adulthood and may be responsible for hemoptysis in 10–20% of patients, which may be life threatening. Pulmonary hypertension is found in 25–40% of patients and is one of the most important determinants of the prognosis. Other symptoms include recurrent pulmonary infections, mild dyspnea, or limited tolerance for exercise. Mortality rate is 7% and surgery, either pneumectomy or revascularization, is indicated in up to 15% of patients (Ten Harkel et al. 2002). Chest X-ray shows a small ipsilateral lung, depicted as a diaphragmatic elevation with the heart and mediastinum shifted towards the affected side and contralateral lung hyperinflation (Morgan et al. 1991). The ipsilateral hilum is small or absent and pulmonary vascular markings are grossly diminished, whereas the contralateral

hilum and lung blood volume are frequently increased as they drain the entire right cardiac output. The affected lung may be hyperlucent (with no air-trapping) or show mild to extensive opacities (Fig. 7.9). Although best seen on CT, reticular opacities (and bronchial wall thickening) reflect the systemic arteries to PAs shunts, which may be associated with pleural thickening and evidence of rib notching due to hypertrophied transpleural collateral vessels (Morgan et al. 1991; Ryu et al. 2004). Bronchiectasis or fibrotic changes secondary to recurrent infections may be seen (Fig. 7.9). Differential diagnosis includes fibrosing mediastinitis, Takayasu arteritis, and Swyer-James syndrome. The absence of more distal branches of a PA has been also exceptionally reported (Ryu et al. 2008).

7.3.1.2 Left Pulmonary Artery Sling

Rarely, the left PA originates from the posterior wall of the right PA and then turns to the left, passing between the trachea and the esophagus to join the left hilum, forming a "sling" around the distal trachea. Two types have been described. Type 1 is an isolated anomaly, usually asymptomatic and incidentally discovered in adulthood. Type 2 is diagnosed in children and is associated with tracheal stenosis and cardiovascular or lung anomalies ("ring-sling" complex) (Siripornpitak et al. 1997). Symptoms include stridor, apneic spells, hypoxia, dysphagia, and repeated pulmonary infections. Chest x-ray may be normal. On frontal chest X-ray, the anomalous PA may be seen as a right suprahilar opacity or right mediastinal enlargement in the region of the azygos arch (Fig. 7.10). Repercussions on airways may be seen as a leftward deviation and right-sided compression of the distal trachea, a low carina at the level T5–T7 presenting with "inverted T" flat bronchial division pattern, and hyperinflation or consolidation of the right pulmonary lobes due to right-sided bronchi compression. The left hilum may be located at a lower level than usual because the pulmonary artery reaches the hilum in a more caudal location (Procacci et al. 1993). It should be differentiated from right-sided adenopathy, bronchogenic cyst, or azygo-caval continuation (Procacci et al. 1993). On a lateral view, the detection of a mass located between the distal trachea and esophagus must lead to suspicion of a left PA sling. The most specific finding is seen after opacification of the esophagus on lateral

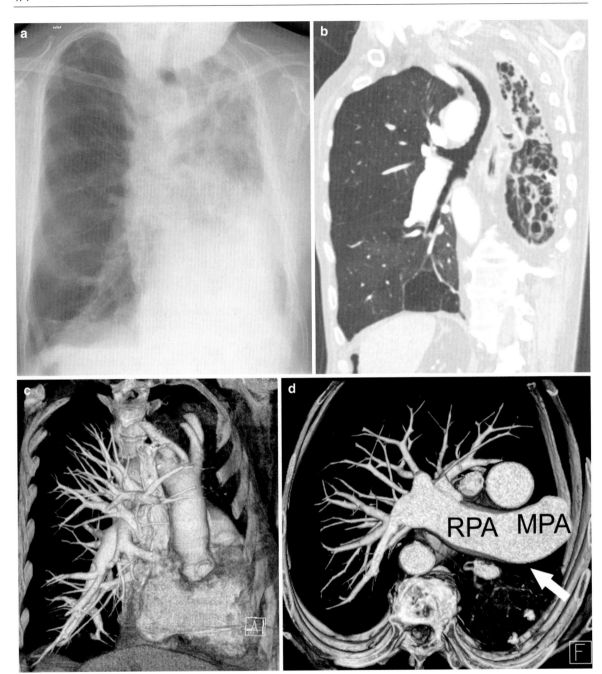

Fig. 7.9 Proximal interruption of the left pulmonary artery. Proximal interruption of the left pulmonary artery in a 75-year-old man presenting with recurrent pulmonary infections in the left lung. Frontal chest X-ray (**a**), multiplanar reformat (**b**), and volume rendering technique frontal (**c**) and axial (**d**) show a small left lung, depicted as left diaphragmatic elevation, with the heart and mediastinum shifted towards the left side, and right lung hyperinflation. The aortic arch is right-sided. The main and right-sided pulmonary arteries are dilated, indicating pulmonary hypertension. The left lung shows extensive fibrotic changes and bronchiectases due to repeated pulmonary infections. The *arrow* in (**d**) indicates the theoretical origin of the absent left pulmonary artery. In (**d**), the *red-colored lacing* in the left lung represents dilated systemic arteries originating from bronchial and nonbronchial systemic arteries. *MPA*, main pulmonary artery; *RPA*, right pulmonary artery

fluoroscopy demonstrating a pulsating mass between the carina anteriorly and esophagus posteriorly. This is different from systemic vascular ring compression that is located posterior to the esophagus (Procacci et al.

1993; Berdon 2000). Differences in PA caliber, flow, and lung perfusion between both sides (up to four times superior for the right side) have been reported (Siripornpitak et al. 1997).

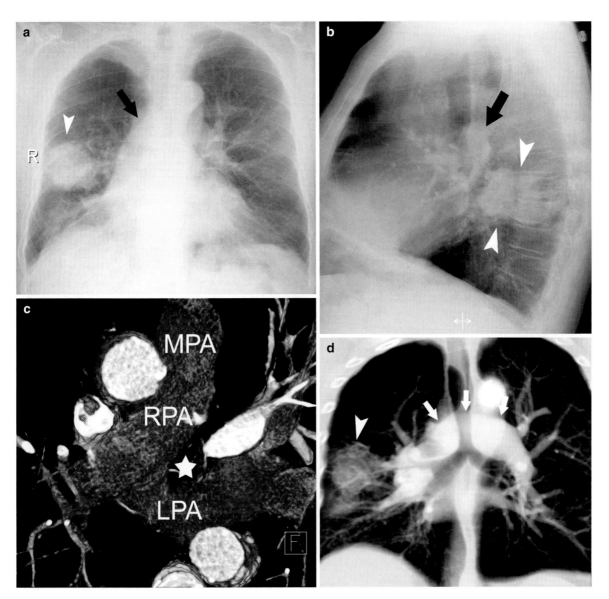

Fig. 7.10 Left pulmonary artery sling. Left pulmonary artery sling in a 75-year-old man investigated for lung cancer. The lung tumor is responsible for the nodular opacity located in the right lower lobe (*arrowheads* in **a**, **b**, and **d**). On axial computed tomography view (**c**) the left pulmonary artery (PA) originates from the posterior aspect of the right PA and then turns to the left, passing between the trachea (indicated by a *star* in **c**) and the esophagus to join the left hilum. On frontal chest X-ray (**a**) the anomalous PA is seen as a right mediastinal enlargement in the region of the azygos arch (*arrow*). The most specific finding is seen on the lateral view (**b**), demonstrating a rounded opacity (*arrow*) posterior to the distal trachea that is slightly compressed posteriorly. The *arrows* on the frontal thick multiplanar reformat (MPR) (**d**) delineate the superior aspect of the left PA. Sagittal thick multiplanar reformat (MPR) reformat (**e**) demonstrates a posterior compression of the distal trachea (*arrowhead*) by the left PA (*arrow*). *LPA*, left pulmonary artery; *MPA*, main pulmonary artery; *RPA*, right pulmonary artery

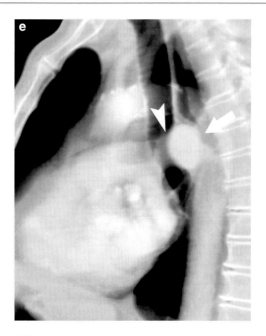

Fig. 7.10 (continued)

7.3.1.3 Idiopathic Dilation of the Main Pulmonary Artery

Idiopathic dilation of the pulmonary arteriys is a rare and probably congenital anomaly that involves abnormal enlargement of the pulmonary trunk, with or without dilatation of right and left PAs. Imaging features are similar to true aneurysm of the main PA found in older patients (Fig. 7.11). It is usually benign and nonprogressive, and patients, mostly young women, are generally asymptomatic (Ring and Marshall 2002). Therefore, it is usually fortuitously found on chest X-ray as a focal bulge of the left middle arc, caudal to the aortic arch and cephalad to the LMB. In some cases, the right and left PAs may be enlarged, but peripheral PA and heart size are normal. Concomitant dilation or hypoplasia of the ascending aorta has been reported (Ugolini et al. 1999). It remains, however, a diagnosis of exclusion; any pulmonary and cardiac diseases have to be excluded (particularly pulmonary valve stenosis), and pressure in the right ventricle and PAs should be normal. Complications including dissection or compression of adjacent structures have been exceptionally reported, confirming that appropriate follow-up is mandatory (Ugolini et al. 1999; Ring

and Marshall 2002). It should be differentiated from other diseases associated with dilation of the main PA, such as pulmonary valve stenosis, pulmonary hypertension, pulmonary embolism, PA tumor, adenopathy, and anterior mediastinal tumor.

7.3.1.4 Pulmonary Arteriovenous Malformations

Pulmonary arteriovenous malformations (PAVMs) are real arteriovenous (right-to-left) shunts, meaning that there is no capillary between the PA and PV. The connection between the PA and PV is frequently dilated (aneurismal sac or dilated and tortuous connection). PAVMs may be congenital (Rendu–Weber–Osler disease or hereditary hemorrhagic telengectasia [HHT] syndrome) or less commonly acquired (i.e., hepatopulmonary syndrome). They may be isolated or multiple, particularly in the HHT disease, and are more frequently found in lower lung zones (Gossage and Kanj 1998). They may be simple, meaning that a single segmental artery feeds the malformation, or complex (multiple segmental feeding arteries). Although the proportions of both types are highly variable in the literature, it is considered that 80–90% is of the simple type (White et al. 1983; Haitjema et al. 1995).

Patients are often asymptomatic but may present with systemic oxygen desaturation, particularly when in the erect position (orthodeoxia), or with heart failure when the shunt is large (Gossage and Kanj 1998). Typically, PAVMS may be associated with complications such as ischemic or infectious paradoxical emboli (notably in the brain) due to absence of pulmonary capillarfilter, or hemorrhage (hemoptysis, hemothorax) due to rupture of the sac.

On chest X-ray, PAVMs manifest as 1- to 5-cm, sharply defined lung nodules, usually with a lobulated contour. The key finding is the demonstration of large serpiginous feeding artery(ies) and draining vein(s) when the PAVMs are peripheral, a finding more difficult to depict in central lesions (Fig. 7.12). Calcifications are exceptional and surrounding tissue is usually normal. CT is the method of choice for the diagnostic workup of PAVMs before treatment by vaso-occlusion. A feeding artery larger than 3 mm in diameter is considered to be an indication for treatment.

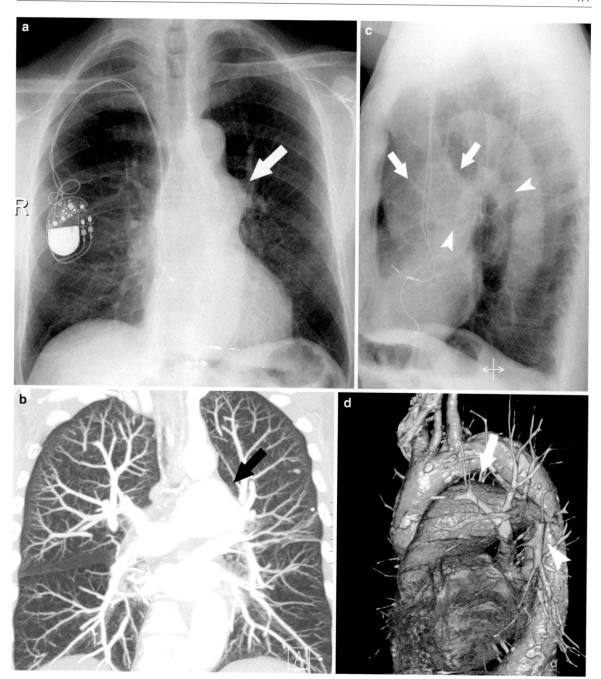

Fig. 7.11 Aneurysm of the main pulmonary artery (PA). Idiopathic dilation of the main PA known for many years in 79-year-old man. Frontal chest X-ray (**a**) demonstrates an abnormal bulge (*arrow*) of the left middle mediastinal arc. Maximum intensity projection frontal view (**b**) shows that dilation of the main PA (*arrow*) is responsible for this bulge. Lateral chest X-ray (**c**) shows an ill-defined opacity in the area of the main PA (*arrows*) whereas the size of right and left PAs is normal (*arrowheads*). Volume rendering technique lateral-view reformat (**d**) confirms abnormal enlargement of the main pulmonary trunk (*arrow*), with only mild dilation of left PAs (*arrowhead*). Pulmonary arterial pressure was normal and no cardiac disease was detected during echocardiography. Note that the retrosternal anterior bulge in (**c**) is due to the ascending aorta

Fig. 7.12 Pulmonary arteriovenous malformations
(PAVMs). Lingular complex
PAVM in a 26-year-old woman.
Close-up view on frontal chest
X-ray (**a**) shows a 3-cm
arteriovenous malformation
(*star*) connected to the left
hilum by two feeding arteries
(*arrow* and *arrowheads*) and
one large draining vein (*thick
arrow*). Findings are confirmed
on the axial computed
tomography sections (**b**),
superior-view three-dimensional
shaded surface display (**c**), and
slightly oblique frontal digital
angiography (**d**)

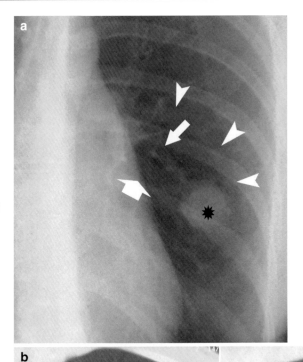

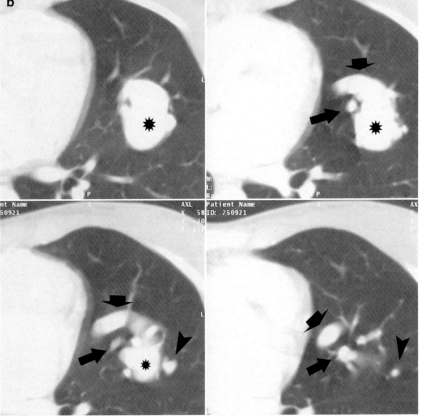

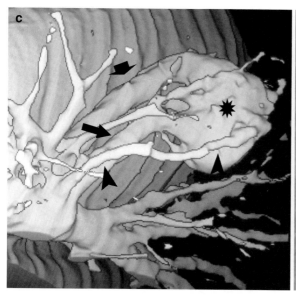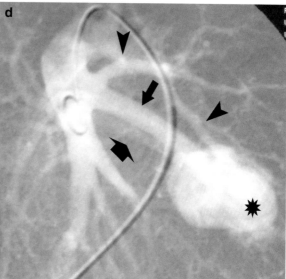

Fig. 7.12 (continued)

7.3.1.5 Anomalies of Pulmonary Veins

Congenital anomalies of the PVs can be conveniently classified into the following categories: (a) anomalous pulmonary venous drainage or return (APVR) with or without abnormal course in the lung, (b) anomalous pulmonary venous course without abnormal connection, or (c) abnormal venous diameters including varicosities, stenoses, and atresia (Remy-Jardin and Remy 1999). Overlapping conditions between categories may exist.

Anomalous Drainage

Partial anomalous pulmonary venous returns (PAPVRs) are congenital malformations in which a portion of the PVs drains into the right atrium or one of its tributaries, resulting in a left-to-right shunt (Ghaye and Couvreur 2009). PAPVRs occur on the right side twice as often as the left. PAPVRs are generally asymptomatic and are discovered incidentally, but some will present with a large left-to-right shunt that requires surgery. Detection is particularly important in patients undergoing contralateral lung surgery; a PAPVR may drain a significant amount of the cardiac output and may require reimplantation. CT is currently considered to be the first-line technique in the workup of PAPVRs because it evidences the anomalous vein and its drainage and shows associated tracheobronchial, lung, or vascular abnormalities, but some may be depicted on the chest X-ray.

Anomalous Drainage Without Anomalous Course

Chest X-ray findings will depend on the configuration of the PAPVR and the degree of the left-to-right shunt. Associated atrial septal defect is not uncommon. Chest X-ray is usually normal but may show the uncommon course, often crescent-shaped, of the anomalous vein that is frequently dilated. The anomalous PV usually drains to the nearest systemic vein, often the superior vena cava (SVC) on the right side and the left brachiocephalic vein on the left. Right-sided PAPVR is easier to detect on chest X-ray because an abnormal mediastinal contour due to dilation of the vein collecting the PAPVR, i.e., the azygos arch or SVC, may be demonstrated (Posniak et al. 1993; Haramati et al. 2003). Left-sided PAPVR draining into the left brachiocephalic vein may mimic a left-sided SVC (Ghaye and Couvreur 2009) (Fig. 7.13). Larger shunts may result in signs of right heart and pulmonary artery enlargement and pulmonary congestion (Kalke et al. 1967; Saalouke et al. 1977).

Anomalous Drainage with Anomalous Course

PAPVRs with anomalous courses are easier to depict than those without anomalous courses. Anomalous drainage in the inferior vena cava (IVC), also known as the *Halasz syndrome,* represents 3–5% of all PAPVRs. The Halasz syndrome often but not always includes a spectrum of associated anomalies: abnormal lobation of the right lung with mediastinal shift to the right (hypogenetic right lung syndrome), dextroposition of

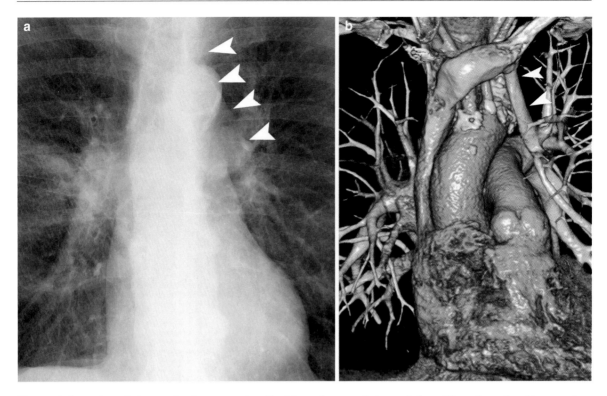

Fig. 7.13 Anomalous drainage of pulmonary veins. Partial anomalous pulmonary venous return of the left upper lobe in a 72-year-old patient. Frontal chest X-ray (**a**) shows an abnormal and oblique left mediastinal border directing upward and crossing the left hilum and the aortic arch (*arrowheads*). Frontal-view volume rendering technique (**b**) confirms that this anomalous border (*arrowheads*) is due to the lateral margin of an anomalous pulmonary venous return of the left upper lobe into the left brachiocephalic vein, which is dilated

the heart, a small right PA and large left PA in half of patients, systemic arterial supply originating from the abdominal aorta, and other tracheal, bronchial, diaphragmatic, or cardiovascular malformations (cysts or diverticula, bronchiectasis) (Mathey et al. 1968; Dupuis et al. 1992).

Halasz syndrome is also known as the *scimitar syndrome* because of the demonstration of the "Turkish curved sword" pattern of the anomalous PV. On frontal chest X-ray, the anomalous PV shows a gently curved tubular shadow from the right mid-lung toward the internal part of the right diaphragm, which gets larger as it progress caudally (Fig. 7.14). The "scimitar sign" on chest X-ray may be absent or overlooked in more than 50% of patients at initial presentation and should be searched for carefully when the right hemithorax is small and hyperlucent (Dupuis et al. 1992). It should be differentiated from the meandering vein that has normal connection with the left atrium.

Anomalous Course Without Anomalous Drainage

Any dilated PV showing an anomalous course in the lung does not represent a PAPVR. In particular, any scimitar-shaped opacity located in the right paracardiac area is not pathognomonic of APVR in the IVC (Blake et al. 1965). The whole right pulmonary venous return may present as a varicose venous dilatation with an anomalous scimitar-like course before entering the left atrium. Such abnormality results in a dilated vessel, which may simulate vascular malformation of a nodule on chest X-ray (Ghaye and Couvreur 2009). It has been called pseudo-scimitar syndrome, but should be better termed "meandering vein" or "wandering vein" to avoid confusion. Such anomaly may nevertheless be associated with other malformations that arealso found in the scimitar syndrome (Agarwal et al. 2004; Furuya et al. 2007). Therefore, scimitar syndrome and meandering vein cannot be differentiated by mean of chest X-ray alone.

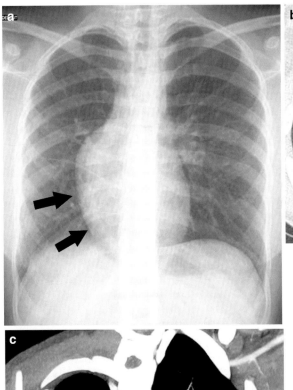

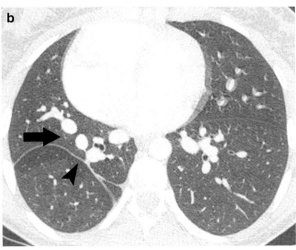

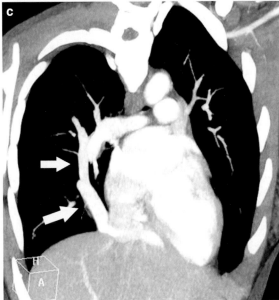

Fig. 7.14 Scimitar syndrome. Partial anomalous pulmonary venous return with abnormal course into the inferior vena cava (Scimitar syndrome) in a 20-year-old woman presenting with palpitations. Frontal chest X-ray (**a**), axial computed tomography (CT) (**b**), and curved-multiplanar reformat (**c**) show a small right hemithorax, small right hilum, and dextroposition of the heart. The anomalous vein (*arrows*) presents with a vertical and oblique course behind the right heart and drains into the supradiaphragmatic part of the inferior vena cava. CT also shows anomalous lobation of the right lung (*arrowhead* in **b**) (Case from the Club Thorax, courtesy of Jacques Giron, Toulouse France)

Anomalous Caliber

Congenital anomalies of the PVs presenting with abnormal diameter can be classified as stenosis, atresia, or varices. Congenital PV stenosis is frequently associated with cardiovascular abnormalities that dominate the imaging pattern in childhood, although cases of primary PV stenosis revealed later in life are reported (Latson and Prieto 2007). Pulmonary varix is defined as a localized enlargement or an aneurysmal dilatation of a segment of a PV that drains normally into the left atrium. Pulmonary varix is generally considered to be congenital, but mitral valvular disease was noted in 26–33% of patients in some studies (Asayama et al. 1984; Andrikakos et al. 2004). Symptoms are unusual, but rare cases of dyspnea or hemoptysis have been reported. Exceptional complications include rupture or systemic embolism consecutive to in situ thrombosis. According to imaging, pulmonary varix can be morphologically classified as saccular, tortuous, and confluent types. Pulmonary varices are preferentially located in the right lower lobe (RLL) (60%). Such a lesion is a fortuitous finding at chest X-ray and appears as a mass with smooth, well-defined, and sometimes lobulated margins, similar to coin lesions of various origins (Andrikakos et al. 2004) (Fig. 7.15). CT and magnetic resonance imaging (MRI) provide the correct diagnosis.

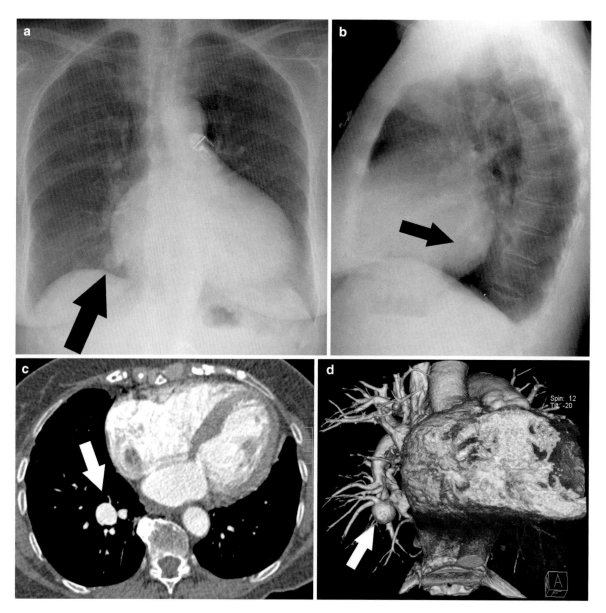

Fig. 7.15 Pulmonary varix. Pulmonary varix in an 83-year-old woman presenting with cardiac failure secondary to persistent atrial fibrillation. The chest X-ray (**a** and **b**) demonstrate an enlarged heart and a 15 mm right paracardiac nodular opacity (*arrow*). Axial contrast-enhanced computed tomography (**c**), and almost frontal view volume rendering technique (**d**) reformatting demonstrate a sacciform vascular structure (*arrows*) measuring 18 mm of great axis that expanded from the inferior root of the right inferior pulmonary vein

7.3.2 Acquired Diseases

Acquired diseases responsible for increased or decreased size of pulmonary vessels are numerous. Some diseases may result in both dilation and stenosis of pulmonary vessels (Tables 7.1 and 7.2). Pulmonary embolism (PE) and pulmonary hypertension are presented in Chap. 18.

Table 7.1

Causes of focal or diffuse dilation of pulmonary vessels
Pulmonary hypertension
Left-to-right shunt (intracardiac, persistant ductus arteriosus, etc.)
Pulmonary valve or pulmonary artery stenosis
Pulmonary embolism
Pulmonary artery aneurysm
Pulmonary artery pseudoaneurysm (mycotic, trauma, etc.)
Dissecting aneurysm
Idiopathic dilation of pulmonary artery
Vasculitis (Takayasu arteritis, Behçet disease, Hughes-Stovin disease, Giant cell arteritis, Williams Syndrome, etc.)
Pulmonary arteriovenous malformations
Pulmonary varice
Pulmonary artery primary tumor or metastasis
Marfan syndrome
Cystic medial necrosis

Table 7.2

Causes of decreased size of pulmonary vessels
Congenital disease resulting in lung hypoplasia
Congenital heart disease (Tetralogy of Fallot, pulmonary atresia, etc.)
Proximal interruption of a pulmonary artery
Compression or invasion (bronchogenic carcinoma, fibrosing mediastinitis, aortic aneurysm, sarcoidosis, etc.)
Pulmonary embolism, particularly chronic
Vasculitis (particularly Takayasu arteritis, Behçet disease, Wegener granulomatosis, connective tissue disorders, etc.)
Ipsilateral bronchial or parenchymal disease
Atelectasis
Postradiofrequency ablation of atrial fibrillation

7.3.2.1 Pulmonary Aneurysm

Aneurysms or pseudoaneurysms are much rarer in PAs than in other locations, e.g., the aorta. Pulmonary aneurysms are focal enlargement of the PAs. Causes of focal or diffuse dilatation of pulmonary vessels are presented in Table 7.1.

Central aneurysms affecting the PAs up to the lobar level may be suggested by an enlarged and lobulated PA or, more generally, an asymmetric hilar enlargement (Fig. 7.11). They may be multiple but are usually asymmetric. Walls may show calcifications. Central PA aneurysms may be found in patients who have primary or secondary pulmonary hypertension, congenital cardiovascular diseases (particularly persistent ductus arteriosus or a bicuspid pulmonary valve), Marfan syndrome, cystic medial necrosis, PA stenosis, trauma, and vasculitis or infections (mycotic aneurysms). A double wall sign (displaced intimal calcifications) should suggest dissection, a life-threatening complication in patients who have pulmonary hypertension.

Peripheral PA aneurysms are elliptical or rounded opacities and present as solitary pulmonary nodules. The location along a PA may be difficult to assess on chest X-ray. Nevertheless, when elliptical, their long axis should parallel the normal course of PAs. They may also be multiple and follow PA trauma, lung infections, or vasculitis.

Pulmonary Pseudoaneurysm

Pseudoaneurysm is dilation of a vessel, formed when bleeding from vascular disruption is contained by surrounding tissues. It may result from any destructive process that erodes the wall of a pulmonary vessel, such as trauma (Swan-Ganz catheter particularly and penetrating or, more rarely, blunt trauma), various infections, tumors or inflammatory diseases. Chest X-ray shows a sharply defined elliptical or round opacity in an area that presented in the previous days with focal consolidation, caused by hemorrhage after PA rupture or the infectious or inflammatory process responsible for the pseudoaneurysm (Ghaye et al. 1997). They are virtually not detectable on chest X-ray when located in a persistent consolidation of the lung parenchyma. Pseudoaneurysms secondary to Swan-Ganz trauma are generally located at the level of the segmental or subsegmental PA. Previous chest X-ray may have shown a Swan-Ganz catheter located too peripherally in the PAs (normally the tip should not be located more than 2 cm from the hilum). Any nodule located in the wall of a cavitary lesion, particularly in the tuberculosis, should raise the suspicion of a mycotic pseudoaneurysm (also called Rasmussen aneurysm) (Remy et al. 1984) (Fig. 7.16). The risks of pseudoaneurysms are enlargement and eventually rupture, resulting in fatal hemoptysis in more than 50% of cases.

7.3.2.2 Pulmonary Valve Stenosis

Pulmonary valve stenosis may be associated with dilation of the PAs, predominantly affecting the main pulmonary trunk and/or the left PA. Pulmonary valve stenosis may be due to commissural fusion of the pulmonary cusps or bicuspid valve or valvular dysplasia (Amplatz and Moller 1993). Elevated pressure in the

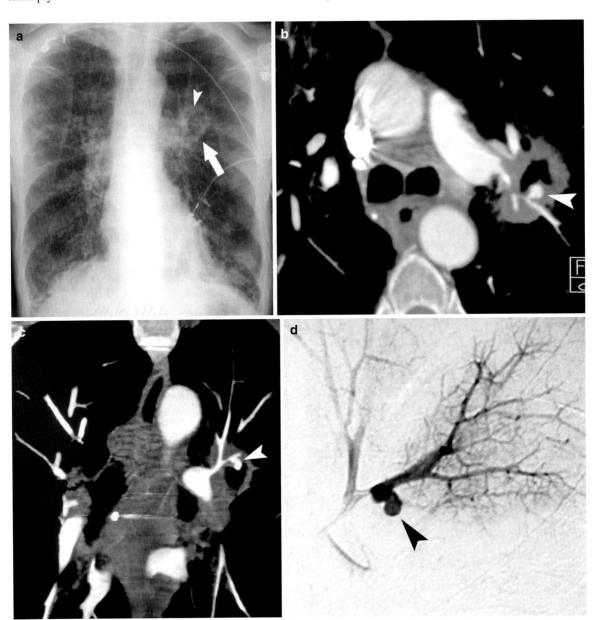

Fig. 7.16 Pulmonary pseudoaneurysm. Pseudoaneurysm in a cavitary lung tumor in a 60-year-old man presenting with haemoptysis. The frontal chest X-ray (**a**) shows a cavitary lesion in the left parahilar area (*arrow*). A nodular contour is suspected on the superior aspect of the lesion (*arrowhead*). Axial maximum intensity projection (**b**), frontal multiplanar reformat (**c**), and digital pulmonary angiography (**d**) show a 4-mm pseudoaneurysm (*arrowheads*) of a subsegmental pulmonary artery of the left upper lobe that required vaso-occlusion with steel coils (Case from the Club Thorax, courtesy of Antoine Khalil, Hôpital Tenon, Paris, France)

right ventricle results in muscular hypertrophy of the ventricle and clockwise rotation of the heart. As a result, increased velocity of the pulmonary outflow produces a jet impact selectively oriented to the wall of the main and left PAs that progressively dilate (Remy and Boroto 2009). Poststenotic dilation mainly occurs in the case of moderate stenosis of the valve; severe stenosis results only in a poor jet through the valve. Chest X-ray will show discrepancy in the size of both hila, with the left being larger (Fig. 7.17). Like other causes of main PA dilation, it may simulate other pathologies responsible for hilar or left middle mediastinal arc enlargement on frontal chest X-ray, including lymphadenopathy, hilar tumor, anterior mediastinal mass, mediastinal pleural mass, or pericardial congenital defect (Cole et al. 1995). Associated dilation of the left PA is a clue to the diagnosis of pulmonary valve stenosis. Furthermore, LUL PAs may appear larger than those of the RUL due to increased blood flow. Calcifications of the pulmonary valve are rare.

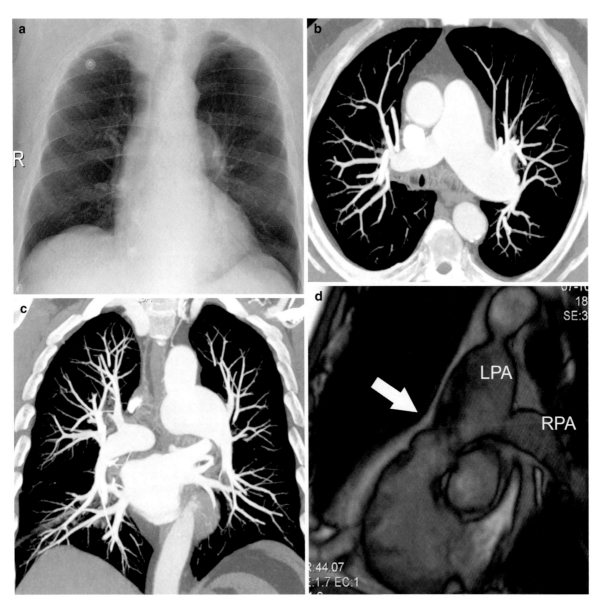

Fig. 7.17 Pulmonary valve stenosis in a 58-year-old patient presenting with increasing dyspnea. Frontal chest X-ray (**a**), axial computed tomograpy (**b**), and frontal maximum intensity projection (**c**) show selective dilation of the left pulmonary artery (LPA) and normal caliber of the right pulmonary artery (RPA). Magnetic resonance imaging (**d**) confirmed a commissural fusion of the pulmonary cusps causing a moderately thickened, dome-shaped valve. The jet flow (*black area – arrow*) is selectively oriented towards the dilated left PA

7.3.2.3 Vasculitis

Behçet disease, Takayasu arteritis, and giant cell arteritis are forms of vasculitides that may affect the central or medium-sized PAs in young or middle-aged patients. They are characterized by wall thickening and stenotic or, less commonly, dilation changes, which can cause peripheral perfusion asymmetry, arterial thrombosis, or thromboembolism with distal pulmonary infarction. Pulmonary aneurysms have also been occasionally reported in other "systemic diseases," including syphilis, ankylosing spondylitis, rheumatoid disease, rheumatic fever, systemic lupus erythematosus, relapsing polychondritis, and Reiter's syndrome (Hartley and al. 1978).

Behçet Disease

Behçet disease is a systemic vasculitis that may involve arteries and veins of any size. It is characterized by recurrent oral and genital ulcerations, ocular and skin lesions, sometimes associated with arthritis, gastrointestinal, and thoracic involvement. Pulmonary involvement is found in 1–10% of cases (Hiller et al. 2004). It consists mainly in vascular complications (20–40%), resulting in aneurysm (65%) or occlusion (35%) of PAs, SVC, and the aorta. PA aneurysms are more frequent with this disease than in other types of vasculitides (Grenier et al. 1981; Tunaci et al. 1995). They may be single or multiple, central or peripheral, frequently rupture, and have a poor prognosis; 30–80% of patients die within 2 years (Hiller et al. 2004; Castaner et al. 2006). Because endovascular thrombosis is frequent, signs of pulmonary infarcts or hemorrhage, oligemic areas, atelectasis, pleural effusion, and ultimately pulmonary hypertension can be seen (Fig. 7.18). Organizing pneumonia, eosinophilic pneumonia, and fibrosis have also been described (Tunaci et al. 1995; Hiller et al. 2004). Therefore, the most common pulmonary parenchymal findings in Behçet disease are subpleural infiltrates and wedge-shaped or ill-defined rounded opacities (Grenier et al. 1981; Tunaci et al. 1995; Ahn et al. 1995). Other patterns of alveolar consolidation may represent pneumonia or lung filling by blood secondary to hemoptysis. Sudden hilar enlargement or apparition of intraparenchymal rounded opacities are signs of PA aneurysm. Poor margins suggest hemorrhage or inflammation around the aneurysm. Disappearance of some aneurysms after steroids treatment has been reported (Tunaci et al. 1995). Mediastinal widening may suggest edema due to thrombosis or stenosis of the SVC (Ahn et al. 1995).

Hughes–Stovin Disease

Hughes–Stovin disease is characterized by the combination of multiple PA aneurysms and deep venous thrombosis. It is currently considered to be a variant of Behçet disease or an incomplete Behçet disease (also called vascular Behçet) because they share similar clinical, radiological, and histopathological findings with Behçet disease (Tunaci et al. 1995; Ketchum et al. 2005; Emad et al. 2007).

Takayasu Disease

Although most frequently found in young Asian women, Takayasu arteritis has a worldwide distribution. This granulomatous arteritis mainly affects the elastic arteries (aorta and its major branches). PAs can be affected in 15%–80%, often as a late manifestation of the disease, and more frequently at the segmental and subsegmental than lobar or main level (Yamada et al. 1992). CT and MRI may show (often smooth) thickening and enhancement of arterial walls in early phases, and mural calcifications, stenosis or occlusion, and collateral vessels in chronic phases (Ferretti et al. 1996). Unilateral occlusion can occur during late phases, whereas aneurysms are more uncommon. Early PA involvement is difficult to detect on chest X-ray, but the late phase may show patchy areas of decreased perfusion, sometimes affecting a single lung, and signs of PA hypertension (Fig. 7.19). Subpleural reticular changes and pleural thickening has been attributed to local thromboembolism (Takahashi et al. 1996). Contrary to PE, upper lung zones seem to be predominantly affected (Yamada et al. 1992). Chest X-ray may show premature calcification of the aorta and branches, as well as rib notching due to formation of collateral vessels in severe stenosis of the aorta. Differential diagnosis includes aortic coarctation, other vasculitis, and fibromuscular dysplasia.

Giant Cell Arteritis

Giant cell arteritis may occasionally affect the central PAs and the aorta (Landrin et al. 1997).

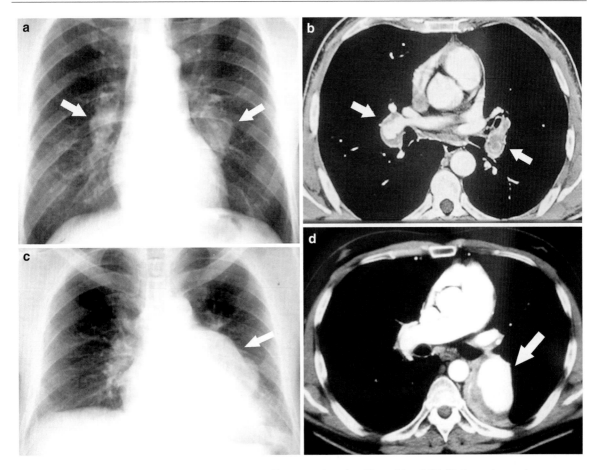

Fig. 7.18 Two examples of patients with Behçet disease. Chest X-ray (**a**) shows lobulated increase of size of both hila, corresponding to aneurysms of pulmonary arteries (*arrows*) on computed tomography (CT) (**b**). CT also shows mural thrombi bilaterally and central filling defects on the left side, responsible for the decrease of perfusion of left lung basis demonstrated on chest X-ray. In another patient chest X-ray (**c**) and CT (**d**) show a huge pulmonary artery aneurysm (*arrow*) on the left side. Prognosis of such a large aneurysm is particularly poor. Indeed, this patient presented with massive hemoptysis secondary to aneurysm rupture 1 week later (Cases from the Club Thorax, courtesy of Mostafa El Hajjam and Pascal Lacombe, Hôpital Ambroise Paré, Paris, France)

Differentiation from Takayasu arteritis or PE may be difficult.

are more frequently peripheral. Lymphangitic carcinomatosis is presented in Chap. 8.

7.3.2.4 Tumor

Tumoral processes affecting the PAs are infrequent and are not commonly detected on chest X-ray. Tumors may involve the pulmonary vasculature in four ways: large central emboli, microscopic emboli, lymphatic dissemination (i.e., lymphangitic carcinomatosis), and a combination of all. They are important to know because they may mimic other conditions such as PE, PA aneurysms, or pulmonary hypertension. Primary tumors are generally central while secondary tumors

Primary Tumor

Most primary tumors of pulmonary vessels are sarcomas (leiomyosarcomas, angiosarcomas, etc.). They mainly affect young and middle-aged adults, around 30–45 years of age, sometimes with history of radiation therapy. Even on CT they mimic acute and chronic PE because they present as an endoluminal mass in the proximal and dilated PA, sometimes associated with distal oligemia or pulmonary infarcts (Fig. 7.20). The diagnosis may be even more difficult because secondary thromboembolic

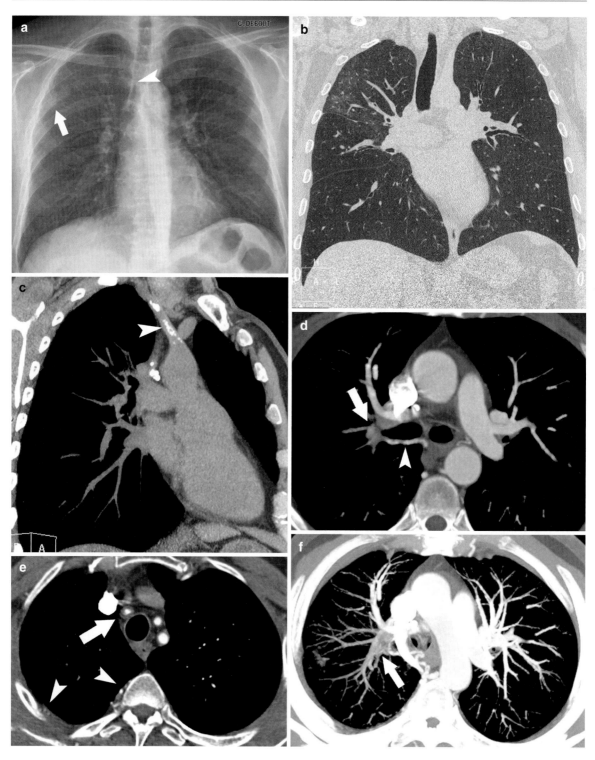

Fig. 7.19 Takayasu arteritis. Thrombosis of posterior segmental pulmonary artery (PA) of the right upper lobe (RUL) in a patient with a history of Takayasu arteritis known for more than 20 years. Chest X-ray (**a**) and frontal (**b**), and oblique (**c**) multiplanar reformats show a chronic ground glass infiltrate in the RUL due to increased systemic vascularisation, ill-defined consolidation probably related to pulmonary infarct (*arrow*), and premature calcifications in the bra-chiocephalic arterial trunk (*arrowhead*). Axial computed tomography (**d** and **e**) and axial maximum intensity projection (**f**) show thrombosis of the posterior segmental PA of the RUL (*arrow* in **d** and **f**), wall thickening and stenosis of supra-aortic vessels (*arrow* in **e**), and collateral vessel development from bronchial arteries and inter-costals vessels (*arrowheads* in **d** and **e**) (Case courtesy of Gilbert Ferretti, University hospital of Grenoble, France)

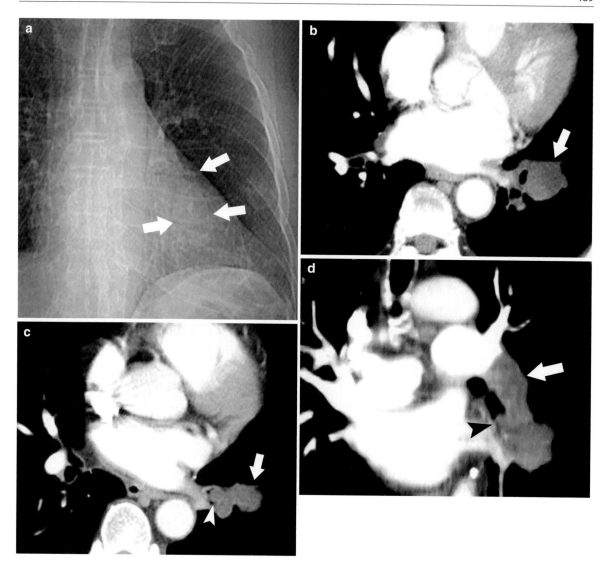

Fig. 7.20 Primary tumor of pulmonary artery (PA). Angiosarcoma of the left lower lobe PA in a 65-year-old man presenting with recurrent infections on the left lower lobe. Close-up view of frontal chest X-ray (**a**) shows a tubular structure (*arrows*) in the left retrocardiac area, oriented along the bronchovascular bundles of the left lower lobe. Axial computed tomography (**b** and **c**) and curved multiplanar reformat (**d**) show an expanding intraluminal process in the left lower lobe PA (*arrows*), invading the neighboring bronchus of the left lower lobe (*arrowheads*). Pathology after fibroscopy showed an angiosarcoma (Case from the Club Thorax, courtesy of Daniel Jeanbourquin, Hôpital Val de Grâce, Paris, France)

events are common and may be the only clinical evidence of tumor at presentation (Engelke et al. 2002). Tumoral process should be suspected when risk factors for PE are absent; there is no dissolution despite the administration of anticoagulation an atypical distribution such as upper lobe predominance or a single large unilateral lesion; a defect occupying the entire section of a central PA; a lobulated or heterogeneous mass that may show enhancement after contrast media injection; and, ultimately, transmural growth in the hilum and mediastinum and lymphadenopathies (Tschirch et al. 2003, Yi et al. 2004). They are differentiated from intravascsular

(IV) metastasis as dilatation of the peripheral PA is not common in sarcoma of PA.

Therefore, chest X-ray is often normal or shows findings that may suggest PE, including dilation of the central PAs containing an endoluminal tumor, sometimes associated with distal oligemia (Westermark sign) or an "Hampton hump" caused by pulmonary infarct, and small- volume pleural effusion. A lobulated pattern of dilated PAs and lung nodules should raise suspicion of a tumoral process. Other differential diagnoses include hilar tumor or adenopathy, fibrosing mediastinitis, or rarely central IV metastasis.

Intravascular Metastasis

IV metastases are not rare at autopsy (3–26%) and are particularly found in solid tumors that tend to invade systemic veins (hepatocellular carcinoma, renal cell carcinoma, stomach, breast, or lung cancer, etc.), but they are not uncommonly seen on medical imaging examinations, even CT or MRI, which are usually normal (Roberts et al. 2003). A ventilation/perfusion lung scan is considered to have the greater diagnostic utility because it demonstrates numerous, symmetric, and distal perfusion defects (Roberts et al. 2003). Most tumor emboli are microscopic and involve peripheral arteries and arterioles, except the right atrial myxoma and renal cell carcinoma that may embolize to the large central and segmental PAs. Symptoms include progressive dyspnea and subacute pulmonary hypertension or a more acute manifestation that simulates PE

(Roberts et al. 2003). On CT they may present as multifocal dilatation or beading of vessels, sometimes with a tree-in-bud appearance (Shepard et al. 1993; Tack et al. 2001) (Fig. 7.21). Areas of mosaic perfusion or pulmonary infarction have been reported (Engelke et al. 2002). Rarely, larger emboli may cause filling defects that mimic acute PE. Such findings are undoubtedly difficult to demonstrate on chest X-ray, which is typically normal. Indeed, a normal chest X-ray with acute or subacute dyspnea and hypoxemia in a patient with a known malignancy should raise the suspicion of IV metastasis. In the advanced stage, signs of PA hypertension, nodular or linear opacities presenting as a vascular distribution, or a branching pattern may be seen (Shepard et al. 1993; Tack et al. 2001). They should be differentiated from PAVMs or filling of a dilated bronchial structure, i.e., mucous plugging in bronchiectasis or intrabronchial growth of a tumor.

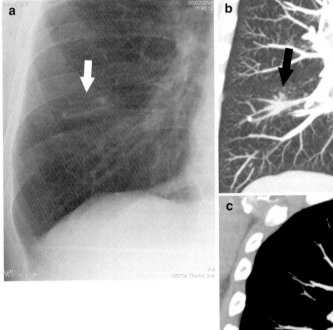

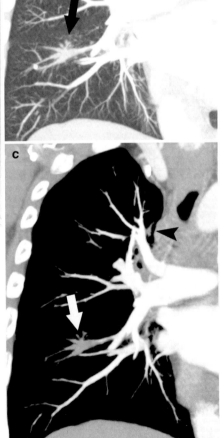

Fig. 7.21 Intravascular (IV) metastasis. In a patient with an uncontrolled neck tumor. Chest X-ray (**a**) shows a linear and branching opacity (*arrow*) in the anterior segment of right lower lobe progressively growing over months. Chest computed tomography was performed because of suspicion of pulmonary embolism since the patient presented with hemoptysis. Maximum intensity projection (**b** and **c**) shows branching intra-arterial filling defects (*arrow*) in a subsegmental pulmonary artery (PA) of A8D, showing a marked dilation of the PA, largely superior to dilation observed in patients who have acute cruoric clots. Beading of small branches representing tree-in-bud pattern is also demonstrated (*arrow* in **b**). Other small peripheral foci of IV metastasis were found (*arrowhead* in **c**). The right ventricle/left ventricle ratio (1:1) was increased compared with a CT performed 8 months earlier, indicating increased pressure in the PA

7.3.2.5 Fibrosing Mediastinitis

Fibrosing mediastinitis is a rare benign disorder caused by proliferation of acellular collagen and fibrous tissue within the mediastinum that may lead to encasement, reduced caliber, and sometimes occlusion of mediastinal structures. Veins and airways are most frequently involved (33–39%); narrowing or obstruction of PAs is reported in 18% and esophageal narrowing is reported in 9% (Sherrick et al. 1994). Two types should be distinguished: The focal type (82%) usually manifests on CT as a localized, partially calcified (63%) mass obliterating normal mediastinal fat planes and encasing adjacent structures in the paratracheal or subcarinal regions of the mediastinum or in the pulmonary hila (Sherrick et al. 1994) (Fig. 7.22). The right side of

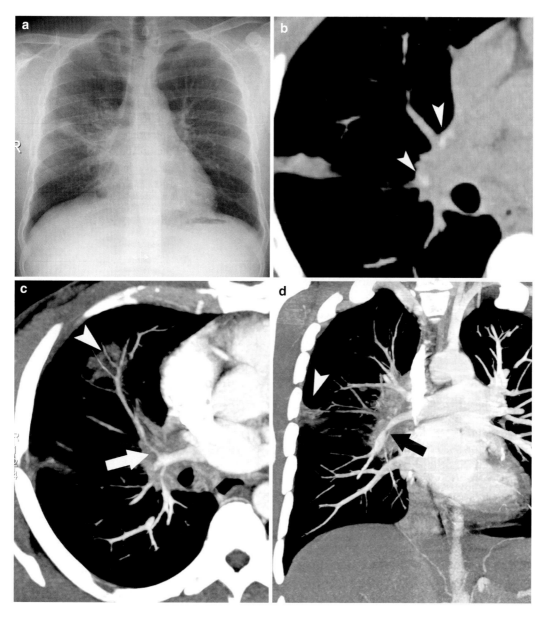

Fig. 7.22 Fibrosing mediastinitis in a 38-year-old man presenting for dyspnea, cough, chest pain, and hemoptysis. Frontal chest X-ray (**a**) shows blurring of the right hilum contour and parahilar parenchymal opacities. Axial computed tomography (**b**) shows calcifications in the right hilum (*arrowheads*). After contrast medium injection, maximum intensity projection (**c** and **d**) demonstrates a "pseudo-tumoral" hilar soft tissue infiltration compressing the pulmonary artery, including the right interlobar pulmonary artery and the internal segmental pulmonary artery of the middle lobe (*arrows*). The infiltrate in the upper lobe corresponds to a pulmonary hemorrhage or infarction (*arrowheads*)

the mediastinum is more commonly involved than the left. It is considered to result from an abnormal immunologic reaction to organisms such as *Histoplasma capsulatum* or tuberculosis and in rare cases to other infectious agents including aspergillosis, mucormycosis, blastomycosis, and cryptococcosis (Rossi et al. 2001). The diffuse type (18%) manifests as a diffusely infiltrating, often noncalcified mass that affects multiple mediastinal compartments. It is mostly due to an autoimmune disease associated with other idiopathic fibroinflammatory disorders such as retroperitoneal fibrosis, sclerosing cholangitis, Riedel thyroiditis, and drug reaction, or it is idiopathic (Sherrick et al. 1994).

Chest X-ray is often normal or underestimates the extent of the disease. It may show a focal or diffuse mediastinal widening and distortion or obliteration of normally recognizable mediastinal interfaces or lines (Rossi et al. 2001). Calcifications may be difficult to assess on chest X-ray. Compression or stenosis of the tracheal or central bronchi is rarely depicted. Secondary signs of vascular (SVC syndrome with dilation of collaterals, i.e., the aortic nipple, pulmonary edema, lung infarction) or bronchial involvement (pneumonitis, atelectasis, hyperlucent area due to hypoxemic vasoconstriction) are more commonly seen. Differential diagnosis is large on chest X-ray, requiring CT or MRI to differentiate the various causes of tumoral or nontumoral mediastinal enlargement or encasement.

7.3.2.6 Postablation Stenosis of Pulmonary Veins

Percutaneous ablation using radiofrequency energy has become a well-established technique for treatment of atrial fibrillation and consists of removing or isolating tissue at the site of the abnormal impulse formation, namely the PVs. The technique is, however, associated with complications, including PV stenosis and, more rarely, PV thrombosis (Ghaye et al. 2003). The incidence of PV stenosis varies from 1% to 5% in experienced hands. Early stenosis is caused by tissue swelling that may regress, or progress to fibrosis and contraction of the venous wall. If a single PV is obstructed, the clinical symptoms may be mild or unrecognized. Pulmonary hypertension is unlikely to develop unless a substantial portion of the pulmonary venous drainage is affected. Multiple PV stenoses are potentially life threatening. Recurrence of stenosis

after treatment is frequent and patients must be followed carefully (Latson and Prieto 2007). Chest X-ray may evidence septal thickening and ground-glass opacities, which may reflect localized pulmonary venous hypertension or focal pulmonary edema. Nodules and wedge-shaped parenchymal consolidation, reflecting venous infarction, can also be seen. CT and MRI are necessary to evidence the stenosis or thrombosis of PV (Ghaye et al. 2003).

7.4 Conclusion

Most pulmonary vessel diseases can be detected with chest X-ray, and a definite diagnosis can be reached using CT or MRI. In an appropriate clinical setting, the awareness of radiologic manifestations of pulmonary vessel diseases can lead to early diagnosis, workup, and treatment, or, on the contrary, can prevent unnecessary examinations in patients with benign congenital diseases.

References

Agarwal PP, Seely JM, Matzinger FR (2004) MDCT of anomalous unilateral single pulmonary vein. AJR Am J Roentgenol 183:1241–1243

Ahn JM, Im JG, Ryoo JW, Kim SJ, Do YS, Choi YW, Oh YW, Yeon KM, Han MC (1995) Thoracic manifestations of Behçet syndrome: radiographic and CT findings in nine patients. Radiology 194:199–203

Amplatz K, Moller JH (1993) Radiology of Congenital Heart Disease. Mosby, St Louis

Andrikakos P, Gallis P, Christopoulos A et al (2004) An asymptomatic pulmonary hilar mass: a case report. Acta Radiol 45:516–518

Andronikou S, Wieselthaler N (2004) Modern imaging of tuberculosis in children: thoracic, central nervous system and abdominal tuberculosis. Pediatr Radiol 34:861–875

Asayama J, Shiguma R, Katsume H et al (1984) Pulmonary varix. Angiology 35:735–739

Berdon WE (2000) Rings, slings, and other things: vascular compression of the infant trachea updated from the midcentury to the millennium – the legacy of Robert E. Gross, MD, and Edward B. D. Neuhauser, MD. Radiology 216: 624–632

Blake HA, Hall RJ, Manion WC (1965) Anomalous pulmonary venous return. Circulation 32:406–414

Castañer E, Gallardo X, Rimola J, Pallardó Y, Mata JM, Perendreu J, Martin C, Gil D (2006) Congenital and acquired pulmonary artery anomalies in the adult: radiologic overview. Radiographics 26:349–371

Cole TJ, Henry DA, Jolles H, Proto AV (1995) Normal and abnormal vascular structures that simulate neoplasms on chest radiographs: clues to the diagnosis. Radiographics 15:867–891

Don C, Hammond DI (1985) The vascular converging points of the right pulmonary hilus and their diagnostic significance. Radiology 155:295–298

Dupuis C, Charaf LA, Breviere GM et al (1992) The "adult" form of the scimitar syndrome. Am J Cardiol 70:502–507

Engelke C, Schaefer-Prokop C, Schirg E, Freihorst J, Grubnic S, Prokop M (2002) High-resolution CT and CT angiography of peripheral pulmonary vascular disorders. Radiographics 22:739–764

Emad Y, Ragab Y, Ael-H S, Gheita T, El-Marakbi A, Salama MH (2007) Hughes-Stovin syndrome: is it incomplete Behçet's? Report of two cases and review of the literature. Clin Rheumatol 26:1993–1996

Felson B (1973) In: Felson B (ed) Chest Roentgenology. Saunders, Philadelphia

Ferretti G, Defaye P, Thony F, Ranchoup Y, Coulomb M (1996) Initial isolated Takayasu's arteritis of the right pulmonary artery: MR appearance. Eur Radiol 6:429–432

Furuya K, Kaku K, Yasumori K et al (2007) Hypogenetic lung syndrome with anomalous venous return to the left inferior pulmonary vein: multidetector row CT findings. J Thor Imag 22:351–354

Genereux GP (1983) Conventional tomographic hilar anatomy emphasizing the pulmonary veins. AJR Am J Roentgenol 141:1241–1257

Ghaye B, Couvreur T (2009) Partial anomalous venous return. In: Remy-Jardin M, Remy J (eds) Integrated cardiothoracic imaging with MDCT. Springer Berlin Heidelberg, pp 307–324

Ghaye B, Szapiro D, Dacher JN, Rodriguez LM, Timmermans C, Devillers D, Dondelinger RF (2003) Percutaneous ablation for atrial fibrillation: the role of cross-sectional imaging. Radiographics 23:S19–S33

Ghaye B, Trotteur G, Dondelinger RF (1997) Multiple pulmonary artery pseudoaneurysms: intrasaccular embolization. Eur Radiol 7:176–179

Gossage JR, Kanj G (1998) Pulmonary arteriovenous malformations. A state of the art review. Am J Respir Crit Care Med 158:643–661

Grenier P, Bletry O, Cornud F, Godeau P, Nahum H (1981) Pulmonary involvement in Behcet disease. AJR Am J Roentgenol 137:565–569

Haitjema TJ, Overtoom TT, Westermann CJ, Lammers JW (1995) Embolisation of pulmonary arteriovenous malformations: results and follow up in 32 patients. Thorax 50: 719–723

Haramati LB, Moche IE, Rivera VT et al (2003) Computed tomography of partial anomalous pulmonary venous connection in adults. J Comput Assist Tomogr 27:743–749

Hartley JP, Dinnen JS, Seaton A (1978) Pulmonary and systemic aneurysms in a case of widespread arteritis. Thorax 33: 493–499

Hiller N, Lieberman S, Chajek-Shaul T, Bar-Ziv J, Shaham D (2004) Thoracic manifestations of Behçet disease at CT. Radiographics 24:801–808

Kalke BR, Carlson RG, Ferlic RM et al (1967) Partial anomalous pulmonary venous connections. Am J Cardiol 20: 91–101

Ketchum ES, Zamanian RT, Fleischmann D (2005) CT angiography of pulmonary artery aneurysms in Hughes-Stovin syndrome. AJR Am J Roentgenol 185:330–332

Landrin I, Chassagne P, Bouaniche M, Dominique S, Doucet J, Nouvet G, Bercoff E (1997) Pulmonary artery thrombosis in giant cell arteritis. A new case and review of literature. Ann Méd Interne 148:315–316

Latson LA, Prieto LR (2007) Congenital and acquired pulmonary vein stenosis. Circulation 115:103–108

Mathey J, Galey JJ, Logeais Y et al (1968) Anomalous pulmonary venous return into inferio vena cava and associated bronchovascular anomalies (the scimitar syndrome). Thorax 23:398–407

Marshall GB, Farnquist BA, MacGregor JH, Burrowes PW (2006) Signs in thoracic imaging. J Thorac Imaging 21:76–90

Morgan PW, Foley DW, Erickson SJ (1991) Proximal interruption of a main pulmonary artery with transpleural collateral vessels: CT and MR appearances. J Comput Assist Tomogr 15:311–313

Nguyen ET, Silva CI, Seely JM, Chong S, Lee KS, Müller NL (2007) Pulmonary artery aneurysms and pseudoaneurysms in adults: findings at CT and radiography. AJR Am J Roentgenol 188:W126–W134

Park CK, Webb WR, Klein JS (1991) Inferior hilar window. Radiology 178:163–168

Posniak HV, Dudiak CM, Olson MC (1993) Computed tomography diagnosis of partial anomalous pulmonary venous drainage. Cardiovasc Intervent Radiol 16:319–320

Procacci C, Residori E, Bertocco M, Di Benedetto P, Andreis IA, D'Attoma N (1993) Left pulmonary artery sling in the adult: case report and review of the literature. Cardiovasc Intervent Radiol 16:388–391

Remy J, Boroto K (2009) Pulmonary valve stenosis. In: Remy-Jardin M, Remy J (eds) Integrated cardiothoracic imaging with MDCT. Springer, Berlin, pp 325–326

Remy J, Lemaitre L, Lafitte JJ, Vilain MO, Saint Michel J, Steenhouwer F (1984) Massive hemoptysis of pulmonary arterial origin: diagnosis and treatment. AJR Am J Roentgenol 143:963–969

Remy-Jardin M, Remy J (1999) Spiral CT angiography of the pulmonary circulation. Radiology 212:615–636

Ring NJ, Marshall AJ (2002) Idiopathic dilatation of the pulmonary artery. Br J Radiol 75:532–535

Roberts KE, Hamele-Bena D, Saqi A, Stein CA, Cole RP (2003) Pulmonary tumor embolism: a review of the literature. Am J Med 115:228–232

Rossi SE, McAdams HP, Rosado-de-Christenson ML, Franks TJ, Galvin JR (2001) Fibrosing mediastinitis. Radiographics 21:737–757

Ryu DS, Spirn PW, Trotman-Dickenson B, Hunsaker A, Jung SM, Park MS, Jung BH, Costello P (2004) HRCT findings of proximal interruption of the right pulmonary artery. J Thorac Imaging 19:171–175

Ryu DS, Ahn JH, Choi SJ, Lee JH, Jung SM, Park MS, Jung BH (2008) Congenital absence of the right interlobar pulmonary artery: HRCT findings. J Thorac Imaging 23:292–294

Saalouke MG, Shapiro SR, Perry LW et al (1977) Isolated partial anomalous pulmonary venous drainage associated with pulmonary vascular obstructive disease. Am J Cardiol 39:439–444

Shepard JA, Moore EH, Templeton PA, McLoud TC (1993) Pulmonary intravascular tumor emboli: dilated and beaded peripheral pulmonary arteries at CT. Radiology 18:797–801

Sherrick AD, Brown LR, Harms GF, Myers JL (1994) The radiographic findings of fibrosing mediastinitis. Chest 106:484–489

Siripornpitak S, Reddy GP, Schwitter J, Higgins CB (1997) Pulmonary artery sling: anatomical and functional evaluation by MRI. J Comput Assist Tomogr 21:766–768

Tack D, Nollevaux MC, Gevenois PA (2001) Tree-in-bud pattern in neoplastic pulmonary emboli. AJR Am J Roentgenol 176:1421–1422

Takahashi K, Honda M, Furuse M, Yanagisawa M, Saitoh K (1996) CT findings of pulmonary parenchyma in Takayasu arteritis. J Comput Assist Tomogr 20:742–748

Ten Harkel AD, Blom NA, Ottenkamp J (2002) Isolated unilateral absence of a pulmonary artery: a case report and review of the literature. Chest 122:1471–1477

Tschirch FT, Del Grande F, Marincek B, Huisman TA (2003) Angiosarcoma of the pulmonary trunk mimicking pulmonary thromboembolic disease. A case report. Acta Radiol 44:504–507

Tunaci A, Berkmen YM, Gökmen E (1995) Thoracic involvement in Behçet's disease: pathologic, clinical, and imaging features. AJR Am J Roentgenol 164:51–56

Ugolini P, Mousseaux E, Sadou Y, Sidi D, Mercier LA, Paquet E, Gaux JC (1999) Idiopathic dilatation of the pulmonary artery report of 4 cases. Magn Reson imaging 17:933–937

White RI Jr, Mitchell SE, Barth KH, Kaufman SL, Kadir S, Chang R, Terry PB (1983) Angioarchitecture of pulmonary arteriovenous malformations: an important consideration before embolotherapy. AJR Am J Roentgenol 140:681–686

Yamada I, Shibuya H, Matsubara O, Umehara I, Makino T, Numano F, Suzuki S (1992) Pulmonary artery disease in Takayasu's arteritis: angiographic findings. AJR Am J Roentgenol 159:263–269

Yamashita H (1978) Roentgenologic Anatomy of the Lung. Igaku-Shoin, New York

Yi CA, Lee KS, Choe YH, Han D, Kwon OJ, Kim S (2004) Computed tomography in pulmonary artery sarcoma: distinguishing features from pulmonary embolic disease. J Comput Assist Tomogr 28:34–39

Interstitial Lung Disease

8

Bart Ilsen, Robert Gosselin, Louke Delrue,
Philippe Duyck, Johan de Mey,
and Cathérine Beigelman-Aubry

Contents

B. Ilsen (✉)
Department of Radiology, Universitair Ziekenhuis Brussel,
Laarbeeklaan 101, 1090, Brussel, Belgium
e-mail: bart.ilsen@uzbrussel.be

R. Gosselin, L. Delrue, and P. Duyck
Department of Radiology, UZ-Gent, De Pintelaan 185,
9000 Gent, Belgium
e-mail: robert.gosselin@uzgent.be
e-mail: louke.delrue@uzgent.be
e-mail: philippe.duyck@uzgent.be

J. de Mey
Department of Radiology, AZ-VUB, Laarbeeklaan 101,
1090 Brussel, Belgium
e-mail: johan.demey@az.vub.ac.be

C. Beigelman-Aubry
Pitié-Salpêtrière Hospital, Paris, France

Abstract

> Interstitial lung disease (ILD), also known as
> diffuse parenchymal lung disease, is a broad
> category of lung diseases that are grouped
> together because of their similar clinical, radio-
> graphic, physiologic, or pathologic manifesta-
> tions. It includes more than 130 disorders
> characterized by scarring (i.e., "fibrosis") and/
> or inflammation of the lungs.

> The traditional approach to radiographic
> assessment of ILD consists primarily of deter-
> mining whether the pulmonary parenchymal
> process is located within the interstitium. This
> is often difficult, although radiographic criteria
> have been established over the past years.
> Therefore, radiologists use a more descriptive
> approach to analyze the predominant pulmo-
> nary pattern, lung volumes, lesion distribution,
> and the presence of associated findings.

> High-resolution computed tomography (HRCT)
> has been widely accepted as the imaging gold
> standard for ILD.

> This chapter reviews the different interstitial
> patterns seen on chest radiograph classified and
> based on their appearance patterns on HRCT.

8.1 Introduction

The term interstitial lung disease (ILD) refers to a
broad category of lung diseases rather than a specific
disease entity. However, the term interstitial is mis-
leading because most of these disorders are also associated with extensive alterations of alveolar and airway

E.E. Coche et al. (eds.), *Comparative Interpretation of CT and Standard Radiography of the Chest*,
Medical Radiology, DOI: 10.1007/978-3-540-79942-9_8, © Springer-Verlag Berlin Heidelberg 2011

architecture. ILD includes a variety of illnesses with various causes, treatments, and prognoses. These disorders are grouped together because of similarities in their clinical presentations, radiographic appearance, and physiologic features.

The interstitium of the lung is normally not visible radiographically because of the summation effect and the low spatial resolution, and radiological findings are nonspecific in most pathologies. High-resolution computed tomography (HRCT) has been widely accepted as the imaging standard of reference when an ILD is suspected. In certain clinical settings, the presence of a typical pattern on HRCT may be sufficient to make a presumptive diagnosis.

8.2 Anatomy

Comprehensive knowledge of lobar, segmental, and subsegmental structures is mandatory to understand CT features of ILD. The differential diagnosis of ILD can be narrowed down when one can decide whether the disease likely is located in or around the airways, the blood vessels, the lymphatics, or the lung interstitium.

The lung is made up of numerous anatomic units much smaller than a lobe or segment. The secondary pulmonary lobule refers to the smallest unit of lung structure and is defined as the portion of lung distal to a lobular bronchiole (Miller 1947). They are irregular polyhedral in shape and their sides are lined by the incomplete interlobular connective tissue septa and their base, which is 1–2 cm in diameter, usually faces the pleural surface of the lung. Lobules that occupy a more central position in the lung are not well defined and are considered to consist of three to five pulmonary acini.

The lung is supported by a network of connective tissue fibers referred to as the *lung interstitium*. For the purpose of interpreting HRCT images and identifying abnormal findings, the interstitium can be thought of as three components that communicate freely: (1) the peripheral connective tissue, (2) the axial connective tissue, and (3) the parenchymal connective tissue (Weibel and Gil 1977; Weibel 1979).

The peripheral connective tissue includes the subpleural space and the interlobular septa of the lung. The interlobular septa are fibrous strands that penetrate deeply as incomplete partitions from the subpleural

space into the lung (Weibel 1979). Hence, the pleura is in anatomic continuity with the different lung septa, including the interlobular septa and the septa between the acini.

The axial connective tissue is a system of fibers that surrounds bronchi and pulmonary arteries, forming a large connective tissue sheath from the lung root to the level of the respiratory bronchiole. It terminates at the center of the acini in the form of a fibrous network that follows the wall of the alveolar ducts and sacs (Weibel 1979).

The parenchymal connective tissue is a network of elastic and collagen fibers that forms a connective tissue mesh between the sacs and alveoli and bridges the gap between the peripheral connective tissue and the axial connective tissue (Weibel 1979).

The arteries of the human lung accompany the airways and their pattern of division is similar to the branching pattern of the airways. The pulmonary veins are formed by the confluence of pulmonary venules at the periphery of the secondary pulmonary lobule and run across the interlobular septa and through the more central connective tissue sheets.

This highly detailed microscopic anatomy is not visible on chest radiograph in a normal situation. Only CT with high-frequency algorithm reconstructions, known as HRCT, is capable of visualizing this complex anatomical structure. Therefore, since the development of HRCT, this method dominates the recent literature about the imaging of ILD (Webb et al. 2009).

The diagnosis of ILD can be suspected initially on the basis of an abnormal chest radiograph, but an accurate diagnosis of ILD is rarely obtained except in some clinical conditions such as pulmonary edema, idiopathic pulmonary fibrosis, complicated silicosis, and end-stage sarcoidosis.

8.3 Patterns of Interstitial Lung Disease

The traditional approach to the radiographic assessment of ILD first involves determining whether the pulmonary parenchymal process is located within the interstitium or in the alveolar spaces. This is often difficult, although radiographic criteria have been established over the past years to make this differentiation. Because of these limitations, a more descriptive approach has been proposed by radiologists for ILD. This takes into account an analysis of the predominant pulmonary pattern, analysis of lung volumes, lesion distribution (focal or multifocal, versus diffuse or disseminated), and finally the appearance of other thoracic structures such as heart, lymph nodes, mediastinum, and ribs.

Pulmonary patterns may be classified as alveolar, interstitial, bronchial, and vascular. Interstitial patterns on chest radiography have been described as linear, reticular, nodular, and reticulonodular. Many attempts have been made to establish criteria for the radiographic recognition of interstitial involvement of the lung on chest radiographs. Often, there is another type of lesion or none at all to account for the shadows. The summation effect and the low spatial resolution are two possible explanations for this phenomenon.

HRCT, however, has been widely accepted as the imaging gold standard for ILD and occupies the middle ground between the vague information provided by chest radiography and the microscopic, but otherwise localized, information obtained from histopathologic examination of a lung biopsy.

Therefore, we present in this chapter the interstitial findings based on their HRCT patterns. For each pattern, the description starts from the viewpoint of chest radiography with a short differential diagnosis based on the radiographic findings. These findings are more accurately and specifically defined on HRCT with a more extensive differential diagnosis. The interstitial patterns on HRCT include linear and reticular pattern, nodular pattern, decreased lung density, and increased lung density.

8.3.1 Linear and Reticular Pattern

Thickening of the interstitial network of the lung by fluid or fibrous tissue, or because of interstitial infiltration by cells or other substances, results in an increase in linear or reticular lung opacities.

On chest radiography, a linear pattern is most commonly caused by thickening of the interlobular septa or thickening of the peribronchial intersitium. However, sometimes parenchymal bands or pleuroparenchymal scars can also lead to line shadows on chest radiographs. A reticular pattern on chest radiography will be the result of a summation of small irregular opacities, cystic spaces, or both.

The distinction between the components responsible for the reticular pattern on a chest radiograph can readily be made on HRCT because of the highly detailed information.

On HRCT, linear or reticular opacities can manifest as peribronchovascular interstitial thickening, interlobular septal thickening, parenchymal bands, subpleural interstitial thickening, intralobular septal thickening, honeycombing, irregular linear opacities, and subpleural lines.

8.3.1.1 Linear Pattern

Chest Radiograph

On chest radiography, a linear pattern is seen when there is a thickening of the interlobular septa or when there is bronchial wall (peribronchial) thickening. (Webb and Higgins. 2004). The interstitial septa of normal lungs are not visible on chest radiographs except in a very small minority of thin patients, and even in this condition only on very high-quality films (Armstrong 2000). The same applies for the normal walls of the bronchi beyond the hila, which are invisible unless they are visualized end-on to the X-ray beam. Thickening of the interlobular septa is caused by infiltration of the lung interstitium by fluid, fibrous tissue, cells, or other materials (Webb 1989). The thickened septa are anatomically divided into deep and peripheral interlobular septa (Ried 1959).

- Kerley B lines (peripheral septal lines) are short, thin lines, 1–2 cm in length. They are perpendicular to the pleural surface and continuous with it and are in direct contact with the pleura. They are readily recognizable laterally at the costophrenic angles on frontal views and in the substernal region on lateral views. They are generally absent along the surfaces of the fissures. The characteristic appearance of Kerley B lines results from the consistent size and regular organization of pulmonary lobules at the lung bases.
- Kerley A lines (deep septal lines) are less often seen. They are longer (at least 2 cm), unbranching lines coursing diagonally from the periphery toward the hila in the inner half of the lungs. They also represent thickened interlobular septa, but their appearance is different from that of B lines because of the

different arrangement of pulmonary lobules in the parahilar regions.

Septal lines must be distinguished from blood vessels on plain radiographs. The identification of septal lines is an extremely useful diagnostic feature because, thickened septal lines occur in few conditions (Table 8.1).

Differential diagnoses of septal lines on chest radiography (Armstrong 2000) include:

- Pulmonary edema (hydrostatic most common, symmetric) (Fig. 8.1)
- Lymphangitic spread of neoplasm (often asymmetric) (Fig. 8.2)
- Congenital lymphangiectasia
- Viral and mycoplasma pneumonia
- Interstitial pulmonary fibrosis from any cause
- Pneumoconiosis
- Sarcoidosis
- Lymphocytic giant-cell interstitial pneumonitis
- Late-stage hemosiderosis
- Lymphangioleiomyomatosis (LAM; and tuberous sclerosis)

When edema or cells infiltrate the peribronchial interstitial space, the combination of the bronchial wall and the thickened interstitium produces so-called bronchial wall thickening (Armstrong 2000). This condition can be seen with edema or neoplastic infiltration. Distinction between lymphangitic carcinomatosis and edema can usually be accomplished on the basis of clinical findings. In cases in which there is a

Table 8.1 Differential diagnosis of septal lines on chest radiograph (Armstrong 2000)

• Pulmonary edema (hydrostatic most common, symmetric) (Fig. 8.1)
• Lymphangitic spread of neoplasm (often symmetric) (Fig. 8.2)
• Congenital lymphangiectasia
• Viral and mycoplasma pneumonia
• Interstitial pulmonary fibrosis from any cause
• Pneumoconiosis
• Sarcoidosis
• Lymphocytic giant-cell interstitial pneumonitis
• Late-stage hemosiderosis
• Lymphangiomyomatosis (LAM) and tuberous sclerosis

doubt, HRCT may be helpful. Peribronchial thickening is also seen in recurrent asthma, allergic bronchopulmonary aspergillosis, bronchiolitis, cystic fibrosis, and bronchiectasis.

HRCT

On HRCT scans, thickened interlobular septa are identified because they are perpendicular to the pleura or by the fact that they form polygonal structures (Johkoh et al. 1999). Only a few septa should be visible in normal patients. Numerous, clearly visible interlobular septa always indicate the presence of an interstitial abnormality.

Peribronchovascular interstitial thickening cannot be distinguished from the underlying opacity of the bronchial wall or pulmonary artery and therefore result in an increased bronchial wall thickness or an increase in diameter of the pulmonary artery branches on unenhanced HRCT.

On HRCT, depending on the cause, smooth, nodular, and irregular thickening of the interlobar septa or peribronchial interstitium can be identified (Webb 1989; Kang et al. 1996).

Smooth Septal Thickening

Smooth septal thickening is seen in patients who have venous, lymphatic, or infiltrative diseases. It may reflect pulmonary edema, congestive heart failure, fluid overload, or hemorrhage (Cassart et al. 1993); pulmonary veno-occlusive disease (Cassart et al. 1993); lymphangitic spread of carcinoma, lymphoma, or leukemia (Munk et al. 1986); lymphoproliferative disease; lymphangiomatosis (Colby and Swensen 1996); amyloidosis; and in some cases pneumonia.

Nodular Septal Thickening

Nodular septal thickening occurs in lymphatic or infiltrative diseases, including lymphangitic spread of carcinoma or lymphoma (Munk et al. 1986), lymphoproliferative disease, sarcoidosis (Lynch et al. 1989; Traill et al. 1997), silicosis or coal worker's pneumoconiosis (Remy-Jardin et al. 1990), and amyloidosis.

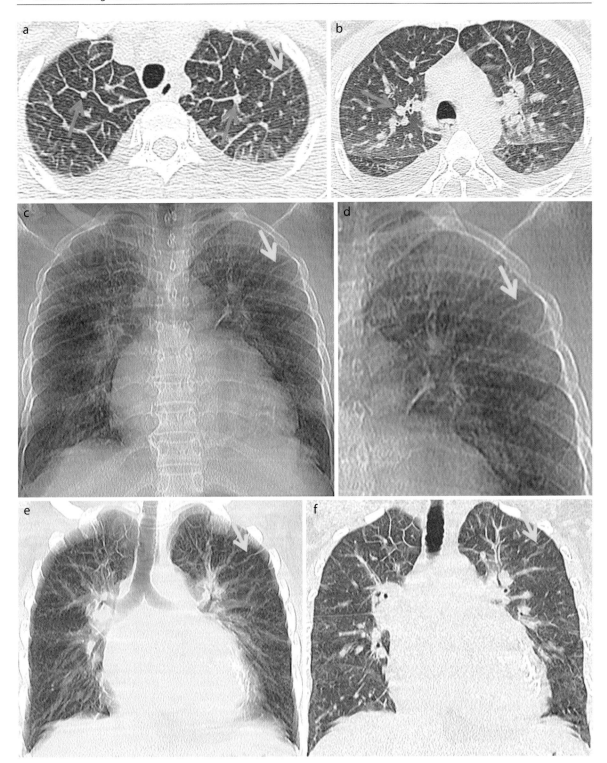

Fig. 8.1 Hydrostatic pulmonary edema in a patient with congestive heart failure. Two successsive axial computed tomography slices (**a** and **b**) demonstrate a nodular thickening of the interlobular septa reflecting the enlarged pulmonary veins (*blue arrows*) with bilateral pleural effusion. Note the peribronchial cuffing on (**b**; *orange arrow*). The chest radiograph equivalent (**c**) and the focused view on the left upper lobe (**d**) show a loss of definition of vascular markings throughout both lungs associated with Kerley lines (*yellow arrows*), reminiscent of interstitial edema. Note the enlargement of the cardiac silhouette. By viewing average coronal slabs (**c–f**) of decreasing slice thickness, Kerley A lines seen on (**f**) corresponding to septal thickening are perfectly understood

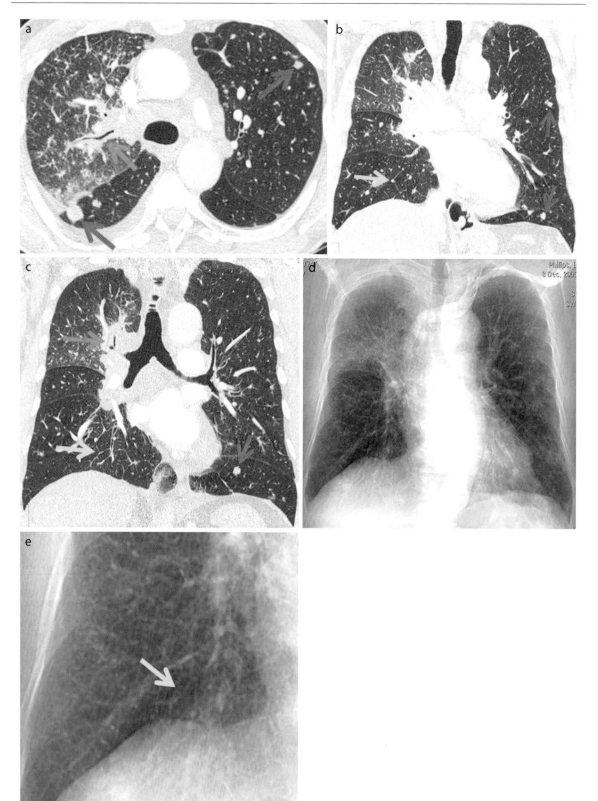

Fig. 8.2 Lymphangitis carcinomatosis from a bronchopulmonary carcinoma. Axial computed tomography slice (**a**) and two successive coronal reformats (**b** and **c**) demonstrate a perilymphatic pattern predominantly located at the level of the right upper lobe. The spiculated nodule that is related to the bronchopulmonary carcinoma and located at the level of the apical segment of the right upper lobe is obviously demonstrated in (**b**). The peribronchovascular thickening (*blue arrows*) and septal lines (*yellow arrows*) are well demonstrated in (**a–c**). Note the pulmonary nodules related to lung metastasis (*orange arrows*) and the ground-glass opacity of the right upper lobe probably related to lymphatic stasis. All these findings are very difficult to individualize on the chest X-ray equivalent (**d**). The linear pattern may be suspected in (**e**)

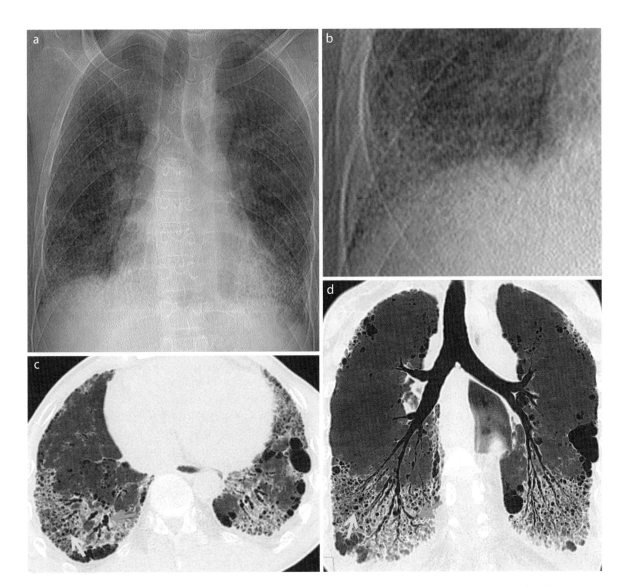

Fig. 8.3 Progressive systemic sclerosis. Chest radiograph equivalent obtained with a thick slab average of 200 mm (**a**) and a focused view at the level of the right lower lobe (**b**) demonstrate bilateral basal fine reticular opacities with honeycombing pattern with a loss of volume of both lower lobes. Axial (**c**) and coronal (**d**) minimum intensity projection (MinIP) slabs of computed tomography (CT) images show bilateral ground-glass opacities, reticulations, traction bronchiectasis (*blue arrows*), and honeycombing (*yellow arrows*). Note the various sizes of the cysts that are impossible to assess on the chest X-ray. Despite the exquisite morphological details offered with CT, a definite diagnosis of fibrotic nonspecific interstitial pneumonia versus usual interstitial pneumonia may not be done with CT

Irregular Septal Thickening

Irregular septal thickening can be seen in patients with fibrosis and honeycombing, although it is usually not a predominant finding (Akira et al. 1990).

8.3.1.2 Reticular Pattern

Chest Radiograph

On chest radiography, a reticular pattern corresponds to a summation of small irregular opacities, cystic spaces, or both. By summation, these lead to an appearance resembling a network (Hansell et al. 2008). The reticular pattern can be subdivided into three subpatterns based on the width of the opacities: a fine reticular pattern (smaller than 3 mm), a medium reticular pattern (3–10 mm), and a coarse pattern (larger than 10 mm). Medium and course reticular patterns are most common and most easily depicted on chest radiographs.

A fine reticular pattern (seen as intralobular linear opacities) may indicate fine lung fibrosis or lung infiltration with fluid or cells. A medium reticular pattern is typical in patients who have pulmonary fibrosis and "honeycombing." Because of its cystic appearance, honeycombing is also discussed in the chapter discussing low attenuation patterns. Honeycombing is the typical feature of usual interstitial pneumonia (UIP). Some cystic lung disease (e.g., Langerhans cell histiocytosis, LAM) result in a coarse reticular pattern because of superimposition of the walls of the cysts. The differential diagnosis of reticular pattern depends upon the acuteness or the chronicity of the process (Table 8.2).

Differential diagnosis of reticular pattern on chest radiograph (Müller et al. 2001):

Acute disease – Acute diseases that produce a reticular pattern include:

- Hydrostatic pulmonary edema (reticular pattern seen in association with septal lines, prominent upper lobe vessels, pleural effusions, and cardiomegaly is common) (Fig. 8.1)
- Acute viral or mycoplasma pneumonia (often in association with segmental consolidation; HRCT shows centrilobular nodules and tree-in-bud pattern)

Table 8.2 Differential diagnosis of a reticular pattern on chest radiograph (Müller et al. 2001)

Acute disease Acute diseases that produce a reticular pattern include:
• Hydrostatic pulmonary edema (reticular pattern seen in association with septal lines, prominent upper lobe vessels, pleural effusions, and cardiomegaly) (Fig.8.1)
• Acute viral or mycoplasma pneumonia (often in association with segmental consolidation; HRCT shows centrilobular nodules and tree-in-bud pattern)
Chronic disease Chronic reticular changes are generally due to:
• Idiopathic pulmonary fibrosis and pulmonary fibrosis associated with connective tissue disease (lower lung zone predominance)
• Asbestosis (lower lung zone predominance; almost always in association with pleural plaques or diffuse pleural thickening)
• End-stage hypersensitivity pneumonia (no zonal predominance)
• Sarcoidosis (coarse reticulation as seen with chronic fibrosis; involves mainly the perihilar region of the middle and upper lung)

Chronic disease – Chronic reticular changes are generally due to:

- Idiopathic pulmonary fibrosis and pulmonary fibrosis associated with connective tissue disease (lower lung zone predominance)
- Asbestosis (lower lung zone predominance; almost always in association with pleural plaques or diffuse pleural thickening)
- End-stage hypersensitivity pneumonia (usually middle and superior or lower lung zone predominance attenuation)
- Sarcoidosis (coarse reticulation as seen with chronic fibrosis; involves mainly the perihilar region of the middle and upper lung)

HRCT

Distinction between the components responsible for a reticular pattern on a chest radiograph is accomplished readily on HRCT scans. A reticular pattern on HRCT can be caused by intralobular linear opacities (thickening of the interstitium within the secondary lobule), irregular thickening of the interlobular septa, honeycombing, and cystic lung disease.

8.3.2 Nodular Pattern

Chest Radiograph

A nodular pattern is characterized by the presence of multiple nodular opacities with a maximum diameter of 3 cm. Generally, the nodules in the pattern range from 1 mm to 1 cm and it may be difficult to discriminate between nodules (Webb et al. 2009). Larger nodules are often the result of the fusion of multiple small nodules. The term "micronodule" usually refers to nodules no larger than 3 mm in diameter (Hansell et al. 2008). The term "miliary pattern" indicates the presence of multiple small (1–3 mm) micronodules with sharp contours distributed throughout most of the lungs (Andreu et al. 2002). On a chest radiograph, the differential diagnosis depends upon the acuteness or the chronicity of the process (Table 8.3).

Differential diagnosis of nodular pattern on chest radiograph (Müller et al. 2001):

Acute disease – Acute diseases that produce a nodular pattern include:

- Miliary tuberculosis or histoplasmosis (diffuse throughout both lungs) (Fig. 8.6)
- Endobronchial spread of tuberculosis (patchy or asymmetrical bilateral distribution)
- Viral infection (diffuse or patchy)

Table 8.3 Differential diagnosis of a nodular pattern on chest radiograph (Müller et al. 2001)

Acute disease Acute diseases that produce a nodular pattern include: • Miliary tuberculosis and histoplasmosis (diffuse throughout both lungs) (Fig.8.6)   • Endobronchial spread of tuberculosis (patchy or asymmetrical bilateral distribution)   • Viral infection (diffuse or patchy)
Subacute of chronic diseases Subacute or chronic changes are generally related to: • Sarcoidosis (usually perihilar and upper lobe predominance; generally associated with hilar and mediastinal lymphadenopathy)   • Hypersensitivity pneumonitis (generalized or middle and upper or lower lung zone predominance)   • Silicosis and coal workers' pneumoconiosis (upper lung zone predominance)   • Metastatic carcinoma (diffuse or lower lung zone predominance)

Subacute of chronic diseases – Subacute or chronic changes are generally related to:

- Sarcoidosis (usually perihilar and upper lobe predominance; generally associated with hilar and mediastinal lymphadenopathy)
- Hypersensivity pneumonitis (generalized or middle and upper or lower lung zone predominance)
- Silicosis and coal workers' pneumoconiosis (upper lung zone predominance)
- Metastatic carcinoma (diffuse or lower lung zone predominance)

HRCT

Because pathologically many nodules involve both the interstitium and alveolar compartments, the distinction between interstitial nodules and airspace nodules is somewhat arbitrary and often difficult (Patti et al. 2004). Hence, the assessment of the distribution of the nodules is generally more valuable to the differential diagnosis than their appearance (Verschakelen and De Wever 2007) .

Compared with chest radiographs, HRCT can accomplish a differential diagnosis based on the distribution of the nodules. In different conditions, nodules can appear perilymphatic in distribution, randomly distributed, or centrilobular (Gruden et al.1999; Lee et al. 1999)

Perilymphatic Distribution

In patients with a perilymphatic distribution, nodules are seen in relation to lymphatics. Lymphatics are found in the axial peribronchovascular connective tissue, the connective tissue around the centrilobular bronchioles and arteries, the interlobular septa, and the subpleural connective tissue. Hence, a nodular pattern with (peri) lymphatic distribution typically shows peribronchovascular nodules, subpleural nodules, nodules in the interlobular septa, and centrilobular nodules (Colby and Swensen 1996; Webb et al. 2009). These nodules are mostly well defined, are of soft-tissue attenuation, and show a patchy distribution. They are most frequently found in sarcoidosis, silicosis, coal worker's pneumoconiosis, lymphangitic carcinomatosis, diffuse amyloidosis, and lymphoproliferative disease (lymphoma,

Table 8.4 Differential diagnosis of perilymphatic nodules on HRCT (Verschakelen and De Wever 2007)

- Sarcoidosis (perihilair, peribronchovascular, subpleural, centrilobular, septal, upper lobes; frequently asymmetric) (Fig.8.4)

- Silicosis and coal worker's pneumoconiosis (subpleural, centrilobular, upper lobes, bilateral, right-sided predominance; Fig.8.5)

- Lymphangitic carcinomatosis (peribronchovascular, subpleural, centrilobular, septal, uni- or bilateral, may be asymmetric)

- Diffuse amyloidosis (subpleural, peribronchovascular, septal, lower lung)

- Lymphoproliferative disease (lymphoma, lymphocytic interstitial pneumonia {LIP}; subpleural, centrilobular, peribronchovascular, septal)

Table 8.5 Differential diagnosis of random distribution of nodules on HRCT (Verschakelen and De Wever 2007)

- Hematogenous metastases (thyroid cancer, renal cancer, melanoma; lower lobe, peripheral, sometimes right-sided predominance)

- Miliary tuberculosis (bilateral symmetrical, uniform distribution) (Fig.8.6)

- Miliary fungal infections (bilateral symmetrical, uniform distribution)

- Sarcoidosis (may mimic this pattern when very extensive)

- Langerhans cell histiocytosis (early nodular stage)

lymphocytic interstitial pneumonia [LIP]) (Verschakelen and De Wever 2007) (Table 8.4).

Differential diagnosis of perilymphatic nodules on HRCT (Verschakelen and De Wever 2007) includes:

- Sarcoidosis (perihilair, peribronchovascular, subpleural, centrilobular, septal, upper lobes frequently asymmetric) (Fig. 8.4)
- Silicosis and coal worker's pneumoconiosis (subpleural, centrilobular, upper lobes, bilateral, right-sided predominance) (Fig. 8.5)
- Lymphangitic carcinomatosis (peribronchovascular, subpleural, centrilobular, septal, uni- or bilateral, may be asymmetric)
- Diffuse amyloidosis (subpleural, peribronchovascular, septal, lower lung)
- Lymphoproliferative disease (Lymphoma, LIP; subpleural, centrilobular, peribronchovascular, septal)

8.3.2.1 Random Distribution

Nodules are randomly distributed relative to structures of the lung and secondary lobule. These nodules are often of a high density with a sharp border. They usually involve the pleural surface and fissures but show a uniform and diffuse distribution. A random distribution of nodules results from a vascular spread. They are characteristically found in hematogenous metastases, miliary tuberculosis, miliary fungal infections, sarcoidosis, and langerhans cell histiocytosis (Hong et al. 1998; Lee et al. 1999) (Table 8.5).

Differential diagnosis of random distribution of nodules on HRCT (Verschakelen and De Wever 2007):

- Hematogenous metastases (thyroid cancer, renal cancer, melanoma; lower lobe, peripheral, sometimes right-sided predominance)
- Miliary tuberculosis (bilateral symmetrical, uniform distribution) (Fig. 8.6)

Table 8.6 Differential diagnosis of centrilobular nodules on HRCT (Verschakelen and De Wever 2007)

Bronchiolar and peribronchiolar diseases

- Infectious bronchiolitis (viral, mycoplasma, aspergillus, bacterial, tuberculosis) and bronchopneumonia (Figs. 8.7 and 8.8)
- Aspiration
- Cystic fibrosis
- Allergic bronchopulmonary aspergillosis
- Hypersensivity pneumonitis (generalized or middle and upper or lower zone predominance)
- Organising pneumonia (lower lobe, peripheral predominance)
- Bronchioloalveolar carcinoma
- Follicular bronchiolitis
- Panbronchiolitis
- Smoking-associated bronchiolar disease (respiratory bronchiolitis in smokers [RB], respiratory bronchiolitis interstitial lung disease [RB-ILD]; upper lobe predominance)
- Early asbestosis (lower lobe peripheral predominance)
- Langerhans cell histiocytosis (upper lobe predominance)

Vascular and perivascular diseases

- Vasculitis (Wegener's granulomatosis, Churg-Strauss syndrome)
- Pulmonary hemorrhage
- Tumour thrombotic microangiopathy
- Metastatic calcification
- Fat embolism

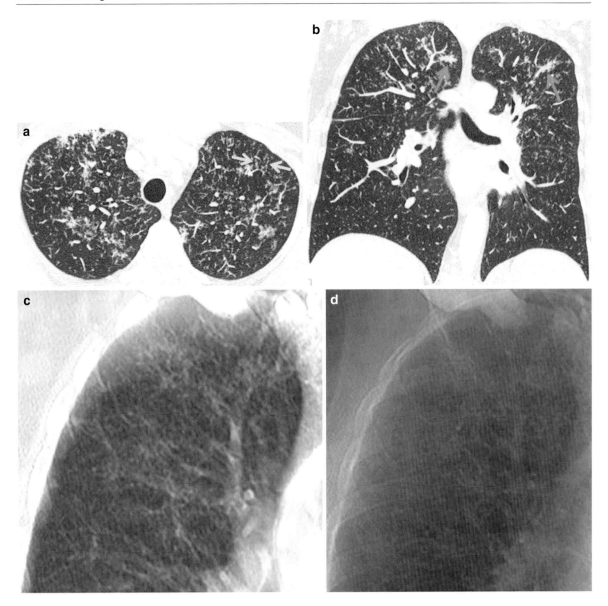

Fig. 8.4 Sarcoidosis. Perilymphatic nodular pattern with multiple, well-defined nodules predominantly located in the upper lobes. Computed tomography on axial view (**a**) and coronal reformat (**b**) shows an extensive nodular involvement along the peribronchovascular bundles (*blue arrows* in **b**), fissures and interlobular septa (*yellow arrows* in **a**). This perilymphatic distribution appears as reticulonodular opacities on average reformats of increasing slab thickness (**c** and **d**) with chest X-ray equivalent (**d**) focused on the right upper lobe

- Miliary fungal infections (bilateral symmetrical, uniform distribution)
- Sarcoidosis (may mimic this pattern when very extensive)
- Langerhans cell histiocytosis (early nodular stage)

8.3.2.2 Centrilobular Distribution

Unlike perilymphatic and random nodules, centrilobular nodules tend to spare the subpleural region and interlobular fissure and tend to surround the surface of small vessels. They are limited to the centrilobular

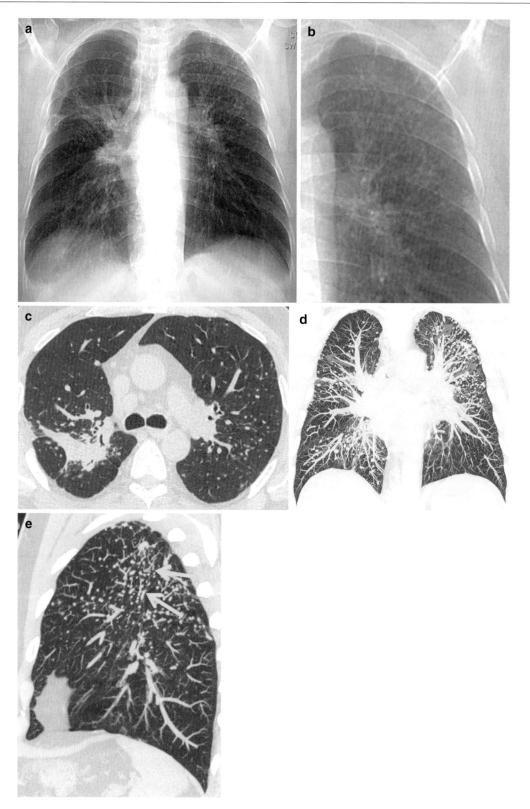

region (Webb 2006) and have a diffuse or patchy distribution. Centrilobular nodular opacities can result from bronchiolar or peribronchiolar and from vascular or perivascular diseases (Table 8.6).

Differential diagnosis of centrilobular nodules on HRCT (Verschakelen and De Wever 2007):

- Bronchiolar and peribronchiolar diseases
- Infectious bronchiolitis (viral, mycoplasma, aspergillus, bacterial, tuberculosis) and bronchopneumonia (Figs. 8.7 and 8.8)
- Aspiration
- Cystic fibrosis
- Allergic bronchopulmonary aspergillosis
- Hypersensivity pneumonitis (generalized or middle and upper or lower zone predominance)
- Organizing pneumonia (lower lobe, peripheral predominance)
- Bronchioloalveolar carcinoma
- Follicular bronchiolitis
- Panbronchiolitis
- Smoking-associated bronchiolar disease (respiratory bronchiolitis [RB] in smokers, respiratory bronchiolitis interstitial lung disease [RB-ILD]; upper lobe predominance)
- Early asbestosis (lower lobe peripheral predominance)
- Langerhans cell histiocytosis (upper lobe predominance)
- Vascular and perivascular diseases
- Vasculitis (Wegener's granulomatosis, Churg–Strauss syndrome)
- Pulmonary hemorrhage
- Tumor thrombotic microangiopathy
- Metastatic calcification
- Fat embolism

When centrilobular nodules are present, the recognition of a "tree-in-bud" pattern is of value to narrow the differential diagnosis. The "tree-in-bud sign" reflects the presence of dilated centrilobular bronchioles with lumina impacted with mucus, fluid, or pus and is often associated with peribronchiolar inflammation (Gruden et al. 1994; Aquino et al. 1996). "Tree-in-bud" describes the appearance of an irregular and often nodular branching structure, most easily identified in the lung periphery. The presence of "tree-in-bud" is indicative of small airway disease and in most cases is associated with airway infection (Table 8.7).

Differential diagnosis of "tree-in-bud" pattern on HRCT (Verschakelen and De Wever 2007):

- Infectious bronchiolitis (bacterial tuberculosis and nontuberculous mycobacteria) and bronchopneumonia (Figs. 8.7 and 8.8)
- Aspiration
- Cystic fibrosis

Table 8.7 Differential diagnosis of "tree-in-bud" pattern on HRCT (Verschakelen and De Wever 2007)

• Infectious bronchiolitis (bacterial tuberculosis and nontuberculous mycobacteria) and bronchopneumonia (Figs. 8.7 and 8.8)
• Aspiration
• Cystic fibrosis
• Bronchiectasis
• Panbronchiolitis
• Allergic bronchopulmonary aspergillosis
• Bronchioloalveolar carcinoma
• Organising pneumonia
• Follicular bronchiolitis (rheumatoid arthritis, Sjögren disease, AIDS)

Fig. 8.5 Complicated silicosis in a dental prothesist. Reticulonodular and nodular interstitial pattern on chest radiograph equivalent (**a**) and on the focused view at the level of the left upper area (**b**) with signs of retraction of the upper lobes predominating (exceptionally) on the left side and with a right hilar mass. Axial computed tomography slice (**c**), coronal 160-mm thick maximum intensity projection (MIP) reformat (**d**), and sagittal 5.70-mm thick MIP (**e**) show numerous small, sharply marginated nodules that have a centrilobular and subpleural predominant distribution (*blue arrows* in **d**) with a posterior and upper lobe predominance (*yellow arrows* in **e**). There is an associated distortion of lung architecture related to lung fibrosis with development of a conglomerated mass on the right side (**c**)

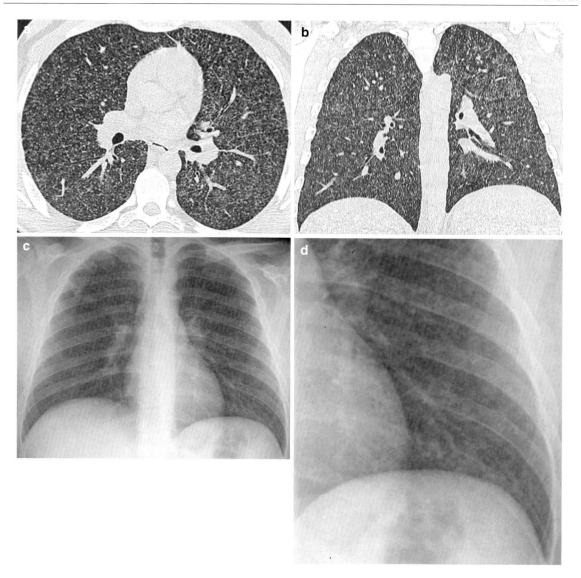

Fig. 8.6 Miliary tuberculosis. Axial computed tomography (**a**) and coronal reformat (**b**) show numerous, well-defined micronodules that are diffuse and uniform in distribution. No predominance may be observed, some nodules having a subpleural or septal distribution, whereas others appear to be located along vessels or everywhere. This is a typical pattern of miliary distribution of hematogenous origin. Micronodules are visualized on the equivalent chest X-ray (**c**) and on the focused view on the left lower area (**d**) despite their small size because of the high profusion of the lesions

- Bronchiectasis
- Panbronchiolitis
- Allergic bronchopulmonary aspergillosis
- Bronchioloalveolar carcinoma
- Organizing pneumonia
- Follicular bronchiolitis (rheumatoid arthritis, Sjögren disease, AIDS)

8.3.3 Decreased Lung Attentuation

Diseases that decrease lung density result in an increased radiolucency on the chest radiograph and decreased attenuation on CT. This can be the result of alteration in pulmonary volume or alteration of pulmonary vasculature.

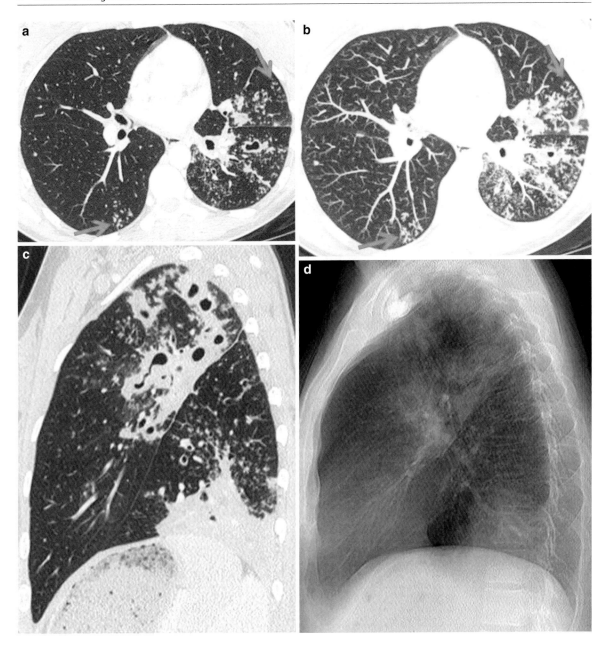

Fig. 8.7 Endobronchial spread of tuberculosis. Axial (**a** and **b**) and sagittal (**c**) images show bilateral micronodules predominating on the left side associated with cavities. The maximum-intensity projection image (**b**) corresponding to the same anatomical level than on (**a**) shows the appearance of tree-in-bud opacities to better advantage (*blue arrows*). Cavities and alveolar consolidation on (**c**) perfectly explain the aspect shown on the equivalent lateral chest X-ray (**d**). This pattern strongly suggests reactivation tuberculosis

8.3.3.1 Alteration of Pulmonary Volume

Alteration of pulmonary volume can be caused by pulmonary emphysema, cystic lung disease, or overinflation (Fraser et al. 2005).

Pulmonary Emphysema

Pulmonary emphysema combines a permanent abnormal enlargement of airspaces distal to the terminal bronchioles and a destruction of the walls of the

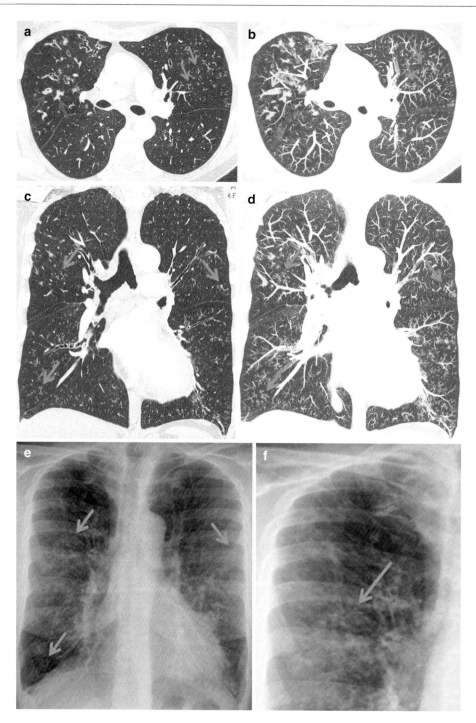

Fig. 8.8 *H. Influenza* infectious bronchiolitis in a patient with bronchiectasis. On the axial computed tomography (CT) slice (**a**) at the level of the middle zones of the lung, the 6.70-mm thick axial maximum intensity projection (MIP) reformat at the same level (**b**), the coronal single reformat (**c**), and the 4-mm thick MIP reformat at the same level (**d**), the centrilobular location of micronodules is recognized because of the respect of 3 mm from adjacent pleural surfaces. The numerous tree-in-bud appearances located within the center of secondary pulmonary lobules are much more obvious in (**b**) than in (**a**) and in (**d**) than in (**c**) (*blue arrows*). Follow-up confirmed complete resolution of the nodules after antibiotherapy.Note the extensive cylindrical bronchiectasies in the right upper lobe associated with mucoid impaction (*orange arrows*), and the small accompanying arteries corresponding to vasoconstriction related to hypoxia (*yellow arrow*). Compared with the heterogeneity of the distribution of micronodules that is well assessed on the chest X-ray equivalent (**e**), the centrilobular distribution is impossible to recognize as done with CT (**f**)

involved airspaces. This will result in an increase of intrapulmonary air and radiologic findings on chest radiographs are related to the diaphragm, the retrosternal space, and cardiovascular silhouette. On HRCT, diagnosis of pulmonary emphysema is based on the recognition of focal areas of very low attenuation that can be easily differentiated from surrounding normal lung..

Cystic Lung Disease

Lung cyst is a nonspecific term used to describe the presence in the lung of a thin-walled, well-defined, and well-circumscribed lesion greater than 1 cm in diameter. Cysts may contain either air or fluid, but this term is used to refer to an air-containing lesion. The most common cause is end-stage pulmonary fibrosis giving rise to honeycombing (air-filled cystic spaces that often predominate in a peripheral subpleural location on HRCT) (Fig. 8.3). Other causes include LAM (Fig. 8.9), langerhans cell histiocytosis, LIP (Sjörgen syndrome, AIDS), and bronchogenic cyst (Verschakelen and De Wever 2007) (Table 8.8).

Differential diagnosis of cystic lung disease on HRCT (Verschakelen and De Wever 2007):

- End-stage pulmonary fibrosis: honeycombing or honeycomb cysts
- LAM: cysts are round and uniform in size
- Langerhans histiocytosis: cysts can have bizarre shapes and different sizes
- LIP: cysts are thin walled and may be multiple
- Bronchogenic cyst

Table 8.8 Differential diagnosis of cystic lung disease on HRCT (Verschakelen and De Wever 2007)

End-stage pulmonary fibrosis (honeycombing or honeycomb cysts)
Lymphangiomyomatosis (LAM): cysts are round and uniform in size
Langerhans histiocytosis: cysts can have bizarre shapes and different sizes
Lymphocytic interstitial pneumonia (LIP): cysts are thin-walled and may be numerous
Bronchogenic cyst

On chest radiographs, cystic lung diseases may result in a reticular pattern, but it is not unusual that the radiograph appears normal. HRCT eliminates the problem of superimposition of multiple thin walls of lung cysts responsible for the interstitial pattern observed on chest radiography and can display the extent and distribution of cystic changes of the wall. Cavitary nodules (cyst-like structures as a result of necrosis in a pre-existing nodule), pneumatoceles (thin-walled, air-filled spaces within the lung), and bullae (emphysematous spaces larger than 1 cm) are other causes of cystic and cyst-like lung changes. Bronchiectasis can also mimic cystic lung disease in certain circumstances.

Overinflation

Overinflation or hyperinflation is an increased expansion of the lungs with air. Overinflation of the lungs must be considered at full inspiration and distinguished from air trapping during expiration. When the overinflation is diffuse (e.g., severe emphysema, asthma, constrictive bronchiolitis, and cystic lung disease), the chest radiograph shows a low position and flattening of the diaphragm, deepening of the retrosternal space, and changes of the cardiovascular silhouette. Isolated hyperinflation is rarely seen on a chest radiograph but can easily be demonstrated on HRCT. On HRCT, a local hyperinflation with and without air trapping (abnormal retention of air in the lungs after expiration) can be differentiated. Overinflation with air trapping results from obstruction of the outflow of air in the affected lung parenchyma (lobar emphysema in infants and bronchial atresia). Overinflation without air trapping is a compensatory process when a part of the lung takes a larger volume than normal in response to loss of volume elsewhere in the thorax. This may occur after surgical resection of lung tissue, or as a result of atelectasis or parenchymal scarring.

8.3.3.2 Alteration in Pulmonary Vasculature

An alteration in the vascular pattern indicates an abnormality of perfusion. Hypoperfusion of a part of the lung may be due to a vascular obstruction (e.g., chronic pulmonary thromboembolism) or regional vasoconstriction resulting from airway disease and abnormal lung ventilation (Fig. 8.10) (Verschakelen and De Wever

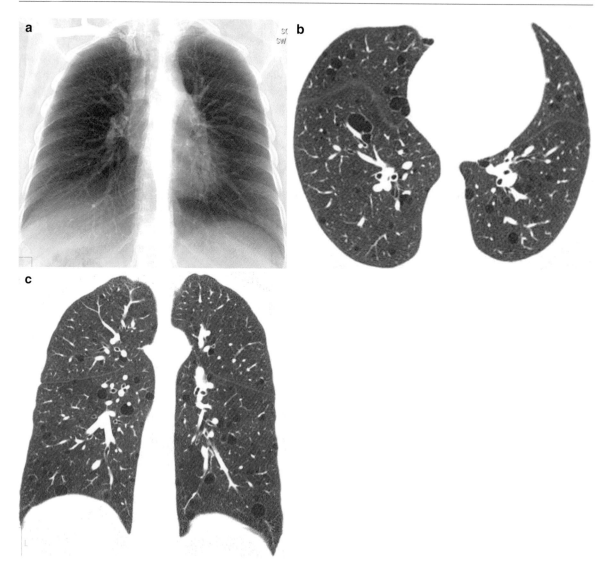

Fig. 8.9 Cystic lung disease suggestive of lymphangioleiomyomatosis in a 31-year-old woman. Thick slab average (**a**) giving a rendering of a chest radiograph does not show any abnormality. Thin axial slice (**b**) and coronal 1.27-thick maximum intensity projection (**c**) demonstrate multiple, thin-walled cysts with normal lung parenchyma between the cystic air spaces. Most cysts are round in shape and uniformly distributed throughout both lungs

2007). On chest radiographs, this hypoperfusion is rarely visible unless the vascular cause is central (e.g., massive pulmonary thromboembolism). The distinction between small airway disease and primary vascular disease requires the use of paired inspiratory/expiratory CT scans.

When the distribution is patchy and when the surrounding normal lung tissue shows an increased attenuation caused by a compensatory hyperperfusion, the term "mosaic perfusion" is used (Lynch et al. 1990; Webb 1994). Often with mosaic perfusion, the pulmonary arteries will be reduced in size in the lucent lung fields, thus allowing mosaic perfusion to be distinguished from ground-glass opacities (GGOs) from other causes.

Mosaic patterning is occasionally seen on HRCT images and is a nonspecific finding.

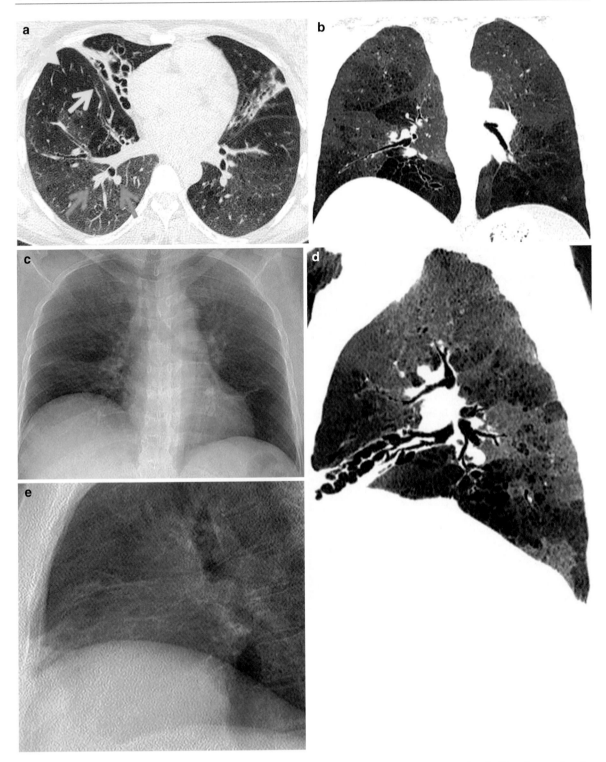

Fig. 8.10 Postinfectious constrictive bronchiolitis. Axial computed tomography slice (**a**), coronal 4.5-mm-thick minimum intensity projection (MinIP) slab (**b**) 200-mm-thick average slab giving a on face chest X-ray equivalent (**c**), sagittal 6-mm-thick MinIP slab (**d**) and lateral chest X-ray equivalent focused on the middle lobe (**e**) show a mosaic perfusion pattern associated with cystic bronchiectasis. The hyperattenuated areas are associated with an increased perfusion (*blue arrows* in **a**) and contrast with hypoattenuated areas that are associated with a decreased perfusion (*yellow arrows*) related to hypoxia. The middle lobe atelectasis with bronchiectasis is very well assessed on (**a**, **d** and **e**). Conversely, the heterogeneity in attenuation is much more difficult to assess on the chest X-ray equivalent (**c**) than on the MinIP slab (**b**). The dilated bronchi within the hypoattenuated areas allow recognition of the airway origin of the mosaic perfusion

8.3.4 Increased Lung Attenuation

Diseases that increase the lung density result in a decreased radiolucency on the chest radiograph and increased attenuation on CT. The degree of parenchymal attenuation depends on the amount or reduction of air in the airspaces and the increase in size and/or volume of the soft tissues (Engeler et al. 1993; Leung et al. 1993; Müller et al. 1987a; Wells et al. 1992). When the changes are limited it will result in a GGO, defined as a hazy increased lung opacity without obscuration of the underlying vessels or bronchial margins on HRCT. On the other hand, when the changes are prominent, the underlying vessels are obscured and this results in a "consolidation" (Webb et al. 1993; Austin et al. 1996; Verschakelen and De Wever 2007).

When GGO is present on HRCT, the chest radiograph may have a variety of appearances. In some cases, the chest radiograph will appear normal. In some cases, the chest radiograph will demonstrate a diffuse alveolar opacity and occasionally it will have an appearance of interstitial opacities. The differential diagnosis of GGO depends upon the acuteness or the chronicity of the process (Table 8.9).

Differential diagnosis of GGO on HRCT (Verschakelen and De Wever 2007):

Acute disease – Acute diseases that produce GGO include:

- Pulmonary infection (bacterial, viral, *Pneumocystis carinii* pneumonia, mycoplasma pneumonia) (Fig. 8.11)
- Pulmonary edema
- Pulmonary hemorrhage
- Adult respiratory distress syndrome
- Acute interstitial pneumonia
- Eosinophilic pneumonia (acute)
- Radiation pneumonitis (acute)

Subacute/chronic disease – Chronic diseases that produce GGO include:

- Hypersensitivity pneumonitis
- Idiopathic pulmonary fibrosis (IPF) and disease associated with UIP (Fig. 8.3)
- Nonspecific interstitial pneumonia (NSIP)

Table 8.9 Differential diagnosis of ground-glass opacities on HRCT (Verschakelen and De Wever 2007)

Acute disease
Pulmonary infection (bacterial, viral, Pneumocystis carinii pneumonia, mycoplasma pneumonia) (Fig.8.11)
Pulmonary oedema
Pulmonary hemorrhage
Adult respiratory distress syndrome
Acute interstitial pneumonia
Eosinophilic pneumonia (acute)
Radiation pneumonitis (acute)
Subacute/chronic disease
Hypersensivity pneumonitis
Usual interstitial pneumonia (UIP): idiopathic pulmonary fibrosis and disease associated with UIP (Fig.8.3)
Nonspecific interstitial pneumonia
Smoking related parenchymal lung disease (respiratory bronchiolitis, respiratory bronchiolitis-interstitial lung disease, desquamative interstitial pneumonia)
Organizing pneumonia
Eosinophilic pneumonia (Fig.8.12)
Bronchioloalveolar carcinoma
Alveolar proteinosis
Asbestosis
Vasculitis (Churg-Strauss syndrome)
Lipoid pneumonia
Sarcoidosis

- Smoking-related parenchymal lung disease RB, RB-ILD, desquamative interstitial pneumonia
- Organizing pneumonia
- Eosinophilic pneumonia (Fig. 8.12)
- Bronchioloalveolar carcinoma
- Alveolar proteinosis
- Asbestosis
- Vasculitis (Churg–Strauss syndrome)
- Lipoid pneumonia
- Sarcoidosis

GGO is a highly significant finding on HRCT because it often indicates the presence of an active and potentially treatable process; active disease is present in more than 80% of patients who show GGOs. Recognition of other HRCT findings can often narrow the differential diagnosis. Because consolidation is due to an alveolar disease, it is not discussed in this chapter.

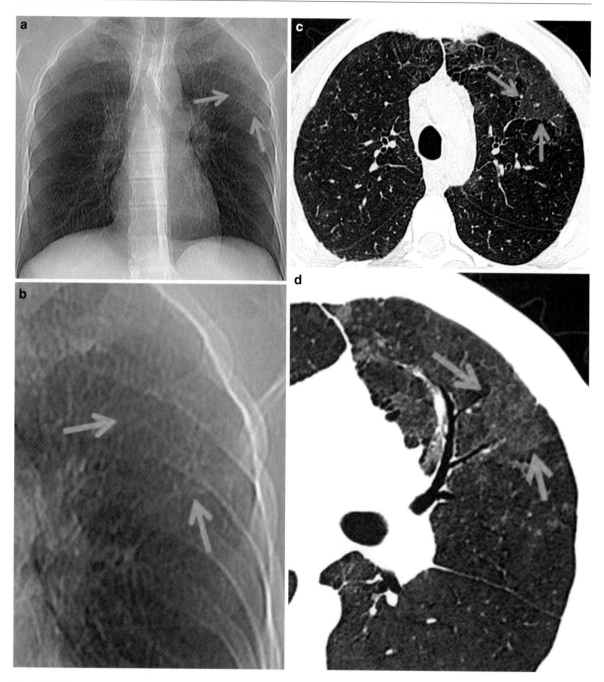

Fig. 8.11 *Pneumocystis carinii* pneumonia in an HIV-positive patient. Chest radiograph (**a**) and the focused view on the left upper area (**b**) shows a subtle ill-defined ground-glass opacity (GGO) in the left axillary area that corresponds on axial computed tomography image (**c**) to patchy areas of GGO with geographic margins (*blue arrows*). The minimum intensity projection (MinIP) on axial oblique view (**d**) and coronal reformat (**e**) reinforce the abnormal contrast between GGO and normal parenchyma and help to guide the bronchioalveolar lavage within the anterior bronchus of the left upper lobe. The equivalent size of pulmonary vessels as demonstrated with maximum intensity projection (MIP) on coronal reformat (**f**) allows exclusion of a mosaic perfusion pattern

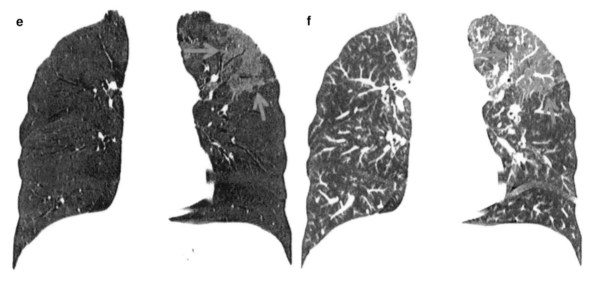

Fig. 8.11 (continued)

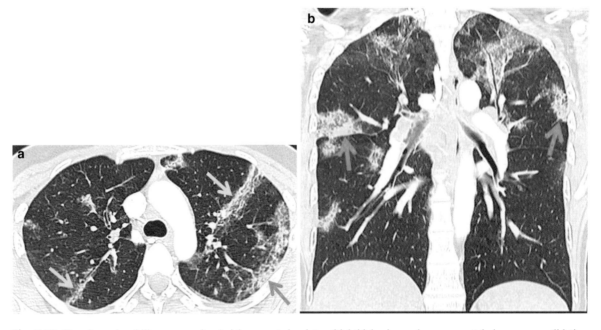

Fig. 8.12 Chronic eosinophilic pneumonia. Axial computed tomography slice (**a**), coronal reformat (**b**), 15-mm-thick slab average (**c**), and 200-mm-thick slab average giving a chest X-ray equivalent (**d**) show ground-glass opacities with intralobular interstitial thickening and nonsegmental airspace consolidation (*blue arrows*) primarily involving the peripheral lung with an upper lobe predominance. Linear bandlike opacities are also present (*yellow arrows*)

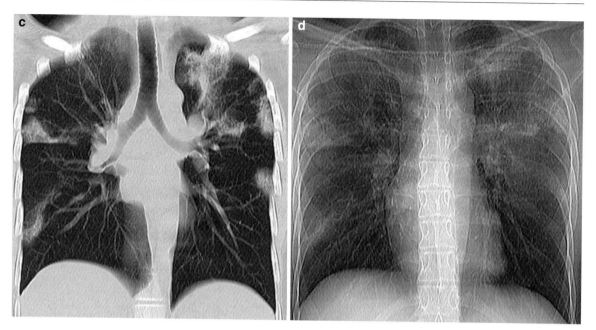

Fig. 8.12 (continued)

8.4 Some Examples of Diseases

When the chest radiograph shows a clear pattern of ILD, a differential diagnosis based on the pattern of parenchymal disease can be suggested. However, difficulties arise when widespread small shadows are difficult to categorize into one group or the other on chest radiography. The next step is to assess which is the predominant pattern, taking into consideration the clinical history and any associated radiographic findings, or to further define the pattern(s) and distribution of disease with HRCT.

In some diseases such as cardiogenic pulmonary edema, idiopathic pulmonary fibrosis, complicated silicosis, or end-stage sarcoidosis, features on a chest radiograph may often lead to the correct diagnosis. However, in the majority of pathologies, radiologic findings are nonspecific and without the use of HRCT only a differential diagnosis can be suggested.

8.4.1 Cardiogenic Pulmonary Edema

Cardiac pulmonary edema results in two principal radiologic patterns related to whether the fluid remains localized in the interstitial space or whether it also occupies the air spaces of the lung. Displacement of fluid into the interstitial space is the first stage of pulmonary edema. When pulmonary venous hypertension is moderate, fluid accumulates within the perivascular interstitial tissue and interlobular septa, which produces a loss of the normal vascular margins and typical thickening of the interlobular septa (Kerley A and B lines) (Fig. 8.1). Evidence for interstitial pulmonary edema is also provided by an increase in the thickness of the wall of bronchi seen in the perihilar zones. However, these are often not the first radiographic signs of cardiogenic pulmonary edema at presentation. Redistribution of blood flow from the lower to the upper zones precedes those interstitial signs (Morgan and Goodman 1991).

When the pulmonary venous hypertension rises, fluid accumulates into the alveolar walls that can give rise to a "haze" (ground glass) with a predominantly lower zone or perihilar distribution. Ultimately, the alveoli become edematous, which leads to an alveolar consolidation pattern on chest radiographs. Besides the interstitial and alveolar pattern, chest radiographs show enlargement of the cardiac silhouette, enlargement of the azygos vein, and sometimes pleural effusion.

Patients with pulmonary edema usually are not imaged with HRCT because their diagnosis is based on a combination of clinical and chest radiographic findings. However, sometimes the diagnosis is not so straightforward and knowledge of the appearance of pulmonary edema on HRCT can be helpful in avoiding misdiagnosis. Image findings on HRCT are bilateral septal thickening and GGOs, perihilar and gravitational distribution predominantly in the dependent lung, cardiomegaly, and pleural fluid.

8.4.2 Idiopathic Pulmonary Fibrosis

IPF has been defined as "a specific form of chronic fibrosing interstitial pneumonia limited to the lung and associated with the histologic appearance of UIP." Peripheral (subpleural) reticular opacities, predominant at the lung bases, are a characteristic finding on the chest radiograph (Fig. 8.3). These opacities are usually bilateral, and often asymmetric (Carrington et al. 1978; McLoud et al. 1983; Müller et al. 1987b; McAdams et al. 1996). As the disease progresses, the abnormalities become more diffuse and assume a coarser reticular or reticulonodular pattern with formation of cysts (honeycombing) associated with progressive loss of volume. Chest radiographs have limited prognostic value, but serial radiographs (including old films) may measure the pace and evolution of the disease.

HRCT findings in UIP are the following: honeycombing consisting of multilayered, thick-walled cysts with predominance in basal and subpleural regions, architectural distortion with traction bronchiectasis caused by fibrosis, and mild mediastinal lymphadenopathy (Müller and Colby 1997). In the presence of a surgical biopsy showing a UIP pattern, the diagnosis of IPF requires exclusion of other known causes of UIP, including drug toxicities, environmental exposures (asbestosis), collagen vascular diseases like rheumatoid arthritis, systemic lupus erythematosus, polyarteritis nodosa, and sclerodermia.

8.4.3 Complicated Silicosis

Silicosis refers to a spectrum of pulmonary diseases caused by inhalation of free crystalline silica (silicon dioxide) and can be classified as acute silicosis, also known as silicoproteinosis, and classic or chronic silicosis.

Acute silicosis follows massive exposure to dust and is a rapidly progressive disease that is often fatal. The chest radiographic appearance mimics pulmonary alveolar proteinosis with alveolar filling opacities and is often nonspecific.

Classic silicosis is an indolent disease that requires more than 10 years of low-dose silica inhalation. Classic silicosis has two forms: simple and complicated silicosis. Simple silicosis refers to a profusion of small (less than 10 mm in diameter) nodular opacities (nodules). The nodules are generally rounded but can be irregular, and are distributed predominantly in the upper lung zones (right sided predominance) with a subpleural or centrilobular distribution (Begin et al. 1987). Their size and opacity vary little. These nodules are calcified in 10–20% of patients and chest radiograph shows a nodular pattern of radiography (Fig. 8.5).

With progression of the disease, the nodules become confluent and form conglomerate masses. The term *complicated silicosis* is used when conglomerate masses are greater than 1 cm in diameter (Webb et al. 2009). The masses can reach 10 cm in diameter and there is associated cicatrization atelectasis of the upper lobes, hilar retraction, bibasilar hyperexpansion, and emphysema. The masses may undergo ischemic necrosis and cavitation. The formation of conglomerate masses is the hallmark of progressive massive fibrosis (PMF) that eventually destroys the lung architecture, and it occurs more frequently in silicosis than in coalworker's pneumoconiosis.

Hilar lymph node enlargement is common and frequently associated with calcifications. The calcifications involve mainly the periphery of the lymph nodes, a finding referred to as eggshell calcifications. Though occasionally seen in other conditions (Gross et al.1980), this pattern is almost pathognomonic of silica-induced disease.

8.4.4 Sarcoidosis

Sarcoidosis is a multisystem, granulomatous disorder of unknown etiology that affects individuals worldwide and is characterized pathologically by the presence of noncaseating granulomas in involved organs. Lung involvement occurs in more than 90% of patients who have sarcoidosis. The stage of pulmonary involvement is based on the chest radiograph. Stage I is defined by the presence of bilateral hilar adenopathy. Stage II consists of bilateral hilar adenopathy and reticular opacities (the latter occurring in the upper more than the lower lung zones). Stage III consists of reticular opacities with shrinking of hilar nodes. Stage IV findings include reticular opacities with architectural distortion, retraction of the hila and the fissures superiorly, cysts and bullae, bronchiectases, honeycombing, and conglomerate masses of progressive fibrosis (end-stage sarcoidosis).

References

Akira M, Yamamoto S, Yokoyama K et al (1990) Asbestosis: high-resolution CT-pathologic correlation. Radiology 176:389–394

Andreu J, Mauleon S, Pallisa E et al (2002) Miliary lung disease revisited. Curr Probl Diagn Radiol 31:189–197

Aquino SL, Gamsu G, Webb WR et al (1996) Tree-in-bud pattern: frequency and significance on thin section CT. J Comput Assist Tomogr 20:594–599

Armstrong P (2000) Basic patterns in lung disease. In: Amstrong P, Wilson AG, Dee P et al (eds) Imaging of diseases of the chest, 3rd edn. Mosby, London, pp 63–132

Austin J, Müller N, Friedman P et al (1996) Glossary of terms for CT of the lungs: recommendations of the nomenclature committee of the Fleischner Society

Begin R, Bergeron D, Samson L et al (1987) CT assessement of silicosis in exposed workers. AJR Am J Roentgenol 148:509–514

Carrington CB, Gaensler EA, Coutu RE et al (1978) Natural history and treated course of usual and desquamative interstitial pneumonia. N Engl J Med 298:801–809

Cassart M, Genevois PA, Kramer M et al (1993) Pulmonary venoocclusive disease: CT findings before and after single-lung transplantation. AJR Am J Roentgenol 160:759–760

Colby TV, Swensen SJ (1996) Anatomic distribution and histopathologic patterns in diffuse lung disease: correlation with HRCT. J Thorac Imaging 11:1–26

Engeler CE, Tashjian JH, Trenkner SW et al (1993) Groundglass opacity of the lung parenchyma: a guide to analysis with high-resolution CT. AJR Am J Roentgenol 160:249–251

Fraser RS, Colman NC, Müller NL et al (2005) Synopsis of diseases of the chest. Saunders, Philadelphia

Gross BH, Schneider HJ, Proto AV (1980) Eggshell calcifications in lymph nodes: an update. AJR Am J Roentgenol 153:1265–1268

Gruden JF, Webb WR, Warnock M et al (1994) Centrilobular opacities in the lung on high-resolution CT: diagnostic considerations and pathologic correlation. AJR Am J Roentgenol 162:569–574

Gruden JF, Webb WR, Naidich DP et al (1999) Multinodular disease: anatomic localization at thin-section CT-multireader evaluation of a simple algorithm. Radiology 210:711–720

Hansell DM, Bankier AA, MacMahon H et al (2008) Fleischner society: glossary of terms for thoracic imaging. Radiology 246:697–722

Hong SH, Im JG, Lee JS et al (1998) High-resolution CT findings of miliary tuberculosis. J Comput Assist Tomogr 22:220–224

Johkoh T, Itoh H, Müller NL et al (1999) Perilobular pulmonary opacities: high-resolution CT findings and pathologic correlation. J Thorac Imaging 14:172–177

Kang EY, Grenier P, Laurent F et al (1996) Interlobular septal thickening: patterns at high-resolution computed tomography. J Thorac Imaging 11:260–264

Lee KS, Kim TS, Han J et al (1999) Diffuse micronodular lung disease: HRCT and pathologic findings. J Comput Assist Tomogr 23:99–106

Leung AN, Miller RR, Müller NL (1993) Parenchymal opacification in chronic infiltrative lung diseases: CT-pathologic correlation. Radiology 188:209–214

Lynch DA, Webb WR, Gamsu G et al (1989) Computed tomography in pulmonary sarcoidosis. J Comput Assist Tomogr 13:405–410

Lynch DA, Brasch RC, Hardy KA et al (1990) Pediatric pulmonary disease: assessment with high-resolution ultrafast CT. Radiology 176:243–248

McAdams HP, Rosado-de-Christenson ML, Wehunt WD et al (1996) The alphabet soup revisited: the chronic interstitial pneumonias in the 1990s. Radiographics 16:1009–1033, discussion 1033–1034

McLoud TC, Carrington CB, Gaensler EA (1983) Diffuse infiltrative lung disease: a new scheme for description. Radiology 149:353–363

Miller WS (1947) The lung. Charles C Thomas, Springfield, pp 39–42

Morgan PW, Goodman LR (1991) Pulmonary edema and adult respiratory distress syndrome. Radiol Clin North Am 29:943–963

Müller NL, Colby TV (1997) Idiopathic interstitial pneumonias: high-resolution CT and histologic findings. Radiographics 17:1016–1022

Müller NL, Guerry-Force ML, Staples CA et al (1987a) Differential diagnosis of bronchiolitis obliterans with organising pneumonia and usual interstitial pneumonia: clinical, functional, and radiologic findings. Radiology 162:151–156

Müller NL, Staples CA, Miller RR et al (1987b) Disease activity in idiopathic pulmonary fibrosis: CT and pathologic correlation. Radiology 165:731–734

Müller NL, Fraser RS, Colman NC et al (2001) Radiologic diagnosis of diseases of the chest. Saunders, Philadelphia

Munk PL, Müller NL, Miller RR et al (1986) Pulmonary lymphangitic carcinomatosis: CT and pathologic findings. Radiology 166:705–709

Patti A, Tognini G, Spaggiari E et al (2004) Diffuse, micronodular lung disease. The high-resolution CT approach. A pictoreal essay. Radiol Med (Torino) 107:139–144

Remy-Jardin M, Degreef JM, Beuscart R et al (1990) Coal worker's pneumoconiosis: CT assessement in exposed workers and correlation with radiographic findings. Radiology 177:363–371

Ried L (1959) The connective tissue septa in the adult human lung. Thorax 14:138–145

Traill ZC, Maskell GF, Gleeson FV et al (1997) High resolution findings of pulmonary sarcoidosis. AJR Am J Roentgenol 152:1179–1182

Verschakelen J, De Wever W (2007) Computed tomography of the lung: a pattern appraoch. Springer, Berlin

Webb WR (1989) High-resolution CT of the lung parenchyma. Radiol Clin North Am 27:1058–1097

Webb WR (1994) High-resolution computed tomography of obstructive pulmonary disease. AJR Am J Roentgenol 169:637–647

Webb WR (2006) Thin-section CT of the secondary pulmonary lobule: anatomy an the Image-The 2004 Fleischner lecture. Radiology 239:322–338

Webb WR, Higgins CB (2004) Thoracic imaging: pulmonary and cardiovascular radiology. Lippincott, Philiadelphia

Webb WR, Müller NL, Naidich DP (1993) Standardized terms for high-resolution computed tomography of the lung: a proposed glossary. J Thorac Imaging 8:167–185

Webb WR, Müller NL, Naidich DP (2009) High-resolution CT of the lung. Lippincott, Philadelphia

Weibel ER (1979) Looking into the lung: what can it tell us? AJR Am J Roentgenol 133:1021–1031

Weibel ER, Gil J (1977) Structure-function relationships at the alveolar level. In: West JB (ed) Bioengineering aspect of the lung. Marcel Dekker, New York, pp 1–81

Wells AU, Hansell DM, Corrin B et al (1992) High resolution computed tomography as a predictor of lung histology in systemic sclerosis. Thorax 47:508–512

The Lung Parenchyma: Radiological Presentation of Alveolar Pattern

José Vilar and Jordi Andreu

9

Contents

Abstract

> The alveolar pattern is the imaging representation of a variety of diseases that tend to occupy the lung airspaces. This pattern is the most common alteration identified in imaging studies of the lungs, and results in an increase in density of the lung parenchyma. The majority can be readily detected in chest radiographs, but some cases will only be detected in CT. The air bronchogram, consolidation, and the silhouette sign are usually detected in plain films. The distribution of the pathology and its temporal presentation can provide clues to specific groups of diseases. Combining the imaging signs and the clinical presentation will narrow the differential diagnosis. Acute airspace disease is usually secondary to pulmonary edema, infectious pneumonia, acute respiratory distress syndrome, pulmonary hemorrhage, and drug-related diseases, whereas subacute and chronic alveolar patterns can be produced by organizing pneumonia, bronchioalveolar cell carcinoma, eosinophilic pneumonia, lymphoma, and radiation pneumonitis. CT can further improve the detection and characterization of airspace disease in the lungs. Specific CT signs of airspace pathology are ground-glass opacities, crazy paving pattern, CT angiogram sign, and the leafless tree sign. The radiologist must be aware of the key points in cases of alveolar disease: morphology, temporal presentation, clinical data, and when to use CT.

J. Vilar (✉)
Hospital Universitario Dr Peset, Gaspar Aguilar 90,
Valencia, Spain, 46017
e-mail: vilarjlu@gmail.com

J. Andreu
Hospital Universitario Vall D'Hebron, Barcelona, Spain
e-mail: jandreus@gmail.com

E.E. Coche et al. (eds.), *Comparative Interpretation of CT and Standard Radiography of the Chest*,
Medical Radiology, DOI: 10.1007/978-3-540-79942-9_9, © Springer-Verlag Berlin Heidelberg 2011

9.1 Introduction

On chest radiography and CT scanning, air attenuation is the main density pattern of the lung. Most pathologic conditions present as an increase in lung density. The air spaces in the lungs correspond anatomically to the most distal areas of the airways, such as the terminal bronchioles, and include the alveolar sacs (Hansell et al. 2008). Airspace occupation is seen as an increase in density that is easily differentiated from density increases secondary to involvement of other structures, such as the alveolar walls, the connective tissue structures, the tissues, surrounding vessels, and bronchi (i.e., the interstitium). The features observed on chest radiographs often are sufficient for the detection and sometimes the characterization of alveolar diseases. CT can provide some signs that allow a more precise diagnosis.

In this chapter we will present the most common signs of the various diseases that manifest as alveolar occupation.

9.2 Basic Features of Alveolar Pattern

9.2.1 Morphology

Airspace occupation can present in a variety of patterns, including consolidation, ground-glass density,

and, more rarely, nodules. There are often combinations of these signs.

9.2.1.1 The Silhouette Sign

On chest radiographs, the silhouette sign is commonly associated with alveolar disease. It consists of obliteration of an anatomic border due to direct contact with an alveolar density (Hansell et al. 2008). The silhouette sign occurs not only in airspace disease, but also in pulmonary collapse, masses, and even some normal variants, such as pectus excavatum (Figs. 9.1–9.3). This sign is a useful localizer of disease; when one of the heart borders is obscured, anterior lung diseases located in middle lobe or lingula should be suspected (Figs. 9.1 and 9.2). The silhouette sign applies also to other structures such as the paraspinal lines or the diaphragm.

9.2.1.2 Pulmonary Consolidation

Consolidation appears as a homogeneous increase in the attenuation of the pulmonary parenchyma that obscures (silhouettes) the margins of vessels and airway walls. The margin of a pulmonary consolidation is usually indistinct, except when in contact with fissures, where it shows a very sharp edge (Fig. 9.4). In most situations, the attenuation characteristics of the consolidated lung are not helpful in the differential

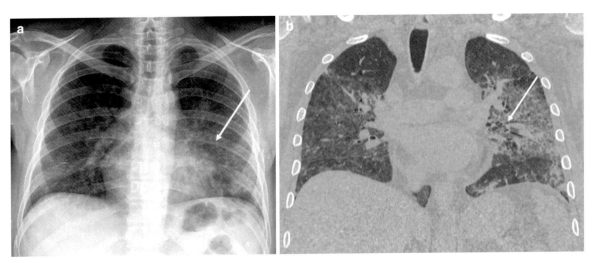

Fig. 9.1 (**a**) Silhouette sign. Posteroanterior chest radiograph. There is an obliteration of the left heart border (*arrow*). (**b**) Coronal CT shows an alveolar consolidation (pneumonia) in the lingula adjacent to the left heart (*arrow*)

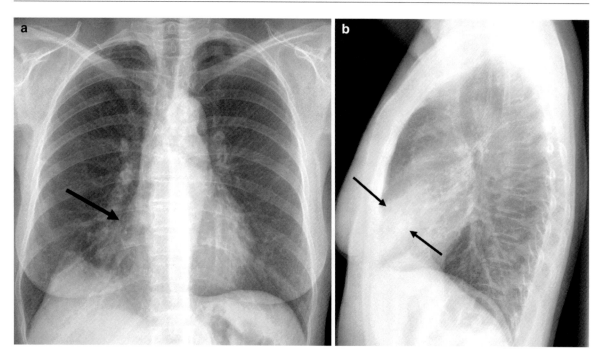

Fig. 9.2 (**a**) Silhouette sign: posteroanterior chest radiograph. The right heart border is obscured (*arrow*). (**b**) Lateral radiograph shows consolidation in middle lobe (*arrows*)

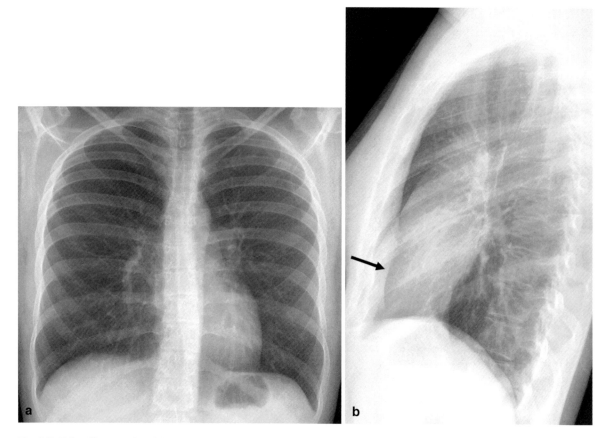

Fig. 9.3 False silhouette sign. The posteroanterior chest radiograph (**a**) shows a loss of the right heart border. The lateral radiograph (**b**) shows a pectus excavatum and absence of pulmonary pathology (*arrow*)

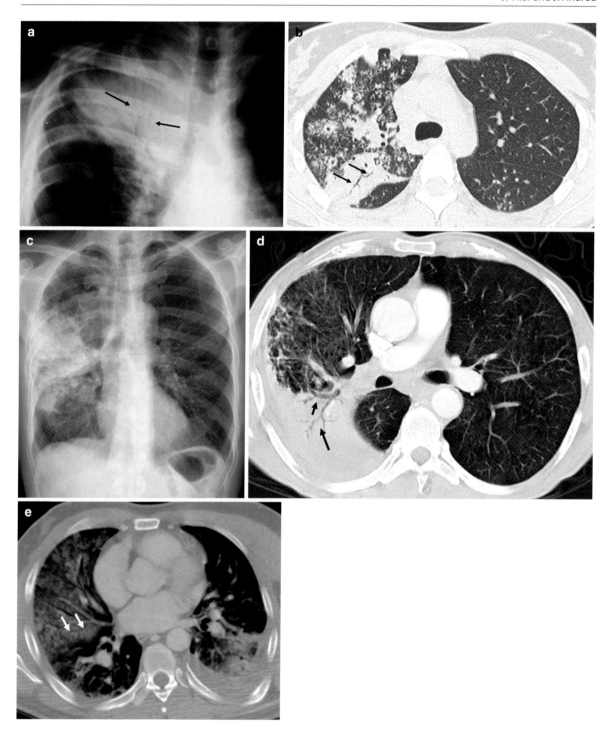

Fig. 9.4 Air bronchogram. (**a**) Chest radiograph shows right upper lobe pneumonia with tubular structures filled with air (*arrows*). (**b**) CT in the same patient shows extensive right upper lobe consolidation with air bronchograms (*arrows*). (**c**) Right upper lobe pneumonia. Ill-defined borders and lobar distribution with small air bronchograms. (**d**) CT of same patient showing branching structures of air bronchograms (*arrows*). (**e**) Pulmonary hemorrhage; the secondary lobules are identified (*arrows*)

diagnosis. However, in bronchoalveolar carcinoma and lipoid pneumonia, there may be a decreased lung attenuation that provides a clue to the diagnosis. In other conditions, such as amiodarone lung, silicoproteinosis, and amyloidosis, consolidation may present with very high lung attenuation (Marchiori et al. 2008). Changes in lung attenuation are usually depicted only on CT.

consolidation and do not obscure the margins of bronchi or vessels (Figs. 9.6 and 9.7) (Hansell et al. 2008). This increased density usually results from partial filling of the alveolar spaces, but can also have other etiologies, such as interstitial thickening, partial collapse of alveolar spaces, increased capillary blood volume, or a combination of these factors.

9.2.1.3 Air Bronchogram

An air bronchogram may be present within a consolidation. This chest radiograph and CT sign is defined as visualization of the air-filled bronchi on a background of opaque, airless lung (Hansell et al. 2008). Air bronchograms are seen in alveolar patterns (Figs. 9.4 and 9.5), but occasionally may appear in extensive interstitial disease.

9.2.1.4 Ground-Glass Opacities

Ground-glass opacities indicate a slight increase in lung density. They show lower attenuation than

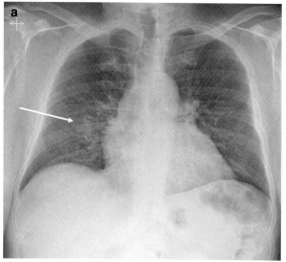

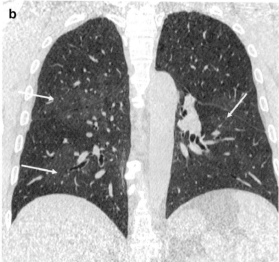

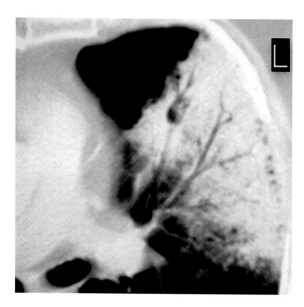

Fig. 9.5 Bronchoalveolar cell carcinoma: leafless tree sign. The air bronchogram shows absence of branching of the bronchi

Fig. 9.6 Ground-glass opacity in *Pneumocystis carinii* pneumonia. (**a**) Chest radiograph shows a slight increase in density in both lungs in a perihilar location (*arrow*). (**b**) CT shows perihilar ground-glass density in both lungs (*arrows*)

9.2.1.5 Nodules

On chest radiographs and CT, alveolar disease can present as a nodular opacity. The lesion characteristically has poorly defined borders on chest radiographs (Figs. 9.7 and 9.8). In some alveolar diseases, CT sometimes shows micronodules with a centrilobular distribution. The micronodules appear as small dot-like or linear opacities in the center of a normal secondary pulmonary lobule (Hansell et al. 2008) (Fig. 9.9).

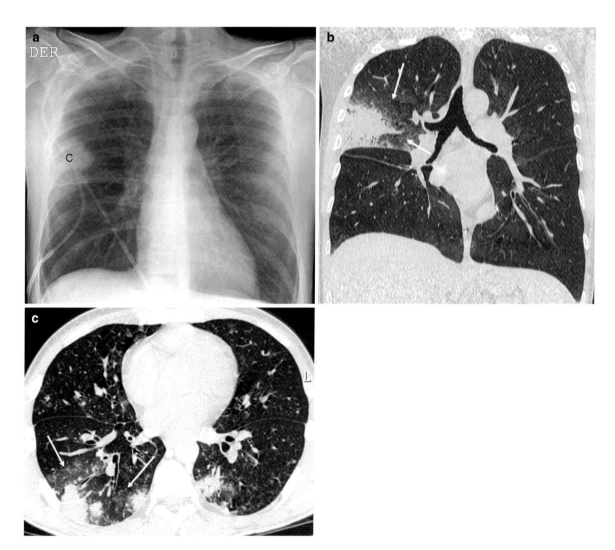

Fig. 9.7 Invasive aspergillosis in a patient with leukemia. (**a**) Chest radiograph demonstrates a right upper lobe consolidation (*C*) with ill-defined margins. (**b**) Coronal CT reconstruction shows a consolidation with a surrounding halo of ground-glass density (*arrows*). (**c**) In another patient with invasive aspergillosis we see multiple poorly defined pulmonary nodules. The loss of definition is produced by the presence of alveolar disease (inflammation and hemorrhage) surrounding the nodules (*arrows*)

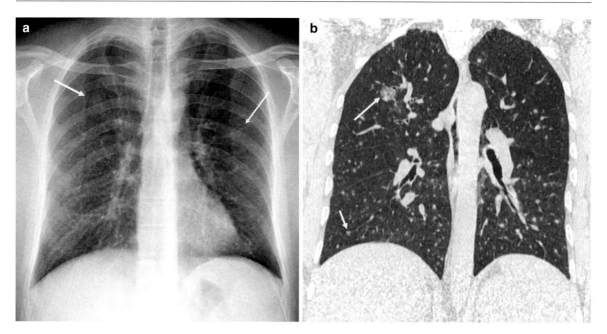

Fig. 9.8 40-year-old man with varicella pneumonia. (**a**) Chest radiograph shows ill-defined densities in both lungs (*arrows*). (**b**) Coronal CT shows multiple nodules with a surrounding halo (*arrows*)

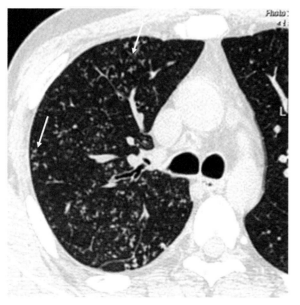

Fig. 9.9 Tuberculosis: acinar nodules on CT with filling of distal bronchioles showing some areas of tree-in-bud pattern (*arrows*)

9.2.1.6 Specific Signs Only Seen on CT

CT has a greater resolution for the visualization of the lung, and therefore some signs will be *better* depicted on CT whereas others signs will be *only* depicted using it. The two CT specific signs of alveolar disease for CT are discussed below.

CT Angiogram

On CT scans after contrast administration, it is sometimes possible to see normal branching lung vessels within a consolidation. This feature is known as the "CT angiographic sign." Two conditions are usually required for this sign to be present manifest: a low-density consolidation and normal pulmonary circulation. The CT angiographic sign has been described as characteristic of bronchoalveolar carcinoma (Fig. 9.10), but can also be observed in other conditions, such as obstructive pneumonia, bacterial

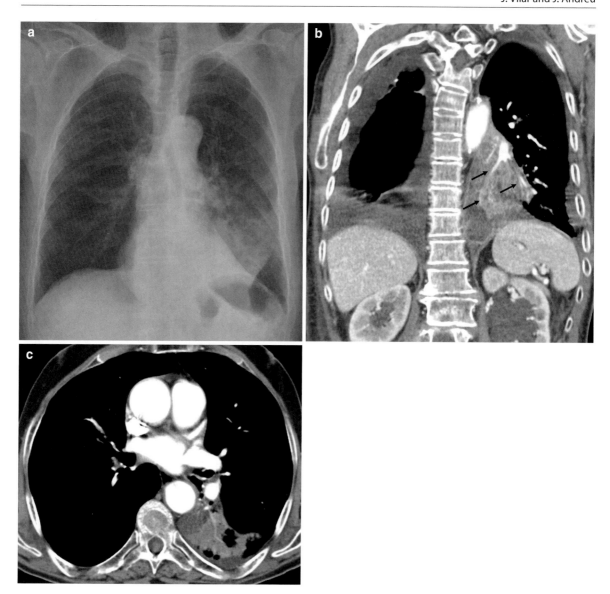

Fig. 9.10 CT angiogram sign in bronchoalveolar cell carcinoma. (**a**) Chest radiograph shows left lower lobe consolidation. (**b, c**) A vessel is seen through the pulmonary consolidation (*arrows*)

pneumonia, pulmonary lymphoma, lipoid pneumonia, and pulmonary edema (Murayama et al. 1993; Maldonado et al.1999; Patsios et al. 2007; Collins 2001).

Crazy Paving

The crazy paving pattern on CT consists of ground-glass attenuation opacity with superimposed interlobular and intralobular thickening, usually in a geographical distribution. Pathologically, this pattern represents mixed involvement of the alveolar and interstitial spaces. Crazy paving was originally reported in patients with alveolar proteinosis, and it is also encountered in other diffuse lung diseases (Frazier et al. 2008; Rossi et al. 2003) (Fig. 9.11).

9.2.2 Distribution

Several distributions of the alveolar pattern have been described, and these are sometimes useful for determining the underlying cause. A central distribution

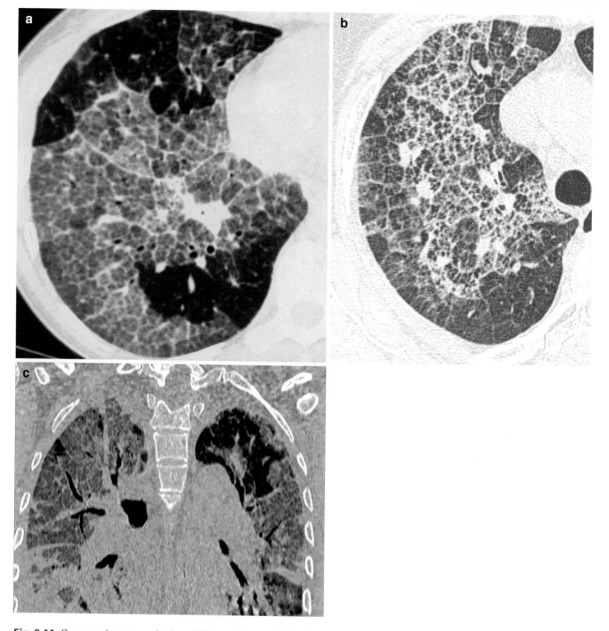

Fig. 9.11 Crazy paving pattern in three different diseases. (**a**) Patient with pulmonary alveolar proteinosis. (**b**) Pulmonary hemorrhage shows an almost identical pattern. (**c**) Acute respiratory distress syndrome

around the hilum with preservation of peripheral lung, known as the "butterfly-wing" or "bat-wing" pattern, is typically present in rapid-onset lung edema (Fig. 9.12). In contrast, a purely peripheral distribution ("anti–butterfly-wing" pattern) (Fig. 9.13) is characteristic of chronic eosinophilic pneumonia. Other diseases, such as bacterial pneumonia and bronchoalveolar carcinoma, show a tendency toward a lobar or segmental distribution (Fig. 9.4).

9.2.3 Evolutive Changes

A useful radiological feature for the differential diagnosis of alveolar patterns is changes occurring over time, which allow them to be divided into acute and subacute/chronic conditions. Acute patterns develop rapidly, in less than a few weeks, whereas subacute/chronic patterns have a slow onset (several weeks) and may remain stable for months.

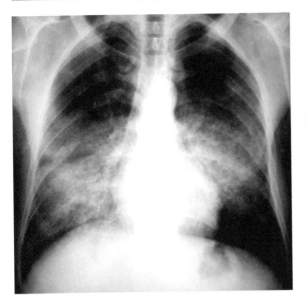

Fig. 9.12 Distribution: Radiograph showing a typical perihilar distribution of pulmonary edema ("bat-wing appearance")

Some diseases migrate; that is, their location in the lungs changes over time. This is a typical finding in chronic eosinophilic pneumonia and organizing pneumonia (Fig. 9.14).

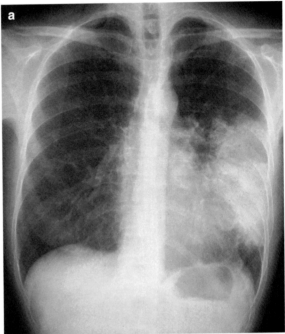

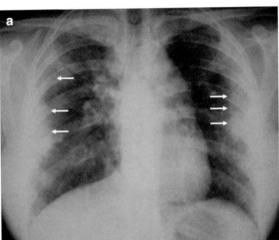

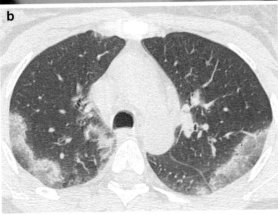

Fig. 9.13 (**a**, **b**) Distribution of "anti–bat-wing" appearance in a patient with chronic eosinophilic pneumonia (*arrows*)

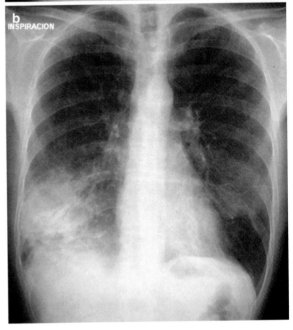

Fig. 9.14 Evolution of COP. (**a**) Chest radiograph shows a left pulmonary consolidation without a lobar or segmental distribution. (**b**) Two months later the consolidation appears in the opposite lung

9.3 Most Relevant Conditions that Present with an Alveolar Pattern

A practical approach to airspace disease should relate to the clinical situation and its translation into imaging. Thus, alveolar diseases can be divided in two groups: those of acute onset and subacute/chronic diseases. The clinical situation is often inconclusive, but the rapid or slow appearance of pulmonary alterations can help the radiologist to identify the underlying disease.

9.3.1 Acute Alveolar Pattern

9.3.1.1 Pulmonary Edema

Pulmonary edema can be classified according to its etiology as cardiogenic or noncardiogenic (Ware and Matthay 2005). On chest radiography, cardiogenic pulmonary edema usually presents with cardiac enlargement and widening of the vascular pedicle (Milne et al. 1985; Aberle et al. 1988). Septal lines and pleural effusion are often present, and there may be thickening of the bronchovascular interstitium and fissures. Air bronchograms are uncommon.

In noncardiogenic edema, the cardiac silhouette and vascular pedicle are usually normal. Pleural fluid and septal lines are generally not seen but air bronchograms are frequent (Milne et al.1985; Aberle et al. 1988).

Cardiogenic pulmonary edema is commonly distributed in the central and lower lobes, but a perihilar distribution (bat-wing appearance) can sometimes be seen, particularly in acute cases (Fig. 9.12) (Gluecker et al. 1999). Cardiogenic edema may be unilateral, caused by emphysema or another disease in one of the lungs (Fig. 9.15). Noncardiogenic edema is patchy and usually shows a peripheral distribution (Fig. 9.16).

Chest radiographs suffice to establish the diagnosis in most cases of pulmonary edema. When CT is performed for another indication, the most common findings are areas of ground-glass attenuation (Fig. 9.16) and septal and peribronchovascular thickening (Storto et al. 1995) (Table 9.1).

A presentation of rapid-onset bilateral airspace occupation should make us think of pulmonary edema. Chest radiographs suffice to distinguish cardiogenic

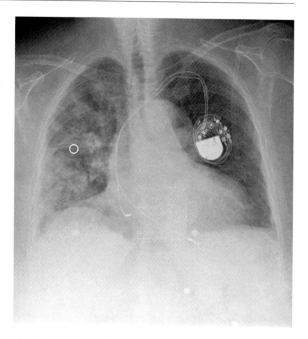

Fig. 9.15 Unilateral right pulmonary edema (*O*) in a patient with cardiac failure

from noncardiogenic pulmonary edema and to monitor the disease's evolution.

9.3.1.2 Infectious Pneumonia

One of the most common causes of airspace occupation is acute pneumonia. Classically, the radiological and histological findings differ between community- and hospital-acquired pneumonia (Franquet 2001). Currently, pneumonia is classified into four groups: community-acquired, aspiration, healthcare-associated, and hospital-acquired pneumonia.

The radiographic patterns of community-acquired pneumonia can vary and are often related to the causative agent. This condition usually manifests as an airspace pattern (Figs. 9.1 and 9.4). Bacterial pneumonia, particularly the disease caused by Gram-positive microorganisms, provokes an inflammatory response in the peripheral lung, and edema quickly spreads through the underlying acini, lobes, segments, and lobules. This rapid spread causes large consolidations. Small lesions, such as centrilobular and tree-in-bud nodules, are limited, and ground-glass areas are seen around the consolidations (Fig. 9.4).

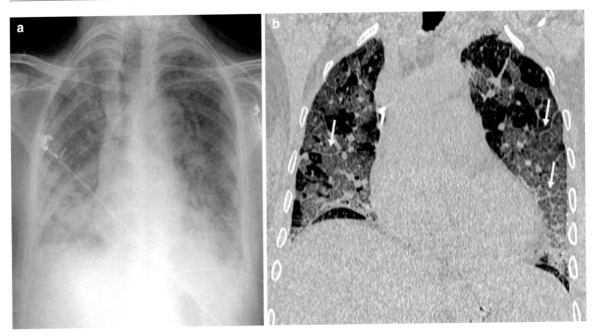

Fig. 9.16 Noncardiac (renal) pulmonary edema. (**a**) Chest radiograph shows bilateral diffuse densities in both lungs. There is no cardiomegaly. (**b**) Coronal CT shows bilateral ground-glass opacities with septal thickening (*arrows*) that result in areas of crazy paving. Note the irregular distribution of the edema

Table 9.1 Chest radiograph in cardiogenic versus noncardiogenic pulmonary edema

Cardiogenic	Noncardiogenic
Lower lobes	Peripheral
Perihilar	Patchy
No air bronchograms	Air bronchograms
Large heart and vascular pedicle	No cardiovascular enlargement
May be asymmetric in COPD	May be asymmetric in COPD[*]

[*] chronic obstructive pulmonary disease

Aspiration pneumonia presents as a bilateral alveolar pattern, usually involving the lower lobes (Figs. 9.17 and 9.18). The radiographic patterns of healthcare-associated and hospital-acquired pneumonia are variable, the most common being diffuse and multifocal involvement with pleural effusion. The diagnosis of pneumonia is based on consistent symptoms and a chest radiograph showing airspace occupation. CT can be used to detect complications and to provide an early diagnosis for immunocompromised patients (Fig. 9.7) (Vilar et al. 2004).

The diagnosis of pneumonia relies on radiographic findings of alveolar disease. In most cases chest radiographs will suffice. CT should be used in unresolved cases or when complications are suspected.

9.3.1.3 Pulmonary Hemorrhage

Several entities can cause pulmonary hemorrhage, such as glomerulonephritis, immunocomplex diseases, basal antimembrane diseases, drug-related causes, bleeding diathesis, and trauma. The bleeding arises from the pulmonary microvasculature and extends to large areas of the lung parenchyma (Green et al. 1996). The clinical presentation is nonspecific and includes cough, chest pain, and dyspnea. More specific findings such as hemoptysis and anemia may also be present. In acute hemorrhage, the hematocrit value can be markedly decreased (Albelda et al. 1985).

The chest radiograph shows nonspecific findings. The usual presentation is that of perihilar or basal airspace disease, mimicking pulmonary edema or an opportunistic pneumonia (Albelda et al. 1985; Witte et al. 1991) (Fig. 9.19a). Initially, pulmonary hemorrhage may have a unilateral distribution (Witte et al. 1991), and there may be an associated reticular pattern. In about 2 weeks' time, the features can evolve

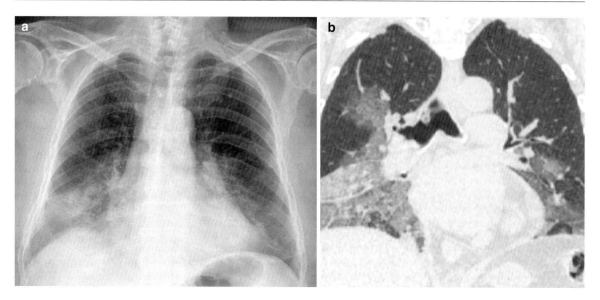

Fig. 9.17 Aspiration pneumonia. (**a**) Chest radiograph shows bilateral lower lobe infiltrates. (**b**) CT, coronal reconstruction, shows consolidations in both lower lobes with areas of ground-glass density

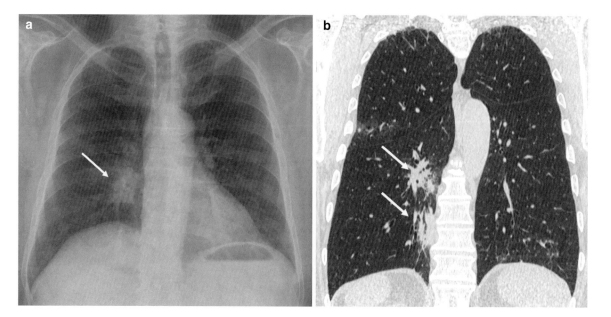

Fig. 9.18 Chronic aspiration in a patient with oral cancer. (**a**) Right lower lobe alveolar consolidation (*arrow*). (**b**) Consolidation with air bronchograms and irregular borders (*arrows*)

toward a normal radiograph. Some pulmonary consolidations migrate during the evolution. There is no associated pleural fluid, lymphadenopathy, or atelectasis.

On CT scans, acute hemorrhage presents as areas of ground-glass attenuation (Cortese et al. 2008) and sometimes consolidations (Fig 9.19b). A "crazy paving" pattern may be seen (Fig. 9.11) (Rossi et al. 2003).

The disease evolves rapidly to resolution, at which time small nodules, uniform in size, can be visualized. These represent partial accumulations of hemosiderin and macrophages with hemosiderin.

Despite the fact that the radiographic changes are similar to those of pulmonary edema or an opportunistic infection, pulmonary hemorrhage should be

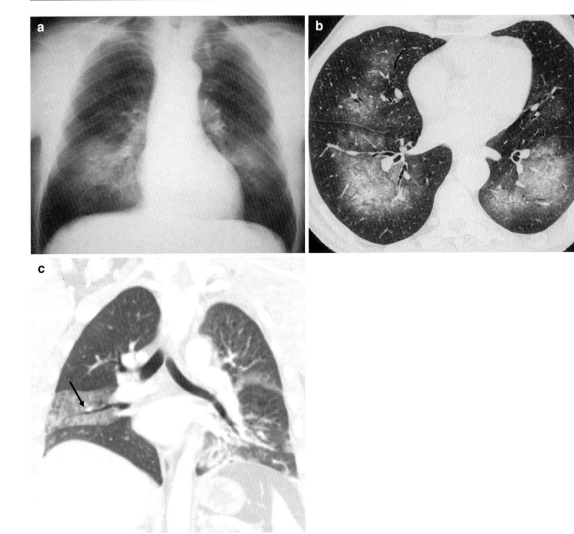

Fig. 9.19 Pulmonary hemorrhage. (**a**) Chest radiograph shows bilateral lower lobe consolidations. (**b**) CT shows that the consolidations have a predominance of ground-glass densities and a perihilar distribution. (**c**) Hemorrhage after thoracic traumatism. An air bronchogram caused by the filling of the alveolar spaces is seen in the middle lobe (*arrow*)

suspected when airspace disease with a rapid evolution is observed, associated with hemoptysis and a low hematocrit value (Table 9.2).

9.3.1.4 Acute Respiratory Distress Syndrome

Acute respiratory distress syndrome (ARDS) is a serious condition related to acute hypoxemia (but not heart failure) that occurs in association with several clinical situations. Chest radiographs show pulmonary opacities that are usually bilateral and are gravity-dependent; thus, they are located in the lung bases (Fig. 9.20) (Table 9.3). On CT scans the alterations can have a homogeneous distribution but frequently show patchy areas of consolidation alternating with areas of ground-glass opacity (Fig. 9.20). Air bronchograms are present in most patients, and small pleural effusions are seen in half of cases.

Respiratory distress can have pulmonary or nonpulmonary causes. In the pulmonary cases, asymmetrical areas of ground-glass density and consolidations are most commonly seen. Extra-pulmonary ARDS is usually symmetrical and ground-glass densities predominate (Goodman et al. 1999). In the initial exudative phases of ARDS, opacities without bronchiectasis are found, whereas the advanced proliferative or fibrotic phases show traction bronchiectasis, a sign of a poor prognosis (Ichikado el al. 2006).

ARDS syndrome should be included in the group of diffuse alveolar diseases. The imaging findings can help to define the causes and the prognosis of the condition (Table 9.4).

Table 9.2 Imaging findings in pulmonary hemorrhage

Features of alveolar pattern
Basal and perihilar (simulates edema)
May be unilateral
Reticular pattern
Rapid change
No pleural fluid
[a]Ground glass
[a]Crazy paving
Nodules

[a]Only seen with CT

Table 9.3 Imaging findings in acute respiratory distress syndrome

Features of alveolar pattern
Bilateral pulmonary opacities
Gravity dependent
Ground glass
Consolidations
Symmetric in extra-pulmonary origin
Asymmetric in pulmonary origin

Table 9.4 Imaging findings in drug-induced lung diseases

Features of alveolar pattern
Uni-or multifocal airspace occupation
Ground glass
Septal thickening

9.3.1.5 Drug-Induced Lung Disease

More than 100 drugs have been reported to produce pulmonary lesions. The pathologic findings of drug-induced lung disease vary and include patterns of diffuse alveolar damage, organizing pneumonia, nonspecific

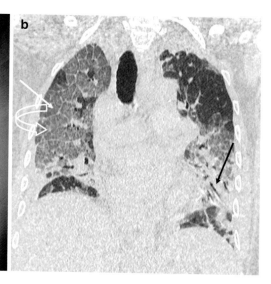

Fig. 9.20 Acute respiratory distress syndrome. (**a**) Portable chest radiograph shows diffuse bilateral pulmonary opacities predominant in the lower lobes. (**b**) Coronal CT in another patient shows a combination of areas of ground-glass attenuation (*curved arrow*), air bronchograms (*black arrow*), consolidations, and thickened septa (*white arrow*)

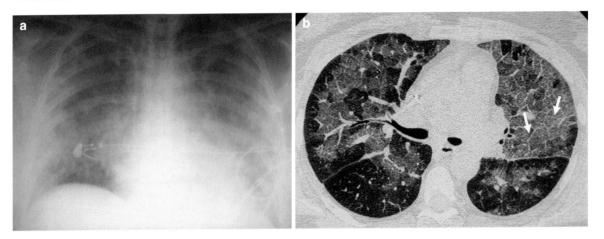

Fig. 9.21 Drug induced pulmonary disease. (**a**) Chest radiograph shows bilateral pulmonary densities. (**b**) High-resolution CT shows areas of ground-glass density and thickened septa (*arrows*) giving a crazy paving appearance

interstitial pneumonia, chronic eosinophilic pneumonia, pulmonary edema, and hemorrhage (Rossi et al. 2000). A single agent can produce several pathologic changes. The clinical and radiologic presentation depends on the pathologic changes. Most patients present diffuse or multifocal airspace occupation. Ground glass and septal thickening are the most common radiological findings (Fig. 9.21) (Akira et al. 2002; Rossi et al. 2000) (Table 9.4).

Often the diagnosis of drug-induced lung disease is made by excluding other diseases that should always be ruled out before making a definitive diagnosis.

9.3.2 Chronic Alveolar Pattern

9.3.2.1 Organizing Pneumonia

Organizing pneumonia (OP) is characterized by a nonspecific pulmonary involvement that may be associated with several conditions, including infection, collagen disease, or aspiration, among others. OP can also be idiopathic, in which case it is known as cryptogenic organizing pneumonia (COP) (Epler 2001); the radiographic presentation is similar in both forms of OP (Lohr et al. 1997; Cazzato et al. 2000; Oymak et al. 2005). Although OP is included in the group of interstitial pneumonias, it involves the airspaces. Pathologically, OP presents as plugs of granulation tissue lying within small airways, alveolar ducts, and alveoli. It is more common during the fifth decade of life and has not been related to smoking. Clinically, OP has an acute or subacute presentation with cough and dyspnea; fever, chest pain, and hemoptysis, as in pneumonia, may also be seen (Oymak et al. 2005).

Chest radiographs of OP show bilateral or, less often, unilateral pulmonary consolidations with a random distribution and preservation of the lung volume, or a focal consolidation simulating a lung mass. Reticular patterns are uncommon, and, when present, are considered to be sign of fibrosis. In one third of cases, the consolidations are migratory on consecutive radiographs (Cazzato et al. 2000; Oymak et al. 2005) (Fig. 9.14).

The CT findings of OP usually include pulmonary consolidations in a subpleural, peribronchial, or bronchial location. The middle and lower lung fields are typically affected. Air bronchograms, bronchial dilatation, and ground-glass areas are common. Other presentations include nodules, masses, and linear patterns (Kim et al.) in a perilobular distribution (Akira et al. 1998; Ujita et al. 2004). Honeycombing is not a typical feature of OP and, when present, is scant. Lymphadenopathy is also infrequent (Souza et al. 2006) (Fig. 9.22).

In approximately 20% of patients, a *reverse halo sign* is observed. This is an area of ground-glass opacity surrounded by an area of consolidation (Fig. 9.22c). The reverse halo sign has been also reported in other conditions (Gasparetto et at. 2005; Benamore et al. 2007; Agarwal et al. 2007; Wahba et al. 2008) and is nonspecific for OP, but within the appropriate clinical context it has a high diagnostic value (Kim et al. 2003).

Organizing pneumonia OP typically responds well to steroids but may recur after the dose is reduced. After treatment of less than 1 year, one third of cases recurred (Epler, 2001).

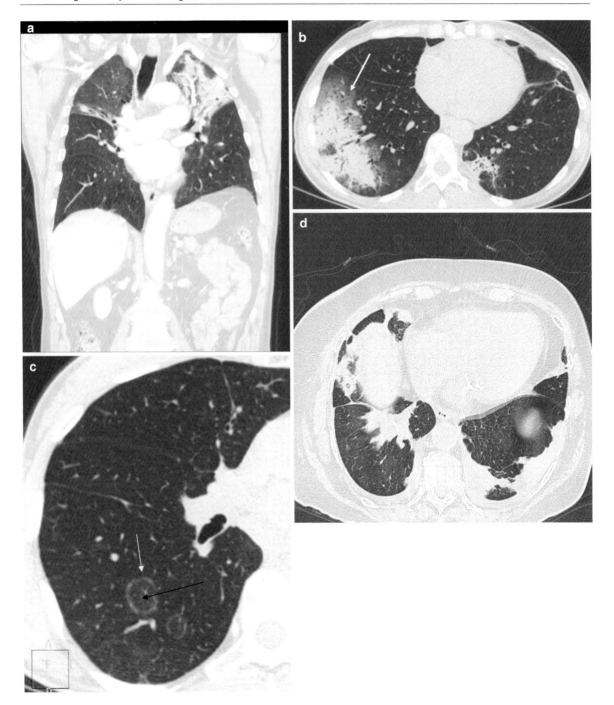

Fig. 9.22 OP: (**a, b**) CT shows several areas of consolidation and others with ground-glass density (*arrow*). (**c**) Note the reverse halo sign seen as a round crescent (*white arrow*) with inner ground-glass density (*black arrow*). (**d**) Radiotherapy-induced OP showing lower lobe consolidations

Table 9.5 Imaging findings in organizing pneumonia

Features of alveolar pattern
Random distribution
50% migratory
Sub pleural and peribronchial
Middle and lower lobes
[a]Reverse halo sign
Response to steroids

[a] Only seen with CT

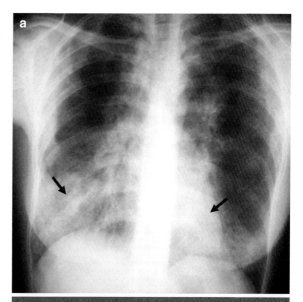

OP should be suspected in patients with multiple pulmonary consolidations that do not respond to antibiotics and show a tendency to migrate (Table 9.5).

9.3.2.2 Pulmonary Alveolar Proteinosis

Pulmonary alveolar proteinosis (PAP) is a rare entity of unknown pathogenesis characterized by occupation of the alveoli by lipoproteinaceous material. PAP may be idiopathic or present in association with some occupation-related diseases, immunodeficiencies, or medications. The condition is more frequent in men (4:1), and usually occurs between the third and fifth decades of life. It has been related to smoking (Seymour and Presneill, 2002).

The symptoms of PAP are mild and include nonproductive cough and progressive dyspnea. Patients rarely present with fever, chest pain, or hemoptysis. Typically, a patient has a very mild clinical presentation compared to the extensive pulmonary involvement seen with chest radiography.

On chest radiographs, bilateral and predominantly perihilar pulmonary consolidations are seen, similar to the findings for pulmonary edema ("bat-wing" pattern), but with the absence of septal lines, pleural effusion, and cardiomegaly (Fig. 9.23) (Frazier et al. 2008). A more diffuse form with a peripheral distribution as well as a unilateral distribution have been described. (Prakash et al. 1987).

CT reveals a geographical distribution and sometimes a more diffuse pattern. The most frequent findings are ground-glass opacities, airspace consolidations, and smooth thickening of the interlobular septa (Holbert et al. 2001). The combination of ground glass and septal thickening gives rise to a "crazy paving" pattern that is highly suggestive of PAP. This pattern can also be present in bronchioalveolar carcinoma,

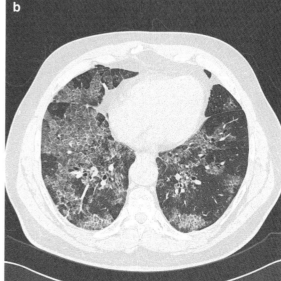

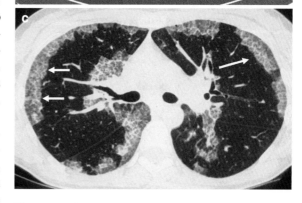

Fig. 9.23 Pulmonary alveolar proteinosis. (**a**) Chest radiograph shows bilateral pulmonary opacities (*arrows*). (**b**) CT shows bilateral central crazy paving pattern. (**c**) Another case of alveolar proteinosis with a subpleural distribution (*arrows*)

pulmonary hemorrhage, and lipoid pneumonia. The ground glass is caused by filling of air spaces with a positive periodic acid-Schiff stain in proteinaceous material. The septal thickening is due to edema and infiltration of the interstitium by lymphocytes and macrophages (Fig. 9.11). Bronchioalveolar lavage may resolve the septal thickening (Trapnell et al. 2003). In 25% of patients, PAP appears as an isolated ground-glass opacity (Frazier et al. 2008). Air bronchograms are infrequent. Few cases progress to fibrosis; thus, signs of fibrosis are not commonly seen on CT scans (Holbert et al. 2001).

Patients with PAP are prone to infections, some of them opportunistic. When a lobar consolidation or cavitation is seen in a patient with alveolar proteinosis, opportunistic infection, frequently *Nocardia,* should be suspected (Holbert et al. 2001)

Pulmonary alveolar proteinosis should be suspected when a patient presents with perihilar consolidations, few clinical symptoms a crazy paving pattern on CT (Table 9.6).

9.3.2.3 Bronchioloalveolar Cell Carcinoma

Bronchioloalveolar cell carcinoma (BAC) is a subtype of adenocarcinoma that has intra-alveolar extension and a lepidic growth pattern through an intact pulmonary structure. It does not invade the vascular or pleural stroma (Travis et al. 1999); hence, the pulmonary architecture is

Table 9.6 Imaging findings in pulmonary alveolar proteinosis

Features of alveolar pattern
Perihilar distribution
No signs of cardiac failure
Ground glass; geographical
[a]Crazy paving
Mild clinical presentation
May have superimposed infection

[a] Only seen with CT

preserved. BAC has been classified into three subtypes: mucinous, nonmucinous, and mixed with adenocarcinoma, but with prominence of BAC. Clinically, BAC presents in a nonspecific form with cough, expectoration, weight loss, dyspnea, hemoptysis, and fever. Occasionally, and rather late in the disease, patients with diffuse disease may show bronchorrhea.

The radiological presentation of BAC is variable. It may present as solitary or multiple nodules, as airspace disease that is segmental, lobar, or diffuse in distribution. Airspace occupation occurs in about 30% of patients and corresponds to the mucinous histological type (Lee et al. 2000; Patsios et al. 2007). On plain films, BAC presents as a lobar or segmental consolidation, often progressive. The differential diagnosis with pneumonia is difficult; thus, there is usually a delay in the diagnosis (Fig. 9.24).

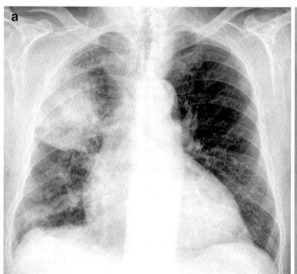
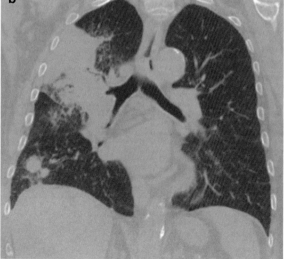

Fig. 9.24 Diffuse bronchoalveolar cell carcinoma. (**a**) Chest radiograph shows several right pulmonary alveolar consolidations. Note bulging of the minor fissure. (**b**) Coronal CT shows consolidation in right upper lobe and additional nodular areas of alveolar disease

On CT scans the consolidations are usually heterogeneous with some cystic areas (Akira et al. 1999; Kim et al. 2006). Air bronchograms are frequent. The bronchi can show stretching, squeezing, or widening and sometimes dilatation (Akira et al. 1999). Other signs include the "leafless tree" sign (Fig. 9.4) and the "CT angiographic" sign (Fig. 9.10), which are seen in one third of patients, although these are nonspecific signs that are present in other diseases, such as infectious pneumonia (Jung et al. 2001). Mucin-producing BAC may increase the volume of the lobe with bulging of the fissures, a finding that has been considered very characteristic of the condition (Fig. 9.24) (Jung et al. 2001). The affected area rarely loses volume and pleural fluid, and lymphadenopathies are infrequent (Akira et al.1999). The diffuse form shows a combination of ground glass areas, consolidations, pulmonary nodules, centrilobular nodules, and air bronchograms with a peripheral distribution, most commonly in the lung bases (Fig. 9.24) (Akira et al.1999). The ground-glass density accompanying the consolidations has a tendency to be intralobular. This explains the straight and undulated borders. Ground-glass areas can appear at a distance from the consolidations, a finding rarely present in other diseases (Akira et al. 1999). Occasionally there is a combination of ground-glass and thickening of the interlobular septa, showing a crazy paving pattern (Aquino et al. 1998; Jung et al. 2001; Rossi et al. 2003). Follow-up studies are useful, showing progression of the disease with increased size of the ground-glass areas and new lesions. Sometimes ground glass will evolve into areas of consolidation (Akira et al. 1999).

Bronchioloalveolar cell carcinoma should be suspected when plain films show chronic pulmonary consolidations. CT can provide imaging findings that indicate the neoplastic nature of the lesion (Table 9.7).

Table 9.7 Imaging findings in bronchioloalveolar cell carcinoma

Features of alveolar pattern
Airspace occupation (30% of cases)
Progressive
Bronchi stretched and widened: Leafless tree sign
Bulging of fissures
[a]CT angiographic sign
Combines ground glass and consolidations
[a]Crazy paving

[a]Only seen with CT

9.3.2.4 Lymphoma

Pulmonary lymphoma may cause airspace occupation. Primary lung lymphomas are very rare. Most of these are bronchus-associated lymphoid tissue (BALT) lymphomas (Maksimovic et al. 2008). Clinically, pulmonary lymphoma can be asymptomatic or present with cough and dyspnea. These tumors have a good prognosis because most of them are a low-grade B-cell, non-Hodgkin type. BALT is associated with immunologic diseases, such as Sjögren, collagen disease dysgammaglobulinemia, and AIDS (Bae et al. 2008).

On chest radiography lymphomas present as isolated or multiple nodules or infiltrates that may be bilateral. The pulmonary consolidations are usually central or peripheral and less often lobar (Figs. 9.25 and 9.26) (Kinsely et al. 1999).

On CT scans, nodules and consolidations without a specific regional predominance can be identified (Lee et al. 2000). The majority have a random distribution. Lymphadenopathy and pleural fluid are uncommon findings. Air bronchograms are often seen in both the nodules and consolidations (Lee et al. 2000) (Figs. 9.25 and 9.26). The CT angiographic sign can also be observed in lymphoma. Some patients present with cystic pulmonary lesions that likely represent dilatation of the distal airways due to bronchiolar obstruction (King et al. 2000; Lee et al. 2000; Bae et al. 2008) (Table 9.8). The pulmonary lesions in lymphoma usually show slow growth and may remain stable through serial studies (Bae et al. 2008).

Pulmonary lymphoma should be suspected when plain films show a slow-growing pulmonary consolidation or nodules with ill-defined borders and air bronchograms. CT can provide some additional imaging findings.

9.3.2.5 Chronic Eosinophilic Pneumonia

Chronic eosinophilic pneumonia is an idiopathic pneumonia with symptoms of progressive pulmonary involvement. It is characterized histologically by eosinophilic and lymphocytic infiltrates in the alveolar space and interstitium, with associated fibrosis. Areas of organizing pneumonia and low-grade vasculitis may appear (Lee 2000; Kim et al. 2006). The clinical presentation is subacute with fever, cough, dyspnea, and weight loss. It may be associated with asthma. An important element in the diagnosis is the presence of

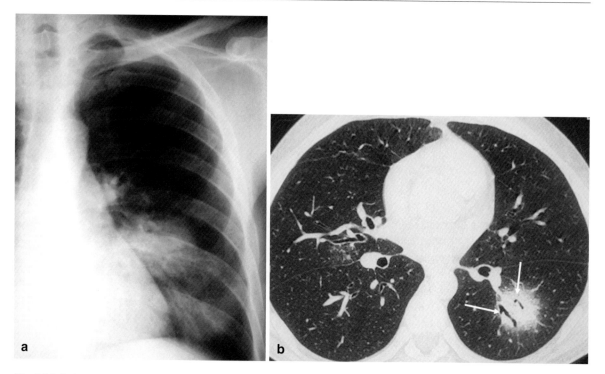

Fig. 9.25 Pulmonary lymphoma. (**a**) Chest radiograph shows a focal pulmonary consolidation seen in the left lower lobe. (**b**) CT of the pulmonary consolidation shows ill-defined borders and an air bronchogram (*arrows*)

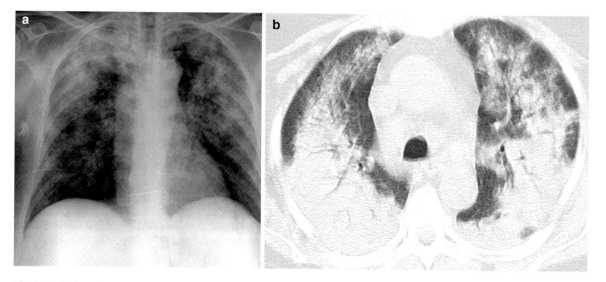

Fig. 9.26 Patient with angioimmunoblastic lymphoma. (**a**) Bilateral pulmonary consolidations are present. (**b**) CT shows extensive alveolar disease with air bronchograms

peripheral eosinophilia, which is usually mild or moderate, but sometimes severe (Jeong et al. 2007).

The chest radiographic findings include peripheral lung consolidations that are nonlobar, nonsegmental and usually subpleural. There is a predominance of upper lobe distribution. This pattern has been called a photographic negative of pulmonary edema, and is seen in half of cases (Fig. 9.13) (Gaensler and Carrington. 1977; Mayo et al. 1989; Jeong et al. 2007). Pleural effusion is rare.

Table 9.8 Imaging findings in pulmonary lymphoma

Features of alveolar pattern
Solitary or multiple consolidations and nodules
Not lobar
Central or peripheral
Air bronchograms in consolidations and nodules
[a]CT angiographic sign
Cysts (rare)

[a]Only seen with CT

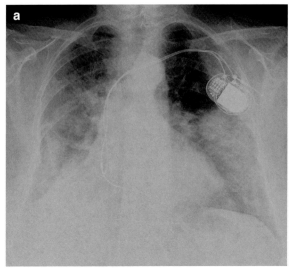

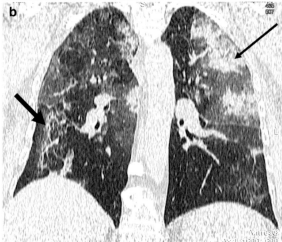

CT images show subpleural consolidations. In advanced stages there will be ground-glass opacities, nodules, and reticular densities (Fig. 9.27) (Johkoh et al. 2000). The infiltrates respond readily to steroids but may reappear when the dose is reduced or the treatment changed.

Chronic eosinophilic pneumonia should be suspected in a patient with eosinophilia and pulmonary consolidations distributed peripherally in the lungs (Johkoh et al. 2000) (Table 9.9).

9.3.2.6 Radiation Pneumonitis

Radiation therapy of the thorax may harm the lung and give rise to airspace disease. This can occur with doses above 30 Gy and particularly with doses above 40 Gy. The lung involvement has two phases. Pneumonitis occurs 1–3 months after the completion of treatment, and fibrosis predominates in the later phase, at 6–12 months after treatment (Choi et al. 2004). Chemotherapy may enhance the negative effects of radiation in these patients.

On the chest radiograph, pulmonary consolidations are seen in the areas of the radiation field. Areas outside of this zone are rarely affected. In the fibrotic phase, volume loss and bronchiectasis are observed (Fig. 9.28).

CT during the initial phase shows pulmonary consolidations and areas of ground-glass attenuation. In the fibrotic phase, traction bronchiectasis and atelectasis may be seen (Fig. 9.28). OP associated with radiation has been described and may simulate other

Fig. 9.27 Chronic eosinophilic pneumonia. (**a**) CT shows a typical peripheral distribution. (**b**) Another case of chronic eosinophilic pneumonia shows a combination of ground-glass areas (*thin arrow*), subpleural lines (*thick arrow*), and opacities

Table 9.9 Imaging findings in chronic eosinophilic pneumonia

Features of alveolar pattern
Peripheral
Patchy upper lobes
Ground glass
Reticular opacities
Response to steroids

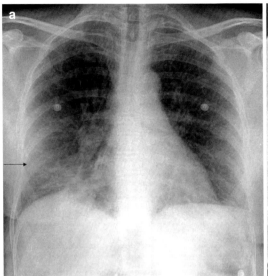
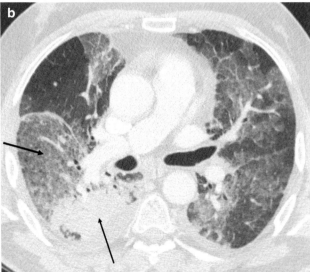

Fig. 9.28 Radiation pneumonitis. (**a**) Chest radiograph shows a right lower lobe opacity (*arrow*) caused by radiation pneumonitis in a patient with right breast cancer 3 months after being treated with radiotherapy. (**b**) CT of another patient shows fibrotic changes as well as areas of ground-glass density following the radiation field (*arrows*)

airspace processes, especially pneumonia or recurrence (Fig. 9.22) (Bayle et al. 1995).

The diagnosis of radiation pneumonitis should be made when focal pulmonary disease coincides with the areas of the radiation field (Table 9.10).

Table 9.10 Imaging findings in radiation pneumonitis

Features of alveolar pattern
Lesions in radiation field
Airspace 1–3 months
Fibrosis 6–12 months
Organizing pneumonia may appear

References

Aberle DR, Wiener-Kronish JP, Webb WR et al (1988) Hydrostatic versus increased permeability pulmonary edema: diagnosis based on radiographic criteria in critically ill patients. Radiology 168:73–79

Albelda SM, Gefter WB, Epstein DM et al (1985) Diffuse pulmonary hemorrhage: a review and classification. Radiology 154: 289–297

Agarwal R, Aggarwal AN, Gupta D (2007) Another cause of reverse halo sign: Wegener's granulomatosis. Br J Radiol 80: 849–850

Aquino SL, Chiles C, Halford P (1998) Distinction of consolidative bronchioloalveolar carcinoma from pneumonia: do CT criteria work? AJR Am J Roentgenol 171:359–363

Akira M, Atagi S, Kawahara M et al (1999) High-resolution CT findings of diffuse bronchioloalveolar carcinoma in 38 patients. AJR Am J Roentgenol 173:1623–1629

Akira M, Yamamoto S, Sakatani M (1998) Bronchiolitis obliterans organizing pneumonia manifesting as multiple large nodules or masses. AJR Am J Roentgenol 170:291–295

Akira M, Ishikawa H, Yamamoto S (2002) Drug-induced pneumonitis: thin-section CT findings in 60 patients. Radiology 224:852–860

Bae YA, Lee KS, Han J et al (2008) Marginal zone B-cell lymphoma of bronchus-associated lymphoid tissue: imaging findings in 21 patients. Chest 133:433–440

Bayle JY, Nesme P, Bejui-Thivolet F, Loire R, Guerin JC, Cordier JF (1995) Migratory organizing Pneumonitis primed by radiation therapy. Eur Respir J 8:322–326

Benamore RE, Weisbrod GL, Hwang DM et al (2007) Reversed halo sign in lymphomatoid granulomatosis. Br J Radiol 80: 162–166

Cazzato S, Zompatori M, Baruzzi G et al (2000) Bronchiolitis obliterans-organizing pneumonia: an Italian experience. Respir Med 94:702–708

Choi YW, Munden RF, Erasmus JJ et al (2004) Effects of radiation therapy on the lung: radiologic appearances and differential diagnosis. Radiographics 24:985–997

Collins J (2001) CT signs and patterns of lung disease. Radiol Clin North Am 39:1115–1135

Cortese G, Nicali R, Placido R (2008) Radiological aspects of diffuse alveolar haemorrhage. Radiol Med 113:16–28

Epler GR (2001) Bronchiolitis obliterans organizing pneumonia. Arch Intern Med 161:158–164

Franquet T (2001) Imaging of pneumonia: trends and algorithms. Eur Respir J 18:196–208

Frazier AA, Franks TJ, Cooke EO et al (2008) From the archives of the AFIP: pulmonary alveolar proteinosis. Radiographics 28:883–899

Gaensler EA, Carrington CB (1977) Peripheral opacities in chronic eosinophilic pneumonia: the photographic negative of pulmonary edema. AJR Am J Roentgenol 128:1–13

Gasparetto EL, Escuissato DL, Davaus T et al (2005) Reversed halo sign in pulmonary paracoccidioidomycosis. AJR Am J Roentgenol 184:1932–1934

Goodman LR, Fumagalli R, Tagliabue P et al (1999) Adult respiratory distress syndrome due to pulmonary and extrapulmonary causes: CT, clinical, and functional correlations. Radiology 213:545–552

Green RJ, Ruoss SJ, Kraft SA et al (1996) Pulmonary capillaritis and alveolar hemorrhage update on diagnosis and management. Chest 10:1305–1316

Gluecker T, Capasso P, Schnyder P et al (1999) Clinical and radiologic features of pulmonary edema. Radiographics 19:1507–1531

Hansell DM, Bankier AA, MacMahon H et al (2008) Fleischner society: glossary of terms for thoracic imaging. Radiology 246:697–722

Holbert JM, Costello P, Li W et al (2001) CT features of pulmonary alveolar proteinosis. AJR Am J Roentgenol 176:1287–1294

Ichikado K, Suga M, Muranaka H et al (2006) Prediction of prognosis for acute respiratory distress syndrome with thin-section CT: validation in 44 cases. Radiology 238:321–329

Im JG, Han MC, Yu EJ et al (1990) Lobar bronchioloalveolar cell carcinoma: angiogram sign on CT scans. Radiology 176:749–753

Jeong YJ, Kim KI, Seo IJ et al (2007) Eosinophilic lung diseases: a clinical, radiologic, and pathologic overview. Radiographics 27:617–637

Johkoh T, Müller NL, Akira M et al (2000) Eosinophilic lung diseases: diagnostic accuracy of thin-section CT in 111 patients. Radiology 216:773–780

Jung JI, Kim H, Park SH et al (2001) CT differentiation of pneumonic-type bronchioloalveolar cell carcinoma and infectious pneumonia. Br J Radiol 74:490–494

Kim SJ, Lee KS, Ryu YH et al (2003) Reversed halo sign on high-resolution CT of cryptogenic organizing pneumonia: diagnostic implications. AJR Am J Roentgenol 180:1251–1254

Kim TH, Kim SJ, Ryu YH et al (2006) Differential CT features of infectious pneumonia versus bronchioloalveolar carcinoma (BAC) mimicking pneumonia. Eur Radiol 16:1763–1868

King LJ, Padley SP, Wotherspoon AC et al (2000) Pulmonary MALT lymphoma: imaging findings in 24 cases. Eur Radiol 10:1932–1938

Kinsely BL, Mastey LA, Mergo PJ et al (1999) Pulmonary mucosa-associated lymphoid tissue lymphoma: CT and pathologic findings. AJR Am J Roentgenol 172:1321–1326

Lee DK, Im JG, Lee KS et al (2000) B-cell lymphoma of bronchus-associated lymphoid tissue (BALT): CT features in 10 patients. J Comput Assist Tomogr 24:30–34

Lohr RH, Boland BJ, Douglas WW et al (1997) Organizing pneumonia. Features and prognosis of cryptogenic, secondary, and focal variants. Arch Intern Med 157:1323–1329

Marchiori E, Franquet T, Gasparetto TD et al (2008) Consolidation with diffuse or focal high attenuation: computed tomography findings. J Thorac Imaging 23:298–304

Maksimovic O, Bethge WA, Pintoffl JP et al (2008) (2008) Marginal zone B-cell non-Hodgkin's lymphoma of mucosa-associated lymphoid tissue type: imaging findings. AJR Am J Roentgenol 191:921–930

Maldonado RL (1999) The CT angiogram sign. Radiology 210:323–324

Mayo JR, Müller NL, Road J et al (1989) Chronic eosinophilic pneumonia: CT findings in six cases. AJR Am J Roentgenol 153:727–730

Milne EN, Pistolesi M, Miniati M et al (1985) The radiologic distinction of cardiogenic and noncardiogenic edema. AJR Am J Roentgenol 144:879–894

Murayama S, Onitsuka H, Murakami J et al (1993) "CT angiogram sign" in obstructive pneumonitis and pneumonia. J Comput Assist Tomogr 17:609–612

Oymak FS, Demirbaş HM, Mavili E et al (2005) Bronchiolitis obliterans organizing pneumonia. Clinical and roentgenological features in 26 cases. Respiration 72:254–262

Patsios D, Roberts HC, Paul NS et al (2007) Pictorial review of the many faces of bronchioloalveolar cell carcinoma. Br J Radiol 80:1015–1023

Prakash UB, Barham SS, Carpenter HA et al (1987) Pulmonary alveolar phospholipoproteinosis: experience with 34 cases and a review. Mayo Clin Proc 62:499–518

Rossi SE, Erasmus JJ, McAdams HP et al (2000) Pulmonary drug toxicity: radiologic and pathologic manifestations. Radiographics 20:1245–1259

Rossi SE, Erasmus JJ, Volpacchio M et al (2003) "Crazy-paving" pattern at thin-section CT of the lungs: radiologic-pathologic overview. Radiographics 23:1509–1519

Seymour JF, Presneill JJ (2002) Pulmonary alveolar proteinosis: progress in the first 44 years. Am J Respir Crit Care Med 166:215–235

Storto ML, Kee ST, Golden JA et al (1995) Hydrostatic pulmonary edema: high-resolution CT findings. AJR Am J Roentgenol 165:817–820

Souza CA, Müller NL, Lee KS et al (2006) Idiopathic interstitial pneumonias: prevalence of mediastinal lymph node enlargement in 206 patients. AJR Am J Roentgenol 186:995–999

Travis WD, Colby TV, Corrin B et al (1999) World Health Organization International Histological Classification of Tumors. 3rd edn. Histological typing of lung and pleural tumors. WHO, Berlin, pp 34–38

Trapnell BC, Whitsett JA, Nakata KN (2003) Pulmonary alveolar proteinosis. Engl J Med 349:2527–2539

Ujita M, Renzoni EA, Veeraraghavan S et al (2004) Organizing pneumonia: perilobular pattern at thin-section CT. Radiology 232:757–761

Vilar J, Domingo ML, Soto C et al (2004) Radiology of bacterial pneumonia. Eur J Radiol 51:102–113

Wahba H, Truong MT, Lei X et al (2008) Reversed halo sign in invasive pulmonary fungal infections. Clin Infect Dis 46:1733–17337

Ware LB, Matthay MA (2005) Clinical practice acute pulmonary edema. N Engl J Med 353:2788–2796

Witte RJ, Gurney JW, Robbins RA et al (1991) Diffuse pulmonary alveolar hemorrhage after bone marrow transplantation: radiographic findings in 39 patients. AJR Am J Roentgenol 157:461–464

The Respiratory Tract

Walter De Wever

10

Contents

Abstract

> Airways may be affected by a variety of diseases. Diseases of the large airways can result from abnormalities of the wall (intrinsic abnormalities) or from compression from adjacent structures (extrinsic abnormalities). Intrinsic abnormalities are classified as either focal or diffuse, depending on the extent of involvement of the airways. The diffuse abnormalities are less common and usually benign, most of the time caused by autoimmune illnesses or multisystem disorders. Focal abnormalities include tumors, infections, granulomatous diseases, and iatrogenic disorders. Focal disease tends to produce decreased airway diameter. The diffuse diseases may be divided into those that increase the diameter and those that decrease the diameter of the airway.

> Plain chest radiography remains a convenient first-line investigation for any patient who presents with respiratory symptoms and signs. The air within the trachea and main bronchi gives good, inherent radiographic contrast. Well-penetrated films may demonstrate tracheobronchial pathology: however, abnormalities of the major airways can easily be missed on radiographs. Computed Tomography (CT) has been shown to be superior to conventional radiography in the detection of abnormalities of the airways. The axial CT images are primarily used for diagnostic purposes. Two-dimensional and three-dimensional reformatted images offer a number of advantages, such as a better assessment of the craniocaudal extent of disease and the ability to detect subtle airway stenoses.

W. De Wever
Department of Radiology, University Hospitals Leuven,
Herestraat 49, 3000 Leuven, Belgium
e-mail: walter.dewever@uz.kuleuven.ac.be

E.E. Coche et al. (eds.), *Comparative Interpretation of CT and Standard Radiography of the Chest*,
Medical Radiology, DOI: 10.1007/978-3-540-79942-9_10, © Springer-Verlag Berlin Heidelberg 2011

10.1 Anatomy of the Large Airways

10.1.1 Normal Anatomy

The airways are divided into conducting airways and transitional airways. Conducting airways include the trachea, bronchi, and membranous bronchioles. The primary function of these bronchial structures is to conduct air to the alveolar surface. The transitional airways consist of respiratory bronchioles and alveolar ducts. They conduct air to the most peripheral alveoli (Fraser and Müller 1999).

The trachea is a cartilaginous and fibromuscular tube extending from the inferior aspect of the cricoid cartilage to the carina. Typically, the trachea contains 16–22 cartilaginous rings that help to support the tracheal wall and maintain an adequate tracheal lumen during forced expiration. The posterior tracheal wall or membrane lacks cartilage and is supported by a thin band of smooth muscle, the trachealis muscle.

Airways divide by dichotomous branching, with approximately 23 generations of branches identifiable from the trachea to the alveoli. This dichotomy is asymmetric. Usually the bronchus divides into two branches; however, variation in both number and size of the branches is common (Horsfield and Cumming 1968). The trachea bifurcates into the right and left mainstem bronchi at the carina (Fig. 10.1). The right main bronchus is shorter, wider, and more vertical than the left. The mainstem bronchi divide into their lobar and then segmental bronchi. Bronchi are composed of both cartilaginous and fibromuscular elements. Bronchioles differ from the bronchi in that the bronchi contain cartilage and glands in their walls, whereas the bronchioles do not. The term small airways is generally used to refer to airways that are 3 mm or less in diameter (Stone et al. 2006).

Several systems of bronchial nomenclature have been described. The system described by Jackson and Huber in 1943 has been the most widely accepted and remains the generally accepted terminology. Bronchi are also designated using a numeric system popularized by Boyden (1961) (Table 10.1). It should be remembered, however, that the pattern of bronchial branching described is far from standard because there is considerable anatomic variation (Lee et al. 1991; Naidich et al. 1988). Contrary to the numerous variations of lobar or segmental bronchial subdivisions, abnormal bronchi originating from the trachea or main

bronchi are rare. Major bronchial abnormalities include "tracheal" bronchus and accessory cardiac bronchus (ACB). Minor bronchial abnormalities include variants of tracheal bronchus, displaced bronchi, and bronchial agenesis. By definition, a displaced bronchus is one that arises at another level (most of them a lower level) than normal in the bronchial tree. This same bronchus is considered to be supernumerary if a normal bronchus also supplies the same lung segment (Fig. 10.2). The displaced type is more frequent than the supernumerary type (Kubik and Muntener 1971).

10.1.2 Anatomical Variations and Abnormalities

10.1.2.1 Tracheal Bronchus

A tracheal bronchus was described by Sandifort in 1785 as a right upper lobe bronchus originating from the trachea (Kubik and Muntener 1971) (Fig. 10.2). In recent literature, the term tracheal bronchus encompasses a variety of bronchial anomalies originating from the trachea and main bronchus and directed to the upper lobe region. The right tracheal bronchus has a prevalence of 0.1–2% (Ritsema 1983). The right tracheal bronchus is located at the junction of the middle and distal thirds of the right lateral trachea, is more common in men and children with other congenital anomalies, and may be associated with right main bronchus stenosis (Doolittle and Mair 2002). When the entire right upper lobe bronchus is displaced on the trachea, it is also called a "pig bronchus" and has a reported frequency of 0.2% (Ghaye et al. 2001). The left tracheal bronchus has a prevalence of 0.3–1% (Ghaye et al. 2001).

10.1.2.2 Accessory Cardiac Bronchus

ACB was defined by Brock in 1946 as a "supernumerary bronchus arising from the inner wall of the right main bronchus or intermediate bronchus opposite to the origin of the right upper lobe bronchus." The bronchus progresses conically for 1–5 cm in a caudal direction toward the pericardium, paralleling the intermediate bronchus. Most ACBs have a blind extremity, but they can also develop into a series of small bronchioles, which may end in vestigial or rudimentary bronchiolar parenchymal tissue, cystic degeneration, or a ventilated lobulus. An

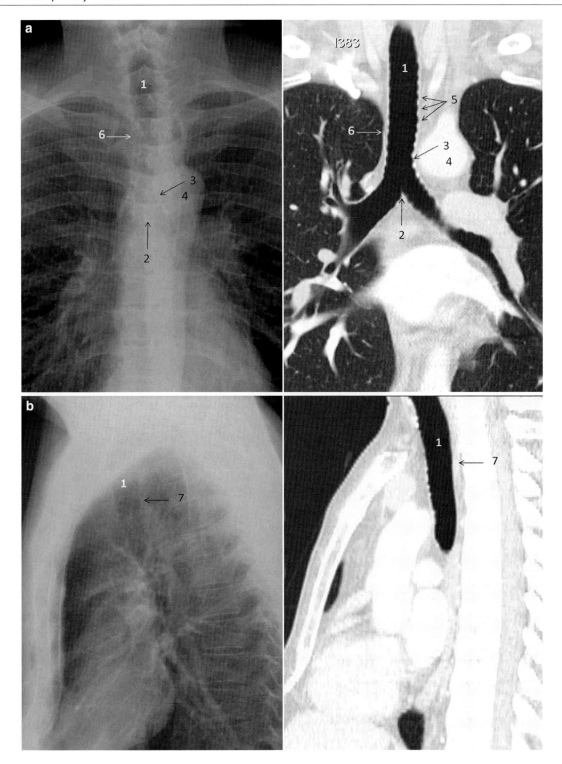

Fig. 10.1 (**a** and **b**) Evaluation of normal trachea. The trachea is a midline structure. The walls of the trachea are parallel except on the left side just above the bifurcation, where the aorta commonly impresses a smooth indentation. The air columns of the trachea have a smoothly serrated contour created by the indentations of the cartilage rings in their walls at regular intervals. The right paratracheal stripe is seen on posteroanterior chest radiographs as a thin, water-density stripe between the air column of the trachea and the adjacent right lung. The posterior tracheal band is a thin band of uniform width consisting primarily of the posterior tracheal wall, which is observed almost constantly in a well-positioned and exposed lateral view of the chest

Table 10.1 Nomenclature of the bronchopulmonary anatomy

Jackson-Huber		Boyden
Right lung		
Upper lobe		
	Apical	B1
	Anterior	B2
	Posterior	B3
Middle lobe		
	Lateral	B4
	Medial	B5
Lower lobe		
	Superior	B6
	Medial basal	B7
	Anterior basal	B8
	Lateral basal	B9
	Posterior basal	B10
Left lung		
Upper lobe		
Upper division		
	Apical-posterior	B1–3
	Anterior	B2
Lingular division		
	Superior	B4
	Inferior	B5
Lower lobe		
	Superior	B6
	Anteromedial	B7–8
	Lateral basal	B9
	Posterior basal	B10

ACB is different from the medial basilar segmental bronchus and does not correspond to proximal migration of this structure, which arises from the right lower lobe bronchus (Ghaye et al. 2001).

10.1.2.3 Bronchial Agenesis

The uncommon agenesis–hypoplasia complex corresponds to arrested development of one lung at different stages: agenesis (absence of bronchus and lung), aplasia (absence of lung with bronchus present), and hypoplasia (bronchus and rudimentary lung present) (Mata and Caceres 1996). Diagnosis is easy when an entire lung or lobe is involved (hypogenetic lung syndrome) but can be more difficult when segmental bronchi are involved. Segmental bronchial agenesis predominates in the right upper lobe (Ghaye et al. 2001).

10.2 Evaluation of Trachea and Bronchial Structures

The plain chest radiograph remains a convenient first-line investigation for any patient who presents with respiratory symptoms and signs. The air within the trachea and main bronchi gives good inherent radiographic contrast. Well-penetrated films may demonstrate tracheal abnormalities (Stone et al. 2006).

Computed tomography (CT) has been shown to be superior to conventional radiography in detecting abnormalities of the airways (Kwong et al. 1992). The axial CT images are primarily used for diagnostic purposes. Two-dimensional and three-dimensional reformatted images offer a number of advantages, such as a better assessment of the craniocaudal extent of disease and the ability to detect subtle airway stenoses (Boiselle 2003).

10.2.1 Evaluation of the Trachea

The trachea is a midline structure. A slight deviation to the right after entering the thorax is a normal finding and should not be misinterpreted as evidence of displacement. The walls of the trachea are parallel except on the left side just above the bifurcation, where the aorta commonly impresses a smooth indentation. The air columns of the trachea have a smoothly serrated contour created by the indentations of the cartilage rings in their walls at regular intervals (Fig. 10.1). Various conditions, including mediastinal masses and vascular anomalies, may bow, displace, or indent the trachea. Such appearances are most commonly seen in patients who have thyroid masses or a right-sided aortic arch. Enlarged nodes do not usually narrow the trachea unless they are much harder than the cartilaginous rings, as occurs in nodular

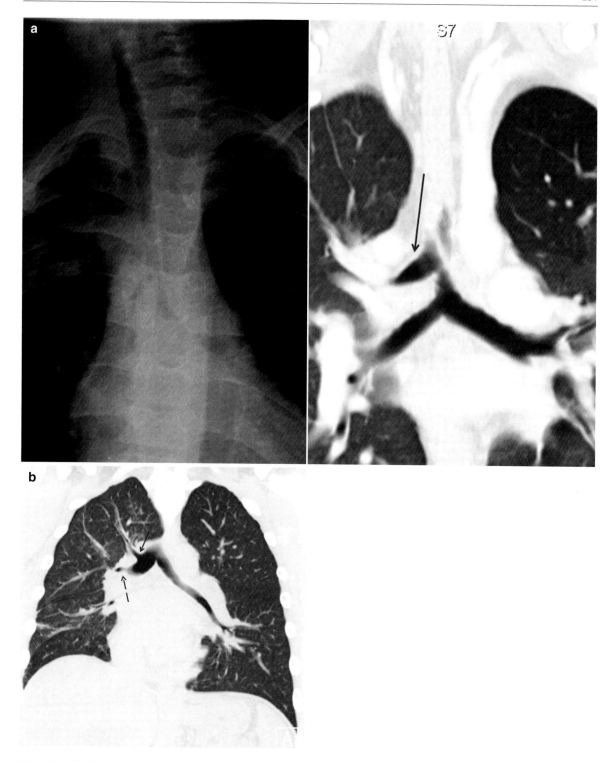

Fig. 10.2 Displaced and supernumerary bronchi. A tracheal bronchus is a right upper lobe bronchus originating from the trachea and main bronchus and directed to the upper lobe region. The right tracheal bronchus is located at the junction of the mid and distal thirds of the right lateral trachea. When the entire right upper lobe bronchus is displaced on the trachea, it is also called a "pig bronchus" (**a**, *arrow*). By definition, a displaced bronchus is one that arises at another level than normal in the bronchial tree. This same bronchus is considered supernumerary (**b**, *arrow*) if a normal bronchus (**b**, *dotted arrow*) also supplies the same lung segment. The displaced type is more frequent than the supernumerary type

sclerosing Hodgkin's disease, or the rings are soft, as it is in children (Dennie and Coblentz 1993).

Important tracheal interfaces include the right and left paratracheal stripes and the posterior tracheal band (PTB). The right paratracheal stripe (RPS) (Fig. 10.1) is seen on posteroanterior chest radiographs as a thin, water-density stripe between the air column of the trachea and the adjacent right lung. The range of width of the RPS is 1–4 mm. An RPS width of 5 mm or more is reliable evidence of disease arising in trachea, mediastinum, or pleura (Savoca et al. 1977). The PTB (Fig. 10.1) is a thin band of uniform width consisting primarily of the posterior tracheal wall that is observed almost constantly in a well-positioned and exposed lateral view of the chest. It is formed by two interfaces: an internal junction line between the inner tracheal wall and air in the lumen, and an external junction line between the adventitial surface of the right posterior wall with paper-thin mediastinal covering and aerated lung in the right retrotracheal recess. Any pathological process in the mediastinum, pleura, or right upper lobe medially that affects the external interface causes an alteration or disappearance of the PTB (Bachman and Teixidor 1975).

The trachea measures 10–12 cm in length in adults, including the extrathoracic trachea (measuring 2–4 cm in length) and the intrathoracic trachea, which measures from 6 to 9 cm (mean, 7.5 ± 0.8 cm) (Gamsu and Webb 1982) beginning at the point where the trachea passes posterior to the manubrium. Anterolaterally, the trachea lies behind the great vessels and adjacent to the aorta. This position accounts for the frequent finding of focal displacement of the trachea to the left, resulting from marked tortuosity of the brachiocephalic artery, and to the right, resulting from tortuosity of the aortic arch. The most common tracheal shape is round, oval, or horseshoe shaped. In men, the upper normal limit for coronal and sagittal diameters is 25 and 27 mm, respectively (Breatnach et al. 1984); in women it is 21 and 23 mm, respectively. The lower normal limit for both dimensions is 13 mm in men and 10 mm in women. The shape of the intrathoracic trachea can change dramatically with expiration as a result of invagination of the posterior membrane, resulting in a crescent-moon-shaped or horseshoe-shaped lumen. The mean anteroposterior diameter of the trachea can decrease by as much as 30% (Stern et al. 1993).

10.2.2 Evaluation of the Carina

The trachea bifurcates into right and left main bronchi at the carina. Many different "normal" values for bifurcation angles exist in the literature. Several factors account for the discrepancies found in the various studies. First, the definition of the term carinal angle is often vague; in some studies it refers to the subcarinal angle, whereas in others it refers to the interbronchial angle (Fig. 10.3) (Haskin and Goodman 1982). The angle of bifurcation varies considerably with a broad range between 35° and 90.5° (mean, 60.8° ± 11.8°) (Haskin and Goodman 1982). Karabulut (2005) found in his study mean values of 77° ± 13° (range, 49°–109°) for the interbronchial angle and 73° ± 16° (range, 34°–107°) for the subcarinal angle. The width of the tracheal bifurcation angle may be of value in recognizing subcarinal masses, lobar collapse, left atrial enlargement, generalized cardiomegaly, or pericardial effusion (Fig. 10.4) (Haskin and Goodman 1982).

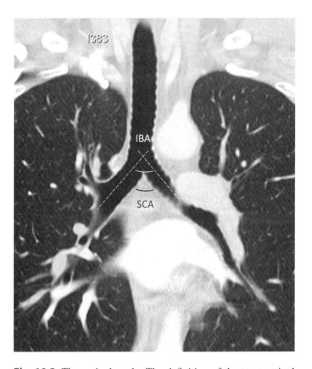

Fig. 10.3 The carinal angle. The definition of the term carinal angle is often vague: in some studies it refers to the subcarinal angle (SCA), whereas in others it refers to the interbronchial angle (IBA)

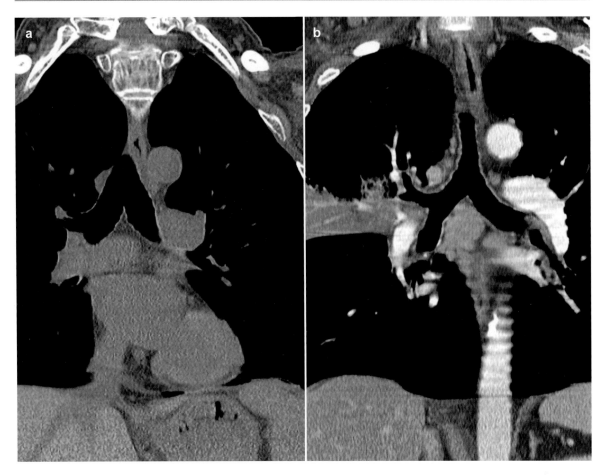

Fig. 10.4 Enlargement of the carinal angle. The width of the tracheal bifurcation angle may be of value in recognizing subcarinal masses, lobar collapse, left atrial enlargement, general-ized cardiomegaly, or pericardial effusion. In (**a**) we see a normal carinal angle. In (**b**) we see an enlargement of the carinal angle due to enlarged subcarinal lymph nodes

10.2.3 Evaluation of the Bronchi

10.2.3.1 Evaluation of the Diameter

Various methods for measuring airway dimensions have been proposed. Subjective visual criteria for establishing the presence of bronchial dilatation are most often used in the interpretation of chest X-ray and CT scans. Bronchial dilatation may be diagnosed by comparing the bronchial diameter to that of the adjacent pulmonary artery branch (i.e., determining the bronchoarterial ratio), by detecting a lack of bronchial tapering, and by identifying airways in the periphery of the lung. In Table 10.2, the approximate diameter of the different generations of airways is listed.

Bronchoarterial Ratio

In most normal subjects, the diameters of bronchi and adjacent pulmonary arteries are nearly the same. Their diameter may be compared by using the bronchoarterial (B/A) ratio (Fig. 10.5a), defined as the internal diameter (luminal diameter) of the bronchus divided by the diameter of the adjacent pulmonary artery. The B/A ratio in normal subjects generally averages from 0.65 to 0.70 (Matsuoka et al. 2003).

Lack of Bronchial Tapering

Lack of bronchial tapering has come to be recognized as an important finding in the diagnosis of bronchus

Table 10.2 Approximate diameter of different generations of airways

Structure	Generation	Diameter (mm)
Trachea	0	25
Main bronchi	1	11–19
Lobar bronchi	2–3	4–13
Segmental bronchi	3–6	4–7
Subsegmental bronchi	4–7	3–6
Bronchi	6–8	1.5–3
Terminal bronchi		1
Bronchioles	9–15	0.8–1
Lobular bronchioles		0.8
Terminal bronchioles	15–16	0.6–0.7
Respiratory bronchioles	17–19	0.4–0.5
Alveolar ducts and sacs	20–23	0.4
Alveoli		0.2–0.3

dilatation. It has been suggested that, for this finding to be present, the diameter of the airway should remain unchanged for at least 2 cm distal to a branching point (Fig. 10.5c and e) (Kim et al. 1997a).

Visibility of Peripheral Airways

The smallest airways normally visible on high-resolution CT or thin-collimation spiral CT techniques have a diameter of approximately 2 mm and a wall thickness of about 0.2–0.3 mm. In normal subjects, airways in the peripheral 2 cm of the lung are not commonly seen (Webb et al. 1988) So, the visibility of airways in the peripheral 1 cm of the lung is a sign of dilatation of the bronchial structure (Fig. 10.5c and d).

10.2.3.2 Evaluation of the Wall Thickness

There is no widespread agreement as to what constitutes bronchial wall thickening or how it should be measured using CT. Various methods have been proposed. Anatomically, the normal thickness of an airway wall is related to its diameter. This relationship may be expressed by using the thickness-to-diameter (T/D) ratio (Fig. 10.5b), which is defined as wall thickness (T) divided by the total diameter of the bronchus (D). This ratio may be measured using CT and averages about

20% for segmental and subsegmental bronchi. Table 10.3 summarizes the T/D ratios for different bronchial structures. The relationship between bronchial wall thickness and bronchial diameter may also be assessed by using the bronchial lumen ratio (BLR), defined as the inner diameter of the bronchus divided by its outer diameter. In essence, the BLR represents $1 - (2 \times T/D)$. At the subsegmental level, the BLR in normal subjects averaged 0.66 ± 0.06 with a range of 0.51–0.86 (Kim et al. 1995).

10.3 Diseases of Trachea and Bronchial Structures

The large airways may be affected by a variety of diseases, producing symptoms such as cough, stridor, dyspnea, or wheezing. Diseases of the large airways can result from abnormalities of the wall (intrinsic abnormalities) or from compression from adjacent structures (extrinsic abnormalities). Intrinsic abnormalities are classified as either focal or diffuse, depending on the extent of involvement of the airways (Table 10.4). The diffuse abnormalities are less common and usually benign, most of the time caused by autoimmune illnesses or multisystem disorders. Focal abnormalities include tumors, infections, granulomatous diseases, and iatrogenic disorders (Kwong et al. 1992). Focal disease tends to produce decreased airway diameter. The diffuse diseases may be divided into those that increase the diameter of the airway and those that decrease the diameter (Table 10.4).

The chest radiograph is usually the first type of image used in the assessment of patients who have airway abnormalities. It is well known, however, that abnormalities of the major airways can easily be missed on radiographs. Chest radiography and CT demonstrate well the degree of widening or narrowing airways, the location and extent of tracheobronchial abnormalities, the presence of associated mediastinal disease, postobstructive atelectasis, and pneumonitis.

10.3.1 Bronchiectasis

Bronchiectasis is most simply defined as irreversible bronchial dilation. It is usually associated with structural abnormalities of the bronchial wall. Chronic or recurrent

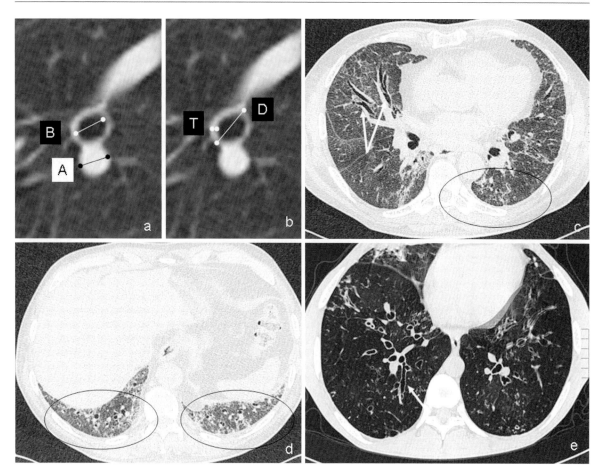

Fig. 10.5 Evaluation of the diameter and wall thickness. The diameter of the bronchial structures may be evaluated by using the bronchoarterial ratio (**a**), defined as the internal diameter of the bronchus divided by the diameter of the adjacent pulmonary artery. For the finding of "lack of bronchial tapering" to be present, the diameter of the airway should remain unchanged for at least 2 cm distal to a branching point (**c** and **e**; *white arrows*). The visibility of airways in the peripheral 1 cm of the lung is also a sign of dilatation of the bronchial structure (**c** and **d**) (circled areas). The normal thickness of an airway wall is related to its diameter. This relationship may be expressed by using the thickness-to-diameter ratio (**b**), defined as wall thickness divided by the total diameter of the bronchus

Table 10.3 Thickness-to-diameter ratios for different bronchial structures

Structure	Generation	Wall thickness	Mean diameter	T/D ratio
Lobar to segmental bronchi	2–4	1.5 mm	5–8 mm	20–30%
Subsegmental bronchi	6–8	0.3 mm	1.5–3 mm	10–20%
Subsegmental bronchi	11–13	0.1–0.15 mm	0.7–1 mm	15%

infection is usually present. Bronchiectasis may occur as a result of various pathologic processes and thus may be a feature of a number of different lung and airway diseases (Barker 2002; Hansell 1998). From a morphological aspect, bronchiectasis has traditionally been subdivided into three categories: cylindrical, varicose, and cystic, each reflecting increasing severity of disease (Fig. 10.6).

Radiologic signs on chest radiographs (Fig. 10.6) (Woodring 1994) are: (1) bronchial dilation, identified by visually comparing bronchial diameters in affected areas with bronchial diameters in normal areas at equal

Table 10.4 Classification of airway diseases

Airway diseases	
Focal diseases	Diffuse diseases
Decreased diameter	Increased diameter
Tracheal strictures	Tracheobronchomegaly (Mounier-Kuhn disease)
Benign neoplasms	Bronchiectasis/bronchiolectasis
Primary malignant neoplasms	Decreased diameter
Secondary malignant neoplasms	Saber-sheath trachea
Infectious disorders	Tracheopathia osteoplastica
	Infectious disorders
	Relapsing bronchitis
	Amyloidosis
	Sarcoidosis
	Wegener granulomatosis
	Tracheobronchitis associated with ulcerative colitis

distances from the hilum; (2) the signet-ring sign, with dilated, thick-walled bronchus adjacent to a smaller accompanying artery; (3) bronchial wall thickening; (4) volume loss; (5) compensatory hyperinflation of surrounding segments or lobes; (6) mucus-or fluid-filled bronchi resulting in tubular structures sometimes presenting as the "finger in glove sign"(Fig. 10.7); and (7) obvious thin-walled cyst formation. By combining these signs, the diagnosis of bronchiectasis is quite obvious. Measurements of the B/A ratio in cases demonstrating the signet-ring sign can be obtained and are useful in validating the signet-ring sign as a relevant sign of bronchiectasis on plain films. Although radiographs are abnormal in 80–90% of patients who have bronchiectasis, findings are often nonspecific and a definitive diagnosis is usually difficult to make except in advanced cases. Overall, the correct diagnosis can be made from chest radiographs in only about 40% of patients (Currie et al. 1987).

CT findings of bronchiectasis can be divided into direct and indirect findings (Table 10.5). A combination of these findings enables an accurate diagnosis for a large percentage of patients. Because bronchiectasis is defined by the presence of bronchial dilation, recognition of increased bronchial diameter is mandatory to the CT diagnosis of this abnormality.

The B/A ratio can be used to evaluate bronchial dilatation (Naidich et al. 1982). The classic signet-ring sign (Fig. 10.8) is very useful in recognizing bronchiectasis and in distinguishing dilated airways from other cystic lung diseases, which tend not to be associated with this finding (Ouellette 1999). Lack of bronchial tapering is another important finding in the diagnosis of bronchiectasis. Visibility of airways in the peripheral 1 cm of the lung is a valuable finding for the diagnosis of bronchiectasis (Kim et al. 1997b). Although bronchial wall thickening is a nonspecific finding seen in various airway diseases, it is usually present in patients who have bronchiectasis. Simply determining the T/D ratio is problematic in the diagnosis of bronchial wall thickening because bronchiectasis increases the bronchial diameter and at the same time the wall becomes thickened. Comparing the bronchial wall thickness with the diameter of the adjacent pulmonary artery is useful as an objective measurement. Bronchial wall thickening is diagnosed if the airway wall is at least 0.5 times the width of an adjacent, vertically oriented pulmonary artery (Reiff et al. 1995).

10.3.2 Focal Diseases

10.3.2.1 Tracheal Stricture

Tracheal stenosis is defined as the cicatricial narrowing of the endotracheal lumen (Fig. 10.9). Endotracheal manipulation (intubation or tracheotomy) remains the most common etiology, followed by inflammatory and collagen vascular diseases. Stenosis can occur many years after the initial insult. Tracheotomy is more troublesome than intubation; the prevalence of stenosis is greater and occurs at the stoma site (Stark 1995). With intubation, it is hypothesized that the cuff pressure in these intubation devices (more than 30 mmHg) may exceed capillary pressure, leading to ischemic necrosis and subsequent fibrosis (Stauffer et al. 1981). In most cases, CT scans better demonstrate the site of narrowing compared with chest radiography. However, because of volume averaging, a web or stenosis that involves a short segment can be missed. CT interpretation may also result in the overestimation of the severity of a fixed stenotic segment and the underestimation of the length of the abnormal trachea.

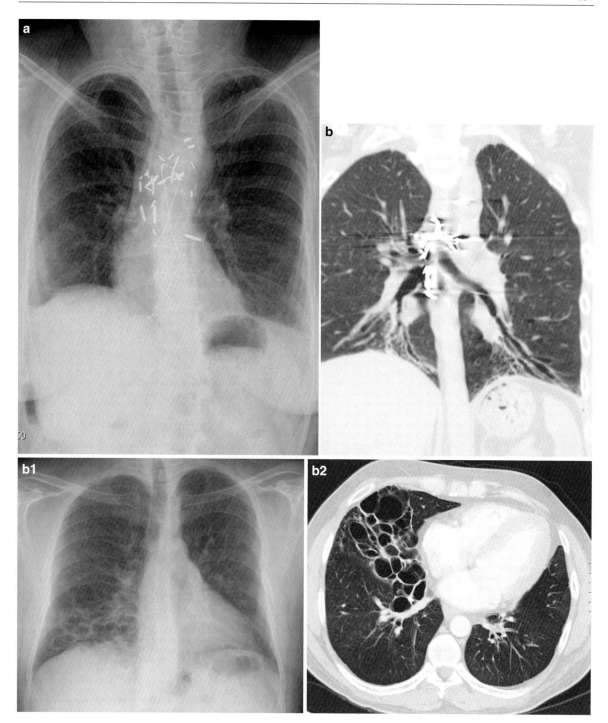

Fig. 10.6 (**a**) Bronchiectasis and (**b**) cystic bronchiectasis. In (**a**) cylindric bronchiectasis are seen in both lower lobes as tubular shadows, resulting in an increase in lung markings. Bronchial wall thickening may be manifested as ring shadows end-on or as tubular shadows en face ("tram lines"; left and right lower lung regions). In (**b**) cystic bronchiectasis are seen in the right middle lobe. These bronchiectasis are seen as ring shadows, cystic lucencies, both on chest radiograph (**b1**) and axial computed tomography images (**b2**)

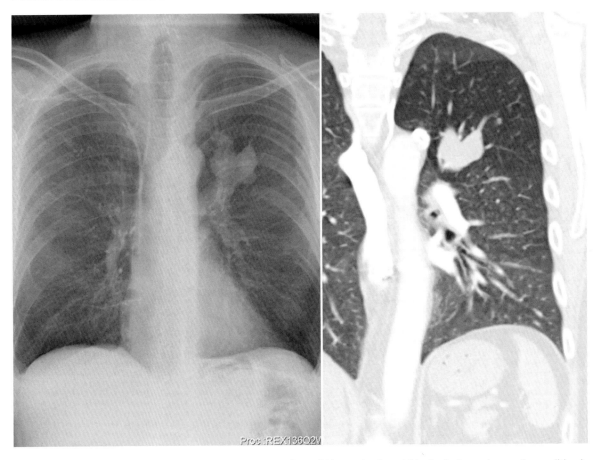

Fig. 10.7 Finger in glove sign. The radiographic appearance of mucoid impaction is variable. In the large airways the condition is classically manifested by tubular or branching opacities that resemble fingers (left upper lobe)

Table 10.5 CT findings in bronchiectasis

Direct signs	Indirect signs
(1) Increased B/A ratio	(1) Bronchial wall thickening
(2) Lack of tapering >2 cm distal to bifurcation	(2) Mucoid impaction
(3) Visibility of peripheral airways within 1 cm of the costal pleura	(3) Centrilobular nodules or tree-in-bud
	(4) Mosaic perfusion
	(5) Air trapping on expiratory scan
	(6) Bronchial artery hypertrophy
	(7) Atelectasis or emphysema

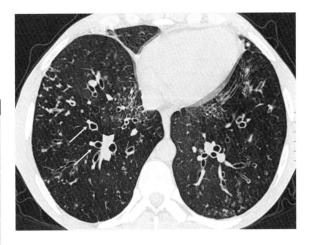

Fig. 10.8 The signet-ring sign. This finding is composed of a ring-shaped opacity representing a dilated bronchus in cross section and a smaller adjacent opacity representing its pulmonary artery, with the combination resembling a signet (or pearl) ring (*arrows*)

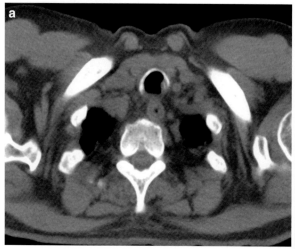

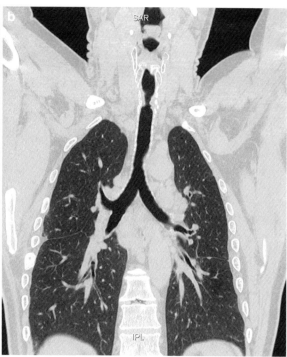

Fig. 10.9 Tracheal stricture: chest X-ray (**a**), CT (**b**) in a 59-year-old man with tracheal stenosis after intubation. Tracheal stenosis is defined as a cicatricial narrowing of the endotracheal lumen. With intubation, the cuff pressure in the intubation devices (more than 30 mmHg) may exceed capillary pressure, leading to ischemic necrosis and subsequent fibrosis. Computed tomography scans better demonstrate, in most cases, the site of narrowing compared with chest radiography

10.3.2.2 Neoplastic Lesions

Tracheal tumors are rare and account for less than 1% of all tumors. In adults, 90% of such lesions are malignant, but in children, 90% are benign. Most malignant lesions are squamous or adenoid cystic carcinomas. The majority of carcinoid tumors (80–90%) arise in lobar, segmental, or proximal subsegmental bronchi, where they appear as polypoidal masses that protrude into the airway lumen (Fig. 10.10). Carcinoid tumors are low-grade malignant tumors of neuroendocrine origin. The endobronchial location is usually easier to appreciate on CT than on plain radiographs and thereby is often associated with atelectasis or obstructive pneumonitis (Fig. 10.11) (Stone et al. 2006).

Benign neoplasms involving the trachea and mainstem bronchi include papillomas, submucosal salivary gland adenomas, and primary mesenchymal tumors such as hamartoma, leiomyoma, schwannoma, and lipoma. They tend to be well circumscribed, round or smooth masses, and less than 2 cm in diameter. CT scans will usually demonstrate the polypoidal configuration and intraluminal location of the mass, which is limited by the tracheal cartilage. Hamartoma may be formally diagnosed using CT if fat can be demonstrated. Tracheobronchial papillomatosis is caused by the human papillomavirus, which is usually acquired at birth from an infected mother. Dissemination of upper airway and laryngeal lesions occurs in 5% of patients and results in multiple nodules projecting into the airways. The papillomas are benign but may undergo malignant transformation to squamous cell carcinoma (Gruden et al. 1994). Chest radiography or CT may reveal intraluminal masses, parenchymal nodules (after distal airway dissemination), air-filled cysts (pneumatocoeles), or thick-walled cavities.

Endotracheal or endobronchial metastases from nonpulmonary tumors are uncommon. The prevalence depends on how they are defined and ranges from approximately 2–50% (Baumgartner and Mark 1980; Kiryu et al. 2001). Four types of development of endotracheal or endobronchial metastases can be found: (1) direct metastases to the bronchus; (2) bronchial invasion by a parenchymal lesion; (3) bronchial invasion by mediastinal or hilar lymph node metastasis; and (4) peripheral lesions extended along the proximal

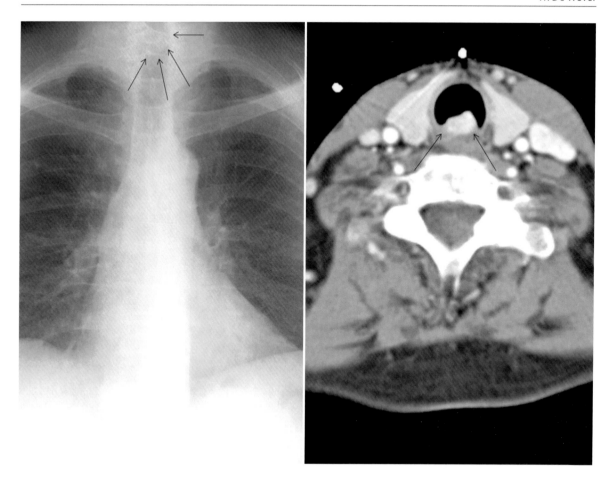

Fig. 10.10 Carcinoid of the trachea: chest X-ray (**a**), CT (**b**). Scans of a 70-year-old man with a polypoid mass into the trachea (*arrows*). The majority of carcinoid tumors arise in lobar, segmental, or proximal subsegmental bronchi, where they appear as polypoidal masses that protrude into the airway lumen. These masses are better visualized on computed tomography imaging (**b**) than on chest radiograph (**a**)

bronchus. The radiographic findings are quite variable. Patients may present with evidence of atelectasis, multiple nodules, hilar masses, mediastinal lymphadenopathy, or a normal chest (Baumgartner and Mark 1980; Braman and Whitcomb 1975). Colletti et al. (1990) reported that CT was more sensitive in detecting and localizing endobronchial neoplasms, including metastatic lesions.

10.3.3 Diffuse Diseases

10.3.3.1 Tracheobronchomegaly

Tracheobronchomegaly is a rare disorder of uncertain etiology, characterized by marked dilatation of the trachea and major bronchi and associated with tracheal diverticulosis, bronchiectasis, and recurrent respiratory tract infections (Fig. 10.12) (Al-Mubarak and Husain 2004). This entity refers to a heterogeneous group of patients who have marked dilatation of the trachea and mainstem bronchi. Conditions that can result in tracheobronchomegaly include congenital disorders such as Mounier-Kuhn's and Ehlers–Danlos syndromes, sarcoidosis and cystic fibrosis, and inflammatory disorders of the airways such as allergic bronchopulmonary aspergillosis (Marom et al. 2001). Tracheobronchomegaly is defined as a transverse and sagittal diameter exceeding 25 or 27 mm, respectively, or the left and right mainstem bronchi exceeding 18 or 21 mm in diameter, respectively, in men. The respective figures for women are 21, 23, 17.4, and 19.8 mm, respectively (Fraser and Müller 1999). Radiologic

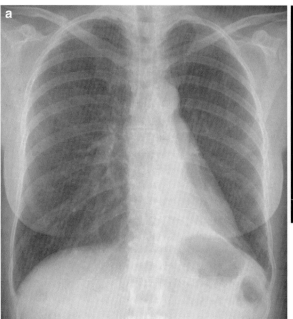

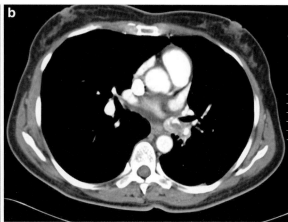

Fig. 10.11 Typical carcinoid of the left main bronchus: chest X-ray (**a**), CT (**b**). Scans of a 56-year-old woman with a tumoral lesion in the left mainstem bronchus. On chest radiograph (**a**), an atelectasis of the left lower lobe is visible. On computed tomography (CT) imaging (**b**) a calcified endobronchial lesion in the left mainstem bronchus is visible. Carcinoid tumors are low-grade malignant tumors of neuroendocrine origin. The endobronchial location is usually easier to appreciate on CT than plain radiographs, and there is often associated atelectasis or obstructive pneumonitis

findings of an irregular air column reflect the "corrugated" effect that is produced when redundant mucosa prolapses through the tracheal rings. Tracheobronchial diverticula and central bronchiectasis occur. CT scans reveal these abnormalities better than chest radiographs. Expiratory studies may reveal collapse of the major airways (Fraser and Müller 1999; Stark 1991).

10.3.3.2 Infectious Tracheobronchitis

A number of infections, both acute and more often chronic, may affect the trachea and proximal bronchi, resulting in focal and diffuse airway disease. The principle abnormalities are bronchial wall thickening and an increase in lung markings (Webb 1997). The latter (sometimes termed "dirty chest" or simply "prominent lung markings") (Fig. 10.13) refers to a general accentuation of markings throughout the lungs associated with loss of definition of the vascular margins (Takasugi and Godwin 1998). Bronchial wall thickening may be manifested as ring shadows end-on or as tubular shadows ("tram lines") (Fraser et al. 1976).

10.3.3.3 Saber-Sheath Trachea

Narrowing of the intrathoracic trachea in the coronal plane with anteroposterior lengthening is characteristic of the "saber-sheath" trachea deformity (Fig. 10.14). This deformity can be symmetric or asymmetric. The condition occurs primarily in middle-aged to elderly men and is rare in women. This structural disorder is strongly associated with chronic obstructive pulmonary disease and may be related to chronic bronchitis (Callan et al. 1988). At least 95% of patients who have saber-sheath trachea show evidence of chronic obstructive pulmonary disease. The saber-sheath appearance is found when mechanical forces of hyperinflated lungs cause the coronal diameter of the intrathoracic trachea to narrow and the sagittal diameter to elongate so that the sagittal-to-coronal diameter ratio exceeds 2:1. The extrathoracic trachea remains normal in configuration. Saber-sheath deformity of the trachea can be identified on chest radiographs, and its characteristic shapes and dimensions can be appreciated on CT (Stark and Norbash 1998). CT may also reveal mild intrathoracic tracheal wall thickening, frequently with

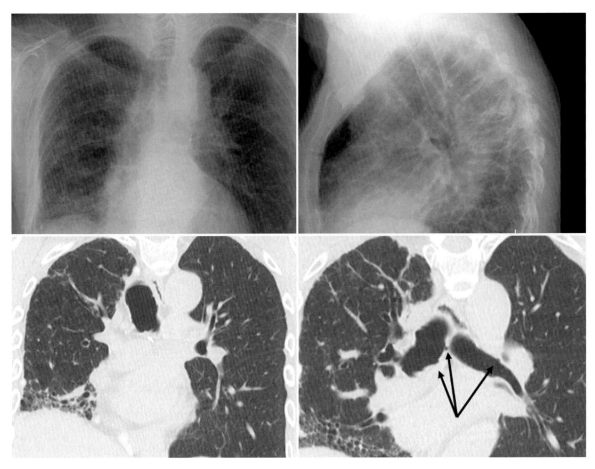

Fig. 10.12 Tracheobronchomegaly: chest X-ray (a), CT (b) in a 57-year-old man. Chest X-ray (**a**) and computed tomography (CT; **b**) show a dilatation of the trachea and the main bronchi. Small diverticles along the main bronchi are also visible due to the mucosa prolapse through the cartilage rings. These diverticles are only seen on the CT images (*black arrows*)

ossification of the trachea rings (Fraser and Müller 1999; Stark 1991).

10.3.3.4 Relapsing Polychondritis

Relapsing polychondritis is an autoimmune connective tissue disease that causes inflammation and destruction of cartilage and other connective tissues. Predominant clinical manifestations include auricular chondritis, polyarthritis, nasal chondritis, ocular inflammation, audiovestibular damage, and respiratory tract chondritis. A relapsing course is characteristic. Airways are involved in 50% of patients and may cause dyspnea, stridor, wheezing, hoarseness, aphonia, and laryngeal or tracheal tenderness (Staats et al. 2002). Recurrent pulmonary infection is the most common

cause of morbidity and mortality in these patients (Fraser and Müller 1999; Michet et al. 1986). Imaging may demonstrate long-segmental tracheobronchial strictures and destruction of the cartilaginous rings with soft tissue thickening, characteristically sparing the posterior membranous portions of the trachea and calcification (Meyer and White 1998; Im et al. 1988). Expiratory collapse of the affected airway may be revealed on fluoroscopy or dynamic CT.

10.3.3.5 Amyloidosis

Primary pulmonary amyloidosis is a rare disorder that can appear in three forms: tracheobronchial, nodular parenchymal, and diffuse parenchymal. Tracheobronchial involvement with amyloids can be local or extensive

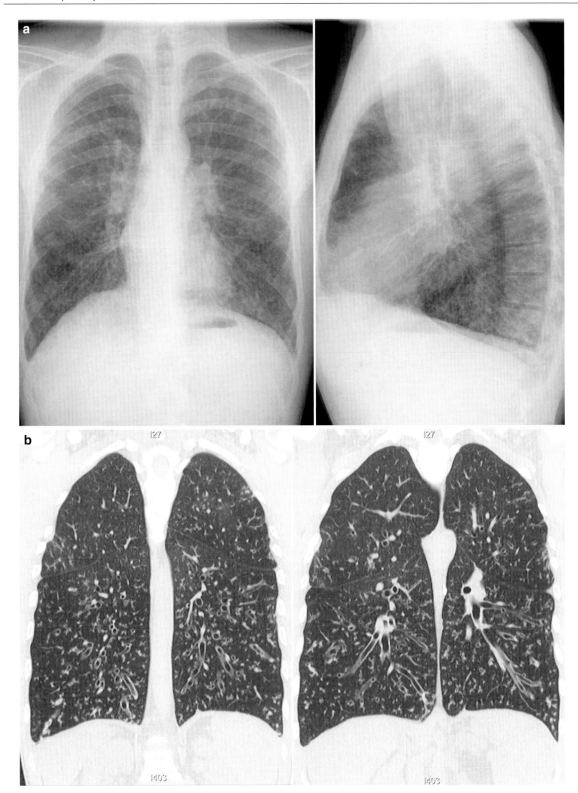

Fig. 10.13 Acute infectious bronchitis: chest X-ray (**a**), CT (**b**). Principle abnormalities of acute bronchial infection are bronchial wall thickening and an increase in lung markings, sometimes termed "dirty chest" or simply "prominent lung markings." It refers to a general accentuation of bronchial structures throughout the lungs associated with loss of definition of the vascular margins (Takasugi anvd Godwin 1998). Bronchial wall thickening may manifest as ring shadows end-on or as tubular shadows on posteroanterior view ("tram lines")

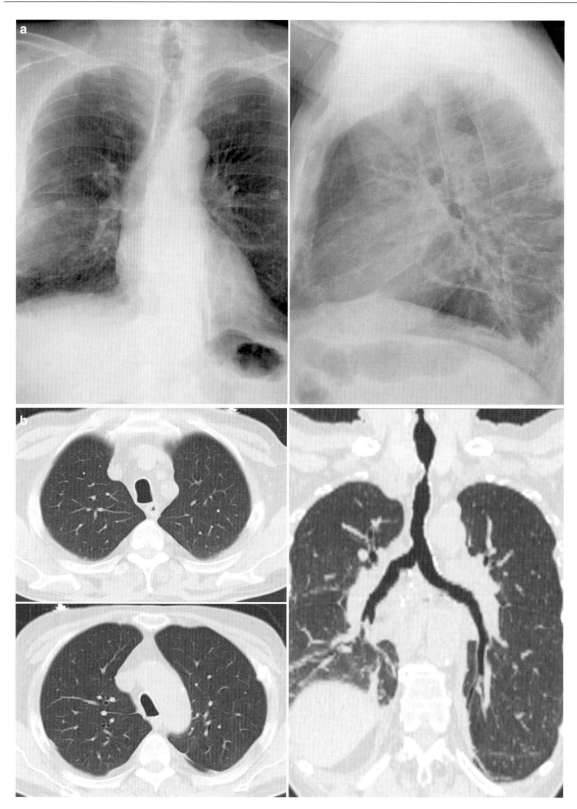

Fig. 10.14 Saber-sheath trachea: chest X-ray (**a**), CT (**b**). Narrowing of the intrathoracic trachea in the coronal plane with anteroposterior lengthening is characteristic of the "saber-sheath" trachea deformity. The saber-sheath appearance is found when the sagittal-to-coronal diameter ratio exceeds 2:1. The extrathoracic trachea remains normal in configuration

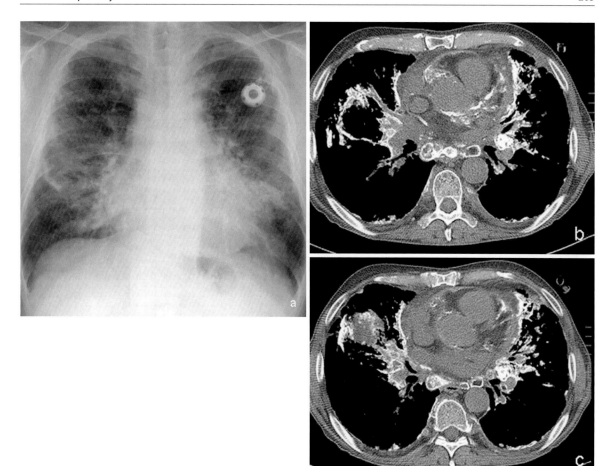

Fig. 10.15 Amyloidosis: chest X-ray (**a**), CT (**b,c**). A 64-year-old man with primary pulmonary amyloidosis. Chest X-ray (**a**) and computed tomography (CT; **b** and **c**) show extensive involvement of the bronchial structures. There is also parenchymal involvement and calcified mediastinal and hilar lymph nodes.

Chest X-ray (**a**) shows a dirty lung image with thickening of the walls of the bronchial structures, especially in the lower lung regions. CT (**b** and **c**) shows calcifications of the bronchial walls with narrowing of the bronchial structures that are filled with mucus

(Fig. 10.15). In extensive disease, CT demonstrates tracheal or bronchial circumferential wall thickening with luminal narrowing and linear calcification of the airway walls. Localized forms of amyloids affecting the airway may appear as plaque-like or tumor-like nodules or masses partially or completely occluding airways and with infiltration of the adjacent paratracheal or bronchial tissue (Kim et al. 1999).

10.3.3.6 Sarcoidosis

Sarcoidosis is a systemic disease of unknown etiology with variable presentation, prognosis, and progression. At diagnosis, about 50% of patients are asymptomatic, 25% complain of cough or dyspnea, and 25% have skin lesions or eye symptoms (Miller et al. 1995). Airway involvement can occur at virtually any location, from the epiglottis to the bronchioles. The trachea is a relatively rare site to be affected by sarcoidosis, occurring in less than 3% of cases (Prince et al. 2002). When present, sarcoidosis has a predilection for the upper trachea. Granulomata within the mucosa or submucosa will appear as a soft-tissue thickening of the tracheal wall. The bronchi can be extrinsically compressed by enlarged lymph nodes or, less frequently, obstructed by endobronchial granuloma (1% of cases) (Freundlich et al. 1970). Scarring and fibrosis lead to bronchiectasis, stenosis, or occlusions (Fraser and Müller 1999). CT is more sensitive than chest radiography in the detection of adenopathy and subtle parenchymal disease (Hamper et al. 1986).

10.3.3.7 Wegener's Granulomatosis

Wegener's granulomatosis induces airway abnormalities in 59% of patients and is seen during bronchoscopy. Endobronchial abnormalities caused by Wegener's granulomatosis include subglottic stenosis, ulcerating tracheobronchitis with or without inflammatory pseudotumor, and tracheal or bronchial stenosis that varies in length from several millimeters to several centimeters without inflammation (Stark 1991; Daum et al. 1995). CT scans depict focal or diffuse wall thickening, which can be concentric or eccentric, and airway narrowing (Screaton et al. 1998). The cartilaginous tracheal rings may calcify. When evaluating tracheal stenosis caused by Wegener's granulomatosis, the larynx should also be included because focal stenosis from this disease most commonly affects the subglottic trachea.

10.3.3.8 Tracheopathia Osteochondroplastica

Tracheopathia osteochondroplastica is a rare disorder of the laryngotracheobronchial tree. The condition is benign and is characterized by submucosal nodules containing combinations of cartilaginous, osseous, and hematopoietic tissue and calcified acellular protein matrix protruding into the bronchial lumen (Fig. 10.16) (Meyer et al. 1997). Tracheopathia osteochondroplastica is distinguished from tracheobronchial amyloidosis or relapsing polychondritis because it does not involve the posterior membranous portion of the trachea. Tracheal irregularity and thickening can be suggested on chest radiographs. Calcification in the nodules can sometimes be seen on a lateral chest radiograph. On CT, focal tracheal thickening, calcification of the tracheal rings, multiple calcified tracheal

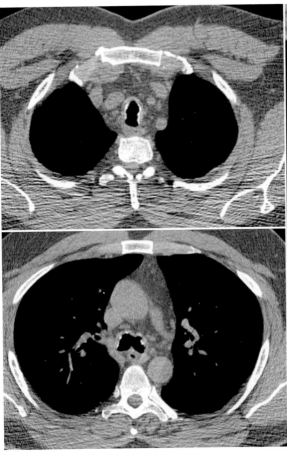
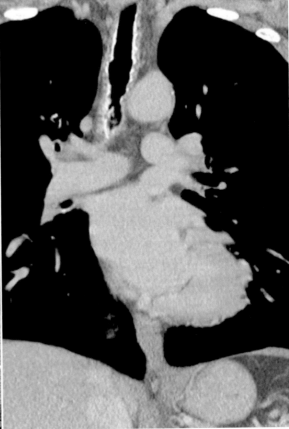

Fig. 10.16 A 40-year-old man with tracheopathia osteochondroplastica presenting with nodular calcified thickening of the trachea and mainstem bronchi. On computed tomography focal tracheal thickening, calcification of the tracheal rings, multiple calcified tracheal nodules, and long-segment tracheal narrowing are typically seen

nodules with or without punctuate calcification, and long-segment tracheal narrowing are typically seen (Manning et al. 1998).

References

Al-Mubarak HF, Husain SA. Tracheobronchomegaly-Mounier-Kuhn syndrome. Saudi Med J. 2004;25(6):798–801

Bachman AL, Teixidor HS. The posterior tracheal band: a reflector of local superior mediastinal abnormality. Br J Radiol. 1975;48(569):352–359

Barker AF. Bronchiectasis. N Engl J Med. 2002;346(18):1383–1393

Baumgartner WA, Mark JB. Metastatic malignancies from distant sites to the tracheobronchial tree. J Thorac Cardiovasc Surg. 1980;79(4):499–503

Boiselle PM. Multislice helical CT of the central airways. Radiol Clin North Am. 2003;41(3):561–574

Boyden EA. The nomenclature of the bronchopulmonary segments and their blood supply. Dis Chest. 1961;39:1–6

Braman SS, Whitcomb ME. Endobronchial metastasis. Arch Intern Med. 1975;135(4):543–547

Breatnach E, Abbott GC, Fraser RG. Dimensions of the normal human trachea. AJR Am J Roentgenol. 1984;142(5):903–906

Brock R. The anatomy of the bronchial tree. London: Oxford University Press; 1946

Callan E, Karandy EJ, Hilsinger Jr RL. "Saber-sheath" trachea. Ann Otol Rhinol Laryngol. 1988;97(5 Pt 1):512–515

Colletti PM, Beck S, Boswell Jr WD, Radin DR, Yamauchi DM, Ralls PW, Balchum OJ. Computed tomography in endobronchial neoplasm's. Comput Med Imaging Graph. 1990;14(4):257–262

Currie DC, Cooke JC, Morgan AD, Kerr IH, Delany D, Strickland B, Cole PJ. Interpretation of bronchograms and chest radiographs in patients with chronic sputum production. Thorax. 1987;42(4):278–284

Daum TE, Specks U, Colby TV, Edell ES, Brutinel MW, Prakash UB, DeRemee RA. Tracheobronchial involvement in Wegener's granulomatosis. Am J Respir Crit Care Med. 1995;151(2 Pt 1):522–526

Dennie CJ, Coblentz CL. The trachea: normal anatomic features, imaging and causes of displacement. Can Assoc Radiol J. 1993;44(2):81–89

Doolittle AM, Mair EA. Tracheal bronchus: classification, endoscopic analysis, and airway management. Otolaryngol Head Neck Surg. 2002;126(3):240–243

Fraser C, Müller, Paré (1999) Synopsis of diseases of the chest. 3rd edn

Fraser RG, Fraser RS, Renner JW, Bernard C, Fitzgerald PJ. The roentgenologic diagnosis of chronic bronchitis: a reassessment with emphasis on parahilar bronchi seen end-on. Radiology. 1976;120(1):1–9

Freundlich IM, Libshitz HI, Glassman LM, Israel HL. Sarcoidosis. Typical and atypical thoracic manifestations and complications. Clin Radiol. 1970;21(4):376–383

Gamsu G, Webb WR. Computed tomography of the trachea: normal and abnormal. AJR Am J Roentgenol. 1982;139(2):321–326

Ghaye B, Szapiro D, Fanchamps JM, Dondelinger RF. Congenital bronchial abnormalities revisited. Radiographics. 2001;21(1):105–119

Gruden JF, Webb WR, Sides DM. Adult-onset disseminated tracheobronchial papillomatosis: CT features. J Comput Assist Tomogr. 1994;18(4):640–642

Hamper UM, Fishman EK, Khouri NF, Johns CJ, Wang KP, Siegelman SS. Typical and atypical CT manifestations of pulmonary sarcoidosis. J Comput Assist Tomogr. 1986;10(6):928–936

Hansell DM. Bronchiectasis. Radiol Clin North Am. 1998;36(1):107–128

Haskin PH, Goodman LR. Normal tracheal bifurcation angle: a reassessment. AJR Am J Roentgenol. 1982;139(5):879–882

Horsfield K, Cumming G. Morphology of the bronchial tree in man. J Appl Physiol. 1968;24(3):373–383

Im JG, Chung JW, Han SK, Han MC, Kim CW. CT manifestations of tracheobronchial involvement in relapsing polychondritis. J Comput Assist Tomogr. 1988;12(5):792–793

Jackson CL, Huber JF. Correlated applied anatomy of the bronchial tree and lungs with a system of nomenclature. Dis Chest. 1943;9:319–326

Karabulut N. CT assessment of tracheal carinal angle and its determinants. Br J Radiol. 2005;78(933):787–790

Kim SJ, Im JG, Kim IO, Cho ST, Cha SH, Park KS, Kim DY. Normal bronchial and pulmonary arterial diameters measured by thin section CT. J Comput Assist Tomogr. 1995;19(3):365–369

Kim JS, Muller NL, Park CS, Lynch DA, Newman LS, Grenier P, Herold CJ. Bronchoarterial ratio on thin section CT: comparison between high altitude and sea level. J Comput Assist Tomogr. 1997a;21(2):306–311

Kim JS, Muller NL, Park CS, Grenier P, Herold CJ. Cylindrical bronchiectasis: diagnostic findings on thin-section CT. AJR Am J Roentgenol. 1997b;168(3):751–754

Kim HY, Im JG, Song KS, Lee KS, Kim SJ, Kim JS, Lee JS, Lim TH. Localized amyloidosis of the respiratory system: CT features. J Comput Assist Tomogr. 1999;23(4):627–631

Kiryu T, Hoshi H, Matsui E, Iwata H, Kokubo M, Shimokawa K, Kawaguchi S. Endotracheal/endobronchial metastases: clinicopathologic study with special reference to developmental modes. Chest. 2001;119(3):768–775

Kubik S, Muntener M. Bronchus abnormalities: tracheal, eparterial, and pre-eparterial bronchi. Fortschr Geb Röntgenstr Nuklearmed. 1971;114(2):145–163

Kwong JS, Muller NL, Miller RR. Diseases of the trachea and main-stem bronchi: correlation of CT with pathologic findings. Radiographics. 1992;12(4):645–657

Lee KS, Bae WK, Lee BH, Kim IY, Choi EW. Bronchovascular anatomy of the upper lobes: evaluation with thin-section CT. Radiology. 1991;181(3):765–772

Manning JE, Goldin JG, Shpiner RB, Aberle DR. Case report: tracheobronchopathia osteochondroplastica. Clin Radiol. 1998;53(4):302–309

Marom EM, Goodman PC, McAdams HP. Diffuse abnormalities of the trachea and main bronchi. AJR Am J Roentgenol. 2001;176(3):713–717

Mata JM, Caceres J. The dysmorphic lung: imaging findings. Eur Radiol. 1996;6(4):403–414

Matsuoka S, Uchiyama K, Shima H, Ueno N, Oish S, Nojiri Y. Bronchoarterial ratio and bronchial wall thickness on high-resolution CT in asymptomatic subjects: correlation with age and smoking. AJR Am J Roentgenol. 2003;180(2): 513–518

Meyer CA, White CS. Cartilaginous disorders of the chest. Radiographics. 1998;18(5):1109–1123. quiz 1241-1102

Meyer CN, Dossing M, Broholm H. Tracheobronchopathia osteochondroplastica. Respir Med. 1997;91(8):499–502

Michet Jr CJ, McKenna CH, Luthra HS, O'Fallon WM. Relapsing polychondritis. Survival and predictive role of early disease manifestations. Ann Intern Med. 1986;104(1): 74–78

Miller BH, Rosado-de-Christenson ML, McAdams HP, Fishback NF. Thoracic sarcoidosis: radiologic-pathologic correlation. Radiographics. 1995;15(2):421–437

Naidich DP, McCauley DI, Khouri NF, Stitik FP, Siegelman SS. Computed tomography of bronchiectasis. J Comput Assist Tomogr. 1982;6(3):437–444

Naidich DP, Zinn WL, Ettenger NA, McCauley DI, Garay SM. Basilar segmental bronchi: thin-section CT evaluation. Radiology. 1988;169(1):11–16

Ouellette H. The signet ring sign. Radiology. 1999;212(1): 67–68

Prince JS, Duhamel DR, Levin DL, Harrell JH, Friedman PJ (2002) Nonneoplastic lesions of the tracheobronchial wall: radiologic findings with bronchoscopic correlation. Radiographics 22(Spec No):S215–S230

Reiff DB, Wells AU, Carr DH, Cole PJ, Hansell DM. CT findings in bronchiectasis: limited value in distinguishing between idiopathic and specific types. AJR Am J Roentgenol. 1995;165(2):261–267

Ritsema GH. Ectopic right bronchus: indication for bronchography. AJR Am J Roentgenol. 1983;140(4):671–674

Savoca CJ, Austin JH, Goldberg HI. The right paratracheal stripe. Radiology. 1977;122(2):295–301

Screaton NJ, Sivasothy P, Flower CD, Lockwood CM. Tracheal involvement in Wegener's granulomatosis: evaluation using spiral CT. Clin Radiol. 1998;53(11):809–815

Staats BA, Utz JP, Michet Jr CJ. Relapsing polychondritis. Semin Respir Crit Care Med. 2002;23(2):145–154

Stark P. Radiology of the trachea. Stuttgart: Thieme; 1991. p. 54–78

Stark P. Imaging of tracheobronchial injuries. J Thorac Imaging. 1995;10(3):206–219

Stark P, Norbash A. Imaging of the trachea and upper airways in patients with chronic obstructive airway disease. Radiol Clin North Am. 1998;36(1):91–105

Stauffer JL, Olson DE, Petty TL. Complications and consequences of endotracheal intubation and tracheotomy. A prospective study of 150 critically ill adult patients. Am J Med. 1981;70(1):65–76

Stern EJ, Graham CM, Webb WR, Gamsu G. Normal trachea during forced expiration: dynamic CT measurements. Radiology. 1993;187(1):27–31

Stone T, Reynolds JH, Williams HJ. Imaging of large and small airway diseases. Imaging. 2006;18:139–150

Takasugi JE, Godwin JD. Radiology of chronic obstructive pulmonary disease. Radiol Clin North Am. 1998;36(1):29–55

Webb WR. Radiology of obstructive pulmonary disease. AJR Am J Roentgenol. 1997;169(3):637–647

Webb WR, Stein MG, Finkbeiner WE, Im JG, Lynch D, Gamsu G. Normal and diseased isolated lungs: high-resolution CT. Radiology. 1988;166(1 Pt 1):81–87

Woodring JH. Improved plain film criteria for the diagnosis of bronchiectasis. J Ky Med Assoc. 1994;92(1):8–13

Pleura

11

Bart Ilsen, Benoît Ghaye, Robert Gosselin,
Louke Delrue, Philippe Duyck, and Johan de Mey

Contents

B. Ilsen (✉)
Department of Radiology, Universitair Ziekenhuis Brussel,
Laarbeeklaan 101, 1090 Brussels, Belgium
e-mail: bart.ilsen@uzbrussel.be

B. Ghaye
Department of Medical Imaging,
University Hospital of Liege, B35 Sart Tilman,
B–4000 Liege, Belgium
e-mail: bghaye@chu.ulg.ac.be

R. Gosselin, L. Delrue, and P. Duyck
Department of Radiology, UZ-Gent, De Pintelaan 185,
9000 Gent, Belgium
e-mail: robert.gosselin@uzgent.be
e-mail: louke.delrue@uzgent.be
e-mail: philippe.duyck@uzgent.be

J. de Mey
Department of Radiology, AZ-VUB, Laarbeeklaan 101,
1090 Brussel, Belgium
e-mail: johan.demey@az.vub.ac.be

Abstract

> Diseases of the pleura and pleural space are common and present a significant contribution to the workload of the chest radiologist. The radiology department plays a crucial role in the imaging and management of pleural disease.

> While a number of different imaging modalities may be used, chest radiography remains the first examination in the initial assessment of these patients. Depending on the clinical context, the optimal imaging technique for further evaluation may be computed tomography (CT), ultrasound (US) or magnetic resonance (MR).

> This chapter reviews chest radiograph findings for some pathologic pleural manifestations by correlating them with their appearance on CT.

E.E. Coche et al. (eds.), *Comparative Interpretation of CT and Standard Radiography of the Chest,*
Medical Radiology, DOI: 10.1007/978-3-540-79942-9_11, © Springer-Verlag Berlin Heidelberg 2011

11.1 Introduction

The thoracic cage is constructed like a vertical cone-shaped bellows, with the diaphragm as the moving part at the bottom. The pleura is a serous membrane that lines the lungs and the thoracic cage. It folds back upon itself to form a two-layered membrane structure, forming the pleural cavity. It normally contains a small amount of pleural fluid that provides a friction-free surface for the lungs to expand and retract against. In other words, the pleural cavity is like a sealed, wet, and stretchable elastic bag inserted between the lung and the thoracic wall.

The pleura and pleural cavity are essential for efficient functioning of the lung, as the pericardium and pericardial cavity are for the heart. Pleural diseases represent a frequent problem in routine clinical practice, representing around 25% of pulmonary unit consultations. The chest X-ray remains the imaging modality of choice for the initial investigation of pleural disease. However, ultrasound, computed tomography (CT), and magnetic resonance imaging may also be helpful. In this chapter, we present the radiologic manifestations of many conditions that primarily or secondarily affect the pleura by comparing chest X-rays and CT findings side by side. Nevertheless, this comparison suffers because of the major drawbacks that X-ray is mainly obtained in an upright position and CT always in a recumbent position, which makes a strict comparison of pleural diseases difficult; their radiological aspects are frequently position dependent.

11.2 Anatomy

The pleura is divided into visceral and parietal pleura. The visceral pleura covers the lungs and the interlobar fissures, while the parietal pleura lines the ribs, diaphragm, and mediastinum. Both are continuous with each other as they reflect around the hilum and the inferior pulmonary ligament. They both consist of a single layer of flattened mesothelial cells that are subtended by layers of fibroelastic connective tissue. The connective tissue component of the visceral pleura is part of the "peripheral" interstitial fiber network and contains small vessels and lymphatic branches. These lymphatics, however, do not connect with the pleural space. The parietal pleura receives its vascular supply from and is drained by the systemic circulation. External to the parietal pleura is a layer of fatty areolar

connective tissue, which separates the pleura from the endothoracic fascia (Collins and Sterns 1999).

A thin film of fluid (pleural fluid) is normally present between the parietal and visceral pleura. The pleural cavity contains a small amount of fluid (approximately 1–10 ml) on each side (Black 1972). A complex balance between fluid production and removal maintains pleural fluid volume. As the thickness of pleural space and visceral and parietal pleura is only 0.2–0.4 mm, they are usually not identified on chest radiographs or CT scans except when outlined by air (or extrapleural fat visible on CT), or where the visceral pleura invaginates into the lung to form the fissures and where the two lungs contact each other at junctional lines (Im et al. 1989).

11.3 Basic Imaging Principles

A peripheral opacity can be located in three different locations related to the pleura:

An *extrapleural opacity* (Fig. 11.1) originates from the chest wall and, when not invading the pleura and lung, it presents with obtuse angles and an internal sharp medial margin.

A *pleural-based opacity* (Fig. 11.2) has margins that are partially or completely well circumscribed, indicating contiguity with a pleural surface, and usually presents with obtuse or right pleural angles.

A *subpleural opacity* (Fig. 11.3) is located in the parenchyma and usually has acute pleural angles and often has irregular internal margins.

11.4 Pleural Effusion

Pleural effusion results from the accumulation of fluid in the pleural space when forces that control the flow in and out of the space are disrupted (Raasch et al. 1982). According to their composition, most pleural effusions can be classified into two categories: transudate and exudate. Pleural transudate is a clear fluid with a protein content of less than 3 g/dl. Pleural exudate is a more opaque fluid with a protein content of more than 3 g/dl. In general, transudates reflect a systemic perturbation (and therefore are commonly bilateral), whereas exudates usually signify underlying local (pleuropulmonary) disease. The more common causes of transudative effusion are congestive heart failure and hypoalbuminemic

Fig. 11.1 Extrapleural opacity – Hodgkin's lymphoma of the rib cage. Frontal chest radiograph (**a**) shows a homogeneous retrocardiac opacity with sharp borders (*black arrow*). Lateral chest radiograph (**b**) shows a posterior opacity, presenting with obtuse angles related to chest wall (*black arrows*). Note a hiatal hernia (*white arrow*). Sagittal reformat in mediastinal (**c**) and lung window (**d**) shows the posterior mass invading the chest wall with rib destruction (*arrows*)

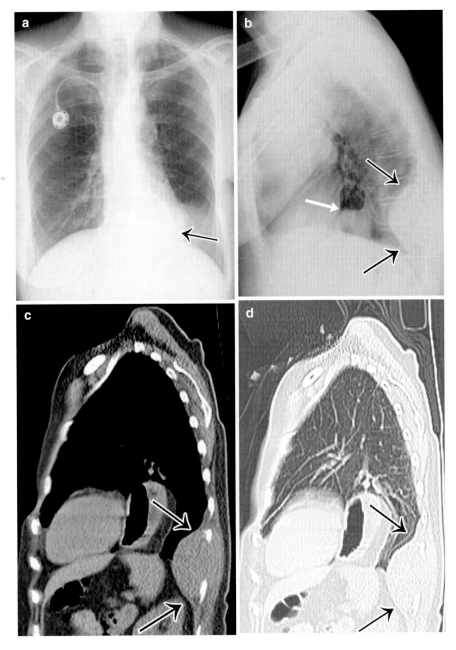

states (e.g., cirrhosis), whereas those of exudative effusions are malignancy, infections (e.g., pneumonia), and inflammatory diseases. Other sorts of pleural effusions include hemothorax, chylothorax, and pancreatic, bilious, and cerebrospinal fluid pleural effusions. The aspect of the effusion depends on patient position and mobility of the effusion (free or constrained to a variable extent) at the time of acquisition.

11.4.1 Distribution of Pleural Effusion in the Erect Patient

The distribution of free pleural fluid depends on patient position because it moves in dependent position due to gravity. In the upright position, the initial site of fluid accumulation is between the base of the lung and the diaphragm, namely the subpulmonic

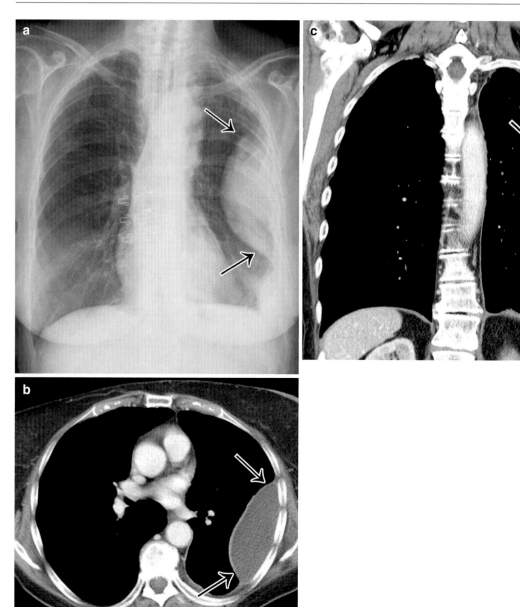

Fig. 11.2 Pleural opacity – Encapsulated pleural effusion. Frontal chest radiograph (**a**) shows a lenticular opacity with smooth borders and obtuse angles related to the chest wall (*black arrows*). Corresponding axial (**b**) and coronal (**c**) images demonstrate clearly the encapsulated pleural effusion (*arrows*)

region, sometimes to a large extent (Fig. 11.4). This represents a diagnostic challenge on posteroanterior and lateral chest radiographs because the upper edge of the fluid mimics the contour of the diaphragm and results in a pattern of only slight hemidiaphragm elevation ("pseudo-diaphragm") (Collins et al. 1972).

As the amount of fluid increases there may be flattening and some inversion of the diaphragm without significant blunting of the lateral costophrenic angle.

Some radiographic signs can suggest a subpulmonary effusion on posteroanterior radiographs of the erect patient (Raasch et al. 1982).

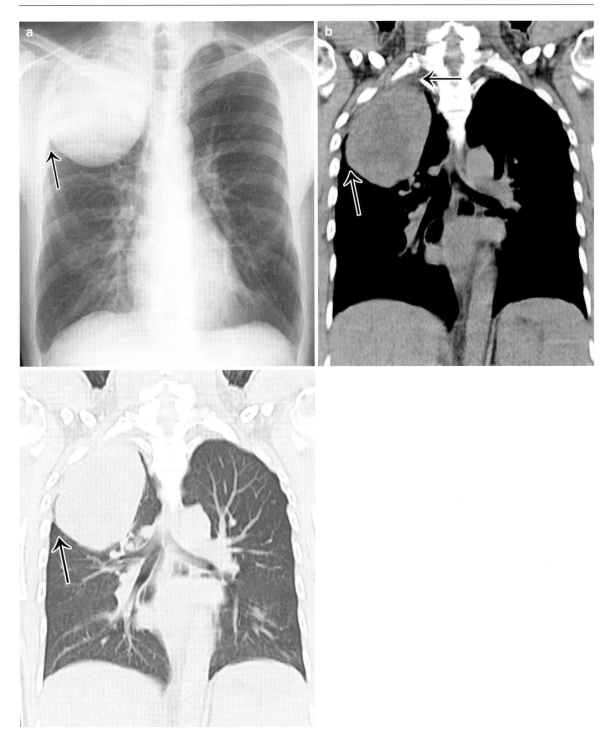

Fig. 11.3 Parenchymal opacity – Adenocarcinoma of the right upper lobe. Frontal chest radiograph (**a**) shows a large mass in the right upper lobe presenting acute angles (*black arrow*) related to the pleura and chest wall. Corresponding coronal reformat in mediastinal (**b**) and lung window (**c**) views

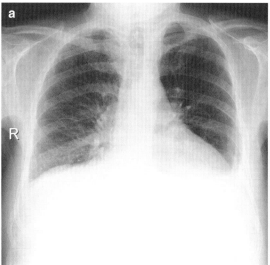 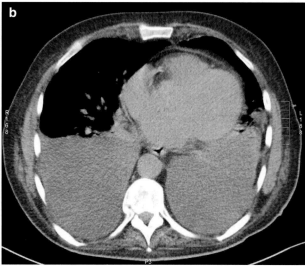

Fig. 11.4 Subpulmonary effusion. Frontal chest radiograph (**a**) shows an elevation of the left and right hemidiaphragm ("pseudo-diaphragm"). There is an obliteration of the retrodia-phragmatic blood vessels. Note blunting of both costophrenic sulci, particularly on the left. The gastric air bubble is not seen. Corresponding axial CT image shows large bilateral effusions (**b**)

- The apex of the "pseudo-diaphragm" is often more lateral than the apex of the normal diaphragm, particularly on expiration films, being situated near the junction of the middle and lateral thirds. Thus, the medial part of the pseudodiaphragm may appear more horizontal (Fig. 11.5 and 11.6).
- Through the "pseudo-diaphragm," the pulmonary blood vessels may be obliterated, but this finding can also be produced by lower lobe disease, abdominal conditions such as ascites, or underexposed films (Fig. 11.4).
- On the left side, the distance between pulmonary air and the gastric air is increased. A distance of more than 2 cm strongly suggests subpulmonic effusion (Fig. 11.6).

The findings on the frontal view are supported by the aspect of a subpulmonary effusion on the lateral view:

- On lateral projection, a characteristic configuration is seen anteriorly where the convex upper margin of the fluid meets the major fissure. In such a condition, the "diaphragmatic" contours anterior and posterior to the fissure are flattened (Fig. 11.7).
- A small amount of fluid is usually apparent in the lower end of major fissure where it joins the infra-pulmonary effusion (Fig. 11.7).

Because the posterior costophrenic sulcus is the deeper part of the pleural cavity, relatively large amounts of

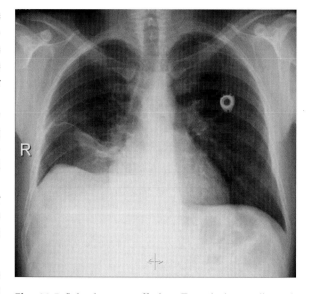

Fig. 11.5 Subpulmonary effusion. Frontal chest radiograph shows a more lateral position of the apex of the right "pseudo-diaphragm," located near the junction of the middle and lateral thirds. A correlation with computed tomography is in this case is almost not possible

pleural fluid may accumulate there without being apparent on the upright posteroanterior view. Accumulation of 200 ml or more of pleural fluid usually leads to blunting of the lateral costophrenic sulcus, although sometimes up to 500 ml or even more may be present without any blunting (Collins et al. 1972). Therefore, because it

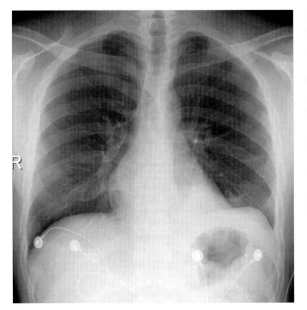

Fig. 11.6 Subpulmonary effusion. Frontal chest radiograph shows an increased distance between the intrapulmonary air and the gastric air, and external displacement of the apex of the left pseudodiaphragm, suggesting a left subpulmonic effusion. There is no correlation with computed tomography

better demonstrates the posterior costophrenic sulcus, the lateral view is more sensitive for the detection of small pleural effusions than the frontal view.

With an increase of the amount of pleural fluid, the typical concave and upward sloping contour of free fluid is known as the meniscus sign (Fig. 11.8). Fluid collects at the base of the pleural space due to gravity. The combination of positive hydrostatic intrapleural pressure at the lung base on the one hand and the elastic recoil of the lung on the other hand act to force some fluid to rise against gravity and surround the lower part of the lung. Because the X-ray beam must therefore penetrate a greater depth of fluid at the periphery of the thorax, the upper fluid margin appears higher at the periphery (Raasch et al. 1982, Davis et al. 1963). Large pleural effusions obscure the contour of the heart and eventually displace the mediastinum contralaterally.

11.4.2 Distribution of Pleural Effusion in the Supine Patient

In the supine patient, free pleural fluid layers posteriorly and produces a hazy increase in opacity without

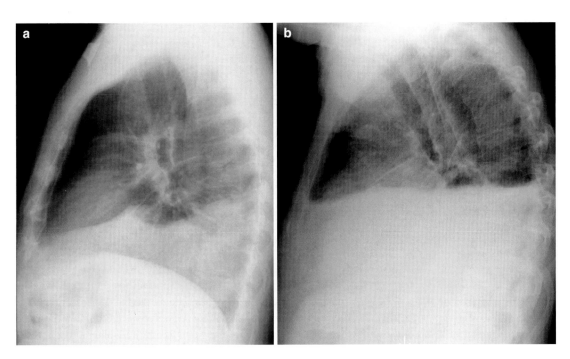

Fig. 11.7 Subpulmonary effusion. Lateral chest radiographs show a small amount of fluid in the major fissure where it joins the subpulmonary effusion in two patients (**a** and **b**). The "dia-phragmatic" contours anterior and posterior to the fissure are flattened (**b**). There is no exact correlation with computed tomography

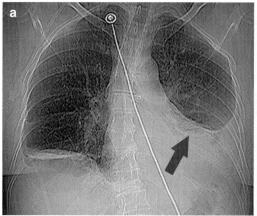
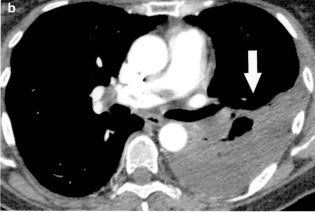

Fig. 11.8 Meniscus sign. When pleural fluid is free, it presents with the typical concave and upward sloping contour (*arrows*) due to association of hydrostatic and elastic recoil forces. Chest radiograph (**a**) and axial CT view (**b**)

obscuration of the bronchovascular markings, which may be difficult to detect, particularly when they are bilateral (Müller 1993). This homogeneous opacity may occupy only the lower part of the pleural cavity, making the lower half of the hemithorax more opaque than the upper. Blunting of the lateral costophrenic sulcus in the supine position occurs when the amount of fluid is sufficient to fill the posterior hemithorax up to the level of the sulcus (Woodring 1984). Other signs include obscuration of the hemidiaphragm, apparent elevation of the hemidiaphragme, decreased visibility of the lower lobe vessels below the level of the apparent dome of the diaphragm, increased opacity of the spleen in a left-sided effusion, and thickening of the minor fissure (Fig. 11.9) (Ruskin et al. 1987; Woodring 1984).

Free pleural fluid can also cap the apex of the lung on supine radiographs, known as the *apical cap sign* (Fig. 11.10). Due to the small capacity of the apex, this is considered to be an early sign as fluid extends tangentially to the X-ray beam to a greater degree between the lung and chest wall at the apex than at the base (Raasch et al. 1982).

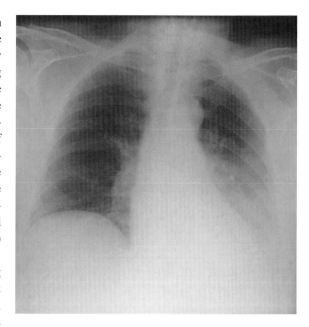

Fig. 11.9 Pleural effusion in a supine patient. Frontal chest radiograph shows a hazy increase in opacity on the lower left side, obscuration of the hemidiaphragm, decreased visibility of the lower lobe vessels, and increased opacity of left hypochondrium

11.4.3 Atypical Distribution and Loculation of Pleural Fluid

Loculation of pleural effusion can occur when adhesions between contiguous surfaces of the pleura develop, often in the case of a pyothorax or hemothorax. When it occurs between two lobes, it can be misdiagnosed as a pulmonary neoplasm on chest radiographs. However, fluid accumulations between two lobes tend to absorb spontaneously and therefore have been called "vanishing tumors" or pseudotumors (Fig. 11.11). Fluid loculated in a fissure may have a distinctive lenticular configuration, frequently on the lateral view, allowing for differentiation from condensation or atelectasis (Fig. 11.12).

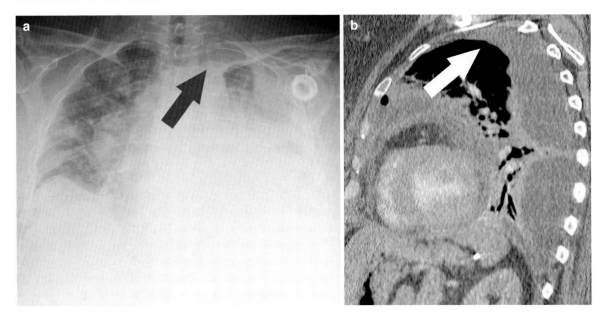

Fig. 11.10 Apical cap sign. Similar to the meniscus sign on erect chest radiographs, the apical cap sign (*arrows*) may be seen in a decubitus chest radiograph (**a**). Due to the association of hydrostatic and elastic recoil forces, fluid may extend tangentially to the X-ray beam at apex. Corresponding sagittal computed tomography view (**b**)

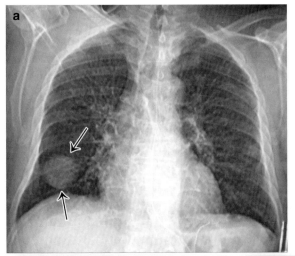

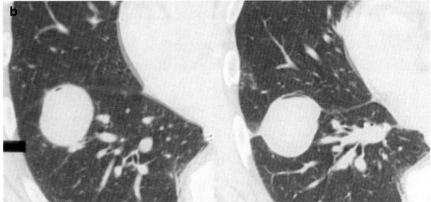

Fig. 11.11 Vanishing tumor or pseudotumor. Frontal chest radiograph (**a**) shows a rounded opacity at the right lung base presenting with smooth borders (*black arrows*). Corresponding axial computed tomography image (two consecutive images) in lung windows (**b**) clearly demonstrate the encapsulated fluid in the major fissure simulating a tumor

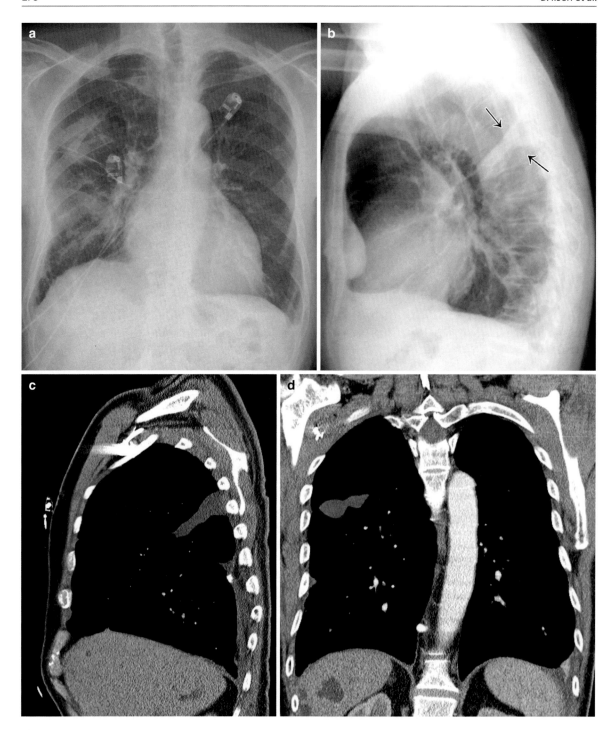

Fig. 11.12 Lenticular configuration of loculated fluid in the fissure. Frontal chest radiograph (**a**) shows an unsharply defined opacity in the upper part of the right hemithorax. Lateral chest radiograph (**b**) shows the loculated fluid in the major fissure (*black arrows*), confirmed on sagittal (**c**) and coronal (**d**) reformatted images on computed tomography

When the elastic recoil of the lung is restricted, the retractility of the lung is modified and the pleural fluid is attracted toward this area (Rigby et al. 1976). Therefore, it must be kept in mind that any atypical distribution of pleural fluid may be a sign of both parenchymal and pleural disease.

11.5 Empyema

Thoracic empyema, or pyothorax, is defined as pus in the pleural cavity. The majority of empyemas follow acute bacterial pneumonia or lung abscesses. Other causes include thoracic surgery, trauma, mediastinitis, and spread from extrapulmonary sites, such as osteomyelitis of the spine and cervical or subphrenic abscesses. Empyemas are associated with an inflammatory pleural reaction and the influx of polymorphonuclear neutrophils, fibrin, and other plasma clotting factors into the pleural space (Sahn 1988). The fibrin coats both the visceral and parietal pleura. If the infection is inadequately treated, organization of this fibrin peel with ingrowths of capillaries and fibroblasts can be seen as early as 7 days from the development of the empyema. The end result is pleural fibrosis that may impede medical or percutaneous treatment (Hanna et al. 1991).

Pleural fluid is often present and is usually unilateral, but when it is bilateral it is substantially greater in volume on the infected side (Hanna et al. 1991). Similar to sterile effusions, nonloculated empyemas are homogeneous in opacity, move with patient position, and have a meniscus sign. When loculated, empyemas should be differentiated from lung abscess, which may be difficult but has important therapeutic consequences. Differentiation is more easily achieved using CT than chest X-ray (Table 11.1). With CT, the visualization of enhancement of the parietal and visceral pleura, thickening of the extrapleural subcostal tissues, and increased attenuation of the extrapleural fat should suggest an empyema (Fig. 11.13). The combination of fluid between the pleural space and thickening of the visceral and parietal pleura is referred to as the *split pleura sign* (Fig. 11.14) (Stark et al. 1983).

Because of overlying lung disease or unfavorable localization and the inability to resolve adequately the pleural-parenchymal interface, differentiation of empyema versus lung abscess often results in

Table 11.1 CT pattern of empyema versus lung abscess (Modified from Stark et al. 1983)

	Empyema	Lung abscess
Shape	Lenticular	Round
Wall	Smooth	Irregular
	Split pleural sign	Dots of air
Wall thickness	Thin	Thick
	Uniform	Nonuniform
Lung compression	Yes	No
Vessels and bronchi	Distorted	Normal or attracted
Chest wall angles	Obtuse	Acute

ambiguous findings on chest X-rays. The features that may help to differentiate an empyema from a lung abscess on chest X-rays are the shape of the collection, their angles and contact with the chest wall, their margins, and the pattern of the air-fluid level (Fig. 11.15). The shape of empyema is ovoid, which makes that dimensions will change with X-ray incidences, whereas lung abscess are more rounded and therefore will not change with various incidences. Similarly, when present, the length of the air-fluid level will change with different projections whereas it is similar on frontal and lateral views of a lung abscess (Hanna et al. 1991; Stark et al. 1983). The angles of the collection related to the chest wall are obtuse for an empyema and acute for a lung abscess. Empyemas present with broader contact to the chest wall and their margins are smooth and regular.

11.6 Pneumothorax

A pneumothorax is the presence of air between the two layers of the pleura, resulting in a partial or complete collapse of the lung (Fig. 11.16). Normally, the pressure in the pleural space is lower than that inside the lungs or outside the chest. When a perforation causes a connection between the pleural space and the lungs or outside the chest, air enters the pleural space until the pressures become equal or the connection closes. Pneumothorax can be divided into spontaneous and traumatic types.

The diagnosis of pneumothorax is usually made on a chest radiograph, which may also detect

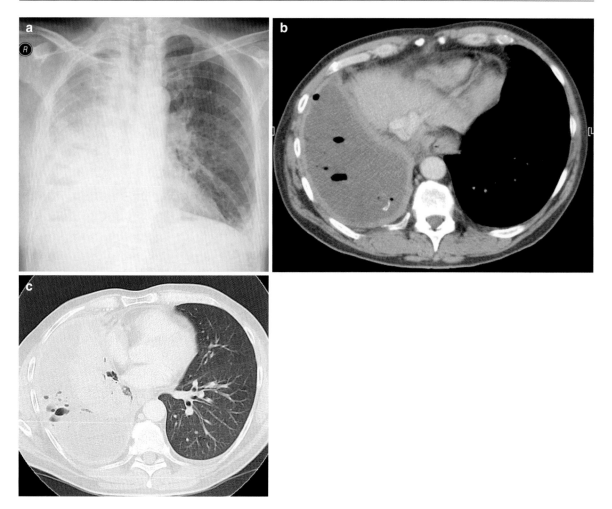

Fig. 11.13 Empyema in a patient who has had cough and fever for 1 week. Chest radiograph (**a**) demonstrates a pleural opacity with multiple air-fluid levels overlying the lower lung. An axial contrast-enhanced computed tomography view in mediastinal (**b**) and lung window (**c**) at the level of the lung base shows thickening and an enhancement of the parietal pleura. Note the multiple air bubbles in the empyema

complications and predisposing conditions. Pneumothorax is seen on chest radiograph as a thin curvilinear opacity corresponding to the visceral pleura separating the vessel-containing lung from the air-containing avascular pleural space (Fig. 11.16). As free air moves to the nondependent part of the chest, difficulties arise when pleural adhesions are present; these can result in a part of the lung being tethered to the thoracic wall, thereby distorting the usual radiographic appearance. As for pleural fluid effusion, the radiographic appearance of a pneumothorax depends on the radiographic projection, the patient's position, and the presence or absence of loculation. Pneumothorax has to be differentiated from other curvilinear shadows caused by hair, clothes, skinfolds,

lines or tubes, and bullae. A complex and distorted radiographic appearance in scans of patients with giant bullous emphysema may hinder the detection of, or even may falsely suggest, a pneumothorax. Air surrounding both sides of the bulla wall, known as the *double-wall sign* on CT, should aid in the triage of those patients (Waitches et al. 2000).

11.6.1 Pneumothorax in the Erect Patient

Fluid falls to the bottom whereas air rises to the apex in the erect position. The apical visceral pleural line is usually readily identifiable. When a pneumothorax

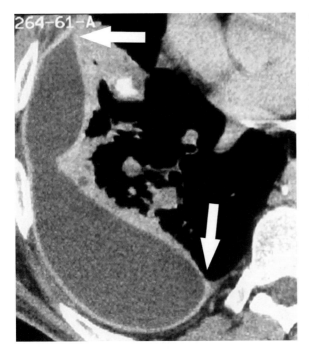

Fig. 11.14 Split pleura sign. An axial contrast-enhanced computed tomography view in mediastinal window at the right base shows a loculated pleural effusion with enhancement and thickening of the visceral and parietal pleura (*arrows*)

is highly clinically suggested but not visualized on the inspiratory chest radiographs, a full expiratory (or more rarely a lateral decubitus chest radiograph with horizontal X-ray beam) should be obtained (Harvey et al. 1989) (Fig. 11.17). A tension pneumothorax is a life-threatening complication that occurs when the pleural tear acts as a one-way valve, responsible for progressively increasing positive intrapleural pressure. Suggestive signs of tension include diaphragmatic contour straightening, contralateral shift of the mediastinum, diaphragmatic flattening, or depression and enlargement of the intercostal spaces. Lung collapse may not be significant in severely diseased lungs (Fig. 11.18).

11.6.2 Pneumothorax in the Supine Patient

When a pneumothorax is present in a patient in supine position, the air rises to the highest point in the hemithorax, which is usually the inferoanteromedial part of the pleural space. Detecting a pneumothorax in a patient in a supine position is challenging because a poorly defined basilar hyperlucency may be the only detectable finding. Depending on its size, a pneumothorax can result in a deep, fingerlike lateral costophrenic sulcus (deep sulcus sign) (Gordon 1980); a visible anterior costophrenic recess seen as an oblique line or interface directed downward and outward over the hypochondrium; the visualization of the inferior surface of the lung or the epipericardic fat pads; and an unusually sharp delineation of the diaphragm or left cardiac apex (Fig. 11.19) (Zitter and Westcott 1981).

The lateral decubitus film (with the involved hemithorax uppermost) is more sensitive than the erect or supine film and can be as sensitive as CT in the detection of pneumothorax (Carr et al. 1992).

11.7 Pleural Fibrosis

Pleural fibrosis or the development of fibrous tissue in the pleura has various origins and can be the result of a primary pleural disease or an inflammatory condition that affects the lungs. It can be either a focal or a diffuse process. In most cases, the fibrosis is localized in a small area and has no clinical impact. Less commonly, the fibrosis is diffuse and functional abnormalities may be apparent if the fibrosis involves the visceral pleura.

11.7.1 Focal Pleural Fibrosis

11.7.1.1 Healed Pleuritis

An organized fibrinous pleuritis or fibrinopurulent pleuritis secondary to pneumonia is the most common cause of localized pleural fibrosis. Because of gravity, the distribution of the pleural thickening related to this cause is usually basal. In the case of obliteration of the costophrenic sulci, differentiation from a small pleural effusion may be difficult (Fig. 11.20).

11.7.1.2 Apical Cap

An apical cap is defined radiographically as a 1- to 30-mm-thick curved soft tissue opacity in the extreme apex of the lung. The lower border is usually sharply

Fig. 11.15 Empyema. Frontal (**a**) and lateral (**b**) chest radiographs show a right pleural effusion and an air-fluid level at the right base. The length of the air-fluid level is twice as long on the lateral view than on the frontal view, suggesting an ovoid shape (as found in pleural collections) rather than a round shape (as in pulmonary abscess). Computed tomography images in three different planes (**c**, **d** and **e**) show the pleural effusion and a loculated empyema with an air-fluid level (*white arrow*). The ovoid form, the large contact with the diaphragm (*black arrows*), the smooth inner wall of the collection, and enhancement of the visceral and parietal pleura further reinforce the pleural origin

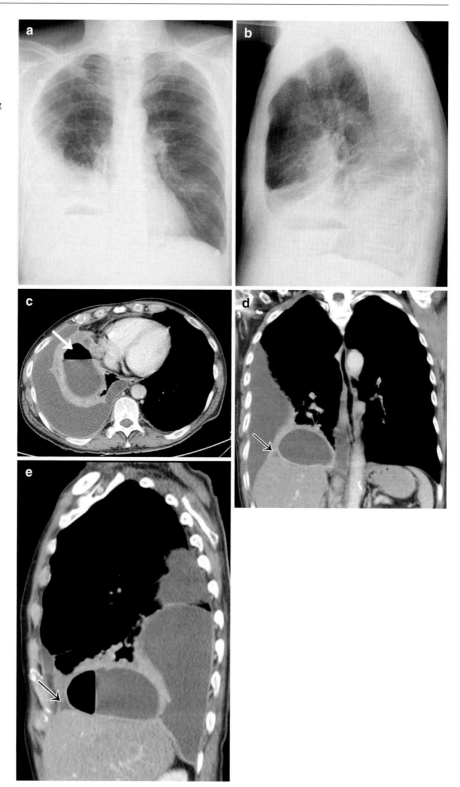

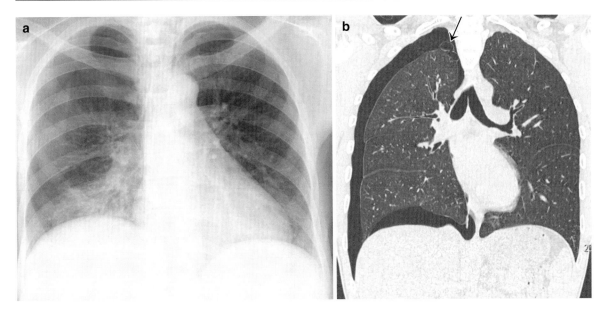

Fig. 11.16 Right pneumothorax in a 19-year-old woman. Frontal chest radiograph (**a**) shows a thin curvilinear opacity corresponding to visceral pleura separating the vessel-containing lung from the air-containing avascular pleural space. Computed tomography image (**b**) demonstrates the same finding and also a ruptured bulla (*black arrow*) as the origin of the pneumothorax

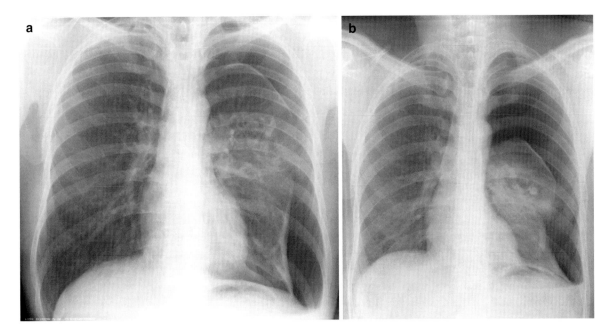

Fig. 11.17 Left pneumothorax in a 25-year-old man. Full inspiratory frontal chest radiograph (**a**) shows an important pneumothorax on the left, accentuated on the full expiratory chest radiograph (**b**)

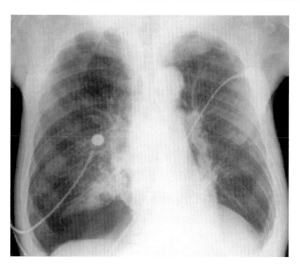

Fig. 11.18 Tension pneumothorax in a 65-year-old man with severely diseased lungs. Frontal chest radiograph shows marked lowering of the right diaphragm, contralateral mediastinal shift, and enlargement of the right intercostal spaces. Note the absence of lung collapse

marginated and may be curvilinear or undulating. Although apical caps are similar in appearance, their clinical significance varies widely. Whether unilateral or bilateral, they are mostly isolated radiographic findings of a benign nature and of no clinical significance due to thickening of extrapleural fat and pleuroparenchymal fibrosis as sequellae of prior infectious disease (Fig. 11.21) (Im et al. 1989). Occasionally, particularly when thick and unilateral, an apical cap may be a sign of a significant lesion arising in the region of the apex of the lung, known as a Pancoast tumor. Comparison with previous films is helpful; otherwise, CT may be recommended.

11.7.1.3 Pleural Plaques

Pleural plaques are a circumscribed accumulation of dense acellular bundles of collagen, which may or may not be calcified. Pleural plaques are the most common manifestation of inhalation of asbestos fibers and are well known as an indication of previous exposure to asbestos fibers, being radiologically seen in 20–60% of workers who have been exposed to high concentrations of asbestos (Schwartz 1991). The prevalence of pleural plaques correlates with the intensity of asbestos exposure and the time interval from initial

exposure. The latency period between exposure to asbestos and development of pleural plaques is approximately 15 years; for radiologically visible calcified pleural plaques, the latency period is at least 20–30 years (Schwartz 1991; Greene et al. 1984).

The plaques involve mainly the posterior and anterolateral aspects of the pleura, following the contours of the posterolateral seventh to tenth intercostal spaces. They spare the lung apices and costrophrenic angles and rarely extend vertically for more than four interspaces. They almost always involve only the parietal pleura but have been rarely described in the interlobar fissures.

Chest radiography has been the primary radiographic method for the detection of asbestos-related pleural disease for a long time. When viewed en face, pleural plaques may be difficult to recognize unless they are large or calcified and are recognized as multiple and bilateral nodular, stippled, irregular, leaflike, or "geographic" opacities (Fig. 11.22). Plaques within fissures can rarely mimic solitary pulmonary nodules. When viewed tangentially, pleural plaques are seen on chest radiographs as focal areas of pleural thickening. Over the diaphragm they produce either curvilinear calcifications or scalloping.

Chest radiography, however, has a relatively low sensitivity for the detection of asbestos-related pleural diseases, and new techniques such as dual-energy digital subtraction chest radiography may improve detection (Gilkeson et al. 2004). Another potential source of difficulty when reading conventional radiographs is the misinterpretation of extrapleural fat as pleural thickening. Subcostal fat may mimic pleural thickening in obese individuals. Typically, it appears as a symmetrical, smooth, sometimes undulating soft-tissue density. It typically extends from the fourth to the eighth ribs.

CT has greater sensitivity and specificity for identifying asbestos-related pleural diseases than conventional radiography (Aberle et al. 1988; Friedman et al. 1987). Pleural plaques appear as well-circumscribed areas of pleural thickening separated from the underlying rib and extrapleural fat by a thin layer of fat. These plaques can look like "table mountains" or mesas. They can have a nodular configuration and can impinge slightly on the adjacent lung parenchyma, in some cases resulting in the formation of a pulmonary subpleural curvilinear line adjacent to the plaque.

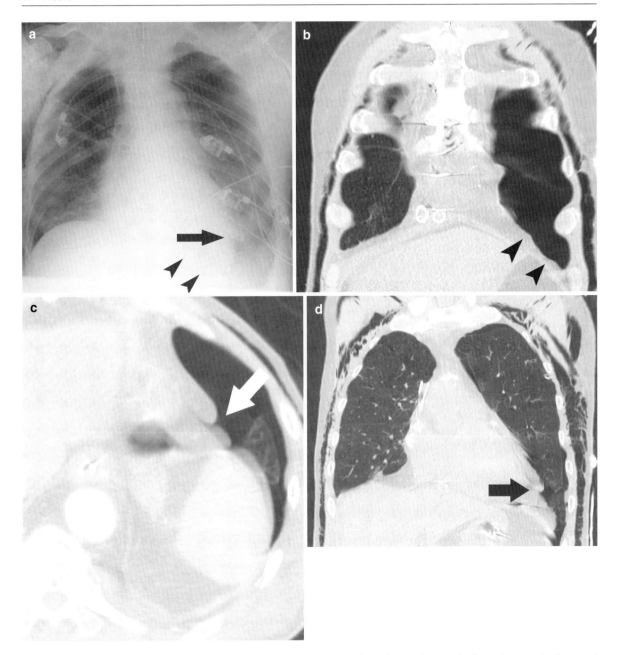

Fig. 11.19 Pneumothorax in a supine patient. Findings on supine chest radiographs (**a**) include an avascular area at the left lung base, a visible anterior costophrenic recess (*arrowheads*), and the visualization of the epipericardic fat pads (*arrow*). Computed tomography views (**b, c,** and **d**) show the anterior costophrenic recess (*arrowheads*) and the epipericardic fat pads (*arrows*)

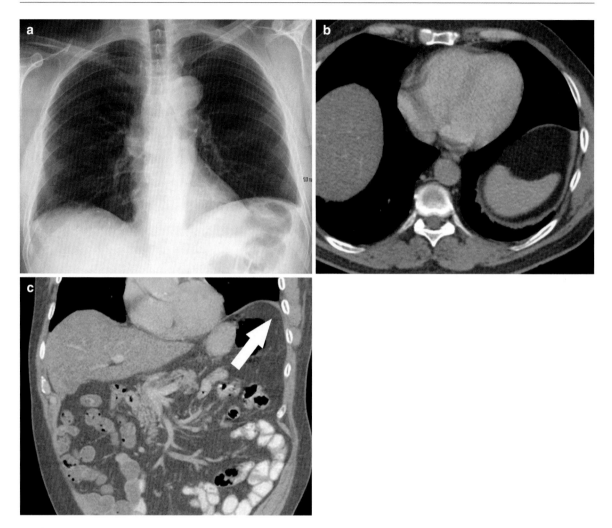

Fig. 11.20 Healed pleuritis in a patient with past history of left pleuritis. Chest radiograph (**a**) and computed tomography scans (**b** and **c**) show lateral pleural adhesion on the left side, resulting in a large contact between the diaphragm and the chest wall. On the chest radiograph, differentiation from a small pleural effusion is difficult

11.7.2 Diffuse Pleural Fibrosis

11.7.2.1 Asbestosis-Related Diffuse Pleural Thickening

Asbestosis-related diffuse pleural thickening is less common than pleural plaques and results in the fusion of visceral and parietal pleura, impairing the pulmonary function (Schwartz 1991). Radiographically, it is considered to be present when a smooth, uninterrupted pleural opacity is seen extending over at least a fourth of the chest wall with or without obliteration of the costophrenic sulci (Lynch et al. 1989). On CT, the abnormality is diagnosed when it extends for more than 8 cm in a craniocaudal direction and 5 cm in a lateral direction and the pleura is more than 3 mm thick (Müller 1993). It is more frequently associated with rounded atelectasis than other types of diffuse pleural thickening (Fig. 11.23).

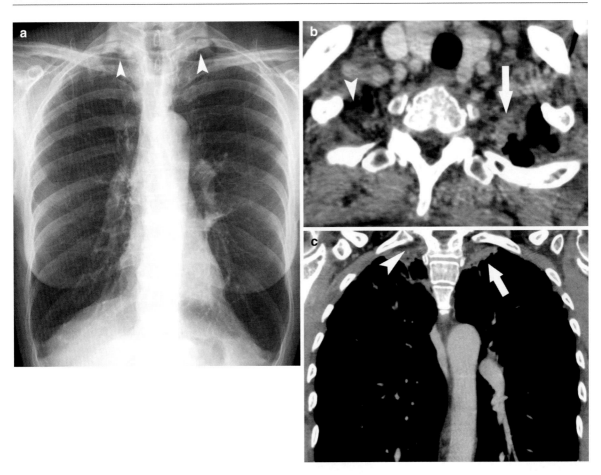

Fig. 11.21 Apical cap. A 10-mm-thick curved soft tissue opacity (*arrowheads*) is demonstrated at both apices on chest radiographs (**a**). Axial and coronal computed tomography views (**b** and **c**) clearly explain the apical cap by the presence of thickened extrapleural fat (*arrowheads*) and pleuroparenchymal fibrosis (*arrows*)

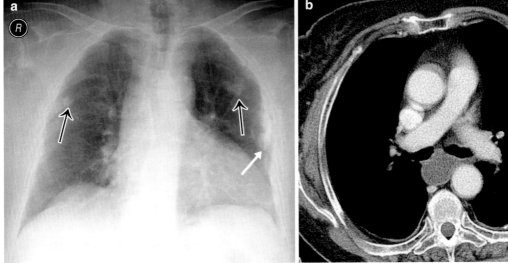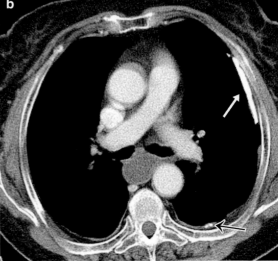

Fig. 11.22 Asbestos-related pleural plaques in a 59-year-old man. Frontal chest radiograph (**a**) shows leaflike or "geographic" opacities when the pleural plaques are viewed en face (*black arrows*). Tangentially viewed, pleural plaques are seen as focal areas of pleural thickening (*white arrows*). Corresponding axial computed tomography image (**b**)

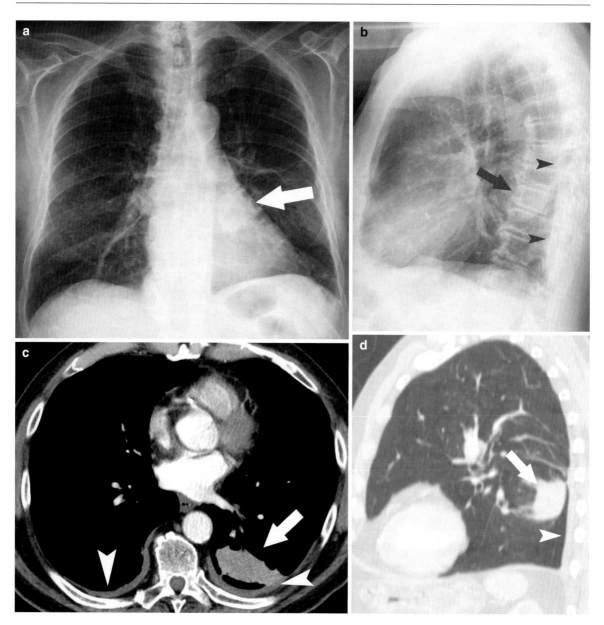

Fig. 11.23 Asbestos-related diffuse pleural thickening in a 55-year-old man. Chest radiographs (**a** and **b**) show an ill-defined opacity (*arrows*) in contact with posterior pleural thickening (*arrowheads*). Note on the frontal view bilateral platelike atelectasis due to hypoventilation secondary to large pleural adhesions. Axial and sagittal computed tomography views (**c** and **d**) show bilateral posterior pleural thickening (*arrowheads*) and a left round atelectasis (*arrows*)

11.7.2.2 Non–Asbestosis-Related Pleural Thickening

Hemorrhagic effusions, tuberculous effusions (Fig. 11.24), other types of empyema, or a complication of various other pleuritic processes often result in an unilateral pleural thickening (Müller 1993; Leung et al. 1989). Diffuse pleural thickening can result in a marked decrease in volume of the affected hemithorax and in marked impaired ventilation of the underlying lung.

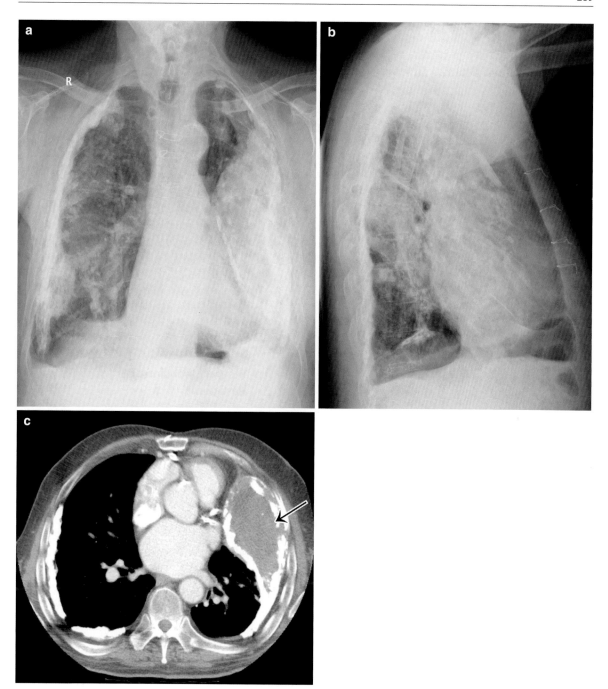

Fig. 11.24 Diffuse pleural thickening in a patient with a history of bilateral tuberculous pleurisy and chronic left tuberculous empyema. Frontal (**a**) and lateral (**b**) chest radiographs show bilateral coarse pleural calcifications and a lenticular and partially calcified pleural opacity in the left hemithorax. Axial contrast-enhanced computed tomography slice (c) shows the bilateral diffuse pleural thickening and a left chronic empyema with soft tissue density centrally and heavy calcifications both in visceral and parietal pleura (*black arrow*)

11.8 Pleural Neoplasms

11.8.1 Localized Pleural Tumors

The most common localized pleural tumors are localized fibrous tumors of the pleura, pleural lipomas, and pleural invasions of bronchogenic carcinoma.

11.8.1.1 Localized Fibrous Tumor of the Pleura

Localized fibrous tumor of the pleura is a slowly growing primary pleural neoplasm unrelated to asbestos exposure. It is a relatively uncommon neoplasm, accounting for less than 5% of all pleural tumors (Theros et al. 1977). Due to great diversity of pathologic findings it has been known by a variety of terms, including benign localized mesothelioma, benign pleural fibroma, fibrosing mesothelioma, and pleural fibromyxoma. It has been described in all age groups but has a peak incidence in persons older than 50 years of age. Approximately 80% arise from the visceral pleura and the majority presents as a pedunculated mass with benign pathologic features (Ferretti et al. 1997).

The radiographic appearance depends on the size of the tumor, which ranges from 1 to 39 cm. A small- to medium-sized tumor usually appears as a solitary, homogeneous, sharply delineated, often lobulated nodule or mass arising from the visceral pleura forming obtuse angles with the chest wall (Fig. 11.25). Large tumors can appear as an opacity occupying a considerable portion of one hemithorax and lose their obtuse angle with the chest wall even as pedunculated tumors. In this case, determination of an extrapulmonary origin may not be possible on the chest radiograph. The stalk can be as long as 9 cm, allowing the lesion to move according to the patient's position.

CT imaging shows a well delineated and often lobulated mass (Ferretti et al. 1997). On unenhanced CT scans, they appear with soft-tissue attenuation. Calcification can be present in large tumors and are related to areas of necrosis. Contrast enhancement can be homogeneous and intense as a result of the rich vascularization of the tumor. However, heterogeneous enhancement can be seen due to necrosis, myxoid degeneration, or hemorrhage within the tumor (Ferretti et al. 1997; Lee et al. 1992).

Malignant forms are often larger then 10 cm in diameter and demonstrate central necrosis. Nevertheless, there are no definite radiologic features to differentiate benign and malignant fibrous tumors and therefore surgery is advised in all patients.

11.8.1.2 Pleural Lipoma and Liposarcoma

Pleural lipomas are uncommon tumors, usually asymptomatic and found incidentally on the chest radiograph. Lipomas may be intrathoracic or transmural, with an intrathoracic and extrathoracic component (Buxton et al. 1988). They are accurately diagnosed on CT, where they appear as a well-defined mass of homogeneous fat attenuation presenting with obtuse angles related to the chest wall and displacing the adjacent pulmonary parenchyma (Fig. 11.26) (Buxton et al. 1988). Liposarcoma is an even rarer tumor that usually has a heterogeneous mixture of fat and mainly soft tissue attenuation (Munk et al. 1988).

11.8.1.3 Pleural Extension of Bronchogenic Carcinoma

A bronchogenic carcinoma invading the visceral pleura is classified as a T2 lesion, whereas extention into the parietal pleura upgrades the classification to T3. If the lesion extends into the pleura and chest wall, all the margins of the lesion may be indistinct.

11.8.2 Malignant Mesothelioma

Malignant mesothelioma is an aggressive malignant tumor of serosal surfaces. It most commonly affects the pleura, but occasionally involves other serosa. It was considered a rare disease before about 1960, but has increased dramatically in incidence since that time due to the widespread use of asbestos fibers during the postwar industrial boom. Abundant epidemiologic studies show a close association between asbestos exposure and the development of mesothelioma, reported in 50–90% of patients (Edge and Choudhury 1978; Yates et al. 1997). However, some patients have no recognized exposure to this mineral, and other factors are probably important in occasional cases such as other minerals, infection, genetic factors, and radiation. A latency of 20–40 years is reported from first exposure to asbestos to presentation of the tumor.

Pleural malignant mesothelioma manifests most commonly as multiple tumoral masses that involve the

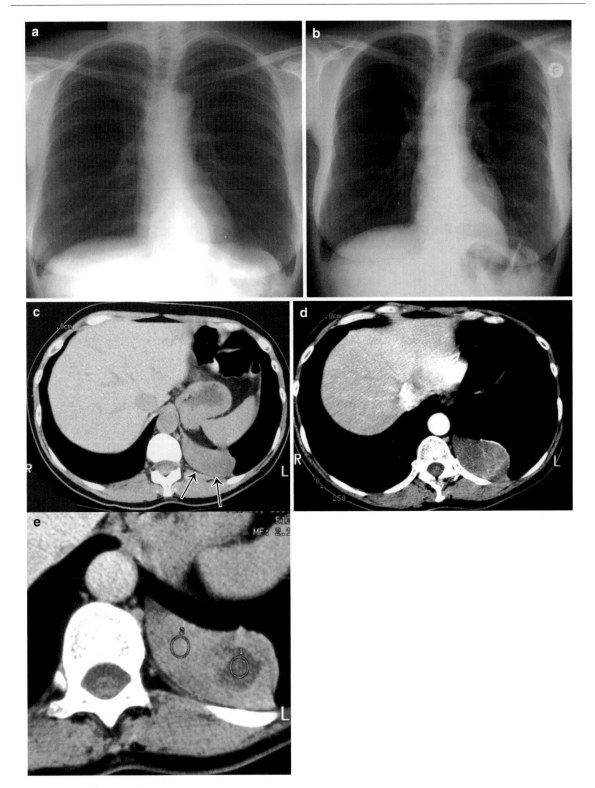

Fig. 11.25 Localized fibrous tumor of the pleura. Two consecutive chest radiographs (**a** and **b**) at 3-year interval show a sharply delineated, slow-growing left retrocardiac mass. Unenhanced axial computed tomography (CT) image (**c**) shows a well-defined homogeneous soft-tissue-density mass. Note the intact subpleural fat (*black arrows*). Enhanced CT images (**d** and **e**) show heterogeneous enhancement corresponding to areas of necrosis (Courtesy of G. Ferretti, Grenoble, France)

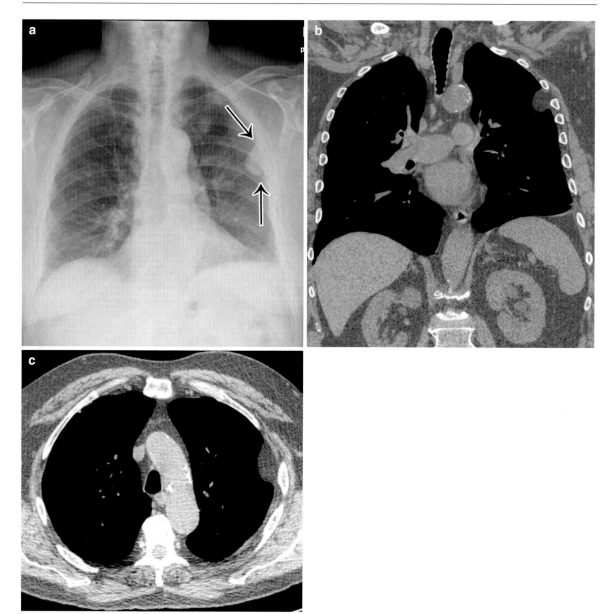

Fig. 11.26 Pleural lipoma in a 79-year-old man. Frontal chest radiograph (**a**) shows a homogeneous peripheral opacity with a sharply defined medial edge (*black arrows*). A coronal reformat computed tomography (CT) view in mediastinal window (**b**) clearly shows the pleural-based lesion (**b**). The axial CT view (**c**) shows the smooth marginated lesion forming obtuse angles with the chest wall. Note the fat attenuation of the pleural-based lesion

parietal and visceral pleural surfaces, with greater involvement of the parietal pleura. Chest wall and mediastinal involvement, including pericardial and cardiac invasion, may occur. The diaphragm is frequently invaded. Tumor extension into the peritoneal cavity is identified in at least one third of autopsies. Tumoral spread across the mediastinum may result in the involvement of the opposite pleural cavity.

The most frequent radiographic manifestation of malignant mesothelioma is unilateral sheetlike of lobulated pleural thickening up to several centimeters thick encasing the entire lung, growing into the fissures, and creating a pleural rind (Fig. 11.27) (Miller et al. 1996). This results in volume loss of the ipsilateral hemithorax with narrowing of the intercostal spaces and elevation of the hemidiaphragm. Less commonly, the tumor

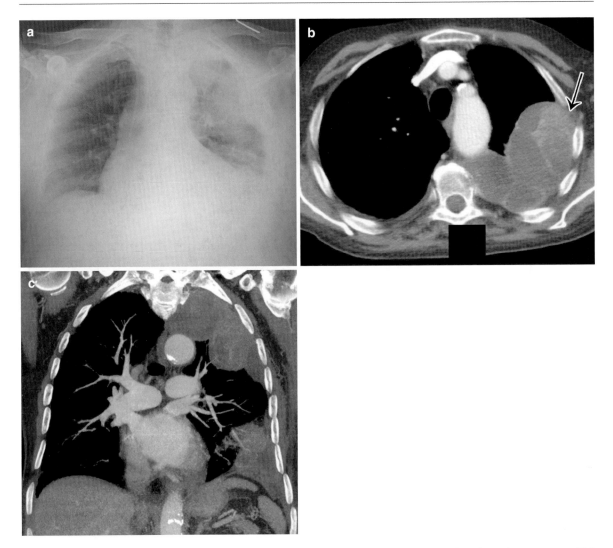

Fig. 11.27 Mesothelioma in a 65-year shipyard employee. Frontal chest radiograph (**a**) shows a unilateral lobulated pleural thickening encasing the entire lung with an associated left pleural effusion. Axial (**b**) and coronal reformatted (**c**) contrast-enhanced computed tomography views demonstrate a thick enhancing pleural tumor involving the left hemithorax. Note the invasion into the subpleural fat (*black arrow*)

manifests as multiple, pleural-based masses. Most of the patients develop a pleural effusion that is typically unilateral, which may obscure underlying pleural thickening or masses. In advanced tumors, chest wall invasion may manifest by a periosteal reaction along the ribs, rib erosion, or rib destruction (Miller et al. 1996). Occasionally, hematogenous metastases to the lung are seen as lung nodules or masses (Krumhaar et al. 1985).

CT is superior to conventional radiography for the identification of early abnormalities, in determining the presence and extent of tumor in the pleura, and in assessing invasion of the mediastinum, chest wall, and upper part of the abdomen. (Fig. 11.27) (Rabinowitz et al. 1982; Alexander et al. 1981). The most common findings are similar to conventional radiography, a pleural thickening and effusion. In a review of 50 patients, the pretreatment CT findings were pleural thickening (92%), thickening of the pleural surface in the interlobular fissures (86%), pleural calcifications (20%), and pleural effusions (74%) (Kawashima et al. 1990). Less common findings include loss of volume of ipsilateral hemithorax, a contralateral shift of the mediastinum, lymph node enlargement, and chest wall invasion. Findings suggestive of chest wall invasion are obscuration of fat planes, infiltration of intercostal muscles, periosteal reaction, and bone destruction. Obliteration of fat planes, nodular pericardial thickening, and direct soft tissue extension are features of mediastinal invasion.

11.8.3 Other Tumors of the Pleura

Other pleural tumors include sarcoma of the pleura (Fig. 11.28), lymphoma (Fig. 11.29), and pleural plasmacytoma. Most of the sarcomas of the pleura are

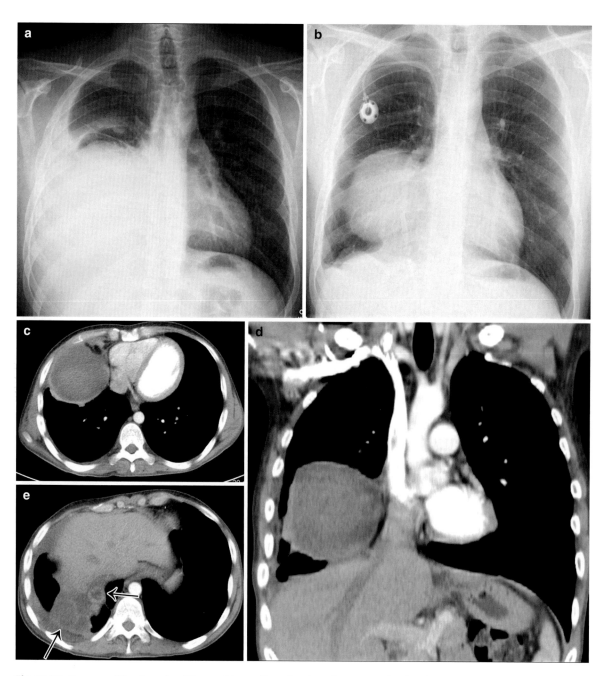

Fig. 11.28 Sarcoma of the pleura in a 33-year-old man. Frontal chest radiograph (**a**) shows a large right pleural effusion at admission. After thoracocentesis, a large opacity in the right lung base is demonstrated (**b**). Axial (**c**) and coronal (**d**) contrast-enhanced computed tomography (CT) views show a hypodense mass developed at the anterior part of the right middle lobe. An axial CT view (**e**) shows several tissular masses located in the pleural cavity (*black arrows*). Pathology revealed a poorly differentiated sarcoma of the pleura

metastatic. Pleural involvement by lymphoma is relatively common; however, a primary pleural lymphoma is more uncommon.

11.8.4 Pleural Metastases

Metastatic disease to the pleura is a frequent finding with intrathoracic or extrathoracic primary tumors because of the rich lymphatic network of the pleura. Almost all cancers can metastasize to the pleura, including, among others, lung or breast tumors, lymphoma, thymoma, or sarcoma (Fig. 11.30). In approximately 10–30% of patients with malignant pleural effusion, the primary site remains unknown. Differentiating primary tumors from metastatic disease sometimes can be difficult because they may mimic primary tumors of the pleura radiologically, clinically, grossly, and histopathologically. The pattern is very close to mesothelioma.

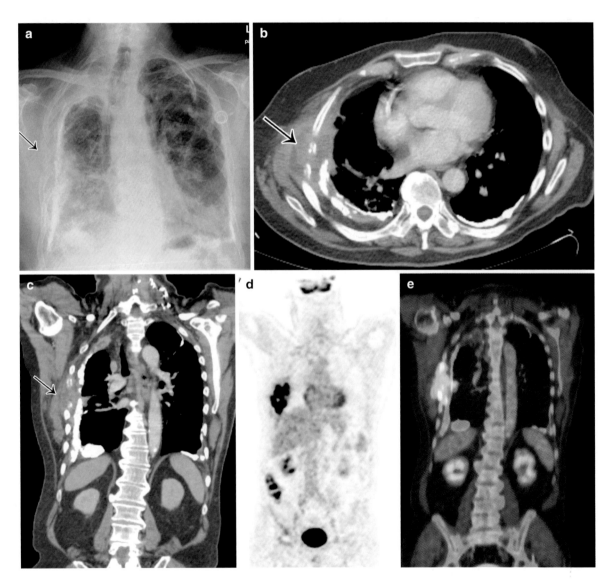

Fig. 11.29 Primary B-cell lymphoma of the pleura in a 63-year-old man with a history of bilateral bilateral tuberculous pleurisy. Frontal chest radiograph (**a**) shows severe bilateral pleural thickening and calcifications. Note the post-tuberculous apical cap on the right. The posterolateral arch of the right ribs 5 and 6 are disrupted, presuming an infiltrating mass (*black arrow*). Axial (**b**) and coronal (**c**) contrast-enhanced computed tomography (CT) views demonstrate the right pleural mass invading the chest wall with rib destruction and extension into the underlying muscles (*black arrows*). Corresponding positron emission tomography (PET) image (**d**) and PET-CT image (**e**) show an important hypermetabolic mass

Fig. 11.30 Pleural metastases of osteosarcoma in a
42-year-old man. Chest
radiograph (**a**) shows an
almost complete opacification
of the left hemithorax and
diffuse calcified pleural
thickening (*black arrows*).
Axial computed tomography
images in mediastinal and
lung windows (**b** and **c**) show
the large pleural calcifications
with associated pleural
effusion. Note the contralateral calcified lung metastases
in the right lower lobe (*white
arrow*). Pathology confirmed
metastases of an osteosarcoma of the humerus (**d**)

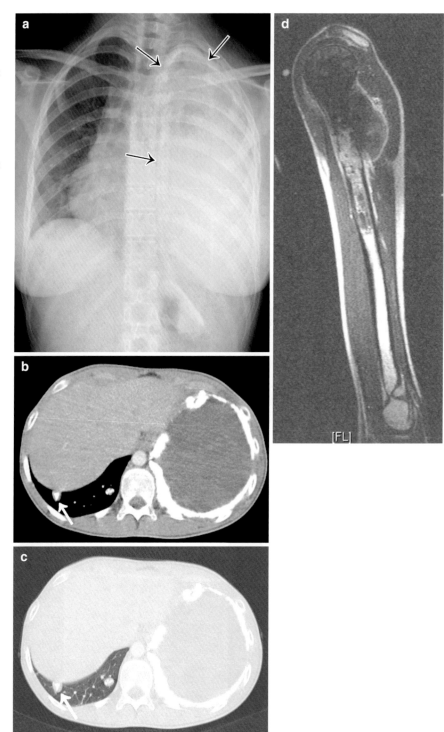

References

Aberle DR, Gamsu G, Sue Ray C (1988) High-resolution CT of benign asbestos-related diseases: clinical and radiographic correlation. AJR Am J Roentgenol 151:883–891

Alexander E, Clark RA, Colley DP (1981) CT of malignant pleural mesothelioma. AJR Am J Roentgenol 137:287–291.

Black LF (1972) The pleural space and pleural fluid. Mayo Clin Proc 47:493–506

Carr JJ, Reed JC, Choplin RH, et al (1992) Plain and computed radiography for detecting experimentally induced pneumothorax in cadavers: implications for detection in patients. Radiology 183:193–199

Collins J, Sterns EJ (1999) Chest radiology: the essentials. Philadelphia: Lippincott

Collins JD, Burwell D, Furmanski S, et al (1972) Minimal detectable pleural effusions: a roentgen pathology model. Radiology 105:51–53

Davis S, Gardner F, Qvist G (1963) The shape of a pleural effusion. Br Med J 1:436–437

Edge JR, Choudhury SL (1978) Malignant mesothelioma of the pleura in Barrow-in-Furness. Thorax 33:26–30

Ferretti GR, Chiles C, Choplin RH (1997) Localized benign fibrous of the pleura. AJR Am J Roentgenol 169:683–686

Friedman AC, Fiel SB, Fisher MS, et al (1987) Asbestos-related pleural disease and asbestosis: a comparison of CT and chest radiography. AJR Am J Roentgenol 150:269–275

Gilkeson RC, Novak RD, Sachs P (2004) Digital radiography with dual-energy substraction: improved evaluation of cardiac calcification. AJR Am J Roentgenol 183:1233–1238

Gordon R (1980) The deep sulcus sign. Radiology 136:25–27

Greene R, Boggis C, Jantsch H (1984) Asbestos-related pleural thickening: effect of threshold criteria on interpretation. Radiology 152:569–573

Hanna JW, Reed JC, Choplin RH (1991) Pleural infections: a clinical-radiologic review. J Thorac Imag 6:68–79

Harvey SG, Dixie JA, Bradley SW (1989) Pneumothorax: appearance on lateral chest radiographs. Radiology 173:707–711

Im JG, Webb WR, Rosen A, et al (1989) Costal pleura: appearances at high-resolution CT. Radiology 171:125–131

Krumhaar D, Lange S, Hartmann C, et al (1985) Follow-up study of 100 malignant pleural mesotheliomas. Thorac Cardiovasc Surg 33:272–275

Lee KS, Im JG, Choe KO, et al (1992) CT findings in benign fibrous mesothelioma of the pleura: pathologic correlation in nine patients. AJR Am J Roentgenol 158:983–986

Leung AN, Müller NL, Miller RR (1989) CT in differential diagnosis of diffuse pleural disease. AJR Am J Roentgenol 154:487–492

Miller BH, Rosado-de-Christenson ML, Mason MC, et al (1996) Malignant pleural mesothelioma: radiologic-pathologic correlation. Radiographics 16:613–644

Müller N (1993) Imaging of the pleura. Radiology 186:297–309

Proto AV (1992) Conventional Chest radiographs: anatomic understanding of newer observations. Radiology 183:593-603

Raasch BN, Carsky EW, Lane EJ, et al (1982) Pleural effusion: explanation of some typical appearances. AJR Am J Roentgenol 139:899–904

Rabinowitz JG, Efremidis SC, Cohen B, et al (1982) A comparative study of mesothelioma and asbestosis using computed tomography and conventional chest radiography. Radiology 144:453–460

Rigby M, Zylak CJ, Wood LDH (1976) Pleural pressure with lobar obstruction in dogs. Respir Physiol 26:239–248

Ruskin JA, Gurney JW, Thorsen MK, et al (1987) Detection of pleural effusions on supine chest radiographs. AJR Am J Roentgenol 148:681–684

Sahn SA (1988) State of the art: the pleura. Am Rev Respir Dis 138:184–234

Schwartz DA (1991) New developments in asbestos-induced pleural disease. Chest 99:191–198

Stark DD, Federle MP, Goodman PC, et al (1983) Differentiating lung abscess and empyema: radiography and computed tomography. AJR Am J Roentgenol 141:163–167

Waitches GM, Stern EJ, Dubinsky TJ (2000) Usefulness of the double-wall sign in detecting pneumothorax in patient with giant bullous emphysema. AJR Am J Roentgenol 174:1765–1768

Woodring JH (1984) Reconnigtion of pleural effusion on supine radiographs: how much fluid is required? AJR Am J Roentgenol 142:59–64

Yates DH, Corrin B, Stidolp PN, et al (1997) Malignant mesothelioma in south east England: clinicopathological experience in 272 cases. Thorax 52:507–512

Zitter FMH, Westcott JL (1981) Supine subpulmonary pneumothorax. AJR Am J Roentgenol 137:699–701

The Diaphragm

Johny A. Verschakelen

Contents

Abstract

> Radiology of the diaphragm may be difficult, mainly because there is no imaging technique that can clearly and entirely visualize the diaphragm. Although we usually speak of the top of the opaque abdominal mass as the diaphragm on a chest X-ray, this is not the diaphragm itself because this structure is only directly visible on this chest X-ray when there is abnormal abdominal air below and normal lung parenchyma above it. Ultrasonography (US), computed tomography (CT), and magnetic resonance imaging (MRI) are the only imaging modalities that can visualize the diaphragm itself, although visualization is usually partial and dependent on the presence of pleural disease when using US and on the presence of subdiaphragmatic fat when using CT and MRI. In general, the aim of the standard chest X-ray for diaphragmatic imaging is threefold: (1) Looking for diaphragmatic pathology, which is often an incidental finding on the chest X-ray. (2) Given the fact that the diaphragm is not directly visible on a chest X-ray, deciding whether the abnormality is indeed located in the diaphragm or whether what is seen is secondary to other disease located adjacent to the diaphragm. (3) Because of the variable presentation of the diaphragm, many changes seen on a chest X-ray are not related to pathology or to "important" pathology, so a decision needs to be made about the importance of the finding and the necessity of performing additional imaging. A complete or

J.A. Verschakelen
Department of Radiology, University Hospitals Leuven,
Herestraat 49, 3000 Leuven, Belgium

E.E. Coche et al. (eds.), *Comparative Interpretation of CT and Standard Radiography of the Chest*,
Medical Radiology, DOI: 10.1007/978-3-540-79942-9_12, © Springer-Verlag Berlin Heidelberg 2011

focal change in the contour delineation of the diaphragm (irregularity, disappearance); a unilateral, bilateral, or focal elevation; and a unilateral, bilateral, or focal depression are the three basic changes of the diaphragm that can be seen on a chest X-ray.

12.1 Introduction

The diaphragm is a thin, flat, musculotendinous structure that has two important functions: (1) it divides the chest from the abdominal cavity and (2) being a respiratory muscle, it has an important role in respiration.

Radiology of the diaphragm is difficult mainly because there is no imaging technique that can clearly and entirely visualize the diaphragm. On conventional chest films, the diaphragmatic muscle is only visible when air is present above and below it (Fig. 12.1). Nevertheless, we usually speak of the top of the opaque abdominal mass (usually composed of the liver, spleen, stomach, or colon with the overlying diaphragm) as

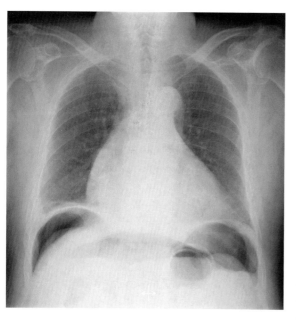

Fig. 12.1 The diaphragm, as such, is only visible on a chest X-ray when there is air above and below it. In this patient with a pneumoperitoneum, the diaphragm presents as thin, 2- to 3-mm thick line between the air-containing lung and the abdominal air

the diaphragm on a chest X-ray. Ultrasonography (US), computed tomography (CT), and magnetic resonance imaging (MRI) are the only imaging modalities that can visualize the diaphragm itself, although visualization is usually partial and dependent on the presence of pleural disease when using US and on the presence of subdiaphragmatic fat when using CT and MRI (Verschakelen et al. 1989; Brink et al. 1994; Gierada et al. 1998). In addition, the radiologic appearance of the diaphragm is related to the function and the integrity of the diaphragmatic muscle, to the thoracic and abdominal volumes, and to the motion and configuration of the ribcage and the abdomen.

In general, the aim of the standard chest X-ray for diaphragmatic imaging is threefold. (1) Look for diaphragmatic pathology that is often an incidental finding on the chest X-ray. (2) Given the fact that the diaphragm is not directly visible on a chest X-ray, try to decide whether the abnormality is indeed located in the diaphragm or whether what is seen is secondary to other disease located adjacent to the diaphragm. (3) Because of the variable presentation of the diaphragm, many changes seen on a chest X-ray are not related to pathology or to "important" pathology, so a decision needs to be made about the importance of the finding and the necessity to perform additional imaging.

The posteranterior (PA) and lateral chest X-rays together with CT are the basic imaging modalities of the chest, and this is also true for the diaphragm (Gierada et al. 1998). As can be deduced from the objectives of diaphragmatic imaging mentioned earlier, a good knowledge of the presentation of the normal and abnormal diaphragm on a chest X-ray is mandatory. This chapter will review the chest X-ray presentation of the normal and abnormal diaphragm and correlate these findings with their CT presentation.

12.2 The Normal Diaphragm

As mentioned in the introduction, the diaphragm, as such, is not normally visualized on a chest X-ray unless there is air present above and below it, as in a patient who has a pneumoperitoneum (Fig. 12.1). The diaphragm then presents as a 2- to 3-mm-thick line between the air-containing lung and the abdominal air. In a normal situation, however, we usually speak of the top of the opaque abdominal mass causing a smooth curved

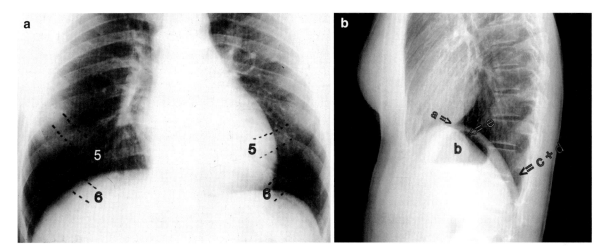

Fig. 12.2 Normal diaphragm on a posteroanterior (PA) and lateral chest X-ray. On deep inspiration PA chest X-rays (**a**), the dome of the right hemidiaphragm is, in the majority of the population, higher than the left dome and located at the level of the fifth or sixth rib interspace (*dotted lines, 5, 6*) anteriorly whereas the left dome is located half an interspace lower. On the lateral view (**b**), both hemidiaphragms project on each other, but usually a correct identification of each leaf is possible. For this, one or more signs can be used: the left diaphragm is obscured anterior by the heart (*arrow a*) and often has an air-distended gastric fundus beneath it (*arrow b*); the leaf nearer to the film is related to the smallest costophrenic angle (*arrow c*) and to the least magnified ribs (*arrow d*) by the diverging beam; the contour caused by the inferior vena cava stops at the level of the right hemidiaphragm (*arrow e*)

contour, as the diaphragm on a chest film. Loss of clarity of this contour occurs when the diaphragm is not tangential to the X-ray beam, but this usually means adjacent pleural or lung disease. However, because the heart is located against the middle part of the diaphragm, the contour is also lost adjacent to this structure.

In this way on a PA chest X-ray, the diaphragmatic contour is divided into two parts: the right and the left hemidiaphragm (Fig. 12.2). Each hemidiaphragm is normally represented on the PA chest X-ray by a smooth, curved line, which is convex upward. The right side is normally higher than the left side, probably because of the underlying liver. After deep inspiration, the dome of the right hemidiaphragm is located at the level of the fifth or sixth anterior rib interspace and the left dome is located half a rib interspace (usually 15 mm) lower (Lennon and Simon 1965; Padovani 1999). It may lie at a lower level in normal young individuals (Fig. 12.3), particularly those of an asthenic build, and at a slightly higher level in the obese, the elderly, and infants. It is also located higher on bedside radiographs when the patient is in a supine position. The lateral attachment to the ribs is represented by the lateral costophrenic recess, which presents as a sharply defined acute angle. Medially the diaphragm meets the heart and the cardiophrenic angle, which is higher than the costophrenic angle and often ill-

defined because of paracardial fat (Tarver et al. 1989).

On the lateral radiograph, each dome makes an acute angle with the ribs posteriorly, approximately at the level of the 12th thoracic vertebral body, to form

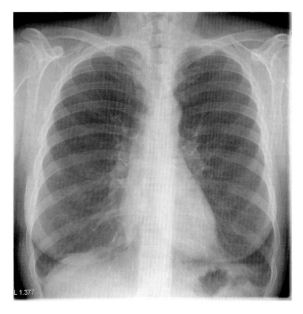

Fig. 12.3 Low position of the diaphragm in a normal young individual taking a very deep breath

the posterior costophrenic recess. The right hemidiaphragm makes an upward curve as it extends anteriorly to the sternum. The anterior part of this hemidiaphragm is often poorly defined because of adjacent fat. The left hemidiaphragm is obscured anteriorly by the heart. This observation helps to differentiate the left and right hemidiaphragm on a lateral chest X-ray (Fig. 12.2b). Other signs that can be helpful are the air-distended gastric fundus beneath the left hemidiaphragm; the hemidiaphragm that is related to the ribs least magnified by the diverging beam or that has the smallest posterior costophrenic angle is nearer to the film and is, in most instances, the left hemidiaphragm; and the contour caused by the inferior vena cava stops at the level of the right hemidiaphragm.

12.3 Pathology of the Diaphragm

Starting from the PA and lateral chest X-rays, pathology of the diaphragm basically can present in three ways:

1. A change in the contour of the diaphragm can occur. This contour can be partially or totally obscured or can become abnormal in shape. An increase in density or a mass-like opacity can project on or below this diaphragmatic contour.
2. The diaphragm can be elevated. This elevation can be bilateral and symmetrical, unilateral or focal. In the latter situation, a focal bulge on the otherwise normal diaphragmatic contour occurs.
3. The diaphragm can be depressed. Again, this depression can be bilateral and symmetric, unilateral or focal. Depression of the diaphragm is often difficult to evaluate because the cause of this depression usually not only causes downward displacement of the entire diaphragm or of a part of it but also obscures it.

12.3.1 Change in Diaphragmatic Contour

As mentioned earlier, the diaphragm, as such, is not visible on a chest X-ray. However, the top of the abdominal mass, which is usually composed of the liver, spleen, fat, stomach, and colon with overlying diaphragm, becomes visible as a sharply defined contour between the air-containing lung above and these abdominal structures that have a density that is higher than air. Localized loss of clarity can occur when the diaphragm is not tangential to the X-ray beam but usually indicates adjacent pleural or pulmonary disease. Typical examples are a pleural effusion that obliterates the costophrenic or costovertebral angles (Fig. 12.4) and a basal lung opacity such as a pneumonia (Fig. 12.5). The diaphragmatic contour can lose its smooth convexity by diaphragmatic pleural adhesions (Fig. 12.6).

12.3.2 Elevation of the Diaphragm

12.3.2.1 Unilateral and Bilateral Symmetrical Elevation of the Diaphragm

The diaphragm can be elevated because it is pushed upward by abdominal structures, i.e., when the abdominal pressure on the diaphragm increases. This is, for example, seen in patients in a supine position, in obese patients, and during pregnancy. It can also be related to abnormal abdominal extension (ascites, intestinal obstruction, and abdominal mass) (Fig. 12.7). In most of these circumstances, the elevation is bilateral and symmetric although the diaphragm can be pushed upward asymmetrically in a patient in a lateral decubitus position when the abdominal pressure increase is highest on the dependent side. Other causes can be a subphrenic mass or infection and gaseous distension of the stomach or colon (Fig. 12.9).

The diaphragm can also be elevated because it is pulled upward by changes in the chest that cause volume loss. Pulmonary fibrosis (Fig. 12.8), pleuropulmonary scarring, lymphangitis carcinomatosa, pulmonary hypoplasia, and pulmonary collapse can be responsible for both unilateral and bilateral elevation of the diaphragm.

Finally, the diaphragm can be elevated because there is a functional disturbance of the diaphragmatic muscle. Bilateral elevation can be seen in painful conditions after abdominal surgery, whereas unilateral diaphragmatic dysfunction and elevation can be the result of pulmonary thromboembolism (Fig. 12.9), adjacent pneumonia or pleurisy, subphrenic infection, and rib fracture or other painful conditions. If none of these causes is present, one should think about phrenic palsy with resulting elevation of the diaphragm, which can be unilateral or bilateral and even focal (see Sect. 12.3.2.2). Paralysis is the result of a lesion somewhere on the "respiratory chain" from the brain to the diaphragm and can be related to trauma (road accidents, birth injury, brachial plexus block, and phrenic crush), irradiation, and a variety of neurological conditions such as poliomyelitis, herpes zoster, and cervical disk degeneration. However, a frequent cause is a lung tumor that is invading or affecting the phrenic nerve. If there is suspicion of phrenic nerve damage, one should carefully look for the site of this involvement. In a small number of patients, no cause can be discovered (Riley 1962). In this group, the right leaf is more commonly affected than the left, and it has been suggested that the palsy is the result of a previous viral neuritis. Paralysis

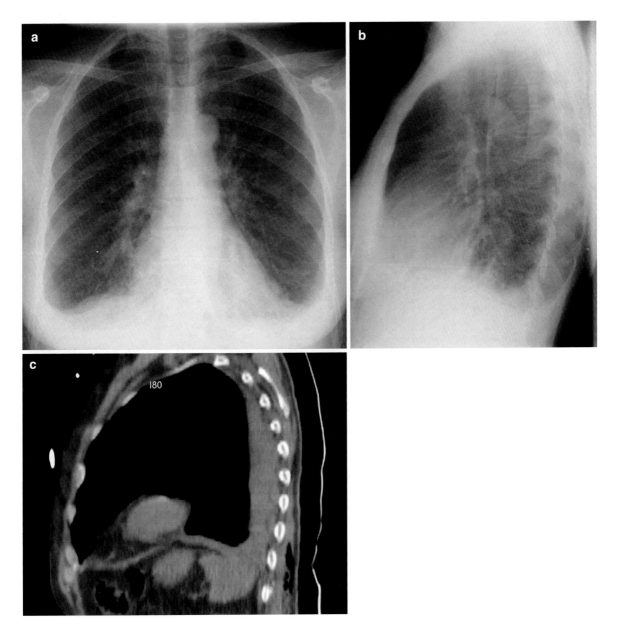

Fig. 12.4 Patient with a pleural effusion causing obliteration of both hemidiaphragms including the costophrenic and costovertebral angles (**a, b**). Computed tomography (**c**) with the patient in a supine body position shows the pleural effusion against the posterior chest wall, filling the posterior costovertebral sinus

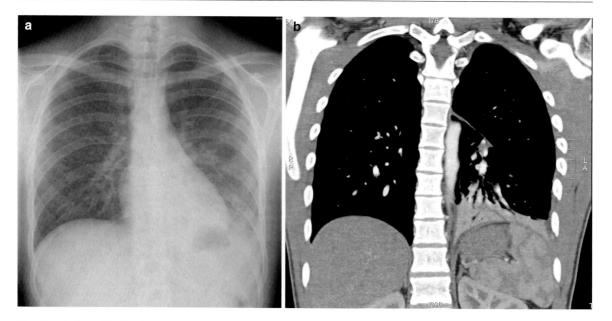

Fig. 12.5 Patient with a basal pneumonia obscuring the left hemidiaphragm. (**a**) Posteroanterior chest radiograph; (**b**) CT coronal view

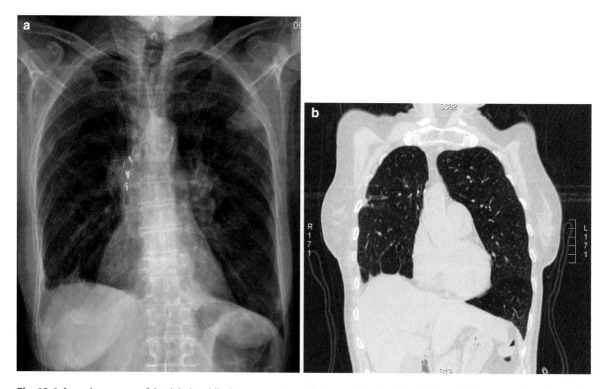

Fig. 12.6 Irregular contour of the right hemidiaphragm caused by diaphragmatic pleural adhesions. (**a**) Posteroanterior chest radiograph; (**b**) CT coronal view

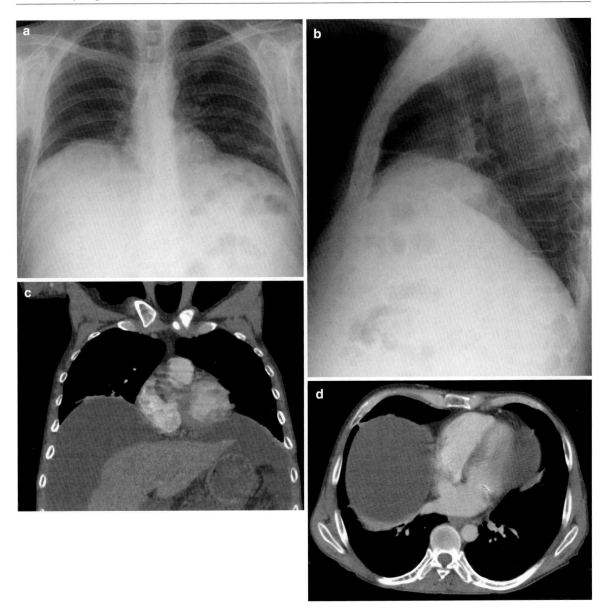

Fig. 12.7 Bilateral symmetrical elevation of the diaphragm caused by ascites, which increases the abdominal pressure. (**a, b**) Posteroanterior and lateral chest radiograph; (**c, d**) CT coronal and axial view

of one hemidiaphragm can be confirmed with fluoroscopy (that should, ideally, be performed in both the anteroposterior and lateral projections with the patient in erect and supine positions) and in a bedside condition with ultrasound by comparing the diaphragmatic motion of the normal and abnormal hemidiaphragm (Houston et al. 1995; Gottesman and McCool 1997; Dorffner et al. 1998). The recognition of diaphragmatic palsy depends on finding a high hemidiaphragm, which exhibits absent, restricted, or paradoxical motion. The latter is well demonstrated during sniffing. Dysfunction of both hemidiaphragms is mostly associated with

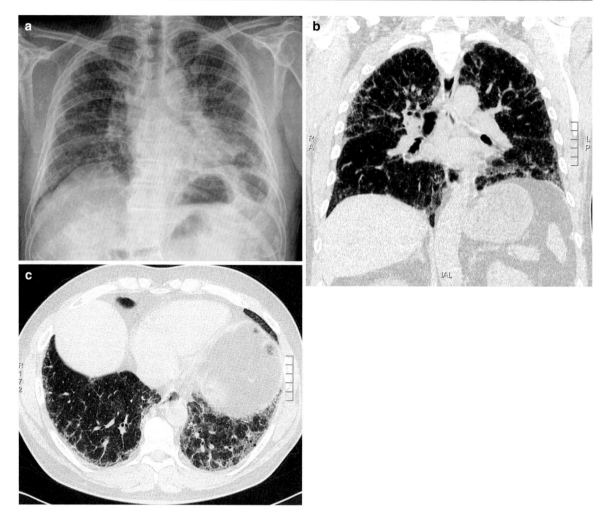

Fig. 12.8 Volume loss of the lung caused by pulmonary fibrosis is responsible for the elevation of the diaphragm. (**a**) Posteroanterior chest radiograph; (**b, c**) CT coronal and axial view

chronic neuromuscular disease and causes severe clinical disability. It may not be recognized by fluoroscopic examination because passive descent of the diaphragm may occur with inspiration (Loh et al. 1977).

It should be emphasized that there are some conditions that can mimic elevation of one hemidiaphragm. These conditions are dorsal scoliosis (Fig. 12.10), a subpulmonic pleural effusion (Fig. 12.11), an encapsulated pleural effusion (Fig. 12.22), a supradiaphragmatic mass in contact with the diaphragm, an important hernia, and a large eventration (see Sect. 12.3.2.2). The differential diagnosis between a subpulmonic pleural effusion and an elevated hemidiaphragm is based on the study of the dome, which has a lateral peak in cases of effusion and a medial peak in cases of paralysis, and

on the lateral downslope of this peak, which is steep when caused by a subpulmonic effusion (Fig. 12.11). When in doubt, ultrasound can be performed. Table 12.1 shows the most frequent causes of a bilateral symmetrical elevation of the diaphragm whereas Table 12.2 shows the causes of an unilateral elevation of the diaphragm.

12.3.2.2 Focal Elevation of the Diaphragm Presenting as a Bulge on the Contour of the Diaphragm

A focal elevation of the diaphragm usually presents as a smooth, focal bulge on the contour, although in some

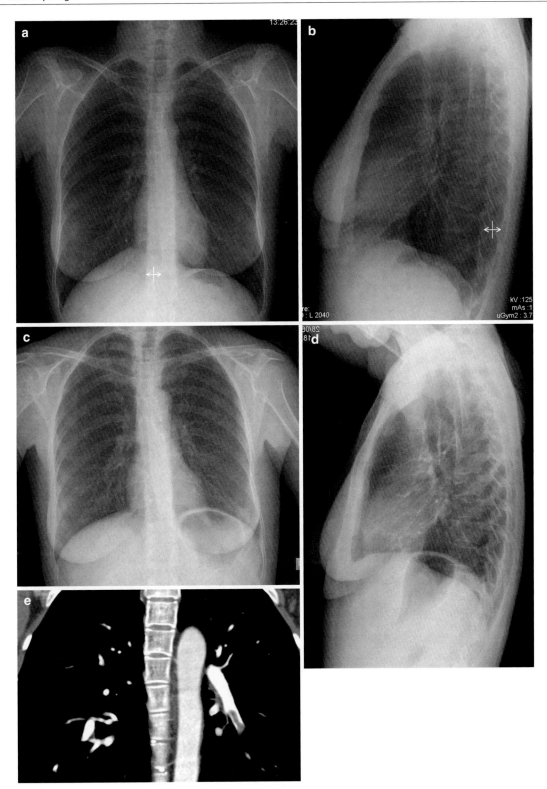

Fig. 12.9 Posteroanterior and lateral chest X-ray in a patient before (**a** and **b**) and after (**c** and **d**) the development of pulmonary embolism in the left pulmonary artery (confirmed with computed tomography (**e**)). Notice the elevation of the left hemidiaphragm, which may, in part, also be related to the gaseous distention of the stomach

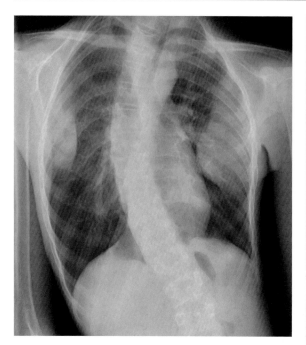

Fig. 12.10 Scoliosis mimicking elevation of the left hemidiaphragm

cases this elevation can have a triangular or irregular shape. The latter situation can occur when the diaphragm is focally pulled up by a fibrous scar (Fig. 12.12). A smooth bulge is seen when the diaphragm is focally pushed upward by a subphrenic process or when there is focal muscular dysfunction or focal absence of the diaphragmatic muscle. In the case of a defect of the diaphragm with herniation of a small amount of abdominal content toward the chest, a focal swelling or mass originating in the diaphragm or a small, well-defined pleural or lung mass adjacent to and in contact with the diaphragm is seen.

The presence of a focal bulge on the contour of the diaphragm is often an incidental finding, and in many cases no further action is required. However, sometimes additional imaging is necessary. The decision whether or not a patient should have additional imaging depends very much on the size of the bulge, whether or not the patient exhibits symptoms, the presence of a pleural effusion or pleural thickening, and whether or not there is a history of diaphragmatic pathology or pathology that can result in diaphragmatic disease, such as cancer or severe trauma to the chest or the abdomen. Table 12.3 lists the causes of a focal elevation of the diaphragm.

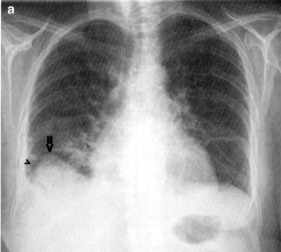

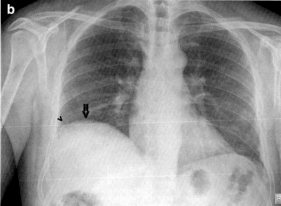

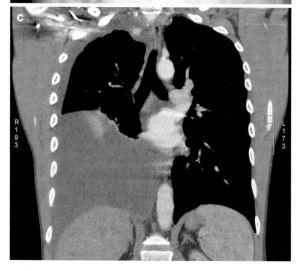

Fig. 12.11 A subpulmonic pleural effusion (**a, c**) can mimic an elevation of the diaphragm (**b**). However, in a subpulmonic pleural effusion, the dome has a more lateral peak than in an elevated hemidiaphragm (*arrows*), whereas the lateral downslope is also more steep in a subpulmonary effusion (*arrowheads*)

Table 12.1 Causes of bilateral symmetrical elevation of the diaphragm

Supine position
Bilateral diaphragmatic paralysis
Poor inspiration
Pregnancy
Obesity
Supine position
Abdominal distension (ascites, intestinal obstruction, abdominal mass)
Lymphangitis carcinomatosa
Disseminated lupus erythematosus
Diffuse pulmonary fibrosis
Bilateral basal pulmonary emboli
Painful conditions (after abdominal surgery)

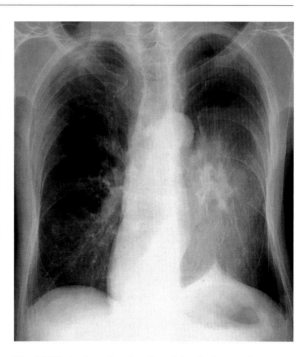

Fig. 12.12 A triangular elevation of the diaphragmatic contour caused by a fibrous scar

Table 12.2 Causes of unilateral elevation of the diaphragm

Gaseous distension of stomach or colon
Posture–lateral decubitus position (dependent side)
Dorsal scoliosis
Eventration
Pulmonary hypoplasia
Pulmonary collapse
Pneumonia or pleurisy
Pulmonary thromboembolism
Rib fracture and other painful conditions
Phrenic nerve palsy
Subphrenic mass
Subphrenic infection

Table 12.3 Causes of focal elevation (bulge) of the diaphragm

Partial eventration
Diaphragmatic tumor
Diaphragmatic hernia
Focal diaphragmatic dysfunction
Focal diaphragmatic adhesions
Pleural tumor
Pulmonary tumor

Focal Diaphragmatic Dysfunction

As mentioned earlier, phrenic palsy can be unilateral or bilateral but also focal. The result is a small weak or paralyzed area of the diaphragmatic muscle. Deep inspiration and contraction of the surrounding normal diaphragmatic muscle causes bulging of the weak area into the chest. Differential diagnosis with eventration can be difficult or even impossible.

Eventration

Eventration of the diaphragm is a disorder in which all or part of the diaphragmatic muscle is replaced by a thin layer of connective tissue and a few scattered muscle fibers. The unbroken continuity differentiates it from a diaphragmatic hernia (Bisgard 1947; Shah-Mirany et al. 1968; Silverman et al. 1992; Tiryaki et al. 2006). Eventration can be partial, unilateral, and bilateral (Rao et al. 1993).

Some authors consider eventration only as a congenital anomaly resulting from a congenital failure of proper muscularization of a part or of the entire diaphragmatic

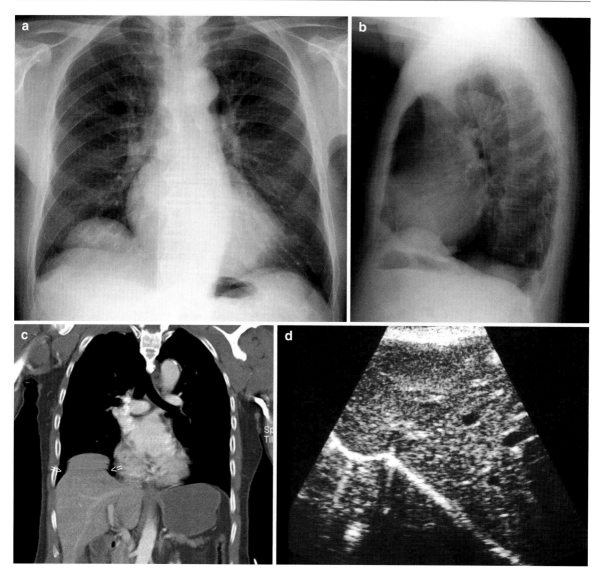

Fig. 12.13 Partial eventration of the right hemidiaphragm presenting as a semicircular homogeneous shadow arising from the anterior part of the right hemidiaphragm (**a, b**). Ultrasound (**d**) and computed tomography (**c**) confirm that this shadow is filled with normal liver tissue. Notice the obtuse angle between the eventration and the normal part of the diaphragm (*arrows*)

leaf. However, most authors use the term eventration not only for diaphragmatic elevation as a result of congenital anomaly but also for total or partial elevation as a result of acquired paralysis (Deslauriers 1998). The idea is that long-lasting paralysis causes atrophy and scarring of the diaphragmatic muscle. That many adults with surgically proven eventration have had previous normal chest films indicates that permanent eventration can be an acquired condition. Total eventration of one hemidiaphragm is more often seen on the left side. Partial eventrations are usually right sided with a predilection for the anteromedial portion. Congenital eventrations are most often isolated and detected incidentally, but they can be associated

with other generic syndromes such as Poland syndrome, cleft palate, congenital heart disease, situs inversus, or undescended testicle (Yazici et al. 2003; Kulkarni et al. 2007).

On conventional chest X-rays, partial eventration presents as a semicircular or semioval homogeneous shadow of soft-tissue density arising from the diaphragm (Fig. 12.13). It becomes more prominent during deep inspiration, when the lateral and dorsal portions of the diaphragm move downward while the convex segment either remains at the same level or perhaps even moves upward. CT (Fig. 12.13c), US (Fig. 12.13d), and MRI can be helpful to differentiate

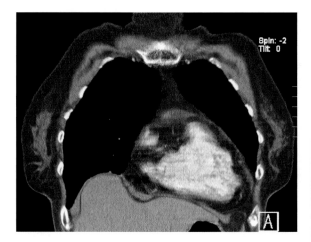

Fig. 12.14 Partial eventration of the right hemidiaphragm. Computed tomography allows for a differential diagnosis of herniation because the intact right hemidiaphragm is seen

this entity from pleural, mediastinal, and pericardial tumors or cysts (Rubinstein and Solomon 1981; Yamashita et al. 1993). Differentiation from a hernia is possible when the presence of bowel or stomach above the diaphragm can be demonstrated. However, differentiation with herniation of liver or fat through an old tear or through the foramen of Morgagni can be difficult (Moore et al. 2001). Differential diagnostic signs on CT can be (1) the angle between the bulge and the normal diaphragm, which is obtuse in eventration (Fig. 12.13c) and sharp in herniation (Fig. 12.17), and (2) direct visualization of the diaphragm overlying the elevated abdominal structure (Fig. 12.14). It can also be difficult to differentiate an eventration, which involves a large portion of a hemidiaphragm, from a paralyzed hemidiaphragm.

Diaphragmatic Hernias

Intrathoracic herniation of abdominal contents occurs through congenital defects in the muscle (Ebbs and McGarry 1952; Clugston and Greer 2007), through traumatic tears or, most commonly, through acquired areas of weakness at the central esophageal hiatus.

Bochdalek Hernia

Bochdalek hernias are the most common manifestation of congenital diaphragmatic herniation and occur when there is a failure of the diaphragm to completely close during development. Large Bochdalek hernias usually become evident during the neonatal period

because they cause respiratory distress. Small asymptomatic Bochdalek hernias are sometimes an incidental finding in adults. These hernias present on lateral chest films as a single, smooth focal bulge centered approximately 4–5 cm anterior to either posterior diaphragmatic insertion (Fig. 12.15a, b). It has been

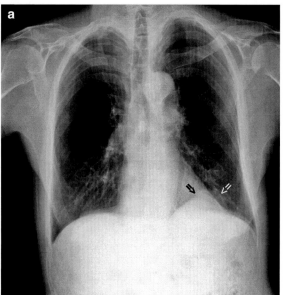

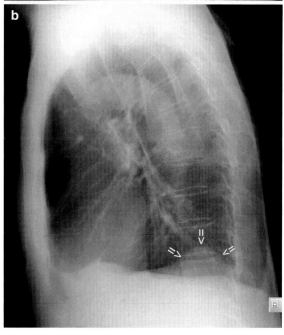

Fig. 12.15 Left-sided Bochdalek hernia presenting as a small, smooth focal bulge on the posterior part of the right hemidiaphragm a few centimeters from the posterior chest wall (*arrows*). Computed tomography shows the defect in the diaphragm with herniation of subdiaphragmatic fat toward the chest. (**a, b**) Posteroanterior and lateral chest radiograph; (**c, d**) CT axial and sagital view

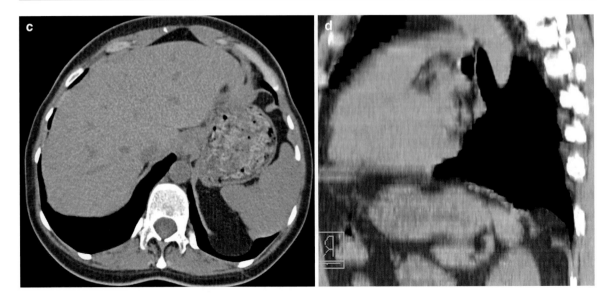

Fig. 12.15 (continued)

shown that asymptomatic small Bochdalek hernias are present in 6% of otherwise normal adults (De Martini and House 1980). On CT, the diagnosis of a Bochdalek hernia can be made when a soft-tissue or fatty mass is seen abutting the upper surface of the posteromedial aspect of either hemidiaphragm (De Martini and House 1980). This mass is in continuity with subdiaphragmatic structures through a diaphragmatic defect presenting as a discontinuity of the soft-tissue line of the diaphragm (Fig. 12.15c, d).

Morgagni Hernia

The Morgagni, retrosternal, or parasternal hernia is characterized by herniation of abdominal contents through the foramina of Morgagni, which are located immediately adjacent to the xyphoid process of the sternum and correspond with small zones between the costal and sternal attachments of the diaphragm (Das et al. 1978). The incidence of Morgagni herniad detected in the neonatal period, because of respiratory symptoms, is low. In older children and adults, a Morgagni hernia is often an incidental finding because there are mostly no symptoms (Machmouchi et al. 2000). Although the weak area is caused by an embryonal failure of muscularization, the herniation of abdominal content to the thorax can be acquired. Increase of intra-abdominal pressure due to severe

effort, trauma, or obesity is probably responsible. In most cases, an acquired Morgagni hernia is right sided because the heart and pericardium cover left-sided defects. On chest films, a Morgagni hernia containing fat or liver presents as a rounded density of varying size in the right (or, rarely, left) anterior cardiophrenic angle (Fig. 12.16a). If the hernia contains bowel, gas shadows can be present (Fig. 12.16c). Herniated liver and bowel can be identified on CT (Fig. 12.16b and d), MRI, or ultrasound (Gale 1986; Yeager et al. 1987; Yildirim et al. 2000).

Esophageal Hiatus Hernia

The frequent occurrence of these hernias in older people compared with their rare occurrence in infants would indicate that these hernias are usually acquired (Caskey et al. 1989). However, congenital hiatal hernias have been described. Diagnosis can be made on conventional PA chest films where the herniated part of the stomach presents as a mass (sometimes with an air-fluid level) projecting through the heart and causing a bulge on the distal part of the paraesophageal line (Tumen et al. 1960). On lateral views, the mass projects behind the heart. A barium study can confirm the presence of the hernia and show complications such as esophagitis or volvulus. Hiatal hernias are often an incidental finding on CT.

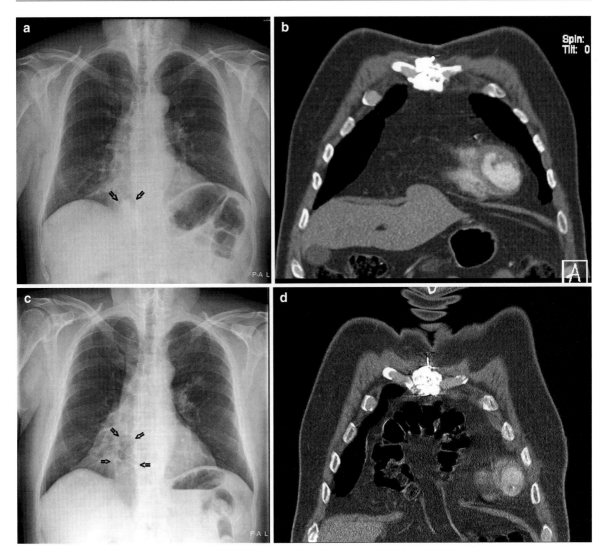

Fig. 12.16 Morgagni hernia with first herniation of liver (**a** and **b**) and later herniation of bowel (**c** and **d**) toward the chest. First chest X-ray (**a**) shows a density in the right anterior cardiophrenic angle (*arrows*), confirmed on computed tomography (CT) (**b**) to be a small amount of liver tissue herniating through a defect in the diaphragm. A few months later bowel also is herniated, presenting on chest X-ray (**c**) as a gas shadow projecting on the heart (*arrows*); on CT (**d**) the defect in the diaphragm and the herniated bowel is clearly shown

Hernia through Traumatic Tear of the Diaphragm

Because diaphragmatic rupture is often associated with thoracic or abdominal injuries that require surgical treatment, the diagnosis is often made during surgery. If surgery is not indicated, a diaphragmatic tear can be missed, especially when it is small and when there is no herniation of abdominal structures into the chest (Shapiro et al. 1996) (Fig. 12.17). Because clinical symptoms are also often very aspecific and because missing a diaphragmatic rupture can have severe consequences when strangulation of herniated viscera occurs, special attention has to be given to small changes in the diaphragmatic contour or basal lung translucency when a conventional chest film of a patient with trauma to the lower chest or the pelvis is interpreted (Sliker 2006). If possible, the posttraumatic thorax should always be compared with previous chest X-rays. Diagnosis is easier when a gas and fluid shadow is seen in the thorax. However, radiologic signs are very often aspecific and can be limited to a

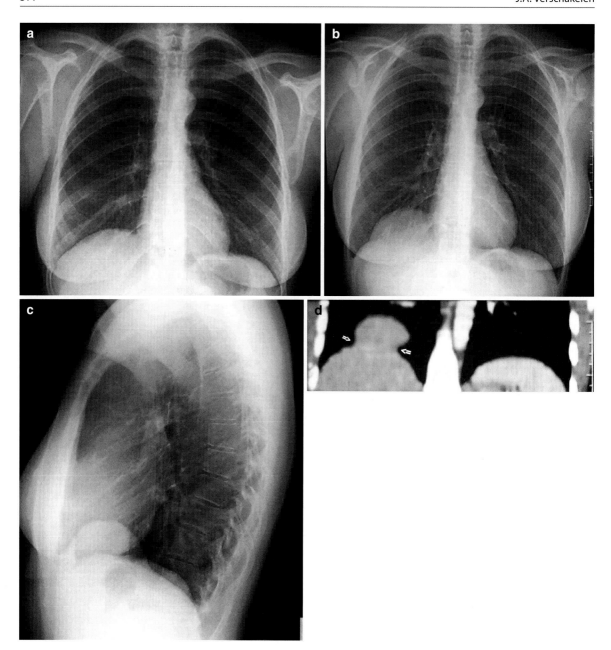

Fig. 12.17 Rupture of the right hemidiaphragm diagnosed 1 year after the trauma. On the chest X-ray 1 month after the trauma (**a**) the rupture was not suspected because no herniation was present. However, 1 year later a chest X-ray was performed because of atypical chest pain that revealed a sharply defined bulge on the contour of the right hemidiaphragm (**b** and **c**) corresponding with herniated liver tissue on a computed tomography scan (**d**). Notice the sharp angle between the herniated liver and the surrounding diaphragm ("collar sign") (*arrows*)

localized density in close relationship to the diaphragm or to a focal bulge on the diaphragmatic contour. Chest films can even appear completely normal. Additional findings that often obscure the delineation of the diaphragm include mediastinal shift, pleural effusion, athelectasis, and consolidation. The position of a nasogastric tube can help to localize the gastric fundus, but it does not reveal anything about the position of the diaphragm, which is essential in the diagnosis of a diaphragmatic tear. On the chest X-ray, the differential diagnosis includes other causes of diaphragmatic elevation and lung contusion, collapse, infection, tension pneumothorax, traumatic pneumatocoele, etc. A follow-up X-ray of an acutely injured patient showing

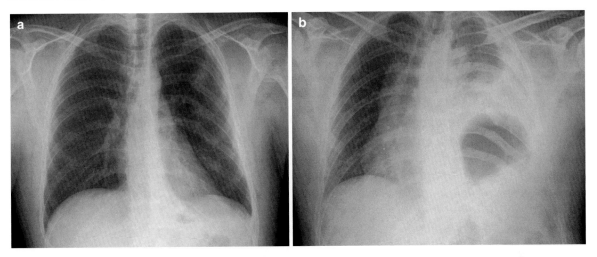

Fig. 12.18 Follow-up chest X-ray of a patient after severe trauma shows the appearance of a gas-filled structure, suggestive of diaphragmatic rupture and herniation of the stomach toward the chest. (**a**) day 30; (**b**) day 65 after the trauma

progressive opacification of one hemithorax by a gas-filled structure is highly suggestive of a diaphragmatic rupture and herniation of stomach or bowel toward the chest (Fig. 12.18).

Barium studies can be helpful in making the correct diagnosis, when an extrinsic narrowing occurs on the border of the stomach or bowel at the point where they pass the diaphragmatic tear. Ultrasound can be diagnostic if both the diaphragm and the herniated organs can be visualized. However, this technique is limited by the oftenminimal visualization of the diaphragm itself, the tenderness over the upper abdomen, and the presence of gas in herniated bowel. Multislice CT is superior because of its high image quality. CT signs of diaphragmatic rupture include discontinuity of the diaphragm with direct visualization of the diaphragmatic injury; herniation of abdominal organs with liver, bowel, or stomach in contact with the posterior ribs ("dependent viscera sign"); thickening of the crus ("thick crus sign"); constriction of the stomach or bowel ("collar sign") (Fig. 12.17); a hypodense band crossing the liver or spleen ("band sign"); active arterial extravasation of contrast material near the diaphragm; and, in cases of a penetrating diaphragmatic injury, depiction of a missile or puncturing instrument trajectory (Heiberg et al. 1980; Murray et al. 1996; Ringler et al. 2003; Stein et al. 2007).

When the rupture is missed at the time of the trauma and the patient has recovered from the associated lesions, a "latent" phase of diaphragmatic rupture can occur (Fig. 12.17). Symptoms and signs are then caused by recurrent herniation of abdominal structures through

the diaphragmatic defect and are again often aspecific. In these circumstances the chest X-ray can show a focal bulge on the contour of the diaphragm caused by herniation of the liver, spleen, or subdiaphragmatic fat through the tear. Differential diagnosis with other causes of focal elevation of the diaphragm may be difficult. For this reason, it is important to check the history of the patient and ask whether a severe trauma to the chest or abdomen has previously occurred. The appearance of a gas-containing shadow in the basal part of the thorax is, in that situation, also suggestive of a missed tear at the time of the trauma, which now appears as herniation of air-containing bowel (Fig. 12.18). CT and MRI can be helpful to further diagnose these missed tears (Holland and Quint 1991).

Tumors of the Diaphragm

Primary tumors of the diaphragm are rare. Both benign and malignant varieties are mostly derived from muscle, fibrous tissue, blood vessels, or fat. Tumors may be cystic (Mayer et al. 2004). They are usually well defined and on the right may mimic an elevated diaphragm, a focal eventration, or herniation. One should think about malignancy when a pleural effusion is accompanies the diaphragmatic change or when the patient has symptoms (Lee et al. 1991; Vade et al. 2000; Froehner et al. 2001).

Secondary tumors are more frequently seen. Metastatic thickening of the diaphragm can present as a focal bulge on the diaphragmatic contour or as a basal opacity (Fig. 12.19). Secondary invasion of the diaphragm by malignant tumors of the lung, pleura, stomach, or pancreas may also occur.

Visualization of the peridiaphragmatic area in frontal or sagittal views with spiral CT or MRI can also give additional information and is particularly helpful in the diagnosis.

12.3.3 Depression of the Diaphragm

The diaphragm can project lower than normal. As mentioned earlier, this can be seen in normal young individuals taking a very deep breath in (Fig. 12.3), particularly those of an asthenic build. The depressed diaphragm is flatter than normal and can be seen when

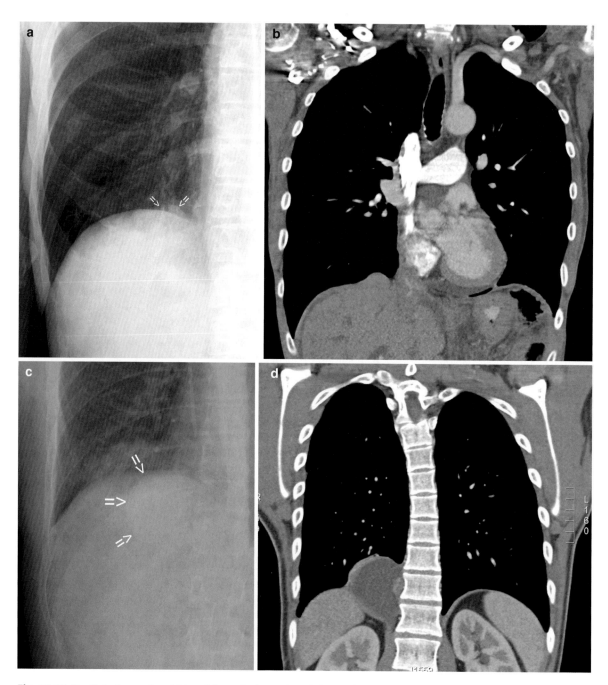

Fig. 12.19 Small (**a** (*arrows*) and **b**) and large (**c** (*arrows*) and **d**) opacity corresponding with metastatic thickening of the diaphragm

the cause of this compression has a low density, i.e., contains air. Typical examples are a tension pneumothorax (Fig. 12.20), which can cause a unilateral downward displacement of the diaphragm. Bilateral depression of the diaphragm is typically seen in patients who have pulmonary emphysema (Fig. 12.21) (Ruel et al. 1998). An important free or encapsulated (Fig. 12.22) pleural effusion and a large mass originating from the lung or pleura can also be responsible for the downward displacement of the diaphragm, but these high-density changes usually obscure the delineation of the diaphragm on the chest X-ray.

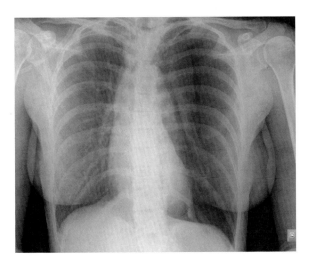

Fig. 12.20 Left-sided diaphragmatic depression in a patient with a tension pneumothorax

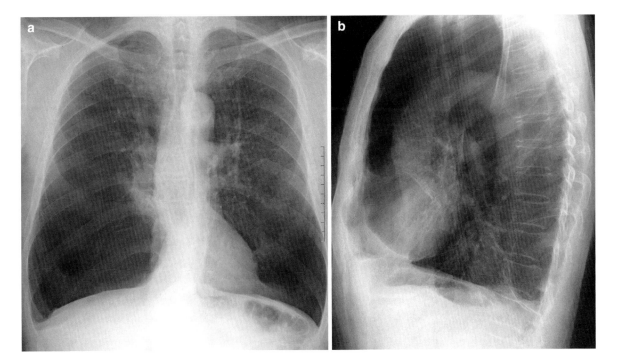

Fig. 12.21 Bilateral diaphragmatic depression in a patient with severe pulmonary emphysema

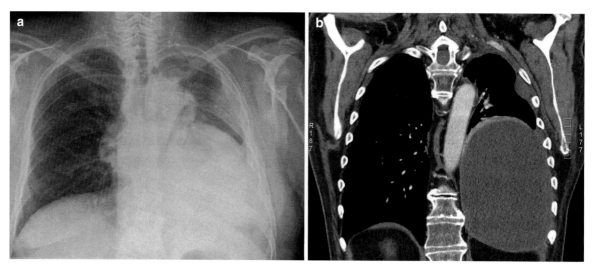

Fig. 12.22 Encapsulated pleural effusion mimicking an elevated left hemidiaphragm (**a**). However, computed tomography (**b**) that the left hemidiaphragm is pushed downward by the fluid

References

Bisgard J (1947) Congenital eventration of the diaphragm. J Thorac Surg 16:484–487

Brink JA, Heiken JP et al (1994) Abnormalities of the diaphragm and adjacent structures: findings on multiplanar spiral CT scans. AJR Am J Roentgenol 163(2):307–310

Caskey CI, Zerhouni EA et al (1989) Aging of the diaphragm: a CT study. Radiology 171(2):385–389

Clugston RD, Greer JJ (2007) Diaphragm development and congenital diaphragmatic hernia. Semin Pediatr Surg 16(2): 94–100

Das PB, Neelaksh, et al (1978) Morgagni hernia: an interesting congenital defect of the diaphragm. Indian J Chest Dis Allied Sci 20(4): 204–207

De Martini WJ, House AJ (1980) Partial Bochdalek's herniation; computerized tomographic evaluation. Chest 77(5): 702–704

Deslauriers J (1998) Eventration of the diaphragm. Chest Surg Clin N Am 8(2):315–330

Dorffner R, Eibenberger K et al (1998) The value of sonography in the intensive care unit for the diagnosis of diaphragmatic paralysis. Rofo 169(3):274–277

Ebbs JH, McGarry HH (1952) Congenital hernia of the diaphragm. Can Med Assoc J 67(2):115–117

Froehner M, Ockert D et al (2001) Liposarcoma of the diaphragm: CT and sonographic appearances. Abdom Imaging 26(3):300–302

Gale ME (1986) Anterior diaphragm: variations in the CT appearance. Radiology 161(3):635–639

Gierada DS, Slone RM et al (1998) Imaging evaluation of the diaphragm. Chest Surg Clin N Am 8(2):237–280

Gottesman E, McCool FD (1997) Ultrasound evaluation of the paralyzed diaphragm. Am J Respir Crit Care Med 155(5): 1570–1574

Heiberg E, Wolverson MK et al (1980) CT recognition of traumatic rupture of the diaphragm. AJR Am J Roentgenol 135(2): 369–372

Holland DG, Quint LE (1991) Traumatic rupture of the diaphragm without visceral herniation: CT diagnosis. AJR Am J Roentgenol 157(1):17–18

Houston JG, Fleet M et al (1995) Comparison of ultrasound with fluoroscopy in the assessment of suspected hemidiaphragmatic movement abnormality. Clin Radiol 50(2):95–98

Kulkarni ML, Sneharoopa B et al (2007) Eventration of the diaphragm and associations. Indian J Pediatr 74(2):202–205

Lee JT, Lee JD et al (1991) Giant malignant schwannoma of the diaphragm: CT and ultrasound findings. Yonsei Med J 32(1): 82–86

Lennon EA, Simon G (1965) The height of the diaphragm in the chest radiograph of normal adults. Br J Radiol 38(456): 937–943

Loh L, Goldman M et al (1977) The assessment of diaphragm function. Medicine (Baltimore) 56(2):165–169

Machmouchi M, Jaber N et al (2000) Morgagni hernia in children: nine cases and a review of the literature. Ann Saudi Med 20(1):63–65

Mayer MP, Janzen J et al (2004) Intrathoracic and intraabdominal locations of a cystic benign tumor: congenital etiology due to embryological diaphragm development? Pediatr Surg Int 19(12):785–788

Moore CM, Mander BJ et al (2001) A case of congenital eventration of the diaphragm mimicking traumatic diaphragmatic rupture. Injury 32(6):508–509

Murray JG, Caoili E et al (1996) Acute rupture of the diaphragm due to blunt trauma: diagnostic sensitivity and specificity of CT. AJR Am J Roentgenol 166(5):1035–1039

Padovani B (1999) Imaging of normal and pathologic diaphragm. Rev Mal Respir 16(Suppl 3):S84–S85

Rao R, Ray R et al (1993) Bilateral congenital eventration of the diaphragm. Indian Pediatr 30(12):1462–1465

Riley EA (1962) Idiopathic diaphragmatic paralysis; a report of eight cases. Am J Med 32:404–416

Ringler L, Lavy R et al (2003) Traumatic rupture of the diaphragm: CT diagnosis. Isr Med Assoc J 5(12):899–900

Rubinstein ZJ, Solomon A (1981) CT findings in partial eventration of the right diaphragm. J Comput Assist Tomogr 5(5):719–721

Ruel M, Deslauriers J et al (1998) The diaphragm in emphysema. Chest Surg Clin N Am 8(2):381–399

Shah-Mirany J, Schmitz GL et al (1968) Eventration of the diaphragm. Physiologic and surgical significance. Arch Surg 96(5):844–850

Shapiro MJ, Heiberg E et al (1996) The unreliability of CT scans and initial chest radiographs in evaluating blunt trauma induced diaphragmatic rupture. Clin Radiol 51(1):27–30

Silverman PM, Cooper C et al (1992) Lateral arcuate ligaments of the diaphragm: anatomic variations at abdominal CT. Radiology 185(1):105–108

Sliker CW (2006) Imaging of diaphragm injuries. Radiol Clin North Am 44(2):199–211, vii

Stein DM, York GB et al (2007) Accuracy of computed tomography (CT) scan in the detection of penetrating diaphragm injury. J Trauma 63(3):538–543

Tarver RD, Conces DJ Jr et al (1989) Imaging the diaphragm and its disorders. J Thorac Imaging 4(1):1–18

Tiryaki T, Livanelioglu Z et al (2006) Eventration of the diaphragm. Asian J Surg 29(1):8–10

Tumen HJ, Stein GN et al (1960) X-ray and clinical features of hiatal hernia. Significance of hiatal hernias of minimal degree. Gastroenterology 38:873–888

Vade A, Bova D et al (2000) Imaging of primary rhabdomyosarcoma of the diaphragm. Comput Med Imaging Graph 24(5):339–342

Verschakelen JA, Marchal G et al (1989) Sonographic appearance of the diaphragm: a cadaver study. J Clin Ultrasound 17(3):222–227

Yamashita K, Minemori K et al (1993) MR imaging in the diagnosis of partial eventration of the diaphragm. Chest 104(1):328

Yazici M, Karaca I et al (2003) Congenital eventration of the diaphragm in children: 25 years' experience in three pediatric surgery centers. Eur J Pediatr Surg 13(5):298–301

Yeager BA, Guglielmi GE et al (1987) Magnetic resonance imaging of Morgagni hernia. Gastrointest Radiol 12(4):296–298

Yildirim B, Ozaras R et al (2000) Diaphragmatic Morgagni hernia in adulthood: correct preoperative diagnosis is possible with newer imaging techniques. Acta Chir Belg 100(1):31–33

Chest Wall

13

Bruno Vande Berg, Frederic Lecouvet,
Paolo Simoni, and Jacques Malghem

Contents

Abstract

> The chest wall comprises the muscles, bones, joints, and soft tissues situated between the neck and the abdomen. Any pathologic process may involve the chest wall, including congenital and developmental anomalies, trauma, inflammatory and infectious diseases, and tumors. The purpose of this chapter is to highlight anatomical variants and lesions that are frequently encountered in the chest wall by providing radiological and cross-sectional imaging correlations.

The chest wall comprises the muscles, bones, joints, and soft tissues situated between the neck and the abdomen. Any pathologic process may involve the chest wall, including congenital and developmental anomalies, trauma, inflammatory and infectious diseases, and tumors. The purpose of this chapter is to highlight anatomical variants and lesions that are frequently encountered in the chest wall by providing radiological and cross-sectional imaging correlations (Kuhlman et al. 1994; Jeung et al. 1999). Disorders affecting the thoracic segment of the spine will be excluded from this chapter because they are not specific to the chest wall and are similar to those observed elsewhere in the spine.

B. Vande Berg (✉), F. Lecouvet, P. Simoni, and J. Malghem
Department of Medical Imaging, Université Catholique
de Louvain, Cliniques Universitaires Saint-Luc,
Avenue Hippocrate 10, 1200 Brussels, Belgium
e-mail: bruno.vandeberg@uclouvain.be

13.1 Normal Variants, Congenital Disorders, and Thoracic Wall Deformities

13.1.1 Rib Variants and Deformities

Lack of visualization of the lower border of the mid-portion of the mid-thoracic ribs is by far the most frequent normal anatomic finding on conventional radiographs that should not be misinterpreted as osteolysis (Fig. 13.1a). When available, computed tomography (CT) images confirm the persistence of normal cortical bone as well as the absence of any soft-tissue mass. On a short axis transverse section of the posterior aspect of the chest wall, the rib is not oval but rather comma shaped, with round upper and thin lower borders (Fig. 13.1b). More medially, near the spine, and more laterally, the rib's shape becomes more oval with a similar round upper and lower cortex (Fig. 13.1c). This occasionally extreme thinning of the lower cortex may cause its focal disappearance on radiographs. Any

similar finding involving any area other than the lower cortex of the mid-portions of the mid-thoracic ribs should be considered abnormal.

Rib notching consists of focal deformation of the lower margin of one or more rib and is generally associated with coarctation of the thoracic aorta (Fig. 13.2). The notches are located bilaterally several centimeters lateral to the costovertebral junction on the ribs 3–9. They result from rib erosion by dilated intercostal arteries taking part in collateral arterial flow. Isolated rib notching may also be due to an intercostal mass like a nerve tumor.

Acquired rib hypertrophy may develop in some rare conditions. Focal rib hypertrophy with cortical thickening is associated with costovertebral joint ankylosis, a frequent finding in diffuse idiopathic skeletal hyperostosis or Forestier's disease (Huang et al. 1993). Altered biomechanics due to joint ankylosis and a subsequent relative increase in mechanical stress on the fused ribs is believed to account for a progressive cortical thickening. Homogeneous rib hypertrophy with cortical thinning can be observed in chronic disorders

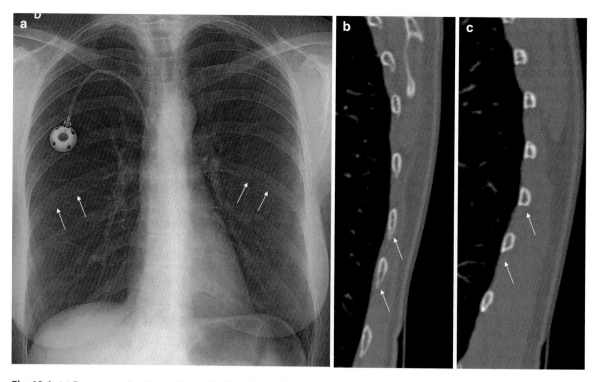

Fig. 13.1 (**a**) Posteroanterior chest radiograph of a patient with breast cancer demonstrates lack of visualization of the lower border of the mid-portion of the mid-thoracic ribs (*arrows*). Compare with upper ribs in which lower cortex is well depicted. (**b**) Sagittal computed tomography (CT) reformat of the mid-portion of the ribs demonstrates the presence of a thin cortical lower margin of the ribs (*arrows*). The shape of the lower cortical margin is different from that of the upper margin. (**c**) Sagittal CT reformat of the paraspinal portion of the ribs (medial to **b**) demonstrates the presence of a thick cortical bone at the round upper and lower rib margins (*arrows*)

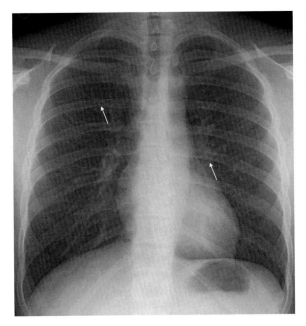

Fig. 13.2 Posteroanterior chest radiograph of a 16-year-old man with thoracic aorta coarctation demonstrates the presence of notches at costal inferior borders (*arrows*)

that are associated with hypertrophy of hematopoietic marrow or in storage disorders and a subsequent increase in medullary space volume (Fig. 13.3). In some cases, extramedullary hematopoiesis that tends to predominantly involve the inner aspect of the ribs, can be present, either alone or in association with paraspinal extramedullary hematopoiesis.

Thoracic wall deformity may develop in association with chronic metabolic bone diseases in which the skeleton is weakened and is subject to plastic deformity, such as in osteomalacia and renal osteodystrophy. Focal deformity of the anterolateral aspect of the chest wall in teenagers is a common cause of clinical concern. Radiographs are generally normal, and ultrasound may demonstrate that the clinical mass is related to asymmetric disposition of the rib cartilage with respect to the sternum and anterior protrusion of one rib cartilage without any intrinsic enlargement of the cartilage, therefore excluding the hypothesis of a tumor (Fig. 13.4). The syrinx syndrome is a clinical syndrome associated with respiratory-associated pain in the lower part of the chest wall. It is believed to be due to a snapping phenomenon between adjacent or superimposed cartilaginous ribs.

Congenital rib anomalies may be found in 1–2% of chest radiographs (Glass et al. 2002; Guttentag and Salwen 1999). Hypoplastic or intrathoracic ribs, bifid or forked ribs, and fused ribs generally lack clinical significance. Associated rib shortening may cause a relative medial displacement of its lateral portion, protruding within the chest, on posteroanterior chest radiographs. Cervical rib generally arises from the

Fig. 13.3 (a) Posteroanterior chest radiograph of a 34-year-old man with thalassemia major demonstrates marked expansion of the medullary cavity of the ribs with homogeneous cortical thinning. (b) Oblique radiograph of the anterior aspect of the ribs better demonstrates soft-tissue masses (*arrows*) on the inner aspects of the ribs corresponding to extramedullary hematopoiesis. (c) Frontal computed tomography reformat illustrates the soft-tissue lesions and rib abnormalities on both sides of the chest

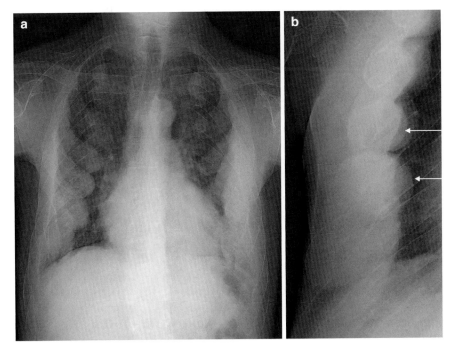

Fig. 13.3 (Continued)

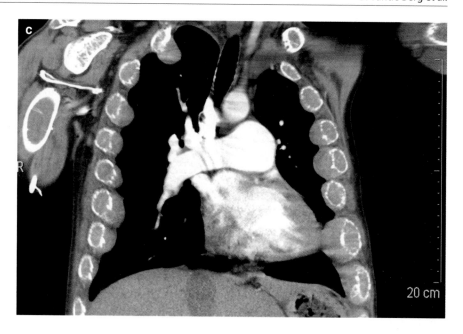

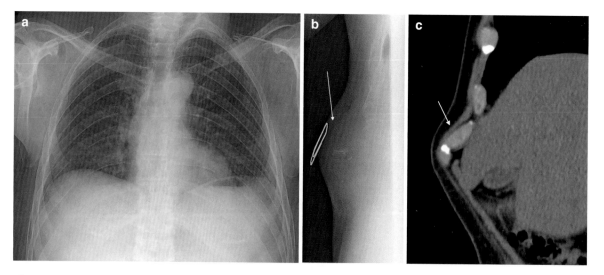

Fig. 13.4 (**a**) Chest radiograph of a 56-year-old man presenting with a mass of the thoracic wall is normal. (**b**) Oblique radiograph demonstrates a mass in the chest wall (*arrow*) in front of a metallic marker. (**c**) Sagittal computed tomography reformat shows that the thoracic wall protrusion is related to an abnormally orientated rib cartilage (*arrow*) without intrinsic costal rib lesion

seventh cervical vertebra in about 0.5% of the population and is frequently bilateral (Guttentag and Salwen 1999). Cervical rib can occasionally cause a thoracic outlet syndrome (upper limb paresthesias, pain, and claudication resulting from pressure on nerves and vessels at the thoracic inlet) but other causes are recognized, including abnormal scalenus muscle and fibromuscular bands (Cotten et al. 1995).

13.1.2 Sternal Deformities

Pectus excavatum, a very common malformation of the chest wall, consists of a depression of the anterior chest wall (Fig. 13.5). It develops progressively as the patient grows, especially during puberty, although it is generally present at birth or shortly thereafter (Fefferman and Pinkney 2005). Pectus excavatum can

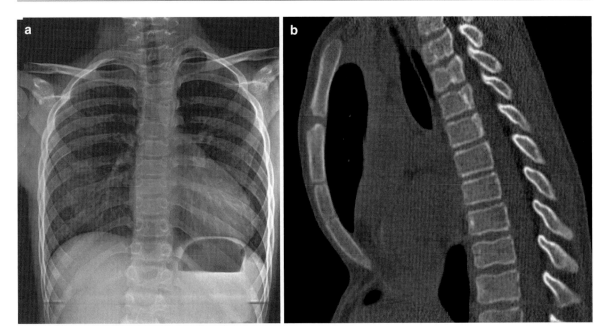

Fig. 13.5 (**a**) Posteroanterior chest radiograph of an 11-year-old boy suggests cardiomegaly. (**b**) Sagittal computed tomography reconstruction demonstrates pectus excavatum with focal depression of the mediastinum by a deformed sternum

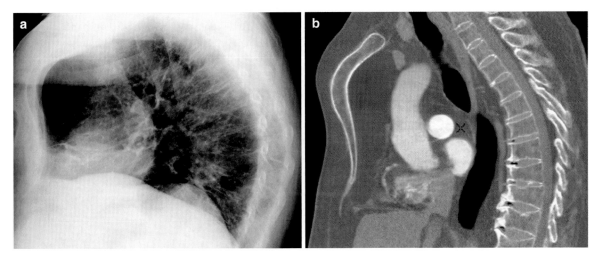

Fig. 13.6 (**a**) Lateral chest radiograph of a 63-year-old man demonstrates anterior bowing of the sternum indicative of pectus carinatum. (**b**) Sagittal computed tomography reformat demonstrates the abnormal shape of the sternum typical of pectus carinatum

be associated with other congenital abnormalities including scoliosis, mitral valve prolapse, osteogenesis imperfecta, and Ehlers-Danlos syndrome. A severe form of pectus excavatum can be observed in the Marfan syndrome. The changes associated with pectus excavatum on the posteroanterior chest radiography are well known: obscuration of the right heart border and apparent cardiomegaly. On lateral chest radiography, the posterior displacement of the lower portion of the sternum is well depicted.

Pectus carinatum is a protrusion deformity of the anterior chest wall consisting of anterior displacement of the sternum that may involve the body of the sternum and, more rarely, the manubrium (Fig. 13.6). Compared with pectus excavatum, it occurs more rarely but it also predominates in male subjects.

13.1.3 Sternal Defect

Sternal hole or defect is a normal variant caused by the lack of or incomplete fusion of the various ossification centers of the body of the sternum during growth. On lateral radiography of the chest, sternal holes may create the disappearance of the anterior and posterior cortex of the sternum in large defects, as in lytic sternal lesions. The lack of a soft-tissue mass and the presence of a cortical border at the upper and lower aspects of the defect on lateral radiography enable recognition of this normal variant. When observed during CT imaging, fat should be present in the bony defect.

13.1.4 Poland Syndrome

Poland syndrome is a rare autosomal recessive condition characterized by unilateral partial or complete absence of the pectoralis major muscle. It is seen more frequently in men than women, and most frequently occurs on the right side. It is associated with multiple bone deformities. Chest radiography usually shows unilateral hyperlucency with the absence of the normal axillary fold on the affected side. Chest ultrasound is the best technique to demonstrate the absence of the pectoralis major muscle.

13.2 Traumatic Lesions of the Chest Wall

Fractures of the chest wall skeleton are extremely frequent and develop either spontaneously or in response to an abnormal external event. Post-traumatic lesions develop when an abnormal stress is suddenly applied to the skeleton, such as in traffic accidents, in sports injuries, or penetrating traumas. Soft-tissue lesions also develop within or around the chest cavity, depending on the causative event.

Spontaneous fractures develop without any external event in different clinical situations. First, spontaneous stress fractures of the thoracic wall develop when a repetitive abnormal biomechanical stimulus is applied on a normal bone. Typically, the involved bone and the fracture topography and orientation depend on the causative event, e.g., fractures of the lateral aspects of the seventh to ninth rib from chronic coughing, or fractures of the posterior aspects of the upper ribs in golf players or deep-sea divers. Second, spontaneous insufficiency fractures of the chest wall develop in response to normal biomechanical stress when the resistance of bone is diffusely decreased, as in metabolic bone disorders. They generally involve the thoracic spine but the ribs and the sternum can also be involved. Finally, spontaneous pathological fractures develop because of focal weakening of bone due to the presence of a focal lytic lesion (Fig. 13.7). The bone involved and the

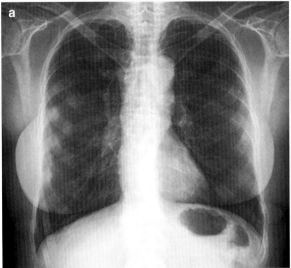
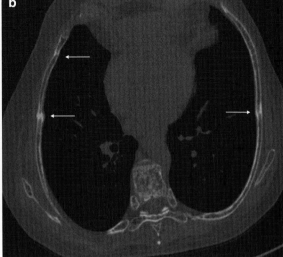

Fig. 13.7 (a) Posteroanterior chest radiograph of a 67-year-old woman with treated multiple myeloma. The anterolateral segments of the ribs demonstrate multiple areas of bone sclerosis. The alignment of these lesions suggests the diagnosis of multiple healed rib fractures. (b) Transverse oblique reconstruction of mid-thoracic ribs demonstrates diffuse bone abnormalities and healed fractures (*arrows*)

topography of the fracture depend on the underlying lesion, except in multiple myeloma, in which bone weakening is diffuse and spontaneous fractures can develop anywhere.

13.3 Inflammatory and Infectious Diseases of the Chest Wall

A wide spectrum of inflammatory and infectious diseases may occur in the bone, muscles, joints, and soft tissues of the chest wall. They derive from hematogenous spreads or, contiguous extension from lung or pleural infection, or are iatrogenic. In western countries, the most common chest wall infection is caused by median sternotomy for cardiac surgery (Templeton and Fishman 1992). Infection may involve presternal and retrosternal soft tissues and can be differentiated from hematoma by the presence of sinus tracts, adjacent fat infiltration, and gas bubbles (Sharif et al. 1990). Sternal osteomyelitis must be suspected when soft-tissue anomalies are associated with bone destruction superimposed on sternotomy-related changes. CT is accurate for the assessment of the extent and depth of infection and can be useful for surgical planning.

Septic involvement of the rib cartilage is an uncommon disorder most frequently observed in drug abusers, although other immunocompromised patients may be involved as well. Cross-sectional images are mandatory for evaluation to demonstrate destruction of the costal cartilage by the infectious process, which is the hallmark of this condition. However, in neoplastic disorders the cartilage is preserved.

Necrotizing fasciitis is a potentially fatal septic condition that can develop either spontaneously or in high-risk patients who are immunocompromised, alcoholic, or diabetic (Fig. 13.8). The process involves the subcutaneous fat and the superficial fascia and should not extend deeper into the adjacent muscles. Magnetic resonance imaging (MRI) may depict the longitudinal and transverse extent of the process, and CT imaging may depict gas formation (Wysoki et al. 1997). In pyomyositis, the muscle is predominantly involved by the process. MRI better displays intramuscular necrosis than CT or ultrasound.

The acronym SAPHO designates a cluster of manifestations including Synovitis, Acne, Palmoplantar pustulosis, Hyperostosis, and Osteitis. SAPHO occurs with

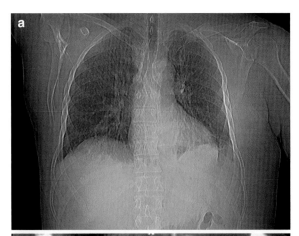

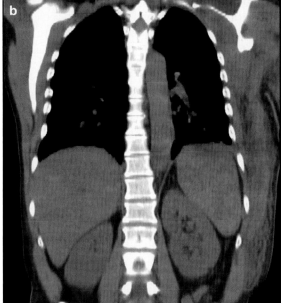

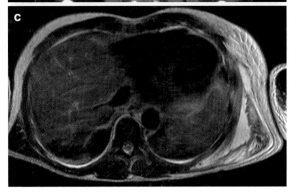

Fig. 13.8 (**a**) Scout view from computed tomography imaging of the chest of a 35-year-old man with a painful and swollen left thoracic wall demonstrates diffuse soft-tissue swelling. (**b**) Coronal CT reconstruction confirms swelling of the lateral soft tissue with deep-seated changes. (**c**) Transverse T2-weighted spin-echo image demonstrates diffuse alteration of the left muscle and infiltration of the subcutaneous and intermuscular fat planes

equal frequency in men and women and most frequently in young and middle-aged adults. The clinical manifestations of SAPHO syndrome vary depending on the age of the patient. Chronic multifocal osteomyelitis and periostitis develop more frequently in young patients without cutaneous abnormalities whereas palmoplantar pustulosis and osteitis develop more frequently in adult and elderly patients (Cotten et al. 1995). Typically, osteitis involves the sternocostoclavicular region. Radiologic manifestations include trabecular and cortical bone sclerosis. In addition to these bone changes, articular manifestations are present and include erosions of the claviculosternal or manubriosternal joint. In some severe forms of palmoplantar pustulosis, a soft-tissue mass adjacent to the bone or the hypertrophic bone itself may cause compression of the venous or nerve structures (Lazzarin et al. 1999). Differential diagnosis includes chronic osteomyelitis and inflammatory spondylitis. These articular changes are also observed in other aseptic inflammatory disorders like ankylosing spondylitis (Laredo 2007). In this latter condition, bone changes are not as extensive as in SAPHO. Finally, in condensing osteitis of the clavicle, an unusual pattern of degenerative disorder of the claviculosternal joint, erosions are better defined and bone sclerosis is limited (Harden et al. 2004). An osteophyte developing at the inferior aspect of the clavicule, at the level of the clavicular costal joint, is usually associated.

13.4 Chest Wall Tumors

Any tissue of the thoracic wall can give birth to benign or malignant tumors. In adults, benign soft-tissue masses are much more frequent than malignant lesions, but malignant bone tumors are more frequent than benign tumors.

13.4.1 Benign Tumors of the Chest Wall

Fibrous dysplasia and osteochondroma are the most common benign bone lesions, but are relatively uncommon among lesions in general. Fibrous dysplasia is a skeletal developmental anomaly in which the medullary bone is replaced by fibrous tissue (Fig. 13.9). It develops sporadically during the period of skeletal growth and may involve any bone of the skeleton. This

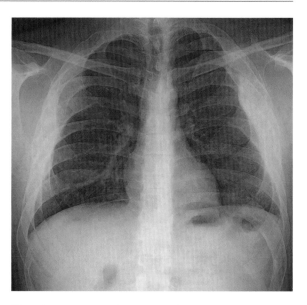

Fig. 13.9 Posteroanterior chest radiograph of a 32-year-old man demonstrates multiple expansile rib lesions. The presence of several normal rib segments (paravertebral and lateral segments) is a keyfinding for the differentiation from disorders related to marrow expansion (compare with Fig. 13.3)

nonhereditary disorder can be either monostotic (80% of cases) or polyostotic. This latter condition may be a part of a McCune-Albright syndrome (fibrous dysplasia, patchy cutaneous pigmentation, and precocious puberty) or Mazabraud syndrome (fibrous dysplastic lesion in close proximity to soft-tissue myxomas) (Kransdorf et al. 1990). The radiographic appearance of fibrous dysplasia includes an osteolytic expansile lesion involving the medullary cavity of the bone with endosteal scalloping. Periosteal reaction should be absent if there is no fracture. The lesion may be surrounded by a rim of sclerotic reactive bone (rim sign). Usually the matrix of the lesion can be well recognized on CT images and shows relatively homogeneous aspect (ground glass appearance) with a moderate increase in Hounsfield units to around 200–250. Irregular areas of sclerosis can be present within the lesions.

Osteochondroma is a frequent benign tumor of the skeleton that consists of a bony outgrowth in continuity with the medullary cavity of the parent bone and that is covered by a thin cartilage layer (Murphey et al. 2000) (Fig. 13.10). Because they are derived from the physeal cartilage, most osteochondromas involve the metaphyseal region of the rib or of the scapula. Osteochondromas may cause a mass effect on adjacent structures, may induce frictional bursitis, and may undergo malignant transformation. Osteochondromas appearing on a chest radiograph show a deformity or expansion of the bone with calcification of the cartilaginous cap. CT or MRI plays a crucial role in the delineation of the extent of the lesions and in the

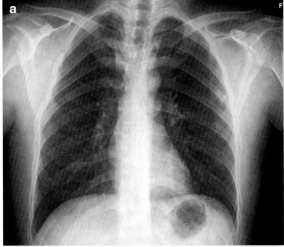

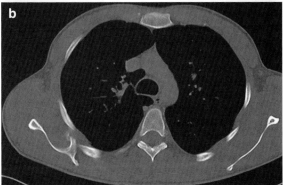

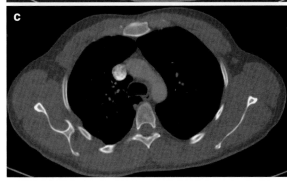

Fig. 13.10 (**a**) Posteroanterior chest radiograph of a 36-year-old man demonstrates alterations of the shape of the right upper thoracic wall. Several ribs demonstrate altered shape and contours. (**b** and **c**) Transverse computed tomography reconstructions demonstrate a bony outgrowth developed on the deep aspect of the right scapula, typical of an enchondroma. The cartilage layer as well as the possible friction bursitis is better seen on magnetic resonance imaging

assessment of the cartilage cap thickness. Actually, in an adult, a cartilage cap thickness greater than 20 mm should indicate malignant transformation, whereas malignancy is unlikely if the cartilage thickness is lower than 10 mm. CT is accurate in the assessment of the cartilage thickness when the lesions develop on the inner side of the chest wall and are in contiguity with the lungs. MRI should be preferred for lesions that extend outward because it enables differentiation between cartilage, bursitis, and muscles.

Benign soft-tissue tumors of the chest wall are relatively uncommon lesions that typically manifest as painless, slow-growing, palpable masses. Lipoma is by far the most frequent benign soft-tissue tumor in adults but other fat-containing masses can also be observed (Kransdorf 1995). Hibernoma, which is derived from brown fat cells, typically develops in the lateral aspects of the chest wall near the axilla (Lee and Collins 2008). Diagnostics and staging of this lesion do not differ in the chest wall from those elsewhere in the body.

Elastofibroma is a relatively common fibroelastic pseudotumor that typically involves the subscapular area (Kransdorf et al. 1992). Lesions are bilateral in 60% of patients and occur in all age groups but occur most frequently in elderly patients. Clinically, patients present with a large, well-circumscribed mass in the subscapular area that becomes more prominent with dorsal flexion and antepulsion of both arms. Its topography is typical as it develops in the area between the latissimus dorsi muscle superficially and the thoracic wall anteriorly, near the lower aspect of the scapula. Ultrasound and radiographic examination of the lesion are relatively nonspecific. CT and MRI reveal the specific intrinsic organization of the lesion related to the presence of alternating planes of adipose and fibrous tissue. The etiology of this lesion is unclear, but repeated trauma caused by mechanical friction of the scapula against the ribs has been suggested to induce the process.

13.4.2 Malignant Tumors of the Chest Wall

13.4.2.1 Bone Metastases

Metastases from carcinoma are the most common malignant tumor involving the skeleton, including the

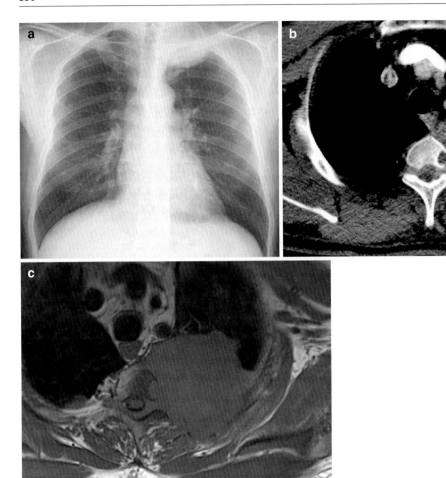

Fig. 13.11 (**a**) Posteroanterior chest radiograph of a 57-year-old man with left upper lobe pulmonary neoplasm demonstrates osteolysis of the posterior aspect of the second rib. (**b**) Transverse computed tomography reconstruction demonstrates the lesion, but its margins are not clearly depicted. (**c**) Transverse T1-weighted spin-echo image better demonstrates neoplastic involvement of the chest wall and vertebral body. Extension of the lesion in the epidural space is also obvious

ribs. Cancers most likely to metastasize to bones originate from the breast, lung, prostate, thyroid, and kidney. The ribs and the sternum are frequently involved because they contain hematopoietic bone marrow in which metastases can grow (Roodman 2004). Chest wall invasion can also occur from contiguous expansion from a pleural or lung cancer (Fig. 13.11). On radiographs, bone metastases may be osteolytic, sclerotic, or mixed. The most common radiographic features include a lytic destructive process in the medullary cavity with poorly delimited margins, erosions of the cortex, and, frequently, extension into the soft tissues. Pathologic fractures are common.

13.4.2.2 Cancers of the Hematopoietic System

Multiple myeloma is a neoplastic proliferation of plasma cells that is characterized by bone destruction and by the presence of an increase in monoclonal immunoglobulins and light-chain proteins in the blood and urine. Radiographically, multiple myeloma typically results in multifocal osteolytic lesions, the pattern of which reflects the space of development of the lesion. A moth-eaten appearance is observed in rapidly growing lesions but, more frequently, small endosteal scalloping with or without rib enlargement may be observed in slow-growing lesions.

In non-Hodgkin lymphomas, the bones of the chest wall can be involved and bone lesion areas are generally mixed lytic and sclerotic with adjacent soft-tissue involvement.

Histiocytosis and other Langerhans cell-derived tumors are lytic lesions that generally develop in children.

13.4.2.3 Chondrosarcoma

Chondrosarcoma is the most common malignant primary tumor of the chest wall in adults and most frequently involve the ribs (Tateishi et al. 2003). Most costal chondrosarcomas arise from the anterior rib or chondrocostal junction, especially along the upper five ribs (Fig. 13.12). Most chondrosarcomas are classified as primary and develop in the medullary cavity of previously normal bone (Murphey et al. 2003). Secondary chondrosarcoma develops in a primary benign chondral tumor such as enchondroma or osteochondroma. Radiographs of costal or sternal chondrosarcoma typically reveal a large mineralized mass with a characteristic ring-and-arches or popcorn pattern of calcification. CT and MRI show a destructive lesion with a large soft-tissue mass. On MRI, nonmineralized areas are isointense relative to skeletal muscle on T1-weighted SE images. On T2-weighted magnetic resonance images, cartilaginous lobules have high signal intensity and are surrounded by septa with low signal intensity. Matrix mineralization manifests as area of low signal intensity on all pulse sequences.

13.4.2.4 Ewing's Sarcoma and Primitive Neuroectodermal Tumor

Ewing's sarcoma are small, round-cell, malignant neoplasms of bone and soft tissues that usually affect patients younger than 30 years. About 40% of Ewing's sarcoma involve flat bones, most commonly the pelvis, scapula, and ribs (Moser et al. 1990). Radiographs and CT images usually show a predominantly osteolytic lesion, although Ewing's tumor can also demonstrate important sclerosis. Cortical destruction, periosteal reaction, ad soft-tissue masses are common associated findings. Ewing's sarcoma of ribs is a typically osteolytic lesion associated with the larger soft-tissue mass that is usually disproportionately large as compared with the extent of bone involvement (Fig. 13.13).

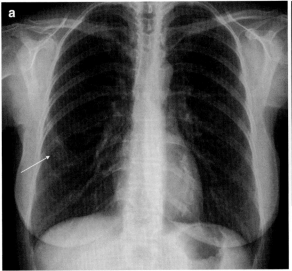
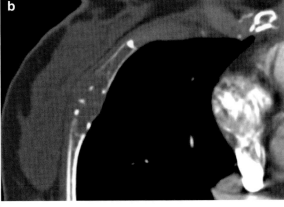

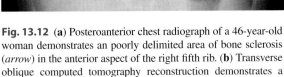

Fig. 13.12 (**a**) Posteroanterior chest radiograph of a 46-year-old woman demonstrates an poorly delimited area of bone sclerosis (*arrow*) in the anterior aspect of the right fifth rib. (**b**) Transverse oblique computed tomography reconstruction demonstrates a lytic lesion with inner calcifications and cortical bone destruction. The osseous borders of the lesion are well delimited, indicating a slow-growing process. A well-differentiated chondrosarcoma was found during histologic analysis of the resected specimen

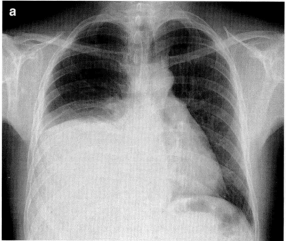
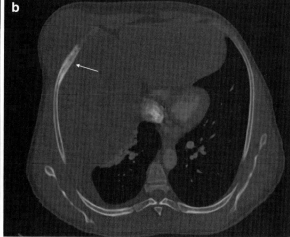

Fig. 13.13 (**a**) Posteroanterior chest radiograph of a 32-year-old man demonstrates the presence of a right mass. (**b**) Transverse computed tomography reconstruction demonstrates a sclerotic lesion (*arrow*) within the anterior aspect of the seventh rib with important extraosseous component. Ewing's tumor was found during histology

References

Cotten A, Flipo RM, Mentre A, Delaporte E, Duquesnoy B, Chastanet P (1995) SAPHO syndrome. Radiographics 15: 1147–1154

Fefferman NR, Pinkney LP (2005) Imaging evaluation of chest wall disorders in children. Radiol Clin North Am 43: 355–370

Glass RB, Norton KI, Mitre SA, Kang E (2002) Pediatric ribs: a spectrum of abnormalities. Radiographics 22:87–104

Guttentag AR, Salwen JK (1999) Keep your eyes on the ribs: the spectrum of normal variants and diseases that involve the ribs. Radiographics 19:1125–1142

Harden SP, Argent JD, Blaquiere RM (2004) Painful sclerosis of the medial end of the clavicle. Clin Radiol 59: 992–999

Huang GS, Park YH, Taylor JA, Sartoris DJ, Seragini F, Pathria MN et al (1993) Hyperostosis of ribs: association with vertebral ossification. J Rheumatol 20:2073–2076

Jeung MY, Gangi A, Gasser B, Vasilescu C, Massard G, Wihlm JM et al (1999) Imaging of chest wall disorders. Radiographics 19:617–637

Kransdorf MJ, Moser RP Jr, Gilkey FW (1990) Fibrous dysplasia. Radiographics 10:519–537

Kransdorf MJ, Meis JM, Montgomery E (1992) Elastofibroma: MR and CT appearance with radiologic-pathologic correlation. AJR Am J Roentgenol 159:575–579

Kransdorf MJ (1995) Benign soft-tissue tumors in a large referral population: distribution of specific diagnoses by age, sex, and location. AJR Am J Roentgenol 164:395–402

Kuhlman JE, Bouchardy L, Fishman EK, Zerhouni EA (1994) CT and MR imaging evaluation of chest wall disorders. Radiographics 14:571–595

Laredo JD, Vuillemin-Bodaghi V, Boutry N, Cotten A, Parlier-Cuau C (2007) SAPHO syndrome: MR appearance of vertebral involvement. Radiology 242:825–831

Lazzarin P, Punzi L, Cesaro G, Sfriso P, De Sandre P, Padovani G et al (1999) Thrombosis of the subclavian vein in SAPHO syndrome. A case-report. Rev Rhum Engl Ed 66:173–176

Lee TJ, Collins J (2008) MR imaging evaluation of disorders of the chest wall. Magn Reson Imaging Clin N Am 16:355–379

Moser RP Jr, Davis MJ, Gilkey FW, Kransdorf MJ, Rosado de Christenson ML, Kumar R et al (1990) Primary Ewing sarcoma of rib. Radiographics 10:899–914

Murphey MD, Choi JJ, Kransdorf MJ, Flemming DJ, Gannon FH (2000) Imaging of osteochondroma: variants and complications with radiologic-pathologic correlation. Radiographics 20:1407–1434

Murphey MD, Walker EA, Wilson AJ, Kransdorf MJ, Temple HT, Gannon FH (2003) From the archives of the AFIP: imaging of primary chondrosarcoma: radiologic-pathologic correlation. Radiographics 23:1245–1278

Roodman GD (2004) Mechanisms of bone metastasis. N Engl J Med 350:1655–1664

Sharif HS, Clark DC, Aabed MY, Aideyan OA, Haddad MC, Mattsson TA (1990) MR imaging of thoracic and abdominal wall infections: comparison with other imaging procedures. AJR Am J Roentgenol 154:989–995

Tateishi U, Gladish GW, Kusumoto M, Hasegawa T, Yokoyama R, Tsuchiya R et al (2003) Chest wall tumors: radiologic findings and pathologic correlation: part 2. Malignant tumors. Radiographics 23:1491–1508

Templeton PA, Fishman EK (1992) CT evaluation of poststernotomy complications. AJR Am J Roentgenol 159:45–50

Wysoki MG, Santora TA, Shah RM, Friedman AC (1997) Necrotizing fasciitis: CT characteristics. Radiology 203:859–863

Selected Diseases with Peculiar Aspect on Chest Radiography

Chronic Obstructive Pulmonary Disease: Comparison Between Conventional Radiography and Computed Tomography

14

Diana Litmanovich, Alexander A. Bankier,
and Pierre Alain Gevenois

Contents

P.A. Gevenois (✉)
Radiology, Hôpital Erasme, Université libre de Bruxelles,
808 Route de Lennik, 1070, Brussels, Belgium

D. Litmanovich and A.A. Bankier
Radiology, Beth Israel Deaconess Medical Center,
Harvard Medical School, 330 Brookline Avenue,
Boston 02215, MA, USA

Abstract

> Traditionally, chronic obstructive pulmonary disease (COPD) includes pulmonary emphysema and chronic bronchitis. This definition of COPD has been recently modified by the Global Initiative for Chronic Obstructive Lung Disease, which has defined it as a disease state characterized by airflow limitation that is not fully reversible. Pathologically, the chronic airflow limitation characteristic of COPD is caused by a mixture of small airway disease and parenchymal lung destruction. Computed tomography (CT) is superior to chest radiography in the detection of emphysema and in the assessment of its distribution and extent. The introduction of multidetector CT (MDCT) allows acquisition of high-resolution scans in a volumetric manner over the entire lung, and this approach has been shown to be suitable for the assessment of emphysema. The inherent limitations of subjective visual scoring, the characteristic CT morphology of emphysema, and the digital nature of the CT dataset have fostered considerable interest in the use of CT as an objective quantification tool for pulmonary emphysema. The evaluation of the airways on chest radiograph is limited, but it provides an ideal contrast in composition for CT image analysis. MDCT now allows for the acquisition of a contiguous thin section. The current techniques for evaluation of COPD increase the importance of MDCT beyond the clinical context toward its truly experimental and preclinical research modality.

E.E. Coche et al. (eds.), *Comparative Interpretation of CT and Standard Radiography of the Chest*,
Medical Radiology, DOI: 10.1007/978-3-540-79942-9_14, © Springer-Verlag Berlin Heidelberg 2011

14.1 Definitions

Traditionally, chronic obstructive pulmonary disease (COPD) includes pulmonary emphysema and chronic bronchitis. Pulmonary emphysema is defined, using histologic criteria, as a condition of the lung characterized by abnormal, permanent enlargement of airspaces distal to the terminal bronchioles, accompanied by destruction of their walls and without obvious fibrosis (Snider et al. 1985). Figures 14.1 and 14.2 show photographs of macroscopic and microscopic samples illustrating the difference between an emphysematous and a normal individual. As a consequence of the histologic definition of pulmonary emphysema, the diagnosis of emphysema during life, without the availability of lung tissue, should always be indirect; however, imaging signs suggestive of pulmonary emphysema can be detected on chest radiograph and on CT scans.

Two types of pulmonary emphysema are recognized: centrilobular emphysema and panlobular emphysema. Centrilobular emphysema results from dilatation or destruction of the respiratory bronchioles and is the type of emphysema most closely associated with cigarette smoking (Snider et al. 1985) (Fig. 14.3). Panlobular emphysema is associated with α_1-antitrypsin deficiency and results in an even dilatation and destruction of the entire acinus (Snider et al. 1985) (Fig. 14.4).

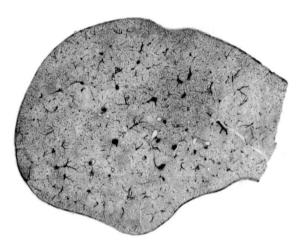

Fig. 14.1 Macroscopic paper-mounted, whole-lung sections illustrating normal lung tissue

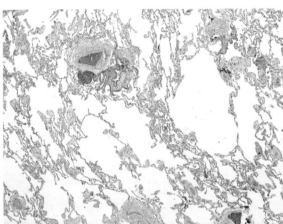

Fig. 14.3 Centrilobular emphysema. Histologic specimen stained with hematoxylin-eosin from a patient with centrilobular emphysema (magnification x20)

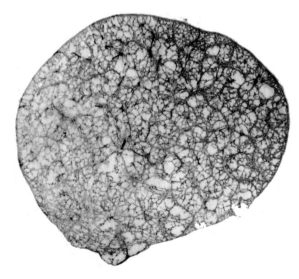

Fig. 14.2 Macroscopic paper-mounted, whole-lung sections illustrating severely emphysematous lung tissue

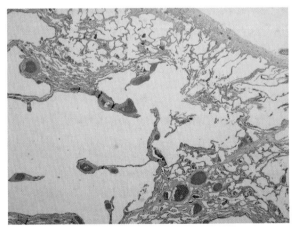

Fig. 14.4 Panlobular emphysema. Histologic specimen stained with hematoxylin-eosin from a patient with α_1-antitrypsin deficiency associated with severe widespread panlobular emphysema (magnification x20)

Chronic bronchitis is defined as a clinical disorder characterized by excessive mucous secretion (of unknown cause) by the bronchial tree, manifested by chronic or recurring productive cough on most days of more than 3 months of each of two successive years (Snider et al. 1985).

The traditional definition of COPD as including pulmonary emphysema on one hand and chronic bronchitis on the other hand has been recently modified. The Global Initiative for Chronic Obstructive Lung Disease (GOLD) – a collaborative project of the US National Heart, Lung, and Blood Institute and the World Health Organization – have prepared a consensus report in which COPD is defined as a disease state characterized by airflow limitation that is not fully reversible (Pauwels et al. 2001). Based on of this definition, the diagnosis of COPD is thus determined with lung function tests, best measured by spirometry, because this is the most widely available and reproducible test of lung function (Calverley 2004).

In GOLD reports, subdivision of COPD into pulmonary emphysema and chronic bronchitis has been removed from the definition of COPD given the overlap between the two conditions and the poor delineation between them (Pauwels et al. 2001; Rabe et al. 2007). The new definition of COPD, as proposed by the GOLD scientific committee, has been rapidly and widely accepted by the medical community and is now used in most major clinical trials. Nevertheless, the possible advance provided by the GOLD classification in our understanding of this complicated and heterogeneous disease is still a matter of debate (Calverley 2004).

The characteristic symptoms of COPD are chronic and progressive dyspnea, cough, and sputum production. A diagnosis of COPD should thus be considered in any patient who has symptoms of cough, sputum production, dyspnea, and/or a history of exposure to risk factors for the disease. The diagnosis is confirmed with spirometry by the presence of a postbronchodilatator FEV_1 < 80% of the predicted value in combination with an FEV_1/FVC < 70% (Pauwels et al. 2001; Rabe et al. 2007). Chronic cough and sputum production may precede the development of airflow limitation by many years. Conversely, significant airflow limitation may develop without chronic cough and sputum production (Rabe et al. 2007).

Pathologically, the chronic airflow limitation characteristic of COPD is caused by a mixture of small airway disease (obstructive bronchiolitis) and parenchymal lung destruction (pulmonary emphysema), the relative

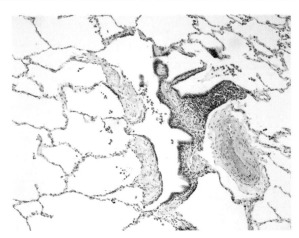

Fig. 14.5 Small airway disease. Histologic specimen stained with hematoxylin-eosin from a patient with COPD. The bronchial wall is thickened and fibrosed. The lumen contains some pigmented macrophages

contributions of which vary from person to person (Rabe et al. 2007). Small airways are defined as smaller than 2 mm in diameter (Hogg et al. 2004). In COPD, the lumen of these small airways is reduced and their wall is thickened (Fig. 14.5).

The only radiographic statement in the GOLD guidelines (Rabe et al. 2007) is that chest radiographs are useful in the identification of alternative diagnoses that can mimic symptoms of an exacerbation. The role of chest radiograph thus seems to be marginal in the diagnosis of COPD. Nevertheless, COPD is so frequent that it is very usual to read chest radiographs and CT scans performed in patients who have COPD. We divide the radiographic and CT imaging features of COPD into two main categories: imaging of the emphysema and imaging of the airways.

14.2 Radiography in Emphysema

The only direct sign of emphysema on plain radiographs is the presence of bullae. However, because of the limited contrast resolution of the chest radiograph, these focal areas of increased lucency can be difficult to detect (Figs. 14.6–14.9) (Müller and Coxson 2002). Indirect signs of lung destruction caused by emphysema, such as focal absence of pulmonary vessels and the reduction of vessel caliber with tapering towards the lung periphery are highly suggestive of emphysema, but their sensitivity is as

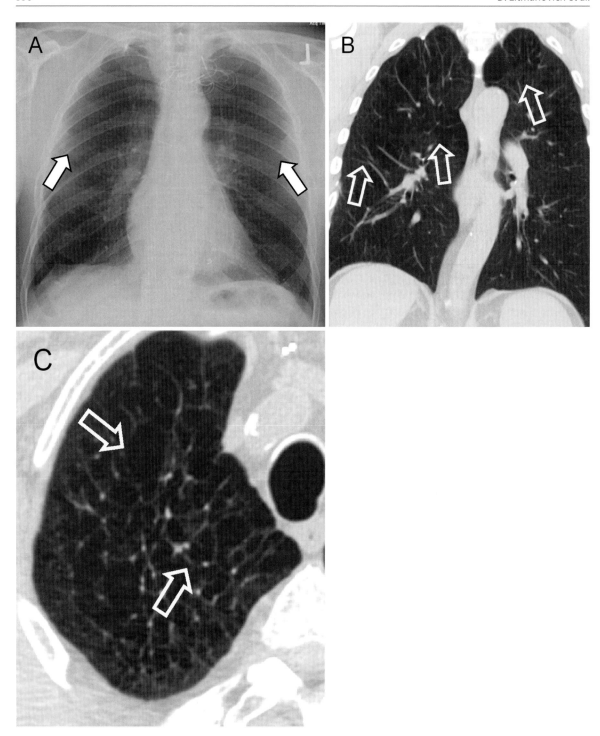

Fig. 14.6 Frontal chest radiograph (**a**), coronal CT reconstruction (**b**), and transverse CT section (**c**, detail) of a patient with severe emphysema. The chest radiograph (**a**) shows no particular abnormalities in the lung apices (*arrows*). Coronal CT reconstruction (**b**) shows extensive bilateral areas of parenchymal destruction (*open arrows*) that were not visible on the chest radiograph. Transverse CT section (**c**) reveals that the emphysema shows a mixed centrilobular–panlobular pattern (*open arrows*)

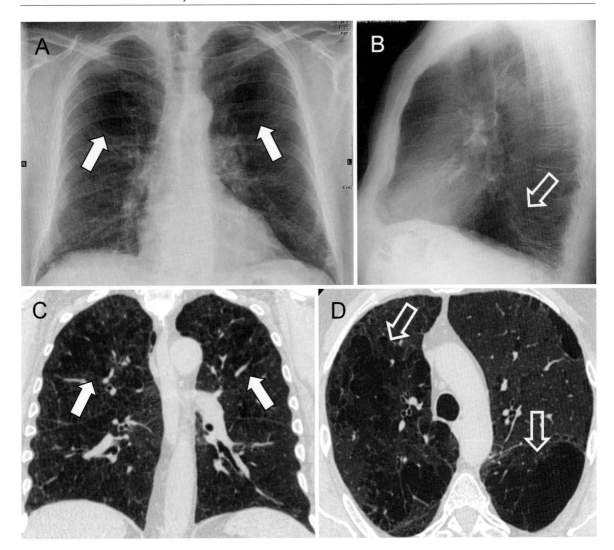

Fig. 14.7 Frontal (**a**) and lateral (**b**) chest radiographs and coronal and transverse CT reconstruction (**c, d**) in a patient with severe emphysema. Hyperlucent zones in both lung apices (*white arrows*) on the frontal chest radiograph (**a**) suggest the presence of emphysema. Flattening of the hemidiaphragm is depicted on the lateral view (**b**; *open white arrow*). The overall extent of the disease, combining centrilobular emphysema predominantly involving lung apices (*white arrows*) with bullous disease (*open white arrows*) can be fully reflected only by CT (**c, d**)

low as 40% (Thurlbeck and Simon 1978). Findings related to overinflation of the lungs include flattening of the diaphragm and an increased retrosternal space on the lateral view (Fig. 14.9). These findings are more common than abnormalities of the vascular pattern, but their specificity is also low (Thurlbeck and Simon 1978). The combined signs of hyperinflation and vascular alterations have been shown to allow the

diagnosis of emphysema in 29 of 30 necropsy-proven and symptomatic patients, but in only 8 of 17 necropsy-proven and asymptomatic patients (Sutinen et al. 1965). The combination of signs of hyperinflation and vascular alterations on radiography allow for the diagnosis of emphysema in the majority of patients who have moderate or severe disease (Müller and Coxson 2002).

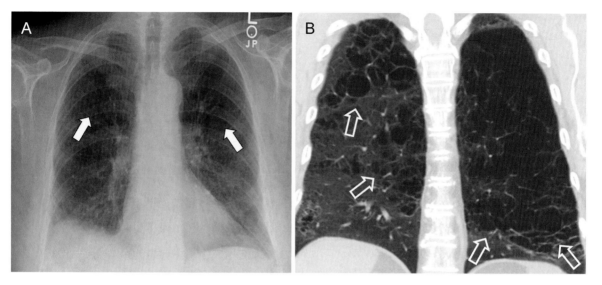

Fig. 14.8 Frontal chest radiograph (**a**) and coronal CT reconstruction (**b**) from a patient with severe emphysema. Subtle hyperlucent zones in both lung apices (*arrows*) on the chest radiograph (**a**) suggest the presence of emphysema. The overall extent of the disease, reflected by subtotal lung destruction (*open arrows*), is visualized only by CT (**b**)

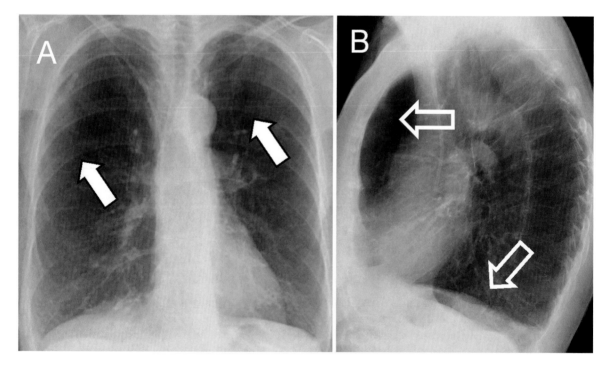

Fig. 14.9 Frontal (**a**) and lateral (**b**) chest radiograph, coronal CT reconstruction (**c**), and transverse CT section (**d**) from a patient who has severe emphysema. The chest radiograph (**a**) shows increased lucency of the lung apices, right more than left, with rarefaction of the lung parenchyma (*white arrows*). *Open white arrows* on the lateral radiograph (**b**) indicate increased retrosternal space and flattening of the diaphragm, consistent with overinflation. Coronal CT reconstruction (**c**) shows extensive bilateral areas of parenchymal destruction (*white arrows*) more visible than on the chest radiograph. Transverse CT section (**d**) reveals that the emphysema shows a panlobular pattern (*white arrow*). Both upper and lower lung zones are affected, which can be better appreciated on coronal reconstructions

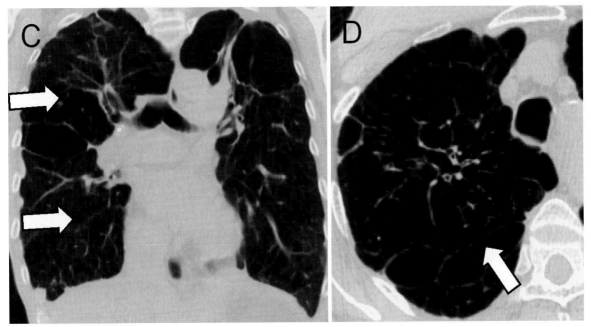

Fig. 14.9 (continued)

Obvious limitations of radiography in the assessment of emphysema include low specificity, low sensitivity in the evaluation of mild disease, considerable interobserver variability in the interpretation of findings, and the inability to quantify the severity of emphysema (Müller and Coxson 2002; Sutinen et al. 1965; Thurlbeck and Simon 1978; Thurlbeck and Müller 1994).

Because emphysema is diagnosed anatomically, only studies comparing radiographs to morphologically proven emphysema are relevant. M.W. Thurlbeck and G. Simon (1978) have extensively compared chest radiographs and paper-mounted whole-lung Gough–Wenthworth sections (Gough and Wentworth 1949) in a vast study including 696 necropsies. They have considered the following radiographic variables: lung length, lung width, diaphragm level, heart size, retrosternal space, and arterial deficiency. Emphysema was considered present when the lung was hypertransparent with diminished or absent vascularity in the outer lung fields (Thurlbeck and Simon 1978). The radiographic findings were compared with the amount of emphysema assessed subjectively on paper-mounted, whole-lung Gough–Wenthworth sections using a standard grading panel, on which the amount of emphysema was scored (Thurlbeck et al. 1970). This very meticulous study revealed that chest radiograph is not a very precise method of diagnosing emphysema.

Occasional patients who have no, trivial, or mild emphysema will indeed be diagnosed as having emphysema, and a fairly high proportion of patients who have severe emphysema will not be diagnosed using the radiologic criterion of arterial deficiency. On the other hand, centrilobular emphysema was usually present when emphysema was diagnosed radiographically in the upper lung zones, and panacinar emphysema was usually present when emphysema was diagnosed in the lower zones. Finally, lung length and the size of the retrosternal space increased, the level of the diaphragm lowered, heart size decreased, and lung width did not change as emphysema became more severe (Thurlbeck and Simon 1978). In accordance with other studies, it is now well established that plain chest radiograph has high accuracy in the diagnosis of severe emphysema using criteria of attenuation of vascular shadows and the presence of bullae with pulmonary overdistension. Moderate emphysema cannot be diagnosed unless the process is locally severe; mild emphysema is rarely diagnosable (Pugatch 1983). These studies clearly reveal the limitation of chest radiography in the diagnosis of pulmonary emphysema on the basis of arterial deficiency, with other signs being nonspecific reflections of hyperinflation that is more precisely investigated through pulmonary function tests (PFTs).

Interestingly, some radiologic studies have reported "increased markings" emphysema (Boushy et al. 1971). Is such emphysema, the vascular markings appear to be increased with irregular small opacities throughout the lungs on the chest radiographs.

Comparisons with CT suggest that these irregular opacities could be explained, at least in part, by the superimposition of the walls of small bullae (Fig. 14.10) and/or by bronchiectases with thickened bronchial walls (Fig. 14.11).

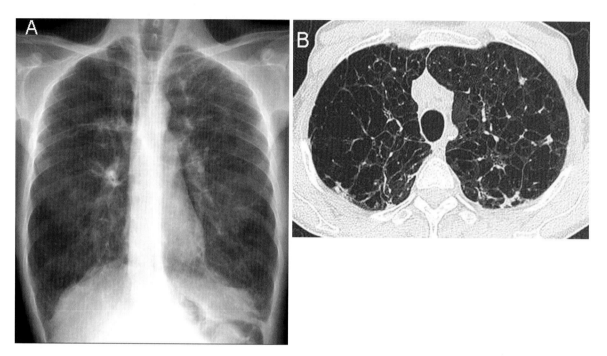

Fig. 14.10 Frontal chest radiograph (**a**) with irregular markings in a patient who has emphysema. CT scan (**b**) suggests that the irregular markings are related to the superimposition of the walls of adjacent bullae

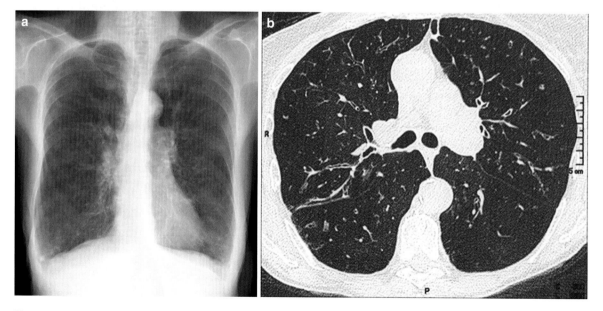

Fig. 14.11 (**a**) Frontal chest radiograph with irregular markings in a patient who has emphysema. (**b**, **c**) CT scans suggest that the irregular markings are related to the superimposition of the thickened walls of dilated bronchi

Fig. 14.11 (continued)

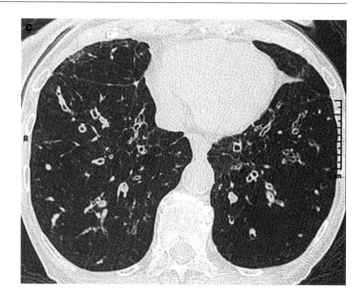

In pulmonary emphysema, the heterogeneity of lung destruction with subsequent heterogeneity in elastic recoil will lead to atelectasis of the less emphysematous parts of the lungs as compared with the more emphysematous parts of the lungs. This heterogeneity in lung elastic recoil may lead to displacement of anatomical structures such as lung fissure, pulmonary hilum (Fig. 14.12), and even irregular opaque bands of atelectatic lung surrounding the most emphysematous areas (Fig. 14.13). It is important to remember that lung parenchyma is an elastic structure that tends to retract. As a consequence, atelectasis adjacent to the emphysematous lung (or bulla) is not the result of any compression by the emphysematous lung (or bulla) against

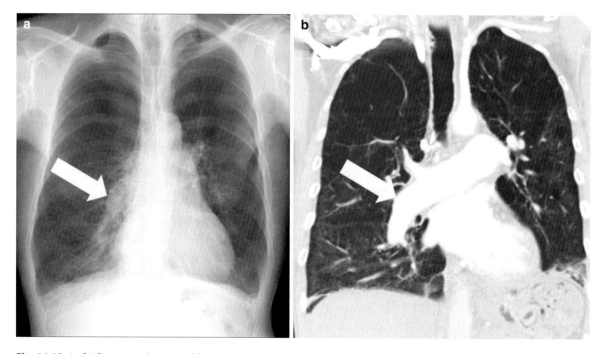

Fig. 14.12 (**a, b**) Severe emphysema with an upper predominance. The heterogeneity of lung destruction leads to heterogeneity in elastic recoil and subsequent downward displacement of anatomical structures such as the right pulmonary artery (*arrows*)

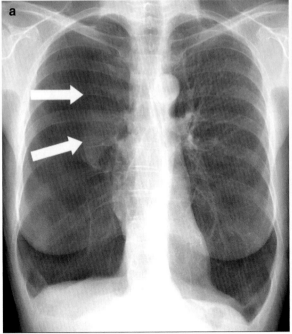

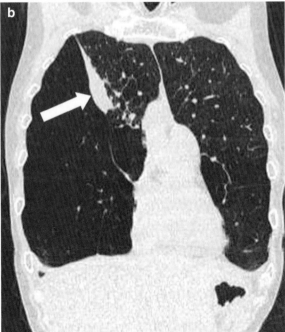

Fig. 14.13 (**a, b**) Severe emphysema with a right and lower predominance. The heterogeneity of lung destruction leads to heterogeneity in elastic recoil and subsequent atelectasis of the less emphysematous parts of the lungs compared with the more emphysematous parts of the lungs. The atelectatic lung appears as opaque bands (*white arrows*)

normal lung. In fact, the normal lung (or the less emphysematous lung) just has a stronger elastic recoil–and thus a stronger tendency to retract—as compared with the neighboring more emphysematous lung (or bulla).

14.3 CT in Emphysema

CT is superior to chest radiography in the detection of emphysema and in the assessment of its distribution and extent. Emphysema will be visible in many conventional CT sections with thicknesses of 5–8 mm. However, it is more readily detected in high-resolution CT (HRCT) sections with thicknesses of 1–2 mm reconstructed with an edge-enhancing algorithm (Kuwano et al. 1990; Miller et al. 1989) (Figs. 14.14–14.16). The introduction of multidetector CT units now allows acquisition of such HRCT in a volumetric manner over the entire lung, and this approach has been shown to be suitable for the assessment of emphysema (Madani et al. 2006). The assessment of mild emphysema can further benefit from the minimum

intensity projection (MinIP) technique (Figs. 14.17 and 14.18), which utilizes dedicated software to identify only areas of lung parenchyma with the lowest attenuation values and simultaneously suppresses normal lung and pulmonary vessels. The technique is based on "slabs" of contiguous HRCT sections through a sample of lung tissue. Comparing MinIP and 1-mm HRCT sections, Remy-Jardin and colleagues (1996) found that the MinIP technique was more sensitive for the detection of subtle emphysema.

On HRCT scans, emphysema is characterized by the presence of areas of low attenuation that contrast with the surrounding lung parenchyma with normal attenuation (Figs. 14.16, 14.19, and 14.20) (Hruban et al. 1987; Webb et al. 1988). Mild to moderate centrilobular emphysema is characterized by the presence of multiple rounded and small areas of low attenuation, which have diameters of several millimeters and usually are predominant in the upper lobe. The lesions have no walls because they are limited by the surrounding lung parenchyma. Sometimes the lesions may appear to be grouped around the center of secondary pulmonary lobules (Figs. 14.16, 14.19, and 14.20)

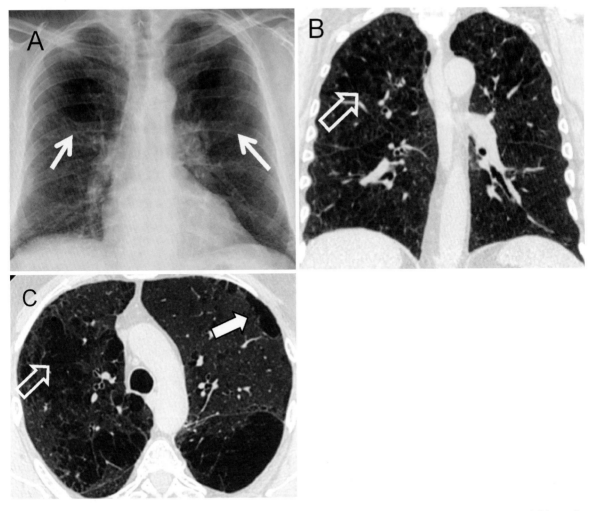

Fig. 14.14 Frontal chest radiograph (**a**), coronal CT reconstruction (**b**), and transverse CT section (**c**, detail) in a patient who has moderate emphysema. The chest radiograph (**a**) shows relatively mild abnormalities in the lung apices (*arrows*). Coronal CT reconstruction (**b**) shows extensive bilateral areas of parenchymal destruction (*open arrows*) that were not visible on the chest radiograph. Transverse CT section (**c**) reveals that the emphysema shows mixed centrilobular–panlobular (*open arrow*) and paraseptal patterns (*white arrow*)

(Murata et al. 1986; Webb et al. 1988). Panlobular emphysema is characterized by uniform destruction of the secondary pulmonary lobule. This leads to widespread and relatively homogeneous patterns of low attenuation (Murata et al. 1989; Webb et al. 1988). Panlobular emphysema can involve the entire lung in a rather homogeneous manner, or it may show lower-lobe predominance.

The accuracy of HRCT in assessing the presence and extent of emphysema has been documented in numerous studies (Gevenois et al. 1995, 1996b; Kuwano et al. 1990; Murata et al. 1986, 1989). In one study based on necropsy specimens, investigators were able to identify even mild centrilobular emphysema (Kuwano et al. 1990). The correlation between the in vitro CT emphysema score and the pathological grade of emphysema was excellent ($r = 0.91$). Because it is difficult to translate the excellent in vitro correlations into an in vivo context, correlations between the in vivo CT assessment and pathological severity range from 0.7 to 0.9 (Gevenois et al. 1995, 1996b), and some authors have noted that very mild emphysema could be missed in vivo (Remy-Jardin et al. 1996). This suggests that the in vivo assessment of the extent

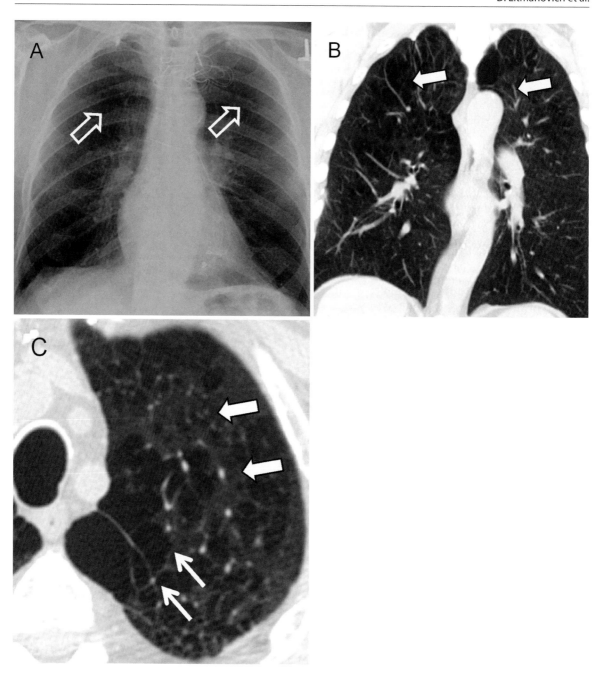

Fig. 14.15 Frontal chest radiograph (**a**), coronal CT reconstruction (**b**), and transverse CT section (**c**, detail) in a patient who has mild to moderate emphysema. The chest radiograph (**a**) shows relatively mild abnormalities in the lung apices (*open arrows*). Coronal CT reconstruction (**b**) shows moderate bilat- eral asymmetric (right more than left) areas of parenchymal destruction (*arrows*) corresponding to increased lucency seen on the chest radiograph. Transverse CT section (**c**) reveals that the emphysema shows a centrilobular (*thick white arrows*) pattern with a paraseptal component (*thin white arrows*)

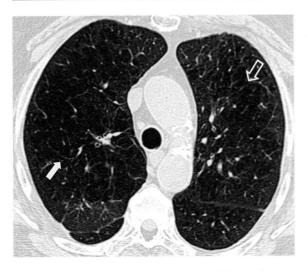

Fig. 14.16 Combined centrilobular and panlobular emphysema seen on a transverse CT section through the upper lobes. The emphysematous pattern in the right lung is centrilobular (*open arrow*); the structure of the secondary pulmonary lobule in the left lung begins to disappear (*solid white arrow*) and the pattern of emphysema becomes more diffuse and thus assumes characteristics of panlobular emphysema

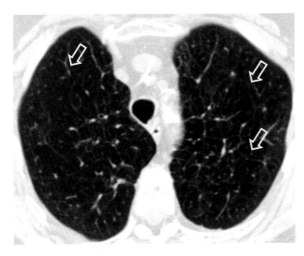

Fig. 14.17 Transverse CT sections through the upper lobes of a patient with normal chest radiograph (not shown). The pattern of destruction seen on a cross-sectional imaging study is focal centrilobular emphysema with the structure of the secondary pulmonary lobule still seen (*open arrows*)

of emphysema is at risk for either under- or overestimation. A computer-assisted method for obtaining objective quantification of horizontal paper-mounted lung sections as a standard of reference was compared with the densitometric evaluation of mean lung

attenuation and to subjective visual assessments by three readers (Bankier et al. 1999). The study found that subjective grading of emphysema was significantly less accurate than objective CT densitometric results when correlated with pathological scores. Moreover, the analysis of visual scoring suggested systematic overestimation of emphysema by all three readers. The majority of studies, however, have shown reasonably good correlations between CT emphysema scores and pathologic specimens, good agreement between expert readers for the assessment of presence and extent of emphysema, and good correlations between subjective and objective assessments of emphysema (Gelb et al. 1998; Müller and Coxson 2002; Müller et al. 1988).

The destruction of lung parenchyma that is present in emphysema can, in practice, lead to atypical appearances of coexisting lung disease. Therefore, CT in patients who have emphysema and coexisting lung disease should be performed early, upon clinical suspicion (Figs. 14.21–14.31)

14.3.1 Objective CT Quantification of Emphysema

The inherent limitations of subjective visual scoring, the characteristic CT morphology of emphysema, and the digital nature of the CT dataset have fostered considerable interest in the use of CT as an objective quantification tool for pulmonary emphysema (Gevenois and Yernault 1995; Madani et al. 2001). Three main approaches have been used to objectively quantify emphysema with CT. First is the use of a threshold density value below which emphysema is considered to be present (threshold technique). Second, the assessment of a range of densities present in a CT section and displayed as a distribution curve. Third, the measurement of the overall CT density of the lung parenchyma.

Hayhurst et al. (1984) showed that the distribution curve of numbers of attenuations was significantly shifted toward lower attenuation values in patients who had emphysema compared with normal individuals. In a CT pathologic correlation study based on microscopic measurements, Gould et al. (1988) showed that the

Fig. 14.18 Diffuse
centrilobular emphysema.
Transverse CT section
through the upper lobes
shows the typical pattern of
diffuse centrilobular
emphysema. Despite the
severity of destruction, the
structure of the secondary
pulmonary lobule is still
visible (*open arrows*)

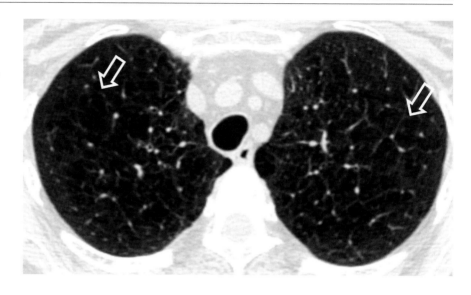

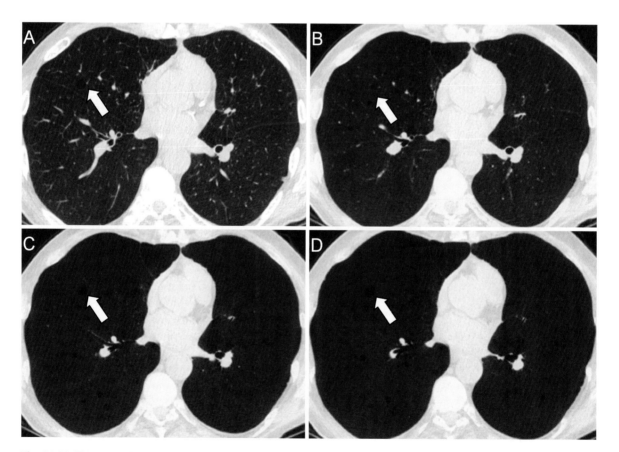

Fig. 14.19 Transverse CT section (**a**) and minimum intensity projections (MinIPs) of 5-mm (**b**), 10-mm (**c**), and 20-mm (**d**) section thickness. Though subtle upper-lobe predominant emphysema can barely be seen on reconstructed image (**a**), it is increasingly well seen with increasing thickness of the MinIPs (**b–d**)

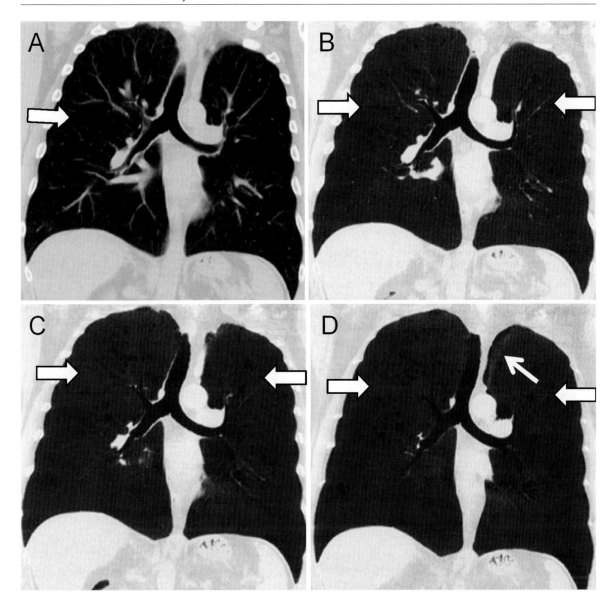

Fig. 14.20 Coronal reconstruction (**a**) and minimum intensity projections (MinIPs) of 5-mm (**b**), 10-mm (**c**), and 20-mm (**d**) section thickness. Though subtle upper-lobe predominant emphysema can barely be seen on the coronal reconstructed image (**a**), it is increasingly well seen with increasing thickness of the MinIPs (**b–d**, *white arrows*). Minimal paraseptal emphysema in the left upper lobe can be seen on the thickest reconstructions (**d**, *small white arrow*, **d**)

lowest fifth percentile of the histogram of attenuation values was significantly correlated with the surface area of the walls of distal airspaces per unit lung volume (AWUV). In 1988, Müller et al. used a commercially available CT program called "Density Mask®" (General Electric Medical Systems, Milwaukee, WI, USA) that highlights pixels within a given attenuation range and automatically calculates the area of highlighted pixels (Müller et al. 1988). In their study, Müller et al. compared the relative area highlighted on a single 1-cm-thick CT section after the injection of contrast material with the corresponding macroscopic section of the fixed lung cut in the same plane as the CT section and graded using a modification of the picture-grading system from Thurlbeck et al. (1970). The highest correlation was observed with attenuation

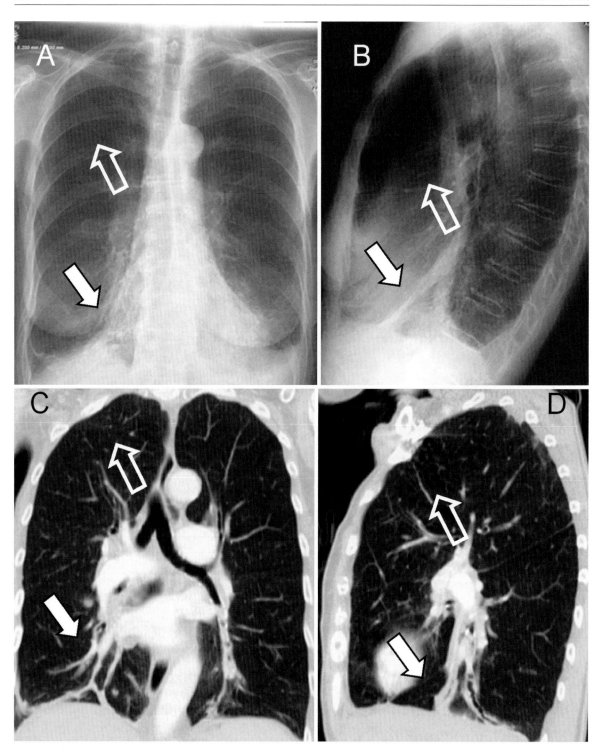

Fig. 14.21 Frontal (**a**) and lateral (**b**) chest radiographs, coronal CT reconstruction (**c**), and sagittal CT section (**d**) in a patient who has centrilobular emphysema. The chest radiographs (**a**, **b**) show increased lucency of the lung apices, with rarefaction of the lung parenchyma and centrilobular emphysema on CT (**c**, **d**; *open arrows*). Both the chest radiographs and the cross-sectional images show bilateral areas of bronchial wall thickening and peribronchial consolidation consistent with bronchopneumonia (*solid arrows*)

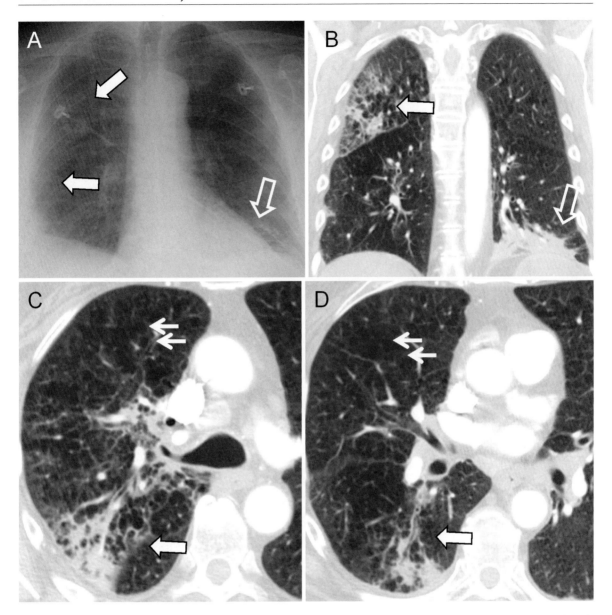

Fig. 14.22 Emphysema and multifocal pneumonia. Three areas of consolidation are difficult to diagnose on chest radiograph (**a**, *open and solid white arrows*) and better seen on CT (**b, c, d**) in a patient who has moderate to severe centrilobular emphysema (**c, d**, *small white arrows*) in right upper and lower lobes (**b, c, d**, *large solid white arrows*) and in left lower lobe, better seen on coronal reconstruction (**d**, *open white arrow*)

values lower than −910 HU; consequently, this threshold was recommended for the identification of emphysema. In an attempt to determine the best attenuation threshold for the recognition of emphysema, Gevenois et al. applied to 1-mm-thick CT sections a program that automatically recognizes the lungs, traces the lung contours, determines histograms of attenuation values, and measures the lung area occupied by pixels included in the predetermined range of attenuation value (Kalender et al. 1991). They showed that the only threshold for which there was no statistically significant difference between the distribution of the CT

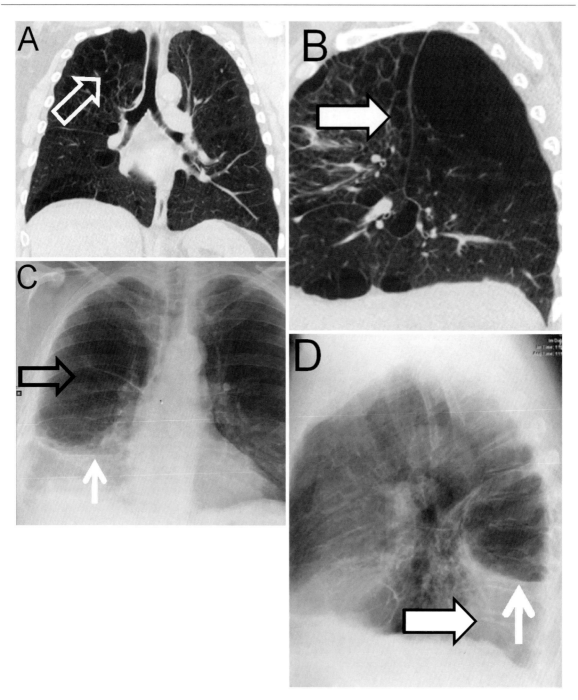

Fig. 14.23 Infected large bulla and surrounding pneumonia in right lower lobe. Severe emphysema (**a**, *open white arrow*) and large right lower lobe bulla car be seen on sagittal reformat (**b**, *white arrow*). The same patient was hospitalized due to non-resolving pneumonia. Posteroanterior and lateral chect radiographs obtained at hospitalization (**c**, **d**) show air-fluid level within the bulla (**e**, *open black arrow*) as well as large right lower-lobe consolidation (**d**, **f**, *thin white arrow*), that can be even better appreciated on CT reformats (**f**, *large white arrow*)

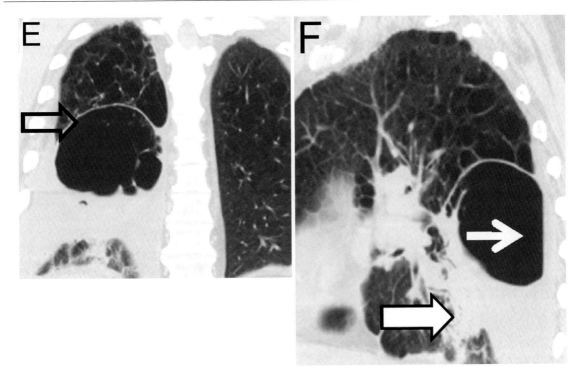

Fig. 14.23 (continued)

measurements and the distribution of macroscopic measurements was −950 HU. Thresholds lower than −950 HU underestimated emphysema, and thresholds above −950 HU overestimated emphysema (Gevenois et al. 1995).

Given that McLean et al. (1992) recommend that pulmonary emphysema should be measured microscopically rather than macroscopically, comparisons between CT and morphometry should also include microscopic measurements and comparisons. Using AWUV as a microscopic measurement of the alveolar wall surface in 28 subjects referred for surgical resection of lung tumors, Gould et al. (1998) reported significant correlations between AWUV and the lowest fifth percentile of the frequency distribution curve of attenuation values calculated on 13-mm-thick CT sections. In a more recent study based on 38 patients who were also referred for lung resection, Gevenois et al. measured the mean interwall distance and mean perimeter and compared the percentage of the surface area of lung occupied by attenuation values lower than the thresholds (range, −900 to −970 HU) to the microscopic indexes. They showed that the highest correlation was obtained with −950 HU. Thus, both

the macroscopic and the microscopic study conducted by Gevenois' group suggest that RA_{950} is a valuable parameter for quantifying emphysema on incremental thin-section CT (Gevenois et al. 1995).

To predict the lung surface to volume ratio from CT attenuation values, Coxson et al. (1999) considered a threshold of −910 HU and compared CT measurements with histologic estimates of surface area. Lung volume was calculated by summing the voxel dimensions in each slice, and lung weight was estimated by multiplying the mean lung attenuation value by the lung volume. This method seemed to be more accurate than the histologic surface area occupied by emphysema because Coxson et al. (1999) observed a reduced surface to volume ratio in mild emphysema whereas surface area and tissue weight were decreased only in severe disease. Finally, Desai et al. (2007) recommended the use of a combined morphologic and functional ("composite") score to assess emphysema.

Overall, the findings from the single-section CT era were an important basis for research about the radiologic/pathologic correlation of emphysema. However, with the advent of multidetector CT units, new challenges have arisen and will be discussed below.

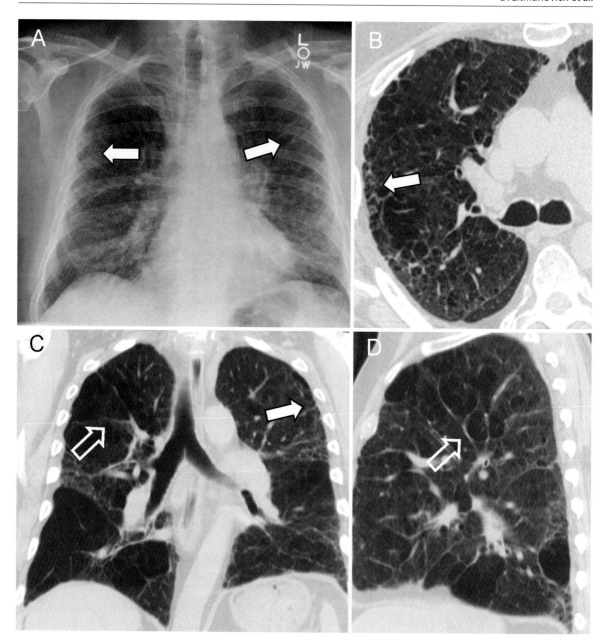

Fig. 14.24 Emphysema and lung fibrosis. Chest radiograph (**a**) demonstrates a slight increase in upper lung lucency corresponding to upper-lobe centrilobular emphysema (**c, d**, *open white arrow*s) in combination with increased subpleural reticulation that can be seen on both chest radiograph and transverse, coronal, and sagittal reformats (**a–c**, *solid white arrow*s)

14.3.2 Tissue Characterization

Quantification of pulmonary emphysema by computer-assisted methods is based on mathematic approaches called metrics, mean lung density, and areas of low attenuation that may be used to describe the heterogeneity of the spatial distribution of the attenuation values within the reconstructed image (Hoffman and McLennan 1997). In order to differentiate normal from emphysematous lungs and normal from emphysematous regions within one lung, Uppaluri et al. (1997) developed an adaptive multiple features method (AMFM) based on textural analysis. The accuracy of AMFM, mean lung

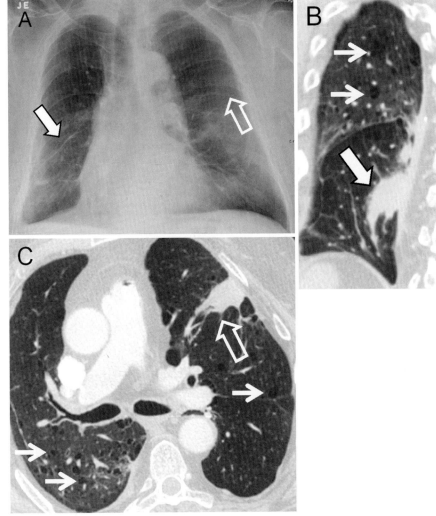

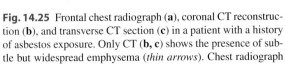

Fig. 14.25 Frontal chest radiograph (**a**), coronal CT reconstruction (**b**), and transverse CT section (**c**) in a patient with a history of asbestos exposure. Only CT (**b, c**) shows the presence of subtle but widespread emphysema (*thin arrows*). Chest radiograph (**a**) shows a right linear opacity (*solid arrow*) and a left ill-defined opacity (*open arrow*). CT (**b, c**) reveals that both lesions correspond to right (**b**, *solid arrow*) and left (**c**, *open arrow*) rounded atelectases

density, and the lowest fifth percentile were 100%, 95%, and 97%, respectively. However, there was no correlation between these three parameters and PFTs. The authors explained this lack of correlation by a too small number of sections per subject and by the absence of patients with mild and moderate emphysema (Hoffman and McLennan 1997; Uppaluri et al. 1997).

In an attempt to detect early emphysema, Mishima et al. (1999a, b) quantified the size distribution of low attenuation–area (i.e., lower than −960 HU) clusters on 2-mm-thick HRCT sections obtained at full inspiration in 30 healthy subjects and 73 COPD patients. All normal subjects had a low attenuation area smaller than 30% of the total lung area; the area size varied from 2.6% to 67.6% in COPD patients. Although the COPD group of patients with a low attenuation area smaller than 30% of total lung area and the normal subjects had similar low attenuation areas, the corresponding D values were significantly smaller among the COPD patients. The authors concluded that 30% could be the critical value of low attenuation areas to discriminate normal and mild from severe COPD patients but that a low attenuation area is

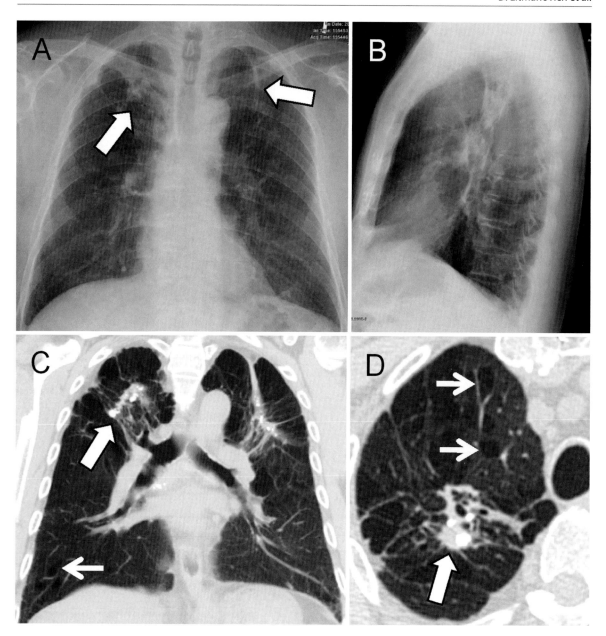

Fig. 14.26 Frontal (**a**) and lateral (**b**) chest radiographs, coronal CT reconstruction (**c**), and transverse CT section (**d**) in a patient with a history of tuberculosis. Bi-apical fibrotic changes and calcifications on chest radiograph (**a**, **b**) and CT (**c**, **d**; thick white arrows in **a**, **c**, and **d**) are obvious. The extent of centrilobular emphysema is underestimated on radiographs, and only CT images (**c**, **d**) show its extent (*thin white arrows*)

not sufficiently accurate to distinguish early emphysematous patients from normal subjects. The value of *D* could be a sensitive parameter for detecting the terminal airspace enlargement that occurs in early emphysema.

More recently, on the basis of an automated technique, Chabat et al. (2003) attempted to distinguish between centrilobular emphysema, panlobular emphysema, constrictive obliterative bronchiolitis, and normal lung tissue. Local texture information was extracted from four regions of interest on thin-section CT images obtained from 33 subjects and represented by first- and second-order measurements. Texture feature segmentation was applied after training and testing steps and

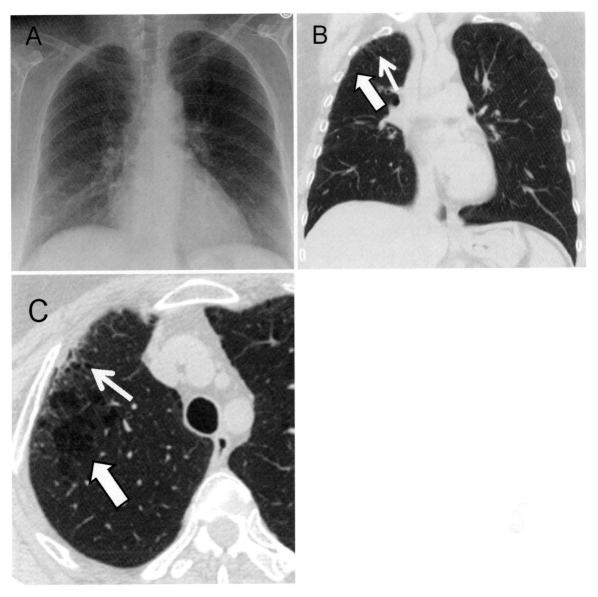

Fig. 14.27 Frontal chest radiograph (**a**), coronal CT reconstruction (**b**), and transverse CT section (**c**) in a patient who has moderate emphysema. The chest radiograph (**a**) shows no abnormalities. Coronal CT reconstruction (**b**) and transverse CT section (**c**) show minimal areas of parenchymal destruction (*thick white arrows*) that were not visible on the chest radiograph. Subtle postradiation changes in a patient with right breast cancer are noted only on the cross-sectional imaging (*thin white arrows* in **b, c**)

based on the visual classification of these four patterns. Given the possible coexistence of both types of pulmonary emphysema in the same individual, the proposed technique discriminated between patterns of obstructive lung disease with sensitivity ranging from 55% to 89%, specificity from 88% to 92%, and positive predictive value from 71% to 77% (Chabat et al. 2003).

14.3.3 Factors Influencing CT Densitometry

Airspace size correlates with age according to morphometric data (Thurlbeck 1967; Gillooly and Lamb 1993). Thus, an increase in airspace size associated with advanced age could potentially influence the CT

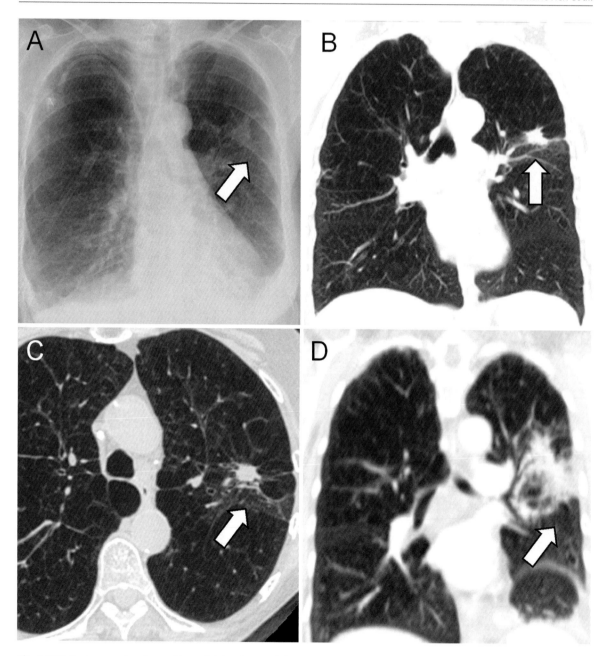

Fig. 14.28 Posteroanterior chest radiograph (**a**) and coronal (**b**) and axial (**c**) CT reformats demonstrate speculated lesion (*white arrow*) in the left upper lobe of a patient who has severe centri-lobular emphysema. This lesion has a radiological appearance highly suspicious of lung cancer. In fact, it represented as a scar-ring formation at the area of pre-existing extensive pneumonia (*white arrow*, **d**) that was shown to be unchanged at 2-year follow-up (not shown)

density parameters and should be taken into account in longitudinal study designs (Gevenois et al. 1996a; Soejima et al. 2000).

Independent from the lung volume at which CT is obtained, the lung size could influence CT parameters. Morphometric studies showed contradictory results, suggesting that the number of alveoli in the human lung either was or was not positively correlated with body length (Dunnill 1982; Gevenois et al. 1996a). Because the structure of the alveolar wall is unrelated to lung size, the dimensions of the airspaces should be bigger in larger lungs than in smaller lungs.

On the basis of image quality, exposure dose, and correlations with lung function tests, Mishima et al.

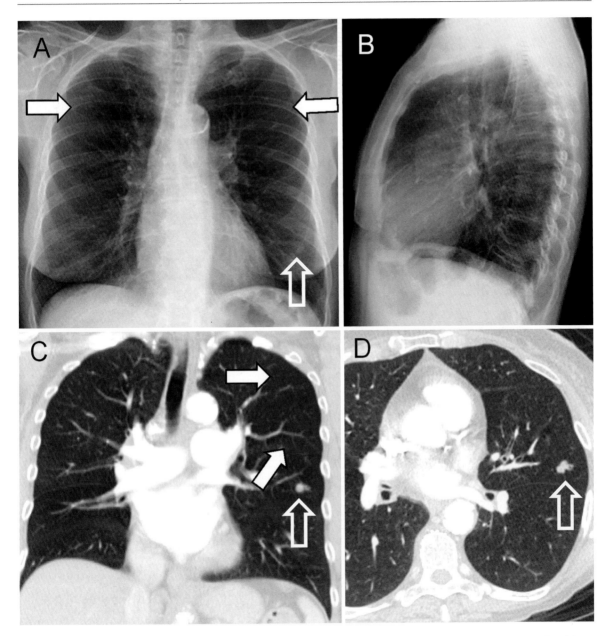

Fig. 14.29 Frontal (**a**) and lateral (**b**) chest radiographs, coronal CT reconstruction (**c**), and transverse CT section (**d**) in a patient with a history of smoking. Chest radiograph (**a**) shows a small subcentimeter nodule in the left lower lobe (*open white arrow*) that on both CT images corresponds to solid lobulated nodule (**c**, **d**, *open white arrow*). Apical hyperlucencies (**a**, **c**, *white arrows*) are suggestive of emphysema that was demonstrated as a mild centrilobular pattern on CT (**c**, **d**)

(1999b) suggested that the following CT parameters: three 2-mm-thick CT sections acquired with 200-mA tube current, are the most appropriate parameters to assess pulmonary emphysema.

Pulmonary emphysema is heterogeneously distributed throughout the lung, and studies based on point-counting have shown that an adequate assessment cannot be obtained from one lung slice alone (Turner and Whimster 1981). Although no CT study has defined the minimum number of images necessary to provide accurate results (Gevenois et al. 1995), Mishima et al. (1999, b) concluded that three slices were sufficient to determine the overall extent of emphysema. Madani and colleagues (2008) have recently demonstrated that sections with 10-mm intervals might be required for precise quantification of emphysema.

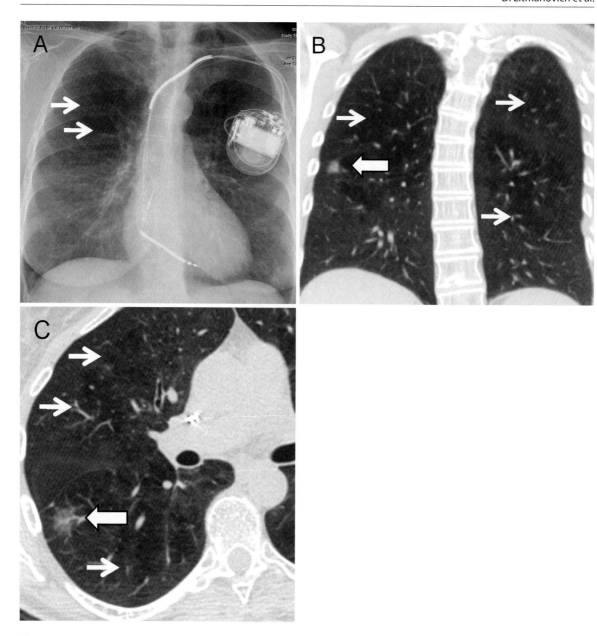

Fig. 14.30 Frontal chest radiograph (**a**), coronal CT reconstruction (**b**), and transverse CT section (**c**) in a patient with a long-standing history of smoking. Chest radiograph (**a**) shows apical hyperlucencies (*thin arrows*) that suggest emphysema, but the true extent of disease is better seen on CT (**b, c**; *thin arrows*). CT also reveals the presence of a subsolid nodule (**b**, **c**; *thick arrows*) that is not visible on the radiograph and later proved to be adenocarcinoma

14.3.4 Spiral and Multidetector CT – New Challenges

14.3.4.1 Density Thresholds

In a recent study, Madani et al. (2006) prospectively compared PFTs and multidetector CT indexes for quantifying pulmonary emphysema with macroscopic and microscopic morphometry. Their study was based on material from 80 patients and on datasets acquired with a four-row multidetector CT unit. They found that for relative lung areas the strongest correlation with macroscopy was seen with a threshold of −970 HU ($r = 0.543$, $P < 0.001$) and with microscopy the strongest correlation was seen at −960 and −970 HU, depending on the index considered ($r = 0.592$, $P < 0.001$ and $r = −0.546$, $P < 0.001$, respectively). For percentiles, the first percentile showed the strongest correlation with both macroscopy ($r = -0.463$, $P < 0.001$) and microscopy ($r = -0.573$, $P < 0.001$; $r = 0.523$, $P < 0.001$ for each microscopic measurement). Forced expiratory volume in 1 s and vital capacity ratio, diffusing capacity of lung for carbon monoxide, and each of the three CT indexes were complementary to predict microscopic indexes. From these observations, Madani et al. (2006) concluded that the relative lung areas with attenuation coefficients lower than -960 or -970 HU and the first percentile were valid indexes to quantify pulmonary emphysema on multidetector row CT scans. Clearly, a nearly identical density threshold can thus be used for quantifying emphysema on both incremental thin-section CT and multidetector CT.

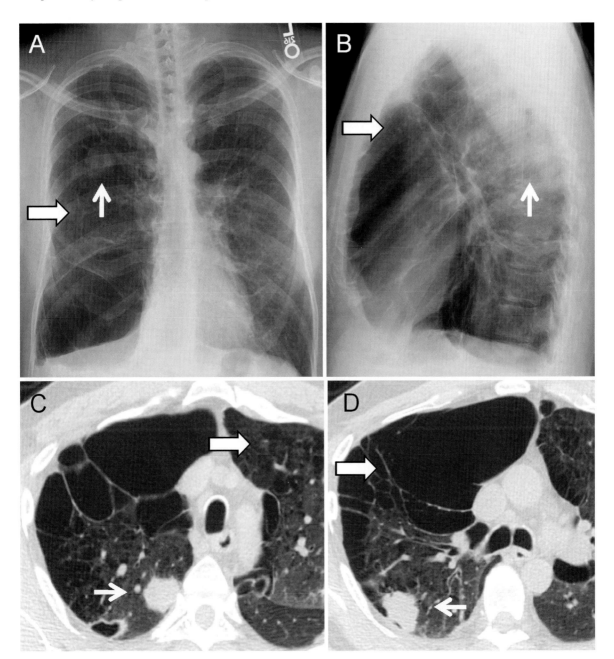

Fig. 14.31 Asymmetric severe panlobular emphysema mostly affecting the right lung. Posteroanterior (**a**) and lateral (**b**) chest radiographs and two transverse sections (**c, d**) through the upper lobes demonstrate severe panlobular emphysema (*thick white arrows*) affecting mostly the right lung with two primary lung cancers (*thin white arrows*)

14.3.4.2 Radiation Dose Exposure

With the advent of multidetector CT, dose reduction has became a more pressing issue (Mayo et al. 2003). Recently, Madani et al. (2007) studied the effects of radiation dose and section thickness on quantitative multidetector CT indexes of pulmonary emphysema. Their study was based on 70 patients and CT datasets acquired with a 4- × 1-mm collimation, 120 peak kilovoltage, and 20–120 effective mAs. At each radiation dose, 1.25-, 5.0-, and 10.0-mm-thick sections were reconstructed at 10-mm intervals. RAs of lung with attenuation coefficients lower than nine thresholds and eight percentiles of the distribution of attenuation coefficients were compared with the histopathologic extent of emphysema, which was measured microscopically using the corrected mean interwall distance and the corrected mean perimeter and macroscopically. The authors found that the first percentile (r range, −0.394 to −0.675; $P < 0.001$) and attenuation coefficients of −980, −970, and −960 HU (r range, 0.478–0.664; $P < 0.001$) yielded the strongest correlations with the macroscopic extent of emphysema, regardless of radiation dose or section thickness. The effects of radiation dose and section thickness on RAs of lung with attenuation coefficients lower than −960 HU ($P = 0.007$ and $P < 0.001$, respectively) and lower than −970 HU ($P = 0.001$ and $P < 0.001$, respectively) were significant. The effect of section thickness on the first percentile was significant ($P < 0.001$), whereas the effect of dose was not ($P = 0.910$). From that the authors concluded that, in CT quantification of pulmonary emphysema, the tube current-time product can be reduced to 20 mAs, but both tube current-time product and section thickness should be kept constant in follow-up examinations (Madani et al. 2007).

14.3.4.3 Potential Role of Expiratory CT

The possible role of CT obtained after deep expiration in the assessment of emphysema was first suggested by Knudson et al. (1991). Gevenois et al. (1995, 1996b) found two different thresholds, respectively validated by comparisons against macroscopy (−910 HU) and microscopy (−820 HU), that were quite different from the threshold found valid for CT images obtained at full inspiration (−950 HU). In addition, multiple regression analysis showed that CT measurements obtained at full expiration did not yield any additional significant information compared with those obtained at full inspiration. In a study based on visual scoring, Nishimura et al. (1998) showed that expiratory CT underestimates the degree of emphysema compared with inspiratory CT. In summary, expiratory CT is not as adequate as inspiratory CT for measuring the extent of pulmonary emphysema. The renewed interest in emphysema, given its contributing role in COPD, could also renew the interest in expiratory CT. Expiratory CT is a key technique for assessing the small airways in vivo, and combined imaging of the parenchyma and the airways with CT during inspiration and expiration, respectively, could open new prospects for a more holistic imaging approach to COPD. Recent studies that found good correlations between expiratory CT and PFTs indeed seem to confirm this prospect.

14.4 Airway Analysis in COPD

The airway exhibits a tree-like structure with almost cylindrical branches of decreasing radius. The evaluation of the airways on chest radiograph is limited. On chest radiograph, signs of overinflation are usually the only signs related to small airway disease, consisting of flattened or even inverted hemidiaphragms, the diaphragm lower than the anterior aspect of the seventh rib, a narrow vertically oriented heart, increased retrosternal space, and a sterno-diaphragmatic angle greater than 90° (Fig. 14.28). With a central air-filled lumen surrounded by higher density mural tissue, proximal airway walls provide an ideal contrast in composition for CT image analysis. The major challenge for quantitative analysis of the airway tree is the partial volume effect that blurs the inner lumen and bronchial wall into an indistinguishable mass with a CT density similar to the lung parenchyma; this is crucial at the level of distal generations.

The advent of multidetector row CT scanning now allows users to acquire thin-slice contiguous images of the lung using a Z dimension that approaches that of the X–Y dimensions with near isotropic voxel resolution and during a single breath-hold (Coxson 2008; Tschirren et al. 2005). A CT scanner with a minimum of 64 detectors is preferable to achieve a 0.5-mm slice thickness, although most studies still use CT slices with a 1- to 1.25-mm slice thickness. If the CT images are acquired using a 1-mm-or-less slice thickness, it is possible for investigators to segment the airway tree in three dimensions, starting in the trachea and projecting out to the fifth or sixth generation (Coxson 2008) (Figs. 14.32 and 14.33). CT slices used to create this three-dimensional reconstruction are contiguous; thus,

airway reformation into a single long tube that is sectioned in a true cross-section of the central axis is also possible. Then, by applying advanced knowledge to the branching pattern of the airway tree, bronchial segments can be labeled (Hasegawa et al. 2006).

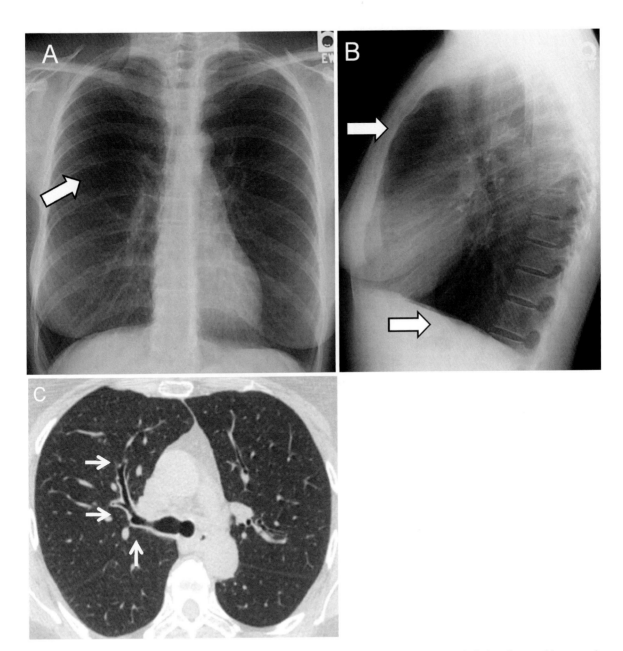

Fig. 14.32 Frontal and lateral chest radiograph in a patient with overinflation of the lungs. Frontal radiograph (**a**) shows increased lung volumes and a relatively large intercostal space (*large white arrows*). On the lateral radiograph (**b**), flattened diaphragms and increased retrosternal and retrocardiac spaces suggest the presence of hyperinflation (*large white arrows*). Transverse CT section at the level of the carina (**c**) obtained from the same patient shows substantial bronchial wall thickening in the right lung and subtle bronchial wall irregularities in the left lung (*small white arrows*)

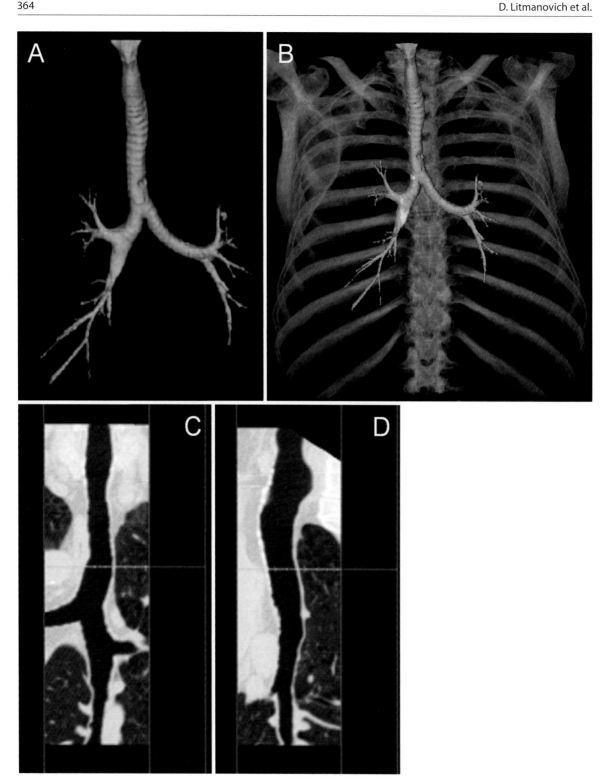

Fig. 14.33 Surface-shaded reconstruction of the trachea, main bronchi, and segmental bronchi. The images (**a, b**) emphasize the potential of CT to visualize these structures in a three-dimensional perspective. Multiplanar reformats of main bronchus with postprocessing technique create "straightened" bronchial structures that can be seen in perpendicular planes (**c, d**), which may allow for easier quantitative comparison during follow-up examinations and between patients

14.4.1 Quantitative CT Assessment of Airway Wall Dimensions

Small airways (<2 mm in diameter) are the known sites of the major airflow limitation in COPD (Hogg et al. 2004). Though there is great interest in CT measurements of airway dimensions, the actual application of these techniques in the studies of COPD is still not widely used. Nakano and colleagues (2000) have analyzed the right apical segmental bronchus and demonstrated that the percentage of the total airway (lumen plus wall) that was airway wall area (wall area percent) correlated with the FEV_1, FVC, and the RV/TLC, but not the DL_{CO}. The results of the study questioned the role of the small airways considered to be the site flow limitation rather than the relatively large apical segmental bronchus (Hogg et al. 2004). This is further backed up by other histologic data that show that in subjects with COPD there is a thickening of the airway wall in the large airways as well as the small airways (Tiddens et al. 1995). More pronounced thickening of the large airways in patients with symptoms of chronic bronchitis and the presence of a significant familial concordance of airway wall thickening with COPD

encourage further research of airway wall parameters (Fig. 14.34) (Orlandi et al. 2005; Patel et al. 2008).

Recently, the potential association between COPD and tracheobronchomalacia has been investigated (Fig. 14.35) (Lee et al. 2009). Anatomic labeling of the bronchial tree is the next step in the evaluation of the segmented bronchial tree. Intersubject variability in airway anatomy, specifically in the small airways, may complicate this stage, although different techniques have shown promising results in achieving more than 90% accuracy in resolution of the right anatomical label up to the fifth generation (Mori et al. 2000).

14.4.2 Clinical Applications and Limitations of Quantitative CT Assessment of Airway Wall Dimension and Three-Dimensional Airway Algorithm

As discussed previously, distal airways that are responsible for the airflow limitation in COPD are below the resolution of the CT scanner. Two studies

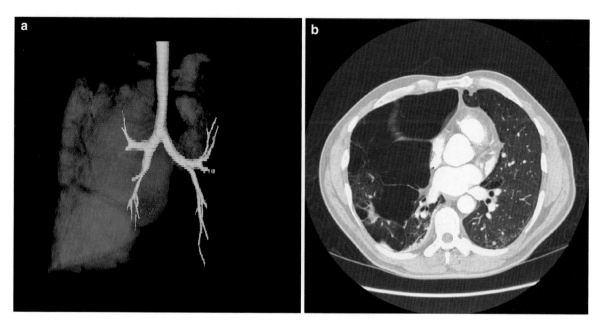

Fig. 14.34 Volume rendering technique for simultaneous three-dimensional evaluation of lung parenchyma (**a, b**) and airways (**c, d**)

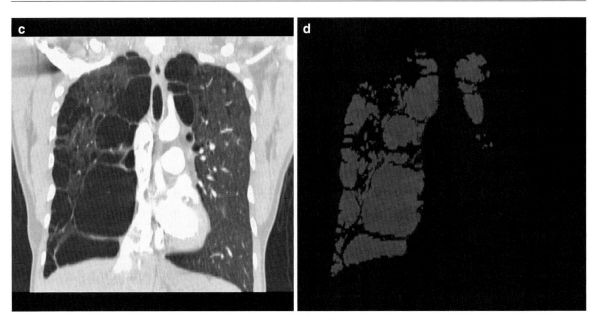

Fig. 14.34 (continued)

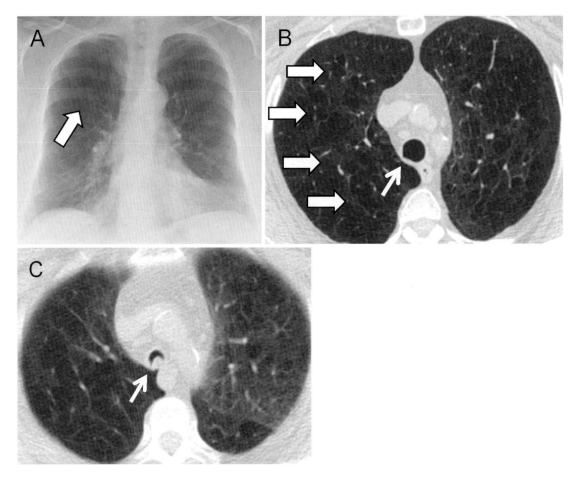

Fig. 14.35 Frontal chest radiograph (**a**), transverse end-inspiration CT section (**b**), and transverse dynamic expiration section (**c**) in a patient with a long-standing history of smoking. Chest radiograph (**a**) shows minimal apical hyperlucencies (*white arrows*) suggesting emphysema, but the true extent of disease is better seen on CT (**b, c**; *thick white arrows*). CT also reveals the presence of a decrease in diameter of the trachea on expiration, a condition known as tracheomalacia (*thin white arrows*)

have examined this problem and have a potential for implication in further clinical practice. Using the two-dimensional approach on trans-axial CT scans, Nakano and coworkers (2005) showed that the wall thickness in the small airways, measured using histology, was correlated with the wall area in the intermediate-sized airways measured with CT. Another study by Hasegawa and colleagues (2006) using three-dimensional reconstructions of the airway walls showed that airway wall dimensions in the smallest airways that were measurable (i.e., sixth generation) had the strongest correlation with FEV_1 compared with larger segmental (third-generation) airways. These studies showed that the sophisticated software measurement of the airways might have future clinical use in general radiologic practice for better understanding of the pathophysiology behind COPD.

Airway analysis still has a long way to go before it becomes practical in the clinical setting. As such, it remains in the research domain and is limited in its applicability.

14.5 Conclusion

Imaging is a robust tool for the analysis of COPD, and the historically important chest radiograph has been mostly replaced by multidetector CT. Cross-sectional imaging provides powerful and reliable measurements regarding not only the lung morphology in COPD, such as the extent and severity of emphysema, lung volumes and density, and airway wall assessment, but it also plays an important role in functional assessment in patients who have COPD. Furthermore, the noninvasive imaging of lung parenchyma and airways has helped with the understanding of the complex interactions between genetics and environmental exposures, and in subdividing the COPD into the major subtypes of predominant airway resistance or predominant increased lung compliance. There are still many challenging aspects of COPD waiting to be investigated, such as relationship between CT lung density and age and gender and ventilation-perfusion abnormalities in COPD. The current spectrum of imaging techniques represents a mixture of mature techniques, such as the evaluation of lung volumes and density, with options still in the "research phase," including airway wall quantitative CT assessment and three-dimensional airway measurements that should be used with

precautions in clinical practice. The current techniques for the evaluation of COPD increase the importance of multidetector row CT beyond the clinical context toward its truly experimental and preclinical research modality.

References

Bankier AA, De Maertelaer V, Keyzer C, Gevenois PA (1999) Pulmonary emphysema: subjective visual grading versus objective quantification with macroscopic morphometry and thin-section CT densitometry. Radiology 211:851–858

Boushy SF, Aboumrad MH, North LB, Helgason AH (1971) Lung recoil pressure, airway resistance, and forced flows related to morphologic emphysema. Am Rev Respir Dis 104:551–561

Calverley PM (2004) The GOLD classification has advanced understanding of COPD. Am J Respir Crit Care Med 170:211–212, discussion 214

Chabat F, Yang GZ, Hansell DM (2003) Obstructive lung diseases: texture classification for differentiation at CT. Radiology 228:871–877

Coxson HO (2008) Quantitative computed tomography assessment of airway wall dimensions: current status and potential applications for phenotyping chronic obstructive pulmonary disease. Proc Am Thorac Soc 5:940–945

Coxson HO, Rogers RM, Whittall KP, D'yachkova Y, Paré PD, Sciurba FC, Hogg JC (1999) A quantification of the lung surface area in emphysema using computed tomography. Am J Respir Crit Care Med 159:851–856

Desai SR, Hansel DM, Walker A, Macdonald SL, Chabat F, Wells AU (2007) Quantification of emphysema: a composite physiologic index derived from CT estimation of disease extent. Eur Radiol 17:911–918

Dunnill MS (1982) The problem of lung growth. Thorax 37:561–563

Gelb AF, Zamel N, Hogg JC, Müller NL, Schein MJ (1998) Pseudophysiologic emphysema resulting from severe small-airways disease. Am J Respir Crit Care Med 158: 815–819

Gevenois PA, Yernault JC (1995) Can computed tomography quantify pulmonary emphysema? Eur Respir J 8:843–848

Gevenois PA, de Maertelaer V, De Vuyst P, Zanen J, Yernault JC (1995) Comparison of computed density and macroscopic morphometry in pulmonary emphysema. Am J Respir Crit Care Med 152:653–657

Gevenois PA, Scilla P, de Maertelaer V, Michils A, De Vuyst P, Yernault JC (1996a) The effects of age, sex, lung size, and hyperinflation on CT lung densitometry. AJR Am J Roentgenol 167:1169–1173

Gevenois PA, Scillia P, de Maertelaer V, Zanen J, Jacobovitz D, Cosio MG, Yernault JC (1996b) Comparison of computed density and microscopic morphometry in pulmonary emphysema. Am J Respir Crit Care Med 154:187–192

Gillooly M, Lamb D (1993) Airspace size in lungs of lifelong non-smokers: effect of age and sex. Thorax 48:39–43

Gough J, Wentworth JE (1949) The use of thin sections of entire organs in morbid anatomical studies. J R Microsc Soc 69:231–235

Gould GA, MacNee W, McLean A, Warren PM, Redpath A, Best JJ, Lamb D, Flenley DC (1988) CT measurements of lung density in life can quantitate distal airspace enlargement – an essential defining feature of human emphysema. Am Rev Respir Dis 137:380–392

Hasegawa M, Nasuhara Y, Onodera Y, Makita H, Nagai K, Fuke S, Ito Y, Betsuyaku T, Nishimura M (2006) Airflow limitation and airway dimensions in chronic obstructive pulmonary disease. Am J Respir Crit Care Med 173:1309–1315

Hayhurst MD, MacNee W, Flenley DC, Wright D, McLean A, Lamb D, Wightman AJ, Best J (1984) Diagnosis of pulmonary emphysema by computerised tomography. Lancet 2: 320–322

Hoffman EA, McLennan G (1997) Assessment of the pulmonary structure-function relationship and clinical outcomes measures: quantitative volumetric CT of the lung. Acad Radiol 4:758–776

Hogg JC, Chu F, Utokaparch S, Woods R, Elliott WM, Buzatu L, Cherniack RM, Rogers RM, Sciurba FC, Coxson HO, Pare PD (2004) The nature of small-airway obstruction in chronic obstructive pulmonary disease. N Engl J Med 350:2645–2653

Hruban RH, Meziane MA, Zerhouni EA, Khouri NF, Fishman EK, Wheeler PS, Dumler JS, Hutchins GM (1987) High resolution computed tomography of inflation-fixed lungs. Pathologic-radiologic correlation of centrilobular emphysema. Am Rev Respir Dis 136:935–940

Kalender WA, Fichte H, Bautz W, Skalej M (1991) Semiautomatic evaluation procedures for quantitative CT of the lung. J Comput Assist Tomogr 15:248–255

Knudson RJ, Standen JR, Kaltenborn WT, Knudson DE, Rehm K, Habib MP, Newell JD (1991) Expiratory computed tomography for assessment of suspected pulmonary emphysema. Chest 99:1357–1366

Kuwano KM, Matsuba K, Ikeda T, Murakami J, Araki A, Nishitani H, Ishida T, Yasumoto K, Shigematsu N (1990) The diagnosis of mild emphysema. Correlation of computed tomography and pathology scores. Am Rev Respir Dis 141:169–178

Lee EY, Litmanovich D, Boiselle PM (2009) Multidetector CT in evaluation of tracheobronchomalacia. Radiol Clin North Am 47:261–269

Madani A, Keyzer C, Gevenois PA (2001) Quantitative computed tomography assessment of lung structure and function in pulmonary emphysema. Eur Respir J 18:720–730

Madani A, Zanen J, de Maertelaer V, Gevenois PA (2006) Pulmonary emphysema: objective quantification at multidetector row CT – comparison with macroscopic and microscopic morphometry. Radiology 238:1036–1043

Madani A, De Maertelaer V, Zanen J, Gevenois PA (2007) Pulmonary emphysema: radiation dose and section thickness at multidetector CT quantification – comparison with macroscopic and microscopic morphometry. Radiology 243:250–257

Madani A, Van Muylem A, de Maertelaer V, Zanen J, Gevenois PA (2008) Pulmonary emphysema: size distribution of emphysematous spaces on multidetector CT images – comparison with macroscopic and microscopic morphometry. Radiology 248:1036–1041

Mayo JR, Aldrich J, Muller NL (2003) Radiation exposure at chest CT: a statement of the Fleischner Society. Radiology 228:15–21

McLean A, Warren PM, Gillooly M, MacNee W, Lamb D (1992) Microscopic and macroscopic measurements of emphysema: relation to carbon monoxide gas transfer. Thorax 47:144–149

Miller RR, Muller NL, Vedal S, Morrison NJ, Staples CA (1989) Limitations of computed tomography in the assessment of emphysema. Am Rev Respir Dis 139:980–983

Mishima M, Hirai T, Itoh H, Nakano Y, Sakai H, Muro S, Nishimura K, Oku Y, Chin K, Ohi M, Nakamura T, Bates JH, Alencar AM, Suki B (1999a) Complexity of terminal airspace geometry assessed by lung computed tomography in normal subjects and patients with chronic obstructive pulmonary disease. Proc Natl Acad Sci USA 96:8829–8834

Mishima M, Itoh H, Sakai H, Nakano Y, Muro S, Hirai T, Takubo Y, Chin K, Ohi M, Nishimura K, Yamaguchi K, Nakamura T (1999b) Optimized scanning conditions of high resolution CT in the follow-up of pulmonary emphysema. J Comput Assist Tomogr 23:380–384

Mori K, Hasegawa J, Suenaga Y, Toriwaki J (2000) Automated anatomical labeling of the bronchial branch and its application to the virtual bronchoscopy system. IEEE Trans Med Imaging 19:103–114

Müller NL, Coxson H (2002) Chronic obstructive pulmonary disease. 4: imaging the lungs in patients with chronic obstructive pulmonary disease. Thorax 57:982–985

Müller NL, Staples CA, Miller RR, Abboud RT (1988) "Density mask". An objective method to quantitate emphysema using computed tomography. Chest 94:782–787

Murata K, Itoh H, Todo G, Kanaoka M, Noma S, Itoh T, Furuta M, Asamoto H, Torizuka K (1986) Centrilobular lesions of the lung: demonstration by high-resolution CT and pathologic correlation. Radiology 161:641–645

Murata K, Khan A, Herman PG (1989) Pulmonary parenchymal disease: evaluation with high-resolution CT. Radiology 170:629–635

Nakano Y, Muro S, Sakai H, Hirai T, Chin K, Tsukino M, Nishimura K, Itoh H, Pare PD, Hogg JC, Mishima M (2000) Computed tomographic measurements of airway dimensions and emphysema in smokers. Correlation with lung function. Am J Respir Crit Care Med 162: 1102–1108

Nakano Y, Wong JC, de Jong PA, Buzatu L, Nagao T, Coxson HO, Elliott WM, Hogg JC, Pare PD (2005) The prediction of small airway dimensions using computed tomography. Am J Respir Crit Care Med 171:142–146

Nishimura K, Murata K, Yamagishi M, Itoh H, Ikeda A, Tsukino M, Koyama H, Sakai N, Mishima M, Izumi T (1998) Comparison of different computed tomography scanning methods for quantifying emphysema. J Thorac Imaging 13:193–198

Orlandi I, Moroni C, Camiciottoli G, Bartolucci M, Pistolesi M, Villari N, Mascalchi M (2005) Chronic obstructive pulmonary disease: thin-section CT measurement of airway wall thickness and lung attenuation. Radiology 234: 604–610

Patel BD, Coxson HO, Pillai SG, Agusti AG, Calverley PM, Donner CF, Make BJ, Muller NL, Rennard SI, Vestbo J, Wouters EF, Hiorns MP, Nakano Y, Camp PG, Nasute Fauerbach PV, Screaton NJ, Campbell EJ, Anderson WH, Pare PD, Levy RD, Lake SL, Silverman EK, Lomas DA (2008) Airway wall thickening and emphysema show independent familial aggregation in chronic obstructive pulmonary disease. Am J Respir Crit Care Med 178:500–505

Pauwels RA, Buist AS, Ma P, Jenkins CR, Hurd SS (2001) Global strategy for the diagnosis, management, and prevention of chronic obstructive pulmonary disease: National Heart, Lung, and Blood Institute and World Health Organization Global Initiative for Chronic Obstructive Lung Disease (GOLD): executive summary. Respir Care 46: 798–825

Pugatch RD (1983) The radiology of emphysema. Clin Chest Med 4:433–442

Rabe KF, Hurd S, Anzueto A, Barnes PJ, Buist SA, Calverley P, Fukuchi Y, Jenkins C, Rodriguez-Roisin R, van Weel C, Zielinski J (2007) Global strategy for the diagnosis, management, and prevention of chronic obstructive pulmonary disease: GOLD executive summary. Am J Respir Crit Care Med 176:532–555

Remy-Jardin M, Remy J, Gosselin BC, Copin MC, Wurtz A, Duhamel A (1996) Sliding thin slab, minimum intensity projection technique in the diagnosis of emphysema: histopathologic-CT correlation. Radiology 200:665–671

Snider GL, Kleinerman JL, Thurlbeck WM, Bengali ZH (1985) The definition of emphysema: report of a National Heart, Lung, and Blood Institute, Division of Lung Disease Workshop. Am Rev Respir Dis 132:182–183

Soejima K, Yamaguchi K, Kohda E, Takeshita K, Ito Y, Mastubara H, Oguma T, Inoue T, Okubo Y, Amakawa K, Tateno H, Shiomi T (2000) Longitudinal follow-up study of smoking-induced lung density changes by high-resolution computed tomography. Am J Respir Crit Care Med 161:1264–1273

Sutinen S, Christoforidis AJ, Klugh GA, Pratt PC (1965) Roentgenologic criteria for the recognition of nonsym-ptomatic pulmonary emphysema. Correlation between roentgenologic findings and pulmonary pathology. Am Rev Respir Dis 91:69–76

Thurlbeck WM (1967) The internal surface area of nonemphysematous lungs. Am Rev Respir Dis 95:765–773

Thurlbeck WM, Müller NL (1994) Emphysema: definition, imaging, and quantification. AJR Am J Roentgenol 163:1017–1025

Thurlbeck WM, Simon G (1978) Radiographic appearance of the chest in emphysema. AJR Am J Roentgenol 130:429–440

Thurlbeck WM, Dunnill MS, Hartung W, Heard BE, Heppleston AG, Ryder RC (1970) A comparison of three methods of measuring emphysema. Hum Pathol 1:215–226

Tiddens HA, Pare PD, Hogg JC, Hop WC, Lambert R, de Jongste JC (1995) Cartilaginous airway dimensions and airflow obstruction in human lungs. Am J Respir Crit Care Med 152:260–266

Tschirren J, Hoffman EA, McLennan G, Sonka M (2005) Intrathoracic airway trees: segmentation and airway morphology analysis from low-dose CT scans. IEEE Trans Med Imaging 24:1529–1539

Turner P, Whimster WF (1981) Volume of emphysema. Thorax 36:932–937

Uppaluri R, Mitsa T, Sonka M, Hoffman EA, McLennan G (1997) Quantification of pulmonary emphysema from lung computed tomography images. Am J Respir Crit Care Med 156:248–254

Webb WR, Stein MG, Finkbeiner WE, Im JG, Lynch D, Gamsu G (1988) Normal and diseased isolated lungs: high-resolution CT. Radiology 166:81–87

Missed Lung Lesions

Nigel Howarth and Denis Tack

15

Contents

Abstract

> Missed lung lesions are one of the most frequent causes of malpractice issues. The clinical value of the chest X-ray is uncontested despite recent advances in technology, in particular multi-detector computed tomography (MDCT). The chest X-ray remains the most frequently requested radiologic examination and plays an important role in the detection of and management of patients with chest diseases. The skills for accurate interpretation of the chest X-ray are often lacking due to the pressures required for mastering and making profitable high technology imaging. Missing a lung lesion, especially lung cancer, can carry medico-legal implications. Many methods have been suggested for correct interpretation of the chest X-ray, but there is no preferred or recommended system. A systematic approach that addresses a clinical question is always helpful and being aware of the areas where mistakes are made is essential. By focusing on a side-by-side comparison of the chest X-ray and MDCT of common missed lung lesions, this chapter aims to provide an understanding of the reasons certain lesions are missed and help to reduce the busy radiologist's error rate.

N. Howarth (✉)
Institut de radiologie, Clinique des Grangettes - Genève,
7, chemin des Grangettes, 1224 Chêne-Bougeries Geneva,
Switzerland
e-mail: nigel.howarth@grangettes.ch

D. Tack
Department of Radiology, RHMS Clinique Louis Caty,
Rue Louis Caty 136, 7331 Baudour, Belgium

15.1 Introduction

Missed lung lesions are one of the most frequent causes of malpractice issues (Berlin 1986, 1995; Potchen and Bisesi 1990). Chest radiography plays an important role in the detection of and management of patients with lung cancer, chronic airway disease, pneumonia, and interstitial lung disease. Among all diagnostic tests, chest radiography is essential to confirm or exclude the diagnosis of most chest diseases. However, numerous lesions of a wide variety of disease processes affecting the thorax may be missed on a chest radiograph. For example, the frequency of missed lung carcinoma on chest radiographs can vary from 12% to 90%, depending on the study design (Quekel et al. 1999). Despite lack of convincing evidence that screening for lung cancer with the chest radiograph improves mortality, chest radiography is still requested for this purpose (Melamed 2000; Marcus 2001). The chest radiograph will also help narrow a differential diagnosis, help to direct additional diagnostic measures, and serve during follow-up. The diagnostic usefulness of the radiograph will be maximized by the integration of the radiologic findings with the clinical features of the individual patient (Aideyan et al. 1995). In this chapter we will review the more important radiologic principles regarding missed lung lesions in a variety of common chest diseases, with a special focus on how correlation with multi-detector computed tomography (MDCT) of missed lung lesions can help improve interpretation of the plain chest radiograph.

15.2 Reasons for Missed Lung Lesions

Conditions contributing to missed lung lesions, especially carcinomas, have been extensively studied (Carmody et al. 1980; Berlin 1986; Potchen and Bisesi 1990; Austin et al. 1992; Quekel et al. 1999; Turkington et al. 2002). Poor viewing conditions, hasty visual tracking, interruptions, inadequate image quality, and observer inexperience are amongst the most important (Carmody et al. 1980; Woodring 1990; Austin et al. 1992; Monnier-Cholley et al. 2001; Krupinski et al. 2003). When looking at nodules, features of lesions themselves, such as location, size, border characteristics and conspicuity, also play a role (Woodring 1990; Austin et al. 1992). Missing lung nodules during initial reading of a chest radiograph are not uncommon. One estimate is that nearly 30% of lung nodules may be overlooked (Samei et al. 1999). Missing a nodule that may represent malignancy will have adverse consequences on patient management, essentially through delayed diagnosis, which may carry medico-legal implications. A number of authors have explored the reasons why lesions are overlooked (Kundel et al.

1989; Samuel et al. 1995; Quekel et al. 2001; Tsubamoto et al. 2002; Shah et al. 2003; Samei et al. 2003). Specific studies have focused on size (Kelsey et al. 1977; Kimme-Smith et al. 1996; Krupinski et al. 2003), contrast gradient (Kundel et al. 1979), conspicuity (Kundel 1975; Revesz and Kundel 1977), and anatomic noise (Kundel and Revesz 1976).

A more recent study (Wu et al. 2008) examined the imaging features of non–small-cell lung carcinoma overlooked during review of digital chest radiography and compared general and thoracic radiologists' performance for lung carcinoma detection. Frontal and lateral chest radiographs from 30 consecutive patients with lung carcinoma that was overlooked during an initial reading and 30 normal controls were submitted to two blinded thoracic radiologists and three blinded general radiologists for retrospective review. The location, size, histopathology, borders, presence of superimposed structures, and lesion opacity were recorded. Interobserver agreement was calculated and detection performance of thoracic and general radiologists was compared. The average size of carcinomas that were missed by the thoracic radiologists was 18.1 mm (range, 10–32 mm). The average size missed by general radiologists was 27.7 mm (range, 12–60 mm). Seventy-one percent (5 of 7) of the missed lesions were obscured by anatomical superimposition. Forty-three percent of lesions were located in the upper lobes, and 63% were adenocarcinomas. Compared with general radiologists, the lesions missed by thoracic radiologists tended to be smaller but also had significantly lower CT density measurements and more commonly had an ill-defined margin. The clinical stage of the overlooked lesions did not differ between the two groups ($p = 0.480$). The authors concluded that the lesion size, location, conspicuity, and histopathology of lesions overlooked on digital chest radiography were similar to those missed on conventional film–screen techniques. Several other studies on the subject have led to similar conclusions (Herman and Hessel 1975; Kundel and Revesz 1976; Kelsey et al. 1977; Bass and Chiles 1990; Aideyan et al. 1995; Sone et al. 2000; Yang et al. 2001).

The detection of carcinoma on a chest radiograph remains difficult, with implications on patient management. Overlooking chronic airway disease, pneumonia, and interstitial lung disease may not have the same potential medico-legal implications, but the consequences on patient care could be critical.

We propose to review how correlations with MDCT of missed lung lesions can help improve interpretation of the plain chest radiograph. During the course of clinical work, when reporting chest CT, every effort should be made to review previous chest radiographs and their reports, thereby providing one of the best learning tools for chest radiograph interpretation.

A CT scan can be performed in patients with a negative chest radiograph when there is a high clinical suspicion of chest disease. CT, especially high-resolution CT (HRCT), is more sensitive than plain films for the evaluation of interstitial disease, bilateral disease, cavitation, empyema, and hilar adenopathy. CT is not generally recommended for routine use because the data for its use in chronic airway disease and pneumonia are limited, the cost is high, and there is no evidence that outcome is improved. Thus, a chest radiograph is the preferred method for initial imaging, with CT reserved for further characterization (e.g., evaluation of pattern and distribution, detection of cavitation, adenopathy, mass lesions, or collections).

Many methods have been suggested for correct interpretation of the chest radiograph. There is no preferred scheme or recommended system. The clinical question should always be addressed. An inquisitive approach is always helpful, and being aware of the areas where mistakes are made is essential. Hidden abnormalities can thus be looked for. The difficult "hidden areas" that must be checked are the lung apex and areas superimposed over the heart, around each hilum, and below the diaphragm. We will concentrate on difficult areas such as lesions at the lung apices or bases and lesions adjacent to or obscured by the hila or heart. For a systematic approach, we will divide the review into three sections representing specific problems: missed nodules, missed consolidations, and missed interstitial lung diseases.

15.3 Specific Problems

Specific problems of missed lung lesions can be divided into missed nodules, missed consolidation, and missed interstitial lung disease. In cases of a missed nodule or missed consolidation, the overlooked pathology may have been detected if special attention was paid to known "difficult areas." The examples that follow will show how a side-by-side comparison of the chest radiograph and CT images improves our understanding of the overlooked lesion. There is no harm done by learning from one's mistakes!

15.4 Missed Nodules

15.4.1 Nodular Lesions – Tumors

Nodular lesions are frequently caused by lung cancer, which may be primary or secondary. Lung cancer is probably one of the most common lung diseases that radiologists encounter in practice. Berbaum (1995) formulated the concept that perception is better if you know where to look and what to look for. Our first example is that of a 53-year-old man who complained of pain in the right axilla for 4 months and underwent chest radiography. The posteroanterior and lateral radiographs were interpreted as showing normal findings (Fig. 15.1a and b). The subsequent MDCT showed a right superior sulcus mass with rib destruction (Figs. 15.1c and d). The coronal and sagittal reformats demonstrated more precisely the lesion delineation (Figs. 15.1e–j). Needle biopsy (Fig. 15.1k) established a diagnosis of bronchogenic carcinoma (adenocarcinoma). Hindsight bias (Berlin 2000) with the information available from the MDCT makes the initial lesion extremely obvious. Careful scrutiny of both apices is essential when reporting a frontal chest radiograph.

Radiologic errors can be divided into two types (Berlin 2001): cognitive, in which an abnormality is seen but its nature is misinterpreted, and perceptual, or the "miss," in which a radiologic abnormality is not seen by the radiologist during initial interpretation. The perceptual type is estimated to account for approximately 80% of radiologic errors (Berlin and Hendrix 1998). Our second example shows how conspicuity influences perception and how this is determined by a combination of size, density, location, and overlying structures rather than any one of these factors alone. A 50-year-old woman with known breast cancer underwent chest radiography as part of a routine follow-up. A single nodule was reported in the right lung (Fig. 15.2a). MDCT showed bilateral nodules; the left upper lobe nodule was "missed" because of the overlying rib (Fig. 15.2b and c). The coronal reformats demonstrated more clearly the position of each nodule on the chest radiograph (Fig. 15.2d and e). The 3-month (Fig. 15.2f) and 6-month (Fig. 15.2g) follow-up chest radiographs after chemotherapy showed a decrease in the size and the density of the right lung nodule and the "disappearance" of the then-known left lung nodule. The follow-up MDCT at 6 months, however, showed that the left lung nodule persisted unchanged (Fig. 15.2h and i). The patient underwent surgical resection of both lesions, with a final

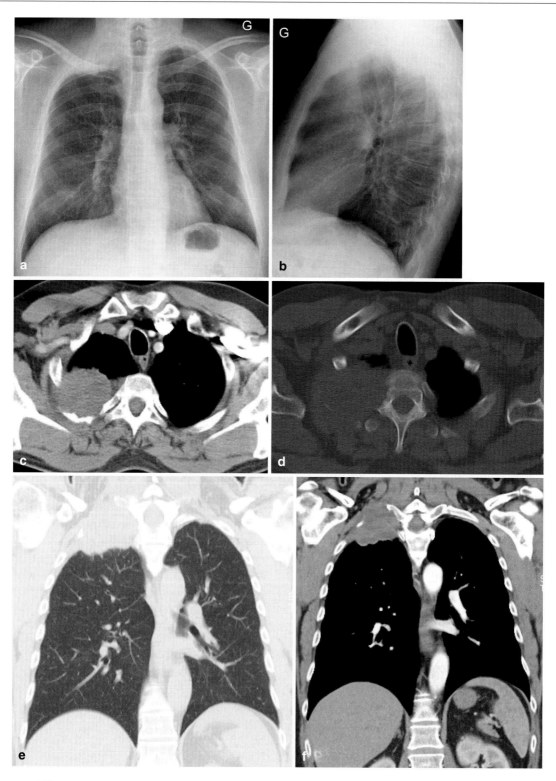

Fig. 15.1 Fifty-three-year-old man who underwent chest radiography for pain in the right axilla. (**a** and **b**) Posterioranterior (**a**) and lateral (**b**) radiographs interpreted as normal. With hindsight bias from multi-detector CT (MDCT), the right apical mass is obvious. (**c** and **d**) MDCT axial images with soft tissue (**c**) and bone (**d**) windows showing a right apical mass with bone destruction. (**e**, **f**, and **g**) Coronal reformats (lung window (**e**), soft tissue window (**f**), magnified view (**g**)) and (**h**, **i**, **j**) Sagittal reformats (lung window (**h**), bone tissue window (**i**), magnified view (**j**)) improve lesion delineation. (**k**) CT-guided needle biopsy established a diagnosis of bronchogenic carcinoma (adenocarcinoma)

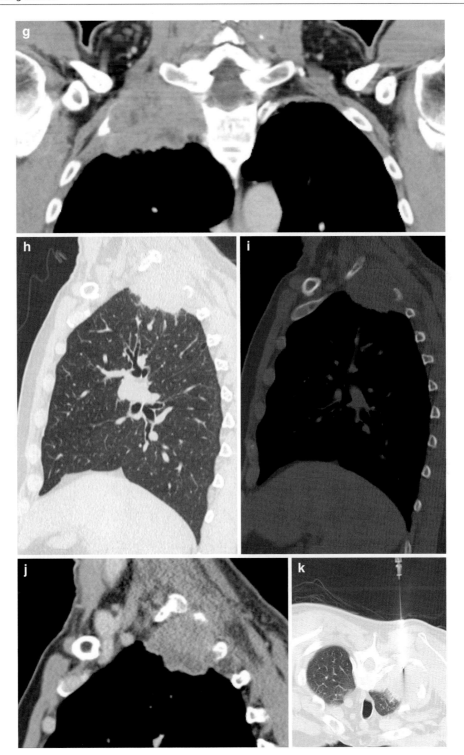

Fig. 15.1 (continued)

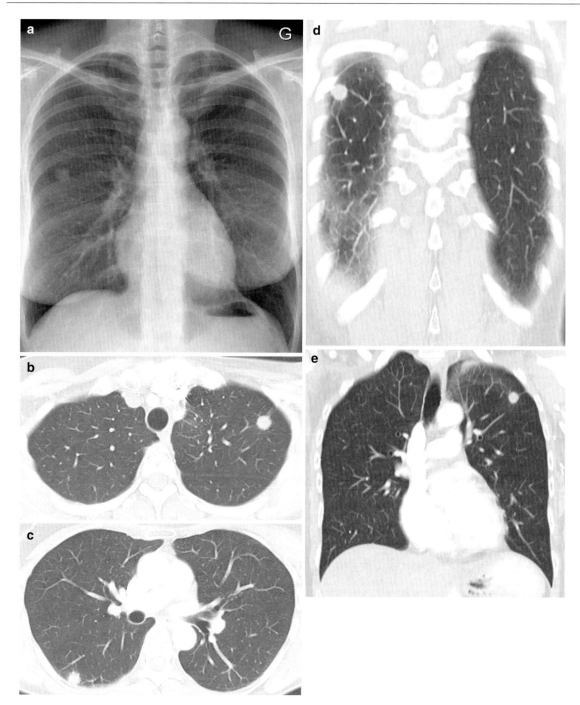

Fig. 15.2 Fifty-year-old woman with known breast cancer who underwent chest radiography as a part of a routine follow-up. (**a**) Posteroanterior radiograph clearly showing a right lung nodule. The left lung nodule is seen overlying the anterior second rib and posterior fifth rib with hindsight after multi-detector CT (MDCT). (**b** and **c**) Two lung nodules are identified by MDCT (axial images, lung window). (**d** and **e**) Coronal reformats (lung window) show the position of each nodule. (**f** and **g**) Posteroanterior radiographs at 3-month (**f**) and 6-month (**g**) follow-up after chemotherapy. The size and density of the right lung nodule have decreased ; the left lung nodule has « disappeared ». (**h** and **i**) Coronal reformats from MDCT at 6-months show that the left lung nodule persists unchanged

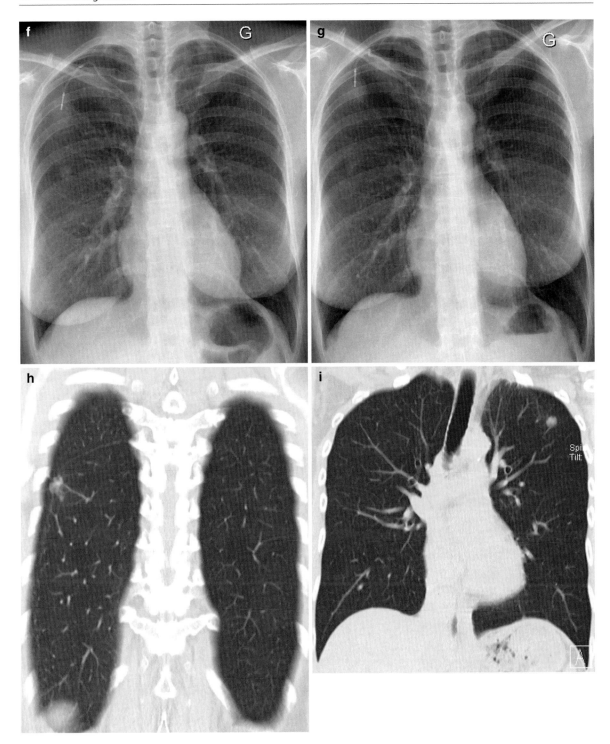

Fig. 15.2 (continued)

histologic diagnosis of breast cancer metastasis in the right lung and fibrous tissue with pleural plaque in the left lung. In this case, "missing" the left lung lesion on the chest radiograph was not so dramatic!

Our third patient illustrates the complexity of the detection of a lung nodule close to the hilum. A 77-year-old man with known prostate cancer underwent chest radiography for right upper quadrant abdominal pain (Fig. 15.3a and b). The radiographs were reported as normal. Subsequent MDCT revealed liver metastases as the cause of the abdominal pain and a 13-mm lung nodule in the superior segment of the lingula (Fig. 15.3c and d). The coronal and sagittal reformats demonstrate the position of the nodule

(Fig. 15.3e and f), which, in hindsight, can be seen clearly on the posteroanterior and lateral chest radiographs.

15.4.2 Nodular Lesions – Infections

Nodular lesions attributed to pulmonary infections are seen most often in nosocomial pneumonias and in immunocompromised patients. They may be caused by bacteria such as *Nocardia asteroides* and *Mycobacterium. tuberculosis,* septic emboli, and fungi. *N. asteroides* causes single or nodular infiltrates with or without

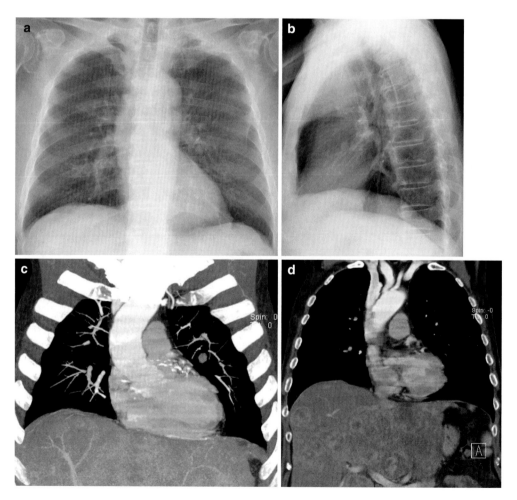

Fig. 15.3 Seventy-seven-year-old man with right upper quadrant pain. (**a**) and (**b**) Posterioranterior (**a**) and lateral (**b**) radiographs interpreted as normal. With hindsight, the 13 mm nodule in the superior segment of the lingula can be seen. (**c** and **d**) Coronal

reformat from multi-detector CT (MDCT) (soft tissue window) shows a nodule in the lingula and multiple liver metastases. (**e**) and (**f**) Coronal (**e**) and sagittal (**f**) reformats (lung window) show the position of the lingular nodule, close to the hilum

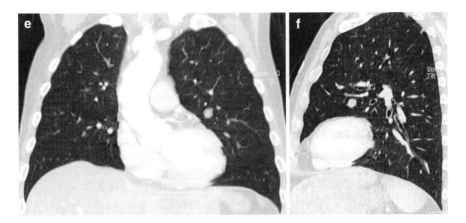

Fig. 15.3 (continued)

cavitation. Invasive pulmonary aspergillosis (IPA), *Mucor*, and *Cryptococcus neoformans* may present with single or multiple nodular infiltrates, which often progress to wedge-shaped areas of consolidation. Cavitation (the "crescent sign") is common later in the course of the infiltrate. In the appropriate clinical setting, CT may aid in the diagnosis of IPA by demonstrating the so-called halo sign. Figure 15.4 shows a scan of a 43-year-old woman with fever after a bone marrow transplant. The posteroranterior radiograph was interpreted as normal (Fig. 15.4a). On hindsight, a subtle infiltrate can be seen at the left apex. Conspicuity is lessened by the overlying clavicle and first rib. Axial CT image (Fig. 15.4b) shows nodular consolidation with crescentic cavitation (the "crescent sign") and surrounding ground-glass infiltrate (the "halo sign"). These characteristic findings of IPA are best identified using CT.

15.4.3 Nodular Lesions – Miscellaneous

A lesion of the chest wall may be mistaken for a parenchymal abnormality, sometimes leading to inappropriate patient care. Figure 15.5 shows a 33-year-old cocaine abuser who presented with a cough. The posteroranterior and lateral radiographs were interpreted as showing right upper lobe consolidation (Fig. 15.5a and b). MDCT was requested after follow-up radiographs showed no change following a course of antibiotics. Coronal and sagittal reformats (Fig. 15.5c and d) and 3-dimensional surface renderings (Fig. 15.5e and f) demonstrate a lesion of the right second rib suggestive of fibrous dysplasia. Such an interpretation can be considered a cognitive error rather than perceptual error (Berlin 2001).

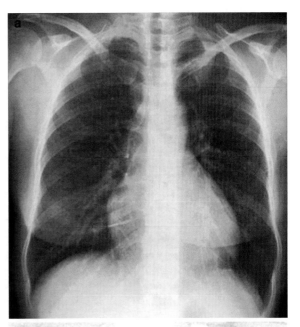

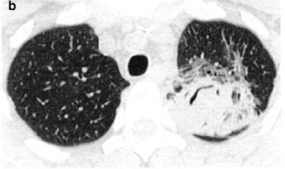

Fig. 15.4 Forty-three-year-old woman with fever after a bone marrow transplant. (**a**) Posteroranterior radiograph interpreted as normal. With hindsight, a subtle infiltrate can be seen at the left apex. Conspicuity is lessened by the overlying clavicle and first rib. Also note the in-dwelling catheter from the left brachial vein to the superior vena cava. (**b**) Axial CT image (lung window) shows nodular consolidation with crescentic cavitation (the « air-crescent » sign) and surrounding ground-glass infiltrate (the « halo » sign)

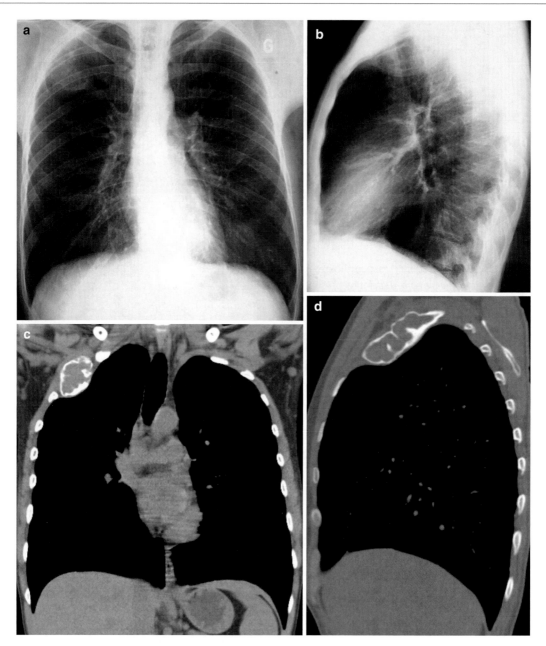

Fig. 15.5 Thirty-three-year-old man with cough and fever. (**a**) and (**b**) Posterioranterior (**a**) and lateral (**b**) radiographs interpreted as showing right upper lobe consolidation (example of a cognitive error). (**c** and **d**) Coronal (**c**) and sagittal (**d**) refor- mats showing a lesion of the right second rib. (**e** and **f**) 3D sur- face renderings clearly demonstrating the bony abnormality of the chest wall

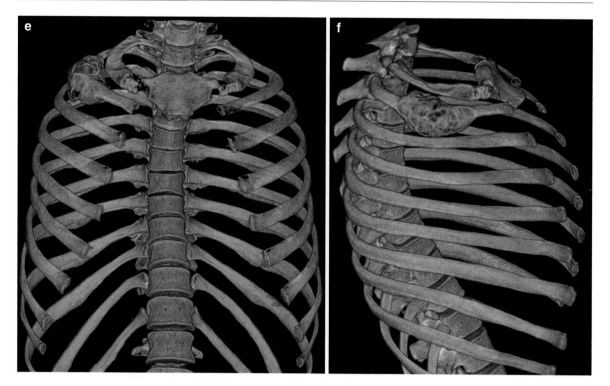

Fig. 15.5 (continued)

15.5 Missed Consolidation

15.5.1 Airspace Disease

Airspace disease is usually caused by bacterial infections. However, airspace disease can be seen in viral, protozoal, and fungal infections as well as malignancies, typically brochioloalveolar carcinoma (Jung et al. 2001). Acute airspace pneumonia is characterized by a mostly homogeneous consolidation of lung parenchyma, well-defined borders, and does not typically respect segmental boundaries. An air bronchogram is common. Progression to lobar consolidation may occur. As with lung nodules, whether consolidation is detected or missed on the plain chest radiograph may be determined by any combination of the same factors of size, density, location, and overlying structures. Location is a significant factor for missed consolidation (Melbye and Dale 1992; Albaum et al. 1996). Consolidation in the middle lobe and both lower lobes can be difficult to diagnose, especially when only the posterioranterior view is obtained (Chotas and Ravin 1994). Figure 15.6 shows a scan of a 46-year-old woman with cough and right-sided chest pain. The posteroanterior radiograph was interpreted as normal (Fig. 15.6a). Because of a clinical suspicion of pulmonary embolism, MDCT was requested and showed consolidation in the anterior segment of the right lower lobe (Fig. 15.6b and c). The coronal and sagittal reformats demonstrate the extent of the consolidation (Fig. 15.6d and e). There were no signs of pulmonary embolism on the contrast media study. A diagnosis of right lower lobe pneumonia was established, and the patient was treated successfully with antibiotics.

Chest radiography is the most frequently performed diagnostic investigation requested by general practitioners in Europe (Woodhead et al. 1996). Chest radiography is considered the gold standard for the diagnosis of pneumonia. Chest radiography can diagnose pneumonia when an infiltrate is present and differentiate pneumonia from other conditions that may present with similar symptoms, such as acute bronchitis. The results of the chest radiograph may occasionally suggest a specific etiology (for example, a lung abscess), and identify a complication (empyema) or coexisting abnormalities (bronchiectasis, bronchial obstruction, interstitial lung disease). Chest radiography remains a valuable diagnostic tool for use in primary care patients who are clinically suspected of having pneumonia and can substantially

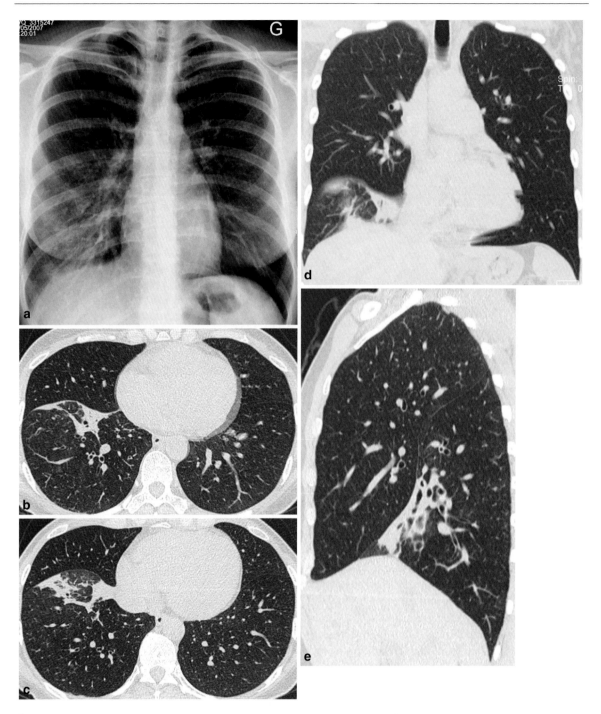

Fig. 15.6 Forty-six-year-old woman with cough and right-sided chest pain. (**a**) Posterioranterior radiograph interpreted as normal. (**b** and **c**) Axial CT images showing consolidation in the anterior segment of the right lower lobe. (**d** and **e**) Coronal (**d**) and sagittal (**e**) reformats showing the extent of the consolidation

reduce the number of patients who are misdiagnosed (Speets et al. 2006). MDCT imaging is useful for patients who have community-acquired pneumonia when there is an unresolved or complicated chest radiograph, and at times is useful for immunocompromised patients who are suspected of having pulmonary infections. MDCT can help to differentiate infectious from noninfectious abnormalities. MDCT may detect empyema, cavitation, and lymphadenopathy when the chest radiograph cannot. MDCT should be performed in immunocompromised patients who are clinically suspected of having pneumonia when the chest radiograph is normal. This is

especially true when the early diagnosis of pneumonia is critical, as is the case in immunocompromised and severely ill patients (Heussel et al. 2004).

Figure 15.7 shows a scan from a 38-year-old immunocompromised man presenting with fever. The posteroanterior and lateral radiographs (Fig. 15.7a and b) were interpreted as showing a perihilar reticular infiltrate with right upper lobe consolidation. MDCT was requested to further characterize the infiltrate, and it revealed ground-glass opacification with bilateral lung cysts (Fig. 15.7c–e). Pneumocystic pneumonia was confirmed by bronchoalveolar lavage.

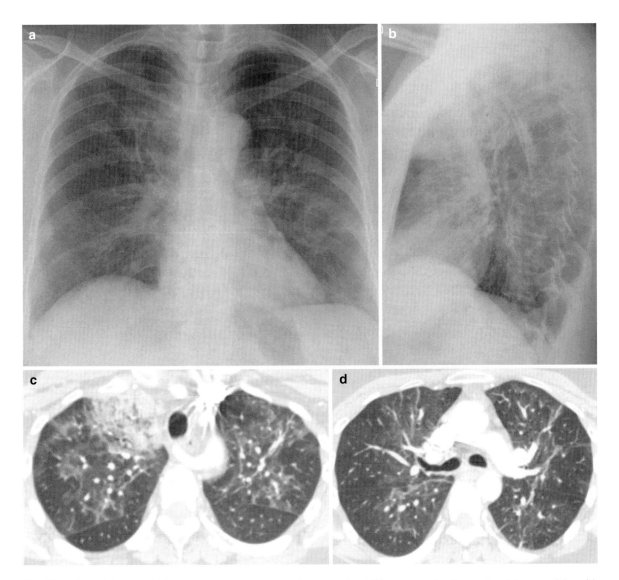

Fig. 15.7 Thiry-eight-year-old immunocompromised man with a fever. (**a** and **b**) Posterioranterior (**a**) and lateral (**b**) radiographs showing a perihilar reticular infiltrate with right upper lobe consolidation. (**c**, **d**, and **e**) Axial CT images showing bilateral lung cysts in addition to consolidation in the right upper lobe with patchy ground-glass opacification in both lungs. Pneumocystis pneumonia was confirmed by bronchoalveolar lavage

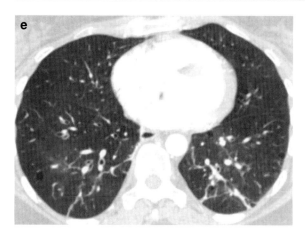

Fig. 15.7 (continued)

15.6 Missed Interstitial Lung Disease

15.6.1 Diffuse (Interstitial or Mixed Alveolar Interstitial) Lung Disease

Diffuse lung disease presenting with widely distributed patchy infiltrates or interstitial reticular or nodular abnormalities can be produced by a number of disease entities. An attempt is usually made to separate the group of idiopathic interstitial pneumonias from known causes such as infections, associated systemic disease, or drugs related. The most common infectious organisms

are viruses and protozoa. In general, the etiology of an underlying pneumonia cannot be specifically diagnosed because the patterns overlap. It is beyond the aim of this chapter to discuss in detail the contribution of MDCT to the diagnosis of diffuse infiltrative lung disease (refer to Chap. 7). The development of HRCT has resulted in markedly improved diagnostic accuracy in acute and chronic diffuse infiltrative lung disease (Mathieson et al. 1989; Grenier et al. 1991; Padley et al. 1991; Webb et al. 2001). The chest radiograph remains the preliminary radiological investigation of patients who have diffuse lung disease, but it is often nonspecific. Pattern recognition in diffuse lung disease has been the subject of controversy for many years. Extensive disease may be required before an appreciable change in radiographic density or an abnormal radiographic pattern can be detected on the plain chest radiograph. At least 10% of patients who ultimately are found to have biopsy-proven diffuse lung disease have an apparently normal chest radiograph (Epler et al. 1978). HRCT and now MDCT have become integral components of the clinical investigation of patients who have suspected or established interstitial lung disease. These techniques have had a major impact on clinical practice (Flaherty et al. 2004; Aziz et al. 2005).

To end with a specific and striking example of the contribution of MDCT to patient management, Fig. 15.8 shows the preoperative chest radiograph (Fig. 15.8a) and subsequent MDCT (Fig. 15.8b–d) of

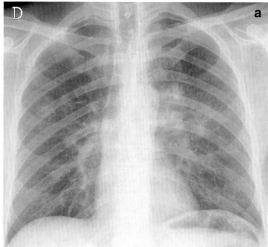

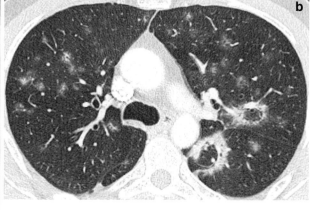

Fig. 15.8 Forty-five-year-old man with renal cancer and no chest symptoms. (**a**) Preoperative posterioranterior radiograph showing bilateral ill-defined nodular ground-glass opacification. (**b**) Axial CT image shows nodular ground-glass opacification, with crescentic or ring-shaped opacities, representing an unusual CT feature encountered in organizing pneumonia. (**c** and **d**) Coronal reformats show the CT feature more clearly, referred to as a reversed halo sign or "atoll" sign. (**e** and **f**) Coronal reformats showing normal lung after six months of corticosteroid therapy

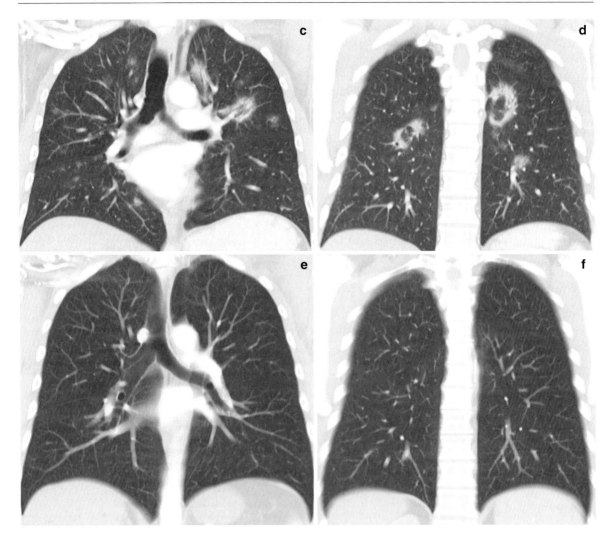

Fig. 15.8 (continued)

a 45-year-old man who was recently diagnosed with renal cancer and had no symptoms of chest disease. On axial CT (Fig. 15.8b), nodular (crescentic or ring-shaped) ground-glass opacities are seen representing an unusual CT feature encountered in organizing pneumonia (Ujita et al. 2004). The reformats (Fig. 15.8c and d) show more clearly this feature, referred to as a reversed halo sign or "atoll" sign (Zompatori et al. 1999). Organizing pneumonia was confirmed by transthoracic needle biopsy of the largest lesion in the apical segment of the left lower lobe. After renal surgery and six months of corticosteroid therapy, the pulmonary infiltrates resolved completely (Fig. 15.8e and f).

15.7 Take Home Messages

Despite the increasing use of CT imaging in the diagnosis of patients who have chest disorders, chest radiography is still the primary imaging method for patients who have suspected chest disease. The presence of an infiltrate on a chest radiograph is considered to be the "gold standard" for diagnosing pneumonia. Extensive knowledge of the radiographic appearance of pulmonary disorders is essential when diagnosing pulmonary disease. Chest radiography is also the imaging tool of choice for the assessment of complications and during the follow-up of patients who have pulmonary diseases.

MDCT plays an increasing role in the diagnosis of chest diseases, especially in patients who have unresolving symptoms. CT will aid in the differentiation of infectious and noninfectious disorders. The role of CT in suspected or proven chest disease can be summarized as follows:

1. CT is valuable in the early diagnosis of chest disease, especially in patient groups in which an early diagnosis is important (immunocompromised patients, critically ill patients).
2. CT may help with the characterization of pulmonary disorders.
3. CT is an excellent tool for the assessment of complications of chest disease.
4. CT is required in the investigation of patients who have a persistent or recurrent pulmonary infiltrate.

A side-by-side comparison of the chest radiograph and MDCT when confronted with a missed lung lesion is very instructive. The radiologist should be able to understand the reasons for missing certain lesions. By adopting this inquisitive approach, both cognitive and perceptual errors could be reduced.

Acknowledgments The authors would like to thank to Ms. Sophie Perrier for assistance in preparing the manuscript. Special thanks go to Professor E. Coche and Dr B. Ghaye for providing help with and material for the chapter.

References

Aideyan UO, Berbaum K, Smith WL (1995) Influence of prior radiologic information on the interpretation of radiographic examinations. Acad Radiol 2:205–208

Albaum MN, Hill LC, Murphy M (1996) Interobserver reliability of the chest radiograph in community-acquired pneumonia. Chest 110:343

Austin JH, Romney BM, Goldsmisth LS (1992) Missed bronchogenic carcinoma: Radiographic findings in 27 patients with a potentially resectable lesion evident in retrospect. Radiology 182:115–122

Aziz ZA, Wells AU, Bateman ED et al (2005) Interstitial lung disease: Effects of thin-section CT on clinical decision making. Radiology 238:725–733

Bass JC, Chiles C (1990) Visual kill: Correlation with detection of solitary pulmonary nodules. Invest Radiol 25:994–998

Berbaum KS (1995) Difficulty of judging retrospectively whether a diagnosis has been "missed." Radiology 194:582–583

Berlin L (1986) Malpractice and radiologists: An 11.5-year perspective. AJR 147:1291–1298

Berlin L (1995) Malpractice and radiologists in Cook County, IL: Trends in 20 years of litigation. AJR 165:781–788

Berlin L (2000) Hindsight bias. AJR 175:597–601

Berlin L (2001) Defending the "missed" radiographic diagnosis. AJR 176:317–322

Berlin L, Hendrix RW (1998) Perceptual errors and negligence. AJR 170:863–867

Carmody DP, Nodine CF, Kundel HL (1980) An analysis of perceptual and cognitive factors in radiographic interpretation. Perception 9:339–344

Chotas HG, Ravin CE (1994) Chest radiography: Estimated lung volume and projected area obscured by the heart, mediastinum, and diaphragm. Radiology 193:403–404

Epler GR, McLoud TC, Gaensler EA et al (1978) Normal chest roentgenograms in chronic diffuse infiltrative lung disease. N Engl J Med 298:934–939

Flaherty KR, King TE Jr, Raghu G et al (2004) Idiopathic interstitial pneumonia: What is the effect of a multi-disciplinary approach to diagnosis? Am J Respir Crit Care Med 170:904–910

Grenier P, Valeyre D, Cluzel P et al (1991) Chronic diffuse interstitial lung disease: Diagnostic value of chest radiography and high-resolution CT. Radiology 179:123–132

Herman PG, Hessel SJ (1975) Accuracy and its relationship to experience in the interpretation of chest radiographs. Invest Radiol 10:62–67

Heussel CP, Kauczor HU, Ullmann AJ (2004) Pneumonia in neutropenic patients. Eur Radiol 14:256–271

Jung JI, Kim H, Park SH et al (2001) Differentiation of pneumonic-type bronchioloalveolar cell carcinoma and infectious pneumonia. Br J Radiol 74:490–494

Kelsey CA, Moseley RD, Brogdon BG et al (1977) Effect of size and position on chest lesion detection. AJR 129:205–208

Kimme-Smith C, Hart EM, Goldin JG et al (1996) Detection of simulated lung nodules with computed radiography: Effects of nodule size, local optical density, global object thickness, and exposure. Acad Radiol 3:735–741

Krupinski EA, Berger WG, Dallas WJ et al (2003) Searching for nodules: What features attract attention and influence detection? Acad Radiol 10:861–868

Kundel HL (1975) Peripheral vision, structured noise and film reader error. Radiology 114:269–273

Kundel HL, Revesz G (1976) Lesion conspicuity, structured noise, and film reader error. AJR 126:233–238

Kundel HL, Revesz G, Toto L (1979) Contrast gradient and the detection of lung nodules. Invest Radiol 14:18–22

Kundel HL, Nodine CF, Krupinski EA (1989) Searching for lung nodules. Visual dwell indicates locations of false-positive and false-negative decisions. Invest Radiol 24:472–478

Marcus PM (2001) Lung cancer screening: An update. J Clin Oncol 19:83S–86S

Mathieson JR, Mayo JR, Staples CA et al (1989) Chronic diffuse infiltrative lung disease: Comparison of diagnostic accuracy of CT and chest radiography. Radiology 171:111–116

Melamed MR (2000) Lung cancer screening results in the National Cancer Institute New York study. Cancer 89:2356–2362

Melbye H, Dale K (1992) Interobserver variability in the radiographic diagnosis of adult outpatient pneumonia. Acta Radiol 33:79–83

Monnier-Cholley L, Arrive L, Porcel A et al (2001) Characteristics of missed lung cancer on chest radiographs: A French experience. Eur Radiol 11:597–605

Padley SPG, Hansell DM, Flower CDR et al (1991) Comparative accuracy of high resolution computed tomography and chest radiography in the diagnosis of chronic diffuse inflitrative lung disease. Clin Radiol 44:222–226

Potchen EJ, Bisesi MA (1990) When is it malpractice to miss lung cancer on chest radiographs? Radiology 175:29–32

Quekel LG, Kessels AG, Goei R et al (1999) Miss rate of lung cancer on the chest radiograph in clinical practice. Chest 115:720–724

Quekel LG, Goei R, Kessels AG et al (2001) Detection of lung cancer on the chest radiograph: Impact of previous films, clinical information, double reading, and dual reading. J Clin Epidemiol 54:1146–1150

Revesz G, Kundel HL (1977) Psychophysical studies of detection errors in chest radiology. Radiology 123:559–562

Samei E, Flynn MJ, Eyler WR (1999) Detection of subtle lung nodules: Relative influence of quantum and anatomic noise on chest radiographs. Radiology 213:727–734

Samei E, Flynn MJ, Peterson et al. (2003) Subtle lung nodules: Influence of local anatomic variations on detection. Radiology 228:76–84

Samuel S, Kundel HL, Nodine CF et al (1995) Mechanism of satisfaction of search: Eye position recordings in the reading of chest radiographs. Radiology 194:895–902

Shah PK, Austin JH, White CS et al (2003) Missed non-small cell lung cancer: Radiographic findings of potentially resectable lesions evident only in retrospect. Radiology 226:235–241

Sone S, Li F, Yang ZG et al (2000) Characteristics of small lung cancers invisible on conventional chest radiography and detected by population based screening using spiral CT. Br J Radiol 73:137–145

Speets AM, Hoes AW, van der Graaf Y et al (2006) Chest radiography and pneumonia in primary care: Diagnostic yield and consequences for patient management. Eur Respir J 28:933–938

Tsubamoto M, Kuriyama K, Kido S et al (2002) Detection of lung cancer on chest radiographs: analysis on the basis of size and extent of ground-glass opacity at thin-section CT. Radiology 224:139–144

Turkington PM, Kennan N, Greenstone MA (2002) Minsinterpretation of the chest x-ray as a factor in the delayed diagnosis of lung cancer. Postgrad Med J 78:158–160

Ujita M, Renzoni EA, Veeraraghavan S et al (2004) Organizing pneumonia: perilobular pattern at thin-section CT. Radiology 232:757–761

Webb WR, Müller NL, Naidich DP (2001) High-resolution CT of the lung, 3rd edn. Lippincott Williams & Wilkins, Philadelphia, PA

Woodhead M, Gialdroni Grassi G, Huchon GJ et al (1996) Use of investigations in lower respiratory tract infection in the community: A European survey. Eur Respir J 9: 1596–1600

Woodring JH (1990) Pitfalls in the radiologic diagnosis of lung cancer. AJR 154:1165–1175

Wu M-H, Gotway MB, Lee TJ et al (2008) Features of non-small cell lung carcinomas overlooked at digital chest radiography. Clin Radiol 63:518–528

Yang ZG, Sone S, Li F et al (2001) Visibility of small peripheral lung cancers on chest radiographs: Influence of densitometric parameters, CT values and tumour type. Br J Radiol 74:32–41

Zompatori M, Poletti V, Battista G et al (1999) Bronchiolitis obliterans with organizing pneumonia (BOOP), presenting as a ring-shaped opacity at HRCT (the atoll sign): A case report. Radiol Med (Torino) 97:308–310

Atelectasis

16

François Laurent, Mathieu Lederlin, Olivier Corneloup,
Valérie Latrabe, and Michel Montaudon

Contents

Abstract

> Atelectasis, or collapse, is used to define an acquired diminution of volume of part of or the whole lung. Proximal or distal bronchial obstruction, adhesion, passivity, compression, cicatrization, and gravity dependence are the various mechanisms involved. The manifestations of atelectasis can be classified into direct and indirect signs. Direct signs include displacement of the interlobar fissures and of bronchi and vessels within the affected part of the lung, and indirect signs include loss of lung volume, pulmonary opacification, and shift of hila and mediastinal, and diaphragmatic structures. Atelectasis can be divided into several types, including lobar, segmental, subsegmental, whole lung, platelike, and round atelectasis. Lobar atelectasis of right upper lobe, right middle lobe, left upper lobe, right lower lobe, and left lower lobe have characteristic patterns on chest films and computed tomography.

F. Laurent (✉), M. Lederlin, and M. Montaudon
Laboratoire de physiologie cellulaire respiratoire, Institut
National de la Santé Et de la Recherche Médicale U885,
Université Victor Ségalen Bordeaux 2, Rue Leo Saignat,
Bordeaux 33000 and
Unité d'imagerie thoracique et cardio-vasculaire, Hôpital du
Haut-Lévêque, Centre Hospitalier Universitaire de Bordeaux,
Avenue de Magellan, 33604 PESSAC

O. Corneloup and V. Latrabe
Unité d'imagerie thoracique et cardio-vasculaire, Hôpital du
Haut-Lévêque, Centre Hospitalier Universitaire de Bordeaux,
Avenue de Magellan, 33604 PESSAC

16.1 Mechanisms

Atelectasis derives from the Greek words *ateles* and *ektasis,* meaning incomplete expansion. Therefore, the term is used to define an acquired diminution of volume of part of or the whole lung (Hansell et al. 2008). Acceptable synonyms are loss of volume and collapse, although the latter usually is reserved for total atelectasis.

Obstruction, adhesion, passivity, compression, cicatrization, and gravity dependence are the various

E.E. Coche et al. (eds.), *Comparative Interpretation of CT and Standard Radiography of the Chest,*
Medical Radiology, DOI: 10.1007/978-3-540-79942-9_16, © Springer-Verlag Berlin Heidelberg 2011

mechanisms that have been proposed for explaining atelectasis (Proto 1996; Woodring and Reed 1996b).

16.1.1 Obstructive or Resorptive Atelectasis

Obstructive or *resorptive atelectasis* comes from the resorption of gas from the alveoli and occurs when communication between the alveoli and the trachea is lacking. Obstruction may involve the large airways or the bronchioles.

When obstruction of a large airway occurs, blood circulating through the capillary bed begins to absorb air, resulting in progressive diminution in size of the alveoli. Complete resorption occurs within 24 h in an otherwise healthy lung unless pneumonitis develops distal to the obstruction. This resorption can be much faster in patients who are receiving 100% oxygen. Diminished alveolar volume is associated with edema fluid drawn from the capillary bed of the atelectatic lung, which diffuses within the collapsed alveoli. When bronchial obstruction is slow, pathologic features are those of a noninfectious process: bronchiectasis with distal mucoid impaction, retention of fluid, and lymphocytic infiltration of the bronchial walls. As the process becomes more chronic, the pathologic condition is termed *cholesterol pneumonia* or *endogenous lipid pneumonia* because the affected lung is filled by collagen and foamy macrophages containing intracytoplasmic lipid. Obstruction does not always result in atelectasis, and collateral air drift between segments or even contiguous lobes separated by an incomplete fissure may keep the lung normally ventilated or even hyperinflated. Uncommonly, a localized collection of air may occur adjacent to the atelectasis (Berdon et al. 1984). The most common cause of obstruction of large airways is bronchogenic carcinoma. Any other type of endobonchial tumor, benign or malignant, as well as infectious or inflammatory conditions that produce endobronchial granulomas or bronchial stenosis, aspirated foreign bodies, mucous plugs, malpositioned endotracheal tubes, and extrinsic compression of the bronchus and lung torsion (Moser and Proto 1987; Shirakusa et al. 1990; Seiler et al. 2008) can result in atelectasis. The middle lobe syndrome refers to chronic atelectasis of the middle lobe caused by granulomatous lymphadenitis with bronchial stenosis from tuberculosis or histoplasmosis.

Obstruction of the small peripheral airways is a common cause of atelectasis because of impairment of mucociliary transport, causing pooling of retained secretions with resultant bronchial and bronchiolar obstruction and distal resorption of air. A number of conditions are known to impair mucociliary clearance, including thoracic and abdominal pain, thoracic or abdominal surgery or trauma, central nervous system depression, general anesthesia, endotracheal intubation and ventilation, inhalation of toxic fumes or smoke, high concentrations of oxygen, chronic changes of airway walls caused by chronic obstructive lung diseases, cystic fibrosis, constrictive bronchiolitis, and pneumonia. Computed tomography (CT) often provides valuable information, particularly with regard to the precise location and extent of the obstructive process. Intravenous contrast material-enhanced CT and magnetic resonance imaging may help to distinguish the proximal obstructing tumor from the collapsed lung.

16.1.2 Adhesive Atelectasis

Adhesive atelectasis is used to describe a type of atelectasis that stems from surfactant deficiency. Surfactant normally acts to reduce the surface tension in the alveoli as their volume decreases. Therefore, the critical closing pressure occurs at a lower volume and distending pressure. Hyaline membrane disease is a typical cause of adhesive atelectasis in neonates. Acute radiation pneumonitis, thromboembolism (Aithan et al. 1994), and acute respiratory distress syndrome are the most common causes in adults. Adhesive atelectasis is common after cardiac surgery and accounts for the marked arteriovenous shunting observed despite a relatively normal chest film. Uremia, prolonged shallow breathing, and smoke inhalation have also been reported as causes.

16.1.3 Passive Atelectasis

In the presence of a pneumothorax, intrapleural pressure becomes atmospheric. Intra-alveolar pressure and intrapleural pressure are equalized, allowing the lung to collapse. The degree of collapse is proportional to the amount of air in the adjacent pleural space. The density of the shrunken lung does not increase so much until it is almost completely collapsed because the reduction in blood volume balances the reduction in lung volume. Paralysis of the diaphragm, congenital weakness of the diaphragm, and pulmonary hypoventilation for full expansion of lungs may lead to similar effects.

16.1.4 Compressive Atelectasis

Any space-occupying lesion of the thorax can compress the lung and squeeze air out of the alveoli. Intrathoracic causes include pleural effusion, tension pneumothorax, empyema, pleural tumors, large pleural masses, large emphysematous bullae, osteophytes, and diaphragmatic hernias. Abdominal causes include distension from obesity, large abdominal tumors, massive ascites, intestinal obstruction, and pregnancy; all these conditions can push the diaphragm upward and compress the lung. Compressive atelectasis is prone to occur in gravity-dependent areas of the lung. The increased attenuation reflects both greater perfusion and decreased alveolar expansion in the dependent areas and is greatest at low lung volume. Any condition that increases lung weight, such as pneumonia, increased blood volume, pulmonary edema, and bedridden hospitalized patients with prolonged shallow breathing, exacerbates atelectasis. On CT, gravity-dependent atelectasis is common in the dependent lung areas and seen as ill-defined areas of increased attenuation; subpleural curvilinear opacities parallel to the pleura and pseudoplaques have been reported. Disappearance when the patient is scanned in the supine position is a clue, but the proper diagnosis can be suspected based on the dependent location of the abnormalities.

16.1.5 Cicatrization Atelectasis

The volume loss is caused by decreased pulmonary compliance due to localized or diffuse fibrosis; the fibrous tissue undergoes retraction. The fibrosis may be localized, such as in cases of long-standing tuberculosis and radiation fibrosis (Davis et al. 1992), or diffuse, as seen in idiopathic pulmonary fibrosis, sarcoidosis, and pneumoconiosis. Increased elastic recoil from the surrounding fibrosis is responsible for dilatation of bronchi and bronchioles, a finding called *traction bronchiectasis* (Westcott and Cole 1986).

It is important to understand the mechanisms and to diagnose atelectasis correctly. In a given patient, however, several mechanisms can work together to cause this condition. For example, in patients who have undergone cardiac bypass surgery, compression of the lower lobe, impaired mucociliary transport, surfactant deficiency, paralysis of the hemidiaphragm, and gravity-dependent changes in the lung can combine to produce lower lobe atelectasis (Wilcox et al. 1988).

16.2 Basic Concepts

The manifestations of atelectasis can be classified into direct and indirect signs. Direct signs are displacement of the interlobar fissures, bronchi, and vessels within the affected part of the lung. Manifestations for compensating for the loss of lung volume, pulmonary opacification, and shift of hila and mediastinal and diaphragmatic structures, are indirect signs. In acute atelectasis, there is a predominance of displacement of mediastinal and diaphragmatic structures, whereas in chronic conditions compensatory overinflation of the nonaffected lung dominates.

16.2.1 Direct Signs

The position and configuration of the displaced fissures are easily recognizable and predictable for a given loss of volume. They will be described later in relation to patterns of specific lobar atelectasis. The earliest indicators of atelectasis are crowding together of the pulmonary vessels and bronchi. Crowded air bronchograms remain visible when increased opacification of the atelectatic lobe results in obscuration of vessels. If the proximal bronchi are occluded or filled with secretions, air within the bronchi can also disappear and displacement of interlobar fissure could be the only sign of atelectasis.

16.2.2 Indirect Signs

Indirect signs of atelectasis include pulmonary opacification; elevation of the diaphragm; shifting of the trachea, heart, and mediastinum; and displacement of the hila.

None of them are constant, and they are more pronounced when the atelectasis is acute. The opacification of a collapsed lobe correlates not only with its degree of volume loss but also with the amount of secretions within the lobe. However, because the lung contains a large amount of air, the lung must be almost completely collapsed before opacification is apparent on a chest radiograph.

The shift of the mediastinum is greater from the more mobile anterior and middle compartments than from the posterior one, and it is well demonstrated by CT. Elevation of the hemidiaphragm is more pronounced in lower than in upper lobes and tends to occur in the area contiguous to the lobe involved. The right dome of the diaphragm is usually 1–2 cm higher than the left. However, in 10% of subjects, both hemidiaphragms are at the same level and, in 2% of subjects, the right hemidiaphragm is more than 3 cm higher than the left. The juxtaphrenic peak is a triangular opacity noted at approximately the mid-portion of the ipsilateral hemidiaphragm, seen in ipsilateral upper lobe atelectasis and caused by the indrawing of diaphragmatic pleura into the inferior accessory fissure as the lower lobe overinflates to compensate for the volume loss. Hilar displacement occurs more commonly in atelectasis of the upper than that of the lower lobes. The left hilum typically lies higher than the right one in 97% of subjects. Because the collapsed lobe obscures the lower lobe artery, a small hilum rather than a depressed hilum is a sign of lower lobe collapse (Proto 1996). A marked lower lobe collapse or an upper lobectomy can be responsible for a reorientation of vessels in a parallel rather than a divergent pattern within the compensatory overinflated lung (Proto 1996). When the upper lobe collapses, the ipsilateral main bronchus is more horizontally oriented than usual and the bronchus intermedius on the right or the left lower lobe bronchus on the left swings outward. On the other hand, the main bronchi are more vertically orientated with an inward swing of the lower lobe bronchi in atelectasis of the lower lobes.

Close approximation of the ribs also may occur but can be caused by poor positioning and is therefore considered an unreliable sign. In segmental and lobar atelectasis, the surrounding lung expands as the affected segment or lobe loses volume, the phenomenon being called compensatory hyperexpansion. A decreased number of visible vessels and wide separation of the vessels are seen in an hyperexpanded lung compared with a normal contralateral lung. The greater the degree of collapse, the greater overinflation is, and the compensatory overrinflated lobe will appear more dark on X-ray. However, changes of vessel direction are considered to be more reliable because technical conditions may be responsible for asymmetric attenuation of hemithoraces. The displacement of a known granuloma, called "shifting granuloma," has also been reported to indicate volume loss (Woodring and Reed 1996a).

16.3 Patterns of Atelectasis

Atelectasis can be divided into several types, including lobar, segmental, subsegmental, whole lung, platelike, and round atelectasis. Lobar atelectasis of the right upper lobe (RUL), right middle lobe (RML), left upper lobe (LUL), right lower lobe (RLL), and left lower lobe (LLL) will be described separately.

16.3.1 Right Upper Lobe Atelectasis

The collapsing RUL moves superiorly, anteriorly, and medially, and the RML and RLL expand proportionally at the same time (Woodring and Reed 1996a). On the frontal view, the minor fissure moves superiorly and medially and often bows in an upward direction, with the lateral portion being typically higher than the medial one (Fig. 16.1a). On the lateral view, the minor fissure moves superiorly and bows in an upward direction while the superior portion of the major fissure moves and bows in the anterior direction. When the lung remains partly aerated, the displaced interlobular fissures, the crowded vessels in the right upper mediastinal border, and a slight upward displacement of the right hilum are visible. Once opacification of the atelectatic lung ensues, the fissures are seen as interfaces between the displaced RML, RLL, and the atelectatic lobe (Fig. 16.1b, c). However, the right upper mediastinal border is obscured by the atelectatic upper lobe (silhouette sign) (Fig. 16.1b). On the lateral view, the collapsing RUL shows a triangular shape with the apex at the hilum and the base at the thoracic apex. The downward bulging of the medial portion of the minor fissure on the frontal view may point out the cause of obstruction by an

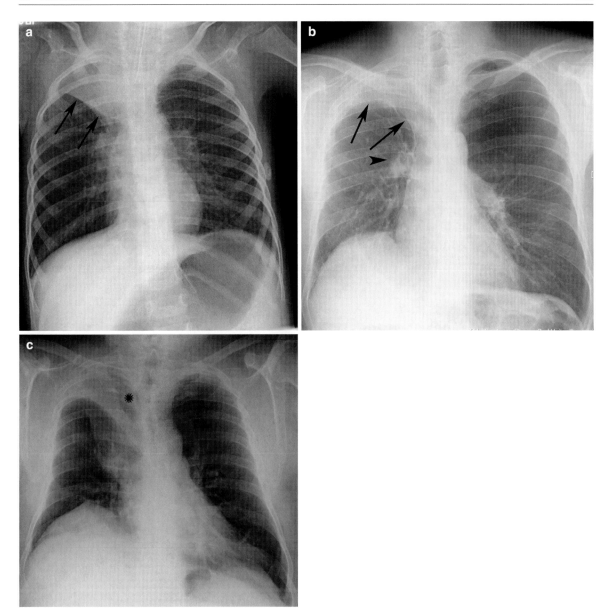

Fig. 16.1 Right upper lobe (RUL) atelectasis. Three different patterns are seen on the frontal chest radiograph. (**a**) Obstructive atelectasis of the RUL in a 8-year-old patient in postoperative status. Opacity of the RUL with upward displacement of the minor fissure (*arrows*). Note the elevated right hilum and the lateral shift of the tracheal tube. (**b**) Chronic atelectasis of the RUL in a 56-year-old patient due to bronchiectasis. Note the major volume loss of the RUL and the marked concavity and elevation of both the minor fissure (*arrows*) and the right hilum (*arrowhead*). (**c**) Peripheral chronic upper lobe atelectasis in a 58-year-old patient. Findings are similar to those seen in (b), but overinflated lung is interposed between the RUL and the mediastinum (*star*)

expanding bronchial mass. This feature is combined with the concave appearance of the lateral aspect of the minor fissure and is known as the Golden S sign. Initially described with RUL atelectasis, this finding is actually applicable to any lobe (Fig. 16.2a, b).

In marked RUL atelectasis, the RUL becomes plastered against the lung apex or upper mediastinum and can be mistaken for an apical pleural thickening or a mediastinal widening on a frontal view (Fig. 16.1b). On a lateral view, the collapsed lobe appears as a triangular shadow with its apex at the hilum and its base contiguous to the parietal pleura and, posterior to the apex of the hemithorax (Fig. 16.2c).

Occasionally, the hyperexpanding superior segment of the RLL or the RML becomes insinuated between the mediastinum and the collapsed RUL. This appearance has been termed *peripheral atelectasis*. The atelectatic lobe lies against the lateral chest wall and mimics a loculated pleural effusion (Fig. 16.1c).

On CT, an atelectatic RUL appears as a triangular soft density lying against the mediastinum and the anterior chest wall (Fig. 16.2a, d, e). When atelectasis is severe, CT shows a band-like configuration plastered against the mediastinum that can be confused with mediastinal disease (Naidich et al. 1983a, b; Khoury et al. 1985).

16.3.2 Right Middle Lobe Atelectasis

The diagnosis is difficult on the frontal chest radiograph and much easier on the lateral view (Woodring and Reed 1996). The projection of the RML is triangular in shape, with its apex against the chest wall and its base against the right border of the heart on the frontal chest radiograph. On the lateral projection the RML is also triangular, with its apex at the hilum and its base against the anterior chest wall. As the RML loses volume it moves inferiorly and medially. A slight downward bowing of the minor fissure is the earliest sign on the frontal view. When opacification of the lobe occurs, it causes obliteration of the right heart border but the right hemidaphragm remains distinct. However, the opacity is so minimal that it is often overlooked (Fig. 16.3a). On the lateral view, a characteristic triangular opacity limited by a minor and inferior portion of the major fissure bowing in opposite directions is visible (Fig. 16.3b). As the RML volume loss increases, the RML lies in an oblique plane and the minor fissure is no longer visible on the posteroanterior view. On the lateral view, the narrow triangular opacity tends to become so thin that it can be mistaken from thickening, a pleural effusion, or a thickened major fissure.

On CT, the RML atelectasis consists of a triangular opacity with the apex directed toward the hilum (Fig. 16.4a, b, c). The anterior border is outlined by the minor fissure displaced downward and the posterior border by the major fissure displaced upward and

forward. The RML bronchus enters the posteromedial corner of the opacity, an important point in the differential diagnosis (Naidich et al. 1983a, b; Khoury et al. 1985).

16.3.3 Left Upper Lobe Atelectasis

The appearance is different from RUL atelectasis because there is no minor fissure on the left. The lobe moves predominantly forward, pulling the expended lower lobe behind it. Therefore, the fissure moves anteriorly and medially. The usual appearance on a frontal chest radiograph is a hazy density extending out from the left hilum, fading laterally and inferiorly. The loss of cardiac contour is a striking feature on the frontal view (Fig. 16.5a). With mild loss of volume, the entire upper mediastinum, cardiac borders, and diaphragm become invisible (Woodring and Reed 1996). Nevertheless, the upper margin of the left mediastinum and the aortic knob remains visible because of the overexpanded superior segment of the upper lobe, called the "Luftsichel sign." Then, the upper segment of the lower lobe inserts itself between the atelectatic upper lobe and the mediastinum, creating a sharp interface with the aortic knob. With further loss of volume, the superior mediastinal contour and left hemidiaphragm reappear and the medial border of the pulmonary opacity becomes sharp because the apex is occupied by the overexpanded upper segment of the LLL (Webber and Davies 1981). On the lateral view, the lateral portion of the major fissure is seen with a concave margin parallel to the anterior chest wall (Fig. 16.5b). Herniation of the opposite lung into the left hemithorax in front of the aorta leads to increased visibility of the aorta on the lateral view. A juxtaphrenic peak on the hemidiaphragm may be seen.

On CT (Fig. 16.5c, d), the atelectatic LUL is seen to abut the anterior chest wall and mediastinum. The major fissure is shifted anteriorly and upward. The posterior margin of the atelectic LUL has a V-shaped contour.

Atelectasis of the upper division of the LUL, sparing the lingula, results in findings similar to those of the RUL atelectasis; lingular atelectasis resembles the RML atelectasis (Fig. 16.6).

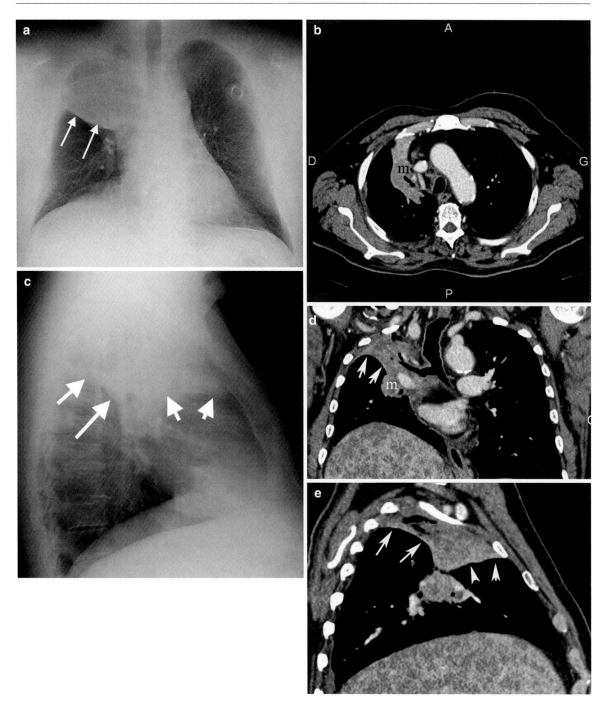

Fig. 16.2 Atelectasis of the right upper lobe (RUL). Bronchogenic carcinoma. The frontal chest radiograph (**a**) shows the RUL opacity outlined inferiorly by the minor fissure displaced upward (*arrows*). Axial computed tomography (CT) section (**b**) shows the anterior and superior displacement of the major fissure, the atelectatic lobe lying against the mediastinum, and a right hilar mass with a focal convexity of the fissure medially (Golden S sign). The lateral view (**c**) and the CT coronal (**d**) and sagittal (**e**) reformation sections show medial and superior displacement of the minor fissure and anterior and superior displacement of the upper part of the right main fissure (*arrows*)

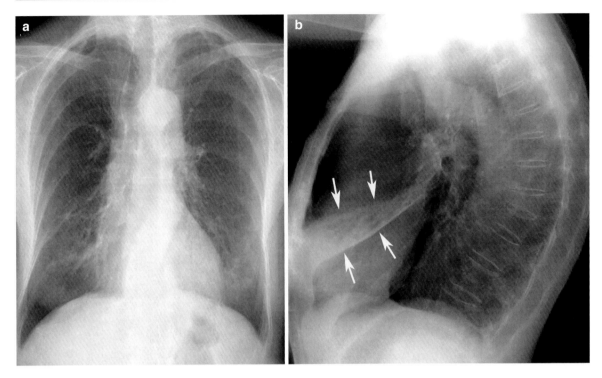

Fig. 16.3 Atelectasis of the middle lobe. The frontal chest radiograph (**a**) shows a poorly defined area of increased attenuation. The lateral view (**b**) shows a triangular area of increased attenuation limited by the downward shift of the minor fissure and the forward shift of the right major fissure (*arrows*). Note the thoracic distension due to chronic obstructive lung disease in this 56-year-old patient

16.3.4 Right Lower Lobe Atelectasis

The RLL, like the left one, is attached to the lower mediastinum and medial hemidiaphragm by the inferior pulmonary ligament. Therefore, when atelectatic, the lobe is displaced medially and posteriorly. On a frontal chest radiograph, the hilum and main bronchus are displaced inferiorly and medially and the interlobar artery is obscured by the surrounding airless lobe (Fig. 16.7a and b). The fissure moves downwards and sagitally. On a lateral view the lobe obscures the posterior part of the hemidiaphragm. When the atelectasis is marked, the only abnormal finding can be a subtle increased opacity of the lower thoracic vertebrae, normally more radiolucent than the upper thoracic vertebrae (Fig. 16.7c and d). On CT, the atelectatic lower lobe occupies the posterior gutter and is limited by the displaced major fissure which the lateral portion demonstrates the greatest mobility (Fig. 16.7e). A lower lobe collapse has a sharply margined triangular opacity that lies over the diaphragm,

presumably due to the attachment of the lobe by the inferior pulmonary ligament to the hemidiaphragm. At times, the inferior pulmonary ligament ends with a free border without attachment to the hemidiaphragm. The adjacent compensatory overinflated lobe places itself between the base of the collapsed lobe and the diaphragm and the atelectasis can then simulate a mass.

16.3.5 Left Lower Lobe Atelectasis

When LLL atelectasis is mild, the lobe is not entirely displaced behind the heart. The superolateral portion of the main fissure, which can be seen in 14% of normal individuals as a curvilinear line in the upper lung area on a frontal chest radiograph, is displaced downward and medially. On the lateral view, the inferior part of the major fissure moves posteriorly and can be seen as an arcuate line projecting posterior to the hilum, whereas the

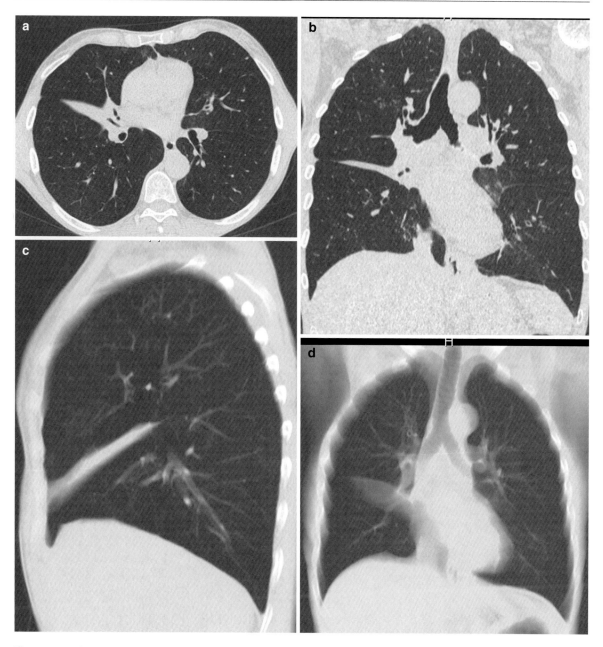

Fig. 16.4 Atelectasis of the middle lobe. The patient was a 50-year-old woman who had persistent cough and fever after an acute pneumonia 3 weeks earlier. Computed tomography multiplanar reformatted (MPR) sections in the axial (**a**), coronal (**b**), and sagittal (**c**) show the characteristic triangular area of consolidation with dilated bronchi. Thick MPR in the coronal plane (**d**) demonstrates the tipped-up configuration of the atelectasis

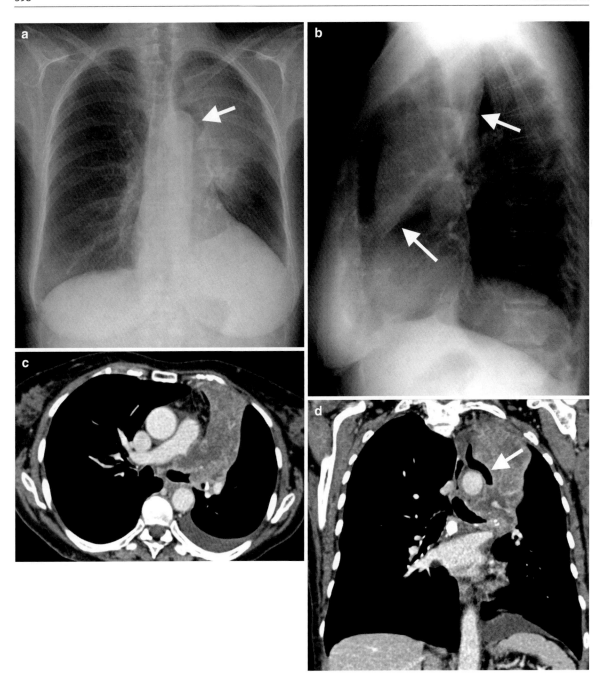

Fig. 16.5 Left upper lobe (LUL) atelectasis. Bronchogenic carcinoma. The frontal chest radiograph (**a**) shows a poorly defined opacity of the left hemithorax with obliteration of the left heart border (silhouette sign) and loss of volume of the left hemithorax. The lateral view (**b**) shows an anterior opacity limited by the forwarded displaced major fissure (*arrows*). Axial (**c**) and coronal (**d**) computed tomography (CT) sections demonstrate an obstructing mass and the distal atelectatic LUL bordered by the left major fissure displaced anteriorly and medially. Note the lucency (*arrow*) visible on the frontal chest radiograph and on the coronal CT section between the atelectasis and the aortic arch (Luftsichel sign) due to the upward displacement of the left upper segment of the left lower lobe. The left hemidiaphragm is obscured on both the frontal and lateral chest radiographs by a left pleural effusion

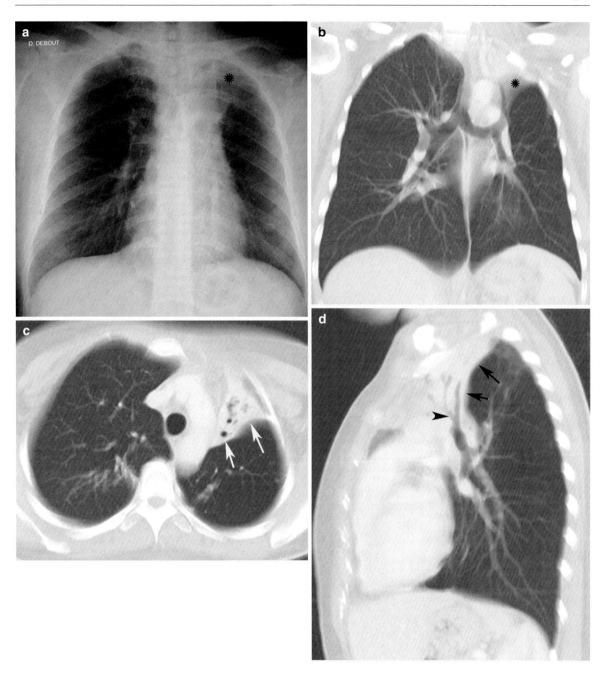

Fig. 16.6 Atelectasis of the upper division of the left upper lobe (LUL) due to chronic bronchiectasis. The chest radiograph (**a**) shows a left apical opacity abutting the apex and the upper mediastinum (*star*). Coronal (**b**), axial (**c**), and sagittal (**d**) multiplanar reformatted thick computed tomography sections depict the opacity of the culmen, the upward and forward displacement of the major fissure (*arrows*), the elevation of the left hilum, the horizontally orientated main right bronchus, and the dilated bronchi without proximal obstruction (*arrowhead*)

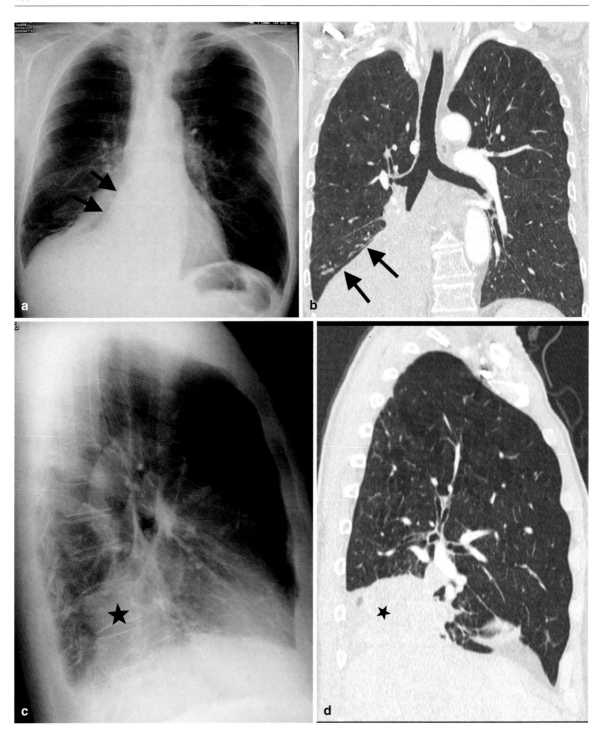

Fig. 16.7 Atelectasis of the right lower lobe (RLL). Broncho-genic carcinoma. The frontal chest radiograph (**a**) and coronal computed tomography (CT) reformation (**b**) show an opacity of the lower part of the right hemithorax sharply limited by the inferiorly displaced right main fissure (*arrows*). The lateral view (**c**) and the sagittal CT reformation (**d**) show the atelectatic lobe (*stars*) lying on the posterior part of the right hemidiaphragm. Axial (**e**) and coronal (**b**) CT sections show the hilar mass (*m*) responsible for the obstruction of the right inferior bronchus and the minor fissure displaced posteriorly, inferiorly, and sagitally (*arrows*)

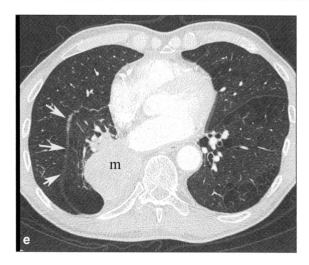

Fig. 16.7 (continued)

superior portion of the major fissure bows inferiorly. When the volume loss is marked, the LLL, with the major fissure as its anterior boundary, moves posteriorly and medially against the lower mediastinum and spine in a fashion similar to that of the RLL (Fig. 16.9a). This results in a triangular opacity visible behind the heart on the frontal view with inferior displacement of the left

hilum and obscuration of the descending branch of the LLL artery. On the lateral view an opacity over the lower thoracic spine is seen, as is blunting of the posterior costophrenic angle. CT typically shows a wedge-shaped opacity against the posterior mediastinum, descending aorta, and thoracic spine (Fig. 16.9c, d).

16.3.6 Combined Middle Lobe and Right Lower Lobe Atelectasis

A single lesion of the bronchus intermedius gives rise to combined atelectasis of these lobes. On the frontal view the atelectatic right middle and lower lobes obscure both the right cardiac border and the right hemidiaphragm. Depression of both major and minor fissures is present and most marked laterally. On the lateral view increased opacity is seen throughout the lower part of the chest. Combined middle lobe and RLL atelectasis can be confused with single RLL atelectasis and subpulmonic effusion. When atelectasis is nearly complete, it is difficult to detect it on the frontal view and the diagnostic should be suspected in patients who have a small hilum and an

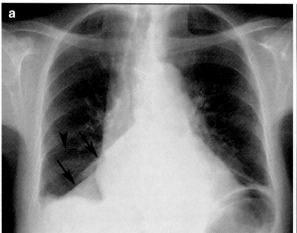

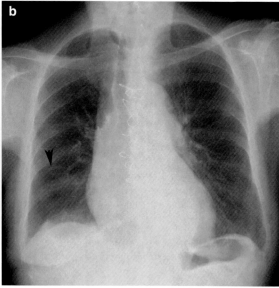

Fig. 16.8 Postoperative resolutive atelectasis of the right lower lobe. The patient was a 72-year-old man who underwent cardiac surgery 1 week previously. Frontal chest radiographs 5 days after cardiac surgery (**a**) shows the downward displacement of

both minor (*arrowhead*) and major fissures (*arrows*). Incomplete resolution occurred at 21 days (**b**) with return to its normal position of the minor fissure (*arrowhead*)

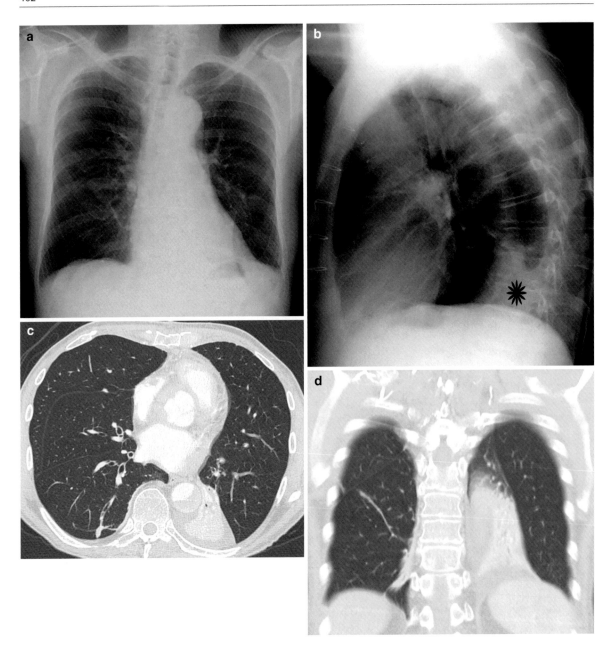

Fig. 16.9 Left lower lobe (LLL) atelectasis. Postoperative status of a 75-year-old man after surgery for aortic dissection. The frontal chest radiograph (**a**) shows a well-defined interface extending obliquely downward and laterally from the left hilum. The lateral view (**b**) shows an ill-defined posterior opacity obscuring the silhouette of the posterior part of the left hemidiaphragm (*star*). Computed tomography (CT) axial section (**c**) shows the sagittally orientated left main fissure bordering the LLL displaced posteriorly and medially. No bronchial obstruction was found. Note the double channel of the descending aorta. Thick CT coronal reformation (**d**) demonstrates the almost entirely opacified atelectatic lobe and the course of the main left fissure. Thick sagittal CT reformation (**e**) shows the atelectatic LLL (*star*) on the posterior part of the hemidiaphragm

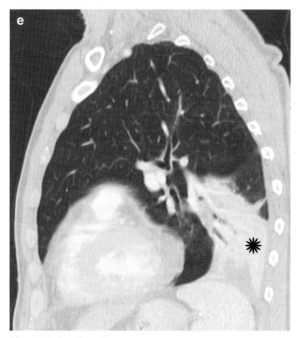

Fig. 16.9 (continued)

The atelectatic right upper and middle lobe can move with changes in the patient's position.

16.3.8 Combined Right Upper and Lower Lobe Atelectasis

Combined atelectasis of right upper and lower lobes is rare. Findings on a frontal chest radiograph are similar to those of isolated atelectasis of each lobe (Fig. 16.10). The middle lobe is overinflated and the minor fissure is higher than normal because of the atelelectasis of the upper lobe; it is more posterior than normal because of the atelectasis of the RLL.

16.3.9 Whole Lung Atelectasis

Whole lung atelectasis on either side leads to opacity of the whole hemithorax. Compensatory phenomena are identical to those that develop with less severe

oligemic hyperexpanded RUL. On CT, the atelectatic lobes occupy the lower hemithorax and abut the right cardiac border medially and the hemidiaphragm anteriorly. The lateral and anteromedial margins of the lobes are bordered by the major and minor fissures, respectively.

16.3.7 Combined Middle and Right Upper Lobe Atelectasis

On a frontal chest radiograph the opacity obscures the outline of the mediastinum and fades laterally. The silhouettes of the ascending aorta and right atrium are usually obscure. On the lateral view the major fissure is displaced anteriorly. Retrosternal radiolucency is caused by herniation of the left lung. On CT the atelectatic lobes cause a wedge-shaped area of soft tissue attenuation abutting the chest wall anteriorly and the ascending aorta and right cardiac border medially. The major fissure is displaced anteriorly and the hyperexpanded lower lobe fills most of the right hemithorax.

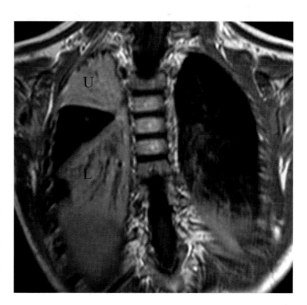

Fig. 16.10 Combined right upper lobe and right lower lobe atelectasis. Gadolinium-enhanced magnetic resonance (MR) coronal section shows triangular opacities of the apex and medial part of the right lung corresponding to upper (*U*) and lower (*L*) lobes, respectively. The patient was a 2-year-old boy undergoing a cardiac MR examination for complex congenital cardiac abnormality

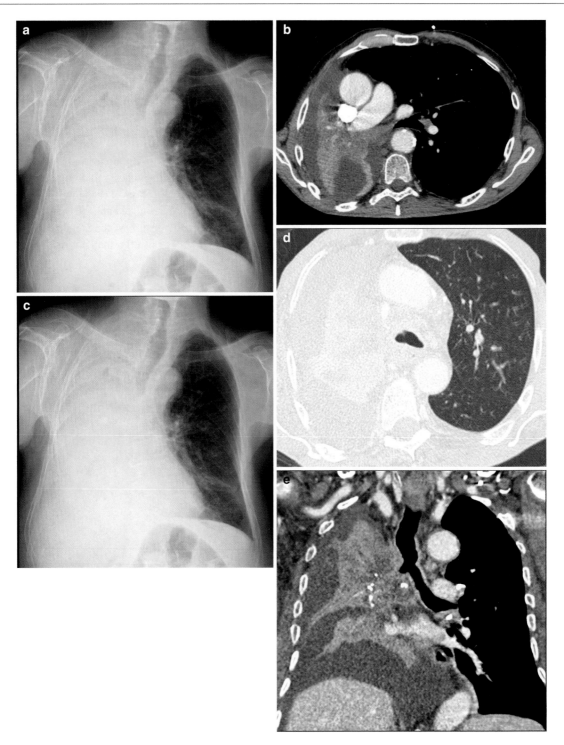

Fig. 16.11 Atelectasis of the whole right lung in two different patients. The chest radiograph (**a**) shows a complete opacity of the right lung with mediastinal shift. Axial computed tomography (CT) (**b**) shows the atelectatic right lung containing necrotic changes. Note that the shift of the mediastinum is mainly caused by anterior and middle part of the mediastinum. In another patient, the chest radiograph (**c**) demonstrates a less pronounced mediastinal shift. This was due to an ipsilateral pleural effusion seen on axial CT (**d**). The coronal CT reformation (**e**) demonstrates a large mass obstructing the main right bronchus that is responsible for the atelectasis

atelectasis. Elevation of the left hemidiaphragm is better recognized on the left side because the stomach bubble indicates its position. The whole mediastinum shifts to the affected side, with the greatest shift occurring anteriorly. The margin of the overinflated lung is usually seen to extend into the affected hemithorax, mostly anteriorly, as CT demonstrates (Fig. 16.11).

16.3.10 Subsegmental Atelectasis

Identification of subsegmental atelectasis can be difficult because many secondary pulmonary lobules within the affected segment may remain aerated while others collapse. In such a case, the degree of volume loss can be very slight and opacification is limited to patchy opacities that resemble bronchopneumonia. They are mostly recognized on CT. Atelectasis of the apical segment stands out as an opacity against the mediastinum or thoracic apex on frontal chest radiograph. The elevated minor fissure usually remains visible. Atelectasis of anterior and posterior segments of the RUL produces opacities that project over the right hilum on the frontal view. On the lateral view they are triangular with the apex directed toward the hilum and the bases directed the anterior or posterior chest wall.

16.3.11 Platelike Atelectasis

Platelike atelectasis, also called linear or discoid atelectasis, is usually located 1–3 cm above the diaphragm and rarely involves the upper lobes. It may be single or multiple, but it invariably extends to the pleural surface. Platelike atelectasis represents sheets of peripheral atelectasis, the formation of which is not dependent on segmental or subsegmental bronchial obstruction. It corresponds to sheets of atelectasis in the subpleural region of the lung extended to the pleural surface and is associated with linear invagination of the overlying pleura (Fig. 16.12). Gravity-dependent alterations in alveolar volume, surfactant deficiency, and hypoventilation seem to be the main predisposing factors to the development of platelike atelectasis. It is known to accompany a variety of thoracic and abdominal conditions, including pulmonary thromboembolism

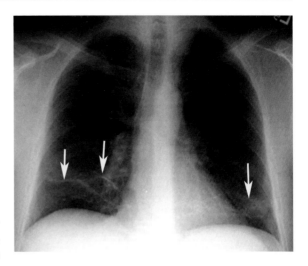

Fig. 16.12 Platelike atelectasis. Frontal chest radiograph shows linear opacities (*arrows*) of both lower hemithoraces in a patient after liver surgery

and infarction, pneumonia, pulmonary edema, diaphragmatic dysfunction, and any cause of hypoventilation (thoracic and abdominal pain, trauma or surgery, general anesthesia, pregnancy, abdominal masses and distension, morbid obesity). Although often unimpressive in appearance, it often indicates more widespread peripheral atelectasis that is radiologically apparent and can be associated with significant disturbances in ventilation and hypoxemia (Westcott and Cole 1985).

16.3.12 Round Atelectasis

Round atelectasis is a loss of volume in the lung in which a portion of the lung turns or invaginates. Various names have been employed to describe this entity, including Blesovsky's syndrome, helical atelectasis, folded lung, pleuroma, atelectatic pseudotumor, and shrinking pleuritis. Two mechanisms have been proposed for the development of round atelectasis. The first relates to the pleural effusion on which a portion of lung floats. The floating lung tilts around a cleft formed at an area of volume loss, and fibrous tissue forms within the cleft and maintains volume loss when the effusion resolves. The second mechanism relates to pleural fibrosis. The adjacent lung loses volume to produce a masslike opacity, which simulates a neoplasm.

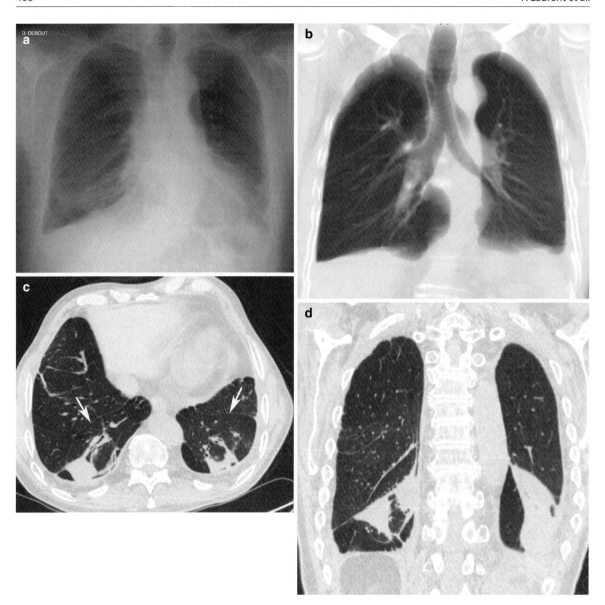

Fig. 16.13 Round atelectasis. Frontal chest radiograph (**a**) and thick multiplanar reformatted computed tomography (CT) (**b**) show the downward orientation of both lower lobe vessels and the downward position of right and left hila indicating a lower lobes volume loss. Axial (**c**) and coronal (**d**) CT reformations show two roughly symmetrical round masses abutting the thick-ened pleura and attracting main fissures downward and medi-ally (*arrows*). Sagittal CT reformation (**e**) through the right hemithorax shows the characteristic curvature of bronchi and vessels (*arrows*) toward the right mass (*m*). Note the thickened pleura and interlobular septae. The patient was a 55-year-old man with high professional exposure to asbestos

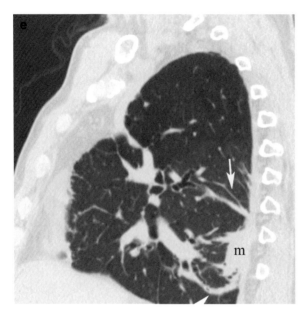

Fig. 16.13 (continued)

Most lesions are located in the lower lobes. CT findings include a peripheral or oval mass, ipsilateral pleural thickening not always immediately adjacent to the mass, and an unsharp central margin of the mass (Hillerdal 1989; McHugh and Blaquiere 1989; Yamaguchi et al. 1997). Fissural, bronchial, and vascular displacements with vessels curving toward the mass are important features (Fig. 16.13).

References

Aithan S et al (1994) Total lung collapse after pulmonary infarction. Thorax 49(9):938–939

Berdon WE et al (1984) Localized pneumothorax adjacent to a collapsed lobe: A sign of bronchial obstruction. Radiology 150(3):691–694

Davis SD et al (1992) Radiation effects on the lung: Clinical features, pathology, and imaging findings. AJR Am J Roentgenol 159(6):1157–1164

Hansell DM et al (2008) Fleischner Society: Glossary of terms for thoracic imaging. Radiology 246(3):697–722

Hillerdal G (1989) Rounded atelectasis. Clinical experience with 74 patients. Chest 95(4):836–841

Khoury MB et al (1985) CT of obstructive lobar collapse. Invest Radiol 20(7):708–716

McHugh K, Blaquiere RM (1989) CT features of rounded atelectasis. AJR Am J Roentgenol 153(2):257–260

Moser ES Jr, Proto AV (1987) Lung torsion: Case report and literature review. Radiology 162(3):639–643

Naidich DP et al (1983a) Computed tomography of lobar collapse: 1. Endobronchial obstruction. J Comput Assist Tomogr 7(5):745–757

Naidich DP et al (1983b) Computed tomography of lobar collapse: 2. Collapse in the absence of endobronchial obstruction. J Comput Assist Tomogr 7(5):758–767

Proto AV (1996) Lobar collapse: Basic concepts. Eur J Radiol 23(1):9–22

Seiler G et al (2008) Computed tomographic features of lung lobe torsion. Vet Radiol Ultrasound 49(6):504–508

Shirakusa T et al (1990) Lung lobe torsion following lobectomy. Am Surg 56(10):639–642

Webber M, Davies P (1981) The Luftsichel: An old sign in upper lobe collapse. Clin Radiol 32(3):271–275

Westcott JL, Cole S (1985) Plate atelectasis. Radiology 155(1):1–9

Westcott JL, Cole SR (1986) Traction bronchiectasis in end-stage pulmonary fibrosis. Radiology 161(3):665–669

Wilcox P et al (1988) Phrenic nerve function and its relationship to atelectasis after coronary artery bypass surgery. Chest 93(4):693–698

Woodring JH, Reed JC (1996a) Radiographic manifestations of lobar atelectasis. J Thorac Imaging 11(2):109–144

Woodring JH, Reed JC (1996b) Types and mechanisms of pulmonary atelectasis. J Thorac Imaging 11(2):92–108

Yamaguchi T et al (1997) Magnetic resonance imaging of rounded atelectasis. J Thorac Imaging 12(3):188–194

Lung Cancer

17

Gilbert R. Ferretti and Adrien Jankowski

Contents

Abstract

> Lung cancer is one of the leading causes of cancer mortality in the world. In clinical practice, lung cancers are divided into non–small cell carcinoma (80% of cases) and small cell carcinoma (20% of cases) due to clinical distinction in presentation, metastatic diffusion, and therapy. Early diagnosis of lung cancer may be associated with better operability and prognosis. Chest X-ray (CXR) remains the most commonly performed test in diagnostic radiology. It is therefore of paramount importance for radiologists to be aware of the radiological presentation of lung cancer because it is often discovered when a CXR is obtained in a patient for another purpose and the frequency of missed lung cancer is high. Because there is a large spectrum of radiologic manifestations of lung cancer, detection of these findings is essential for proper patient management. To highlight the CXR presentation of lung carcinoma, correlations with computed tomography findings in coronal, axial, sagittal, virtual bronchoscopy, and three-dimensional imaging are presented in this chapter.

17.1 Introduction

Lung cancer (bronchogenic carcinoma) is one of the leading causes of cancer mortality in the world. Cigarette smoking is a strong causative factor in the development of lung cancer and accounts for approximately 85% of all cases (Beckett 1993). Although the risk decreases

G.R. Ferretti (✉) and A. Jankowski
CHU Grenoble, Clinique Universitaire de Radiologie et
Imagerie Médicale, 38043, Grenoble cedex 09, France and
INSERM U 823, Institut A. Bonniot, Boulevard de la
Chantourne, 38700 La Tronche, France
e-mail: gferretti@chu-grenoble.fr

E.E. Coche et al. (eds.), *Comparative Interpretation of CT and Standard Radiography of the Chest*,
Medical Radiology, DOI: 10.1007/978-3-540-79942-9_17, © Springer-Verlag Berlin Heidelberg 2011

with smoking cessation, it never completely disappears. The four main cell types of lung cancer are adenocarcinoma, squamous cell carcinoma, small cell carcinoma (SCC), and large cell undifferentiated carcinoma (Brambilla et al. 2001). In clinical practice, however, lung cancers are often divided into non–small cell carcinoma (NSCC) (80% of cases) and SCC (15–20% of cases) due to clinical distinction in presentation, metastatic diffusion, and therapy (Hansell et al. 2005).

As of 2009, surgery remains the only technique that allows for curative treatment of lung carcinoma. However, surgery can only be performed in about 20% of patients who present with lung carcinoma (Scagliotti 2001) either because of histologic type of the tumor (NSCC), diffusion of the disease (local, regional, or diffuse extent), or because of poor clinical status of the patient. Early diagnosis of lung cancer may be associated with better operability and prognosis; therefore, screening by imaging (chest X-ray [CXR] or computed tomography [CT]) has been evaluated for this purpose. Studies performed in the 1970s failed to show the usefulness of CXR in reducing lung cancer mortality (Kubik et al. 1990; Marcus et al. 2000). CT detection of asymptomatic lung cancer in a high-risk population has raised great hope of detecting more and smaller cancers than with CXR, with these cancers being at an earlier stage (Henschke et al. 1999; Swensen et al. 2005). However, early CT detection of lung carcinoma has not yet been proven to decrease lung cancer mortality (Bach et al. 2007). Randomized controled trials are currently being processed (Berg and Aberle 2007).

In clinical practice, CXR remains the most commonly performed test in diagnostic radiology. It is therefore of paramount importance for radiologists to be aware of the radiological presentation of lung cancer since it is often discovered when a CXR is obtained in a patient for another purpose. The frequency of missed lung cancer with CXR is high: 51 of 78 lung cancers (65%) were retrospectively visible 1 year earlier (Heelan et al. 1984), and 25 of 36 central cancers (69%) were retrospectively visible on previous CXR (Muhm et al. 1983). However, improvements in global quality, contrast resolution, and reproducibility have been obtained using digital radiography, which may have modified the ability of CXR to detect lung carcinoma. Reviewing CXRs on a picture archiving and communication system allows comparisons with former CXRs, permitting the detection of subtle abnormalities and small lung carcinomas. Dual energy and temporal subtraction radiography can even enhance

detection of subtle lung abnormalities on radiographs (McAdams et al. 2006). Computer-assisted detection may also increase the radiologist's ability to detect small peripheral cancers (Chen and White 2008). Because there is a large spectrum of radiologic manifestations of lung cancer, detection of these findings is essential for proper patient management. To highlight the CXR presentation of lung carcinoma, correlations with CT findings in coronal, axial, sagittal, virtual bronchoscopy, and three-dimensional imaging are presented in this chapter.

17.2 Clinical Presentations

The majority of patients with bronchogenic carcinoma are symptomatic. Symptoms are related to the local, regional, or general extent of the tumor or due to paraneoplastic syndromes. In less than 20% of cases, lung cancer is discovered fortuitously on a CXR.

17.2.1 Symptomatic Presentation

Approximately 75–85% of patients with bronchogenic carcinoma are symptomatic at the time of diagnosis (Filderman et al. 1986). Patients who have lung cancer are more frequently in the sixth or seventh decade of life. Clinical presentation is often nonalerting in patients with a long history of cigarette smoking and chronic obstructive pulmonary disease (COPD). The site of development of lung cancer, the local and regional extent, and general diffusion create a large variety of presentations. These factors are also strongly correlated with the histologic type of lung cancer (Table 17.1) (Rosado-de-Christenson et al. 1994). Symptoms can be related to the primary tumor involving the central airways (frequent in case of squamous cell carcinoma and SCC) such as cough, hemoptysis, shortness of breath, wheezing, pneumonia, and bronchorrhea. Local extent of lung carcinoma to the mediastinum is responsible for dyspnea, cough, hoarseness, dysphagia, superior vena cava syndrome, and cardiac or pericardial effusion (Spiro et al. 2007). Peripheral tumors can extend to the pleura or chest wall, producing pleuretic or chest wall pain, and are often associated with pleural effusion. Pancoast syndrome is due to the invasion of the superior sulcus. Symptoms can be caused by metastatic

Table 17.1 Typical radiographic manifestations of lung carcinomas according the histologic type (frequent: F; rare: R)

Adenocarcinoma (~35% of lung carcinomas)

Solitary pulmonary nodule or mass (F)

Pleural invasion (F)

Unremarkable chest radiography (small pulmonary nodule, nonsolid and part-solid nodules) (F)

Chronic pulmonary consolidation (R)

Squamous cell carcinoma (~30% of lung carcinomas)

Postobstructive pneumonitis (F)

Atelectasis (lobar, lung) (F)

S-sign of Golden (R)

Localized thickening of the bronchial wall (R)

Enlarged hilum (F)

Dense hilum (R)

Solitary pulmonary nodule or mass (cavitation in about 10% of cases) (F)

Apical mass (the Pancoast syndrome) (R)

Small cell lung carcinoma (~15–25% of lung carcinomas)

Hilar or perihilar mass (isolated or in association with mediastinal enlargement) (F)

Mediastinal widening (associated with hilar mass or isolated) (F)

Lung nodule or mass (R)

Large cell carcinoma (~10–20% of lung carcinomas)

Large (>4 cm) peripheral lung mass

diffusion of the disease to bones, the liver, the central nervous system, or adrenals. Paraneoplastic syndromes are quite common and occur in 10–15% of patients (Beckles et al. 2003). They include those related to secretion of ectopic hormones by the tumor (Cushing syndrome, acromegaly, hypercalcemia, syndrome of inappropriate secretion of antidiuretic hormone) or other manifestations (clubbing and hypertrophic osteoarthropathy, thrombophebitis, and various cutaneous or neurologic syndromes) (Spiro et al. 2007).

17.2.2 Asymptomatic Presentation

Approximately 15–25% of patients have no symptoms at all and the cancer is discovered incidentally; this proportion is currently rising because of an increasing use of CT in patients who have COPD and cardiovascular diseases, and who are at an increased risk of lung cancer (Beckles et al. 2003).

17.3 Radiographic Manifestations of Lung Carcinoma

CXR shows two major types of presentation for bronchogenic carcinoma: centrally located and peripherally located tumors.

17.3.1 Factors That Affect Visualization of Lung Carcinoma on CXR

Five main factors have been described explaining radiographic visualization of lung carcinoma (Brogdon et al. 1983); i.e., the location within the lung, the size, the radiographic attenuation, the presence or absence of parenchyma abnormalities (Sone et al. 1997), and the extent of the tumor, either local or regional. Lung carcinoma can be detected when the contrast between the tumor and the surrounding structures is sufficient, which is limited by either radiographic noise or anatomic noise (Samei et al. 2003). Because of the complexity of adjacent structures to the tumor and the presence of superimposed anatomical details (vessels, ribs, clavicle), pulmonary carcinomas are usually detected when they are 1 cm or greater in diameter.

17.3.2 Location

Pulmonary carcinoma occurs more frequently in the right lung and in the upper lobe, with a frequency of 3:1 and 2:1 as compared with the left lung and the lower lobe, respectively. Regional distribution may be affected by underlying disease; patients who have idiopathic pulmonary fibrosis or asbestosis develop lung carcinoma within the peripheral areas of the lower lobes. Squamous cell carcinoma and SCC occur more frequently in the central part of the airways with a segmental or lobar location whereas adenocarcinoma tends to be more peripheral in distribution. Tumors in the apex of the upper lobes (or Pancoast tumors) are rare, accounting for about 4%; tumors of the trachea are even rarer (less than 1% of cases).

17.3.3 Central Tumors

- Obstructive pneumonitis associated with partial atelectasis is one of the most frequent radiologic presentations of central bronchogenic carcinoma.
- Enlargement or increased opacity of one hilum may be an early sign of lung carcinoma.
- Mediastinal involvement is seen with all histologic types of bronchogenic carcinoma, but bulky mediastinum should raise suspicion for SCC.

Due to their location in the central airways, some of these tumors can be responsible for bronchial obstruction beyond the lesion and subsequent pulmonary collapse or pulmonary consolidation caused by obstructive pneumonitis. Rarely, partial obstruction results in the alteration of regional lung volume with air trapping in expiration. In other cases, these tumors alone or in association with hilar enlarged lymph nodes may appear as an enlarged hilum, increased density of the hilum, or both (Theros 1977).

17.3.3.1 Obstructive Pneumonitis

This is the most common radiographic manifestation of airway obstruction. It is usually associated with atelectasis, bronchiectasis with mucous plugging, and parenchymal consolidation containing lipid-laden macrophages, fibrous tissue, and inflammatory cells. Radiologic patterns of atelectasis are presented in Chap. 16. Not surprisingly, obstructive pneumonitis is more frequently seen to be associated with squamous cell carcinoma (43%) and SSC (50%) than with large cell carcinoma (27%) or adenocarcinoma (29%) (Fraser and Paré 1999). Obstructive pneumonitis affects more commonly a segment or a lobe and more rarely an entire lung.

Obstructive pneumonitis appears on CXR as a homogeneous or patchy pulmonary opacity beyond the bronchial obstruction (Fig. 17.1). The severity of

volume loss is variable, ranging from consolidation without loss of volume (Fig. 17.2) to marked atelectasis (Fig. 17.3). Air bronchogram is rarely visible on CXR but may be seen using CT (Fig. 17.4). Absence of air bronchogram, however, highly suggests a proximal obstruction of the airways by lung carcinoma instead of infectious pneumonia. With obstructive pneumonitis, dilated bronchi filled with mucus are often noticeable in the late contrast-enhanced CT phase (Fig. 17.3). Differentiating centrally located bronchogenic carcinoma from postobstructive pneumonitis may be difficult even when using CT, although this is of clinical relevance for planning radiotherapy.

The "S-sign of Golden" (Fig. 17.5) associates the mass effect of a centrally located tumor with the opacity of a partially collapsed lobe beyond the bronchial obstruction and is highly suspicious for malignancy (Rosado-de-Christenson et al. 1994). CT scan confirms the central tumor, and shows the obstructed or severely narrowed bronchus (Woodring 1988), as well as the consolidation of the lung beyond it with some degree of pulmonary collapse.

17.3.3.2 Unilateral Hilar Enlargement

Unilateral hilar enlargement can be the earliest radiographic manifestation of lung cancer (Fig. 17.6), and was noticed in 38% of patients in a series (Byrd et al. 1969). The hilar mass effect is due to the bronchogenic carcinoma, hilar metastatic enlarged lymph nodes, or the association of both (Fig. 17.7). Such presentation is more common in patients who have squamous cell carcinoma or SCC than in patients who have adenocarcinoma. When enlarged lymph nodes or lung carcinoma are of limited size, they may not enlarge the hilum but appear as an increased opacity of one hilum. In both conditions, contrast-enhanced CT usually shows the primary tumor and the associated lymph nodes.

17.3.3.3 Alteration of Regional Lung Volume

Partial obstruction of main or lobar bronchus lumen may result, in rare cases, in air trapping during expiration. Overinflation of a pulmonary territory due to check valve obstruction is also very uncommon (Fraser and Paré,

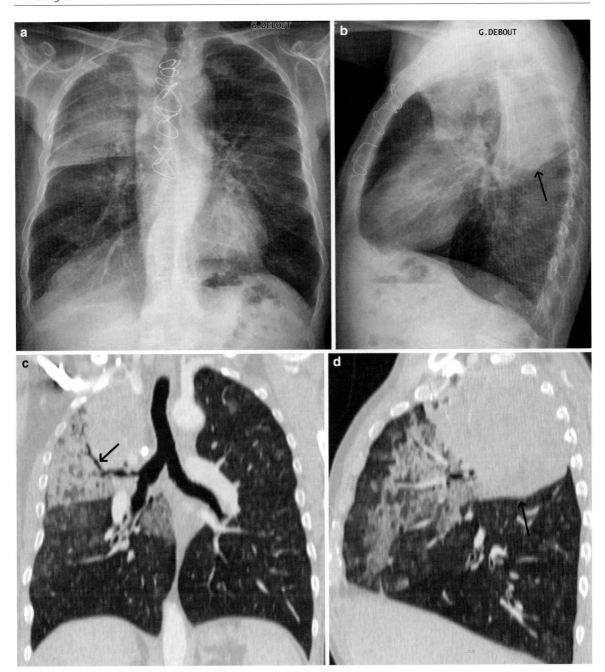

Fig. 17.1 Postobstructive pneumonitis of the upper segment of the right upper lobe (RUL) showing hyperexpansion in a 60-year-old man with RUL squamous cell carcinoma. (**a**) Posteroanterior chest radiograph shows inhomogeneous consolidation of the RUL. (**b**) Lateral chest radiograph demonstrates that the consolidation predominates within the upper and posterior segments of the RUL and is responsible for downward displacement and bulging of the upper part of the major fissure (*arrow*). (**c**) Coronal reformation of contrast-enhanced computed tomography confirms the massive consolidation of the RUL. Air bronchogram is visible within the posterior segmental bronchus (*arrow*). (**d**) Sagittal reformation shows the downward displacement of the upper part of the major fissure due to expansive consolidation of the RUL (*arrow*)

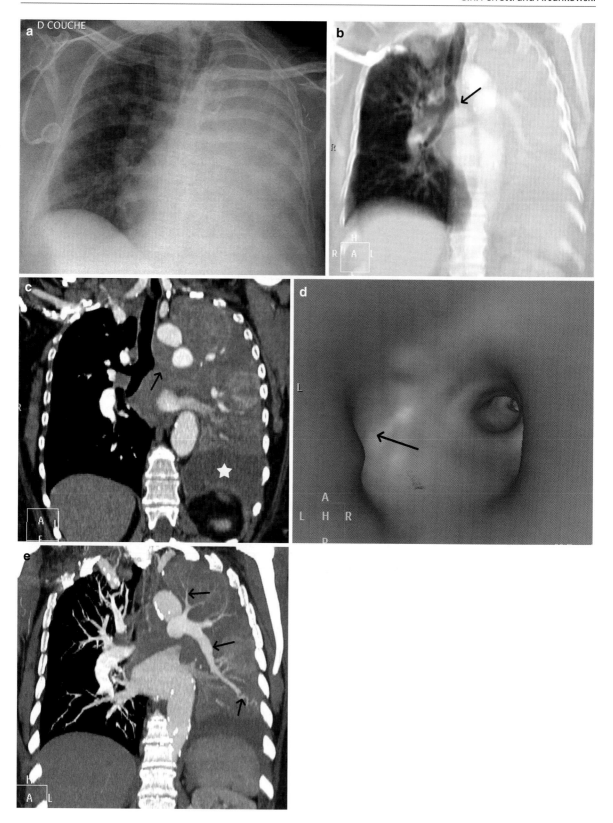

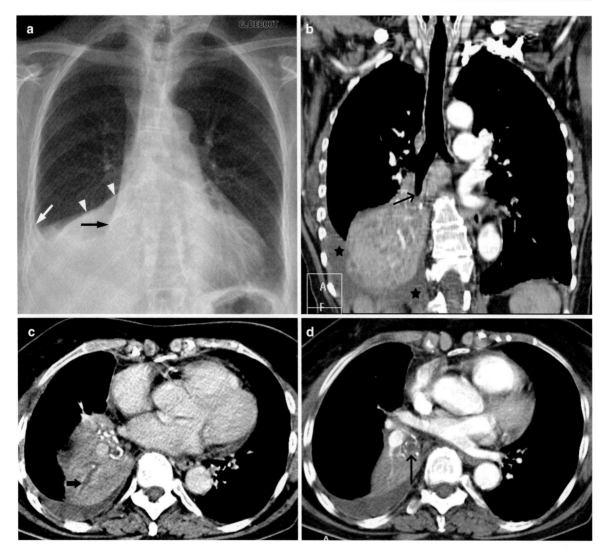

Fig. 17.3 Atelectasis and postobtructive pneumonitis of the right middle lobe and the right lower lobe (RLL), resulting from squamous cell carcinoma of the right intermediate bronchus in a 63-year-old smoking woman. (**a**) Posteroanterior chest radiograph shows combined RLL (*black arrow*) and right main bronchus atelectasis (*arrowheads*) as well as pleural effusion (*white arrow*). (**b**) Coronal reformation of contrast-enhanced computed tomography (CT) at the level of the central airway demonstrates complete obstruction of the intermediate bronchus (*arrow*) with resulting atelectasis and obstructive pneumonitis. Note the right pleural effusion (*stars*). (**c**) Axial CT shows bronchi filled with mucous within the atelectasis (*arrow*). Notice the absence of air bronchogram. (**d**) Axial CT shows the obstruction by a soft tissue tumor of the intermediate bronchus (*arrow*)

←

Fig. 17.2 Postobstructive pneumonitis of the left lung in a 65-year-old woman with a history of carcinoma of the left breast. (**a**) Anteroposterior chest radiograph shows a complete opacification of the left lung with shift of the mediastinum to the right. (**b**) Coronal average reformation (40-mm thick) shows obstruction of the left main bronchus (LMB) (*arrow*) and lack of air bronchogram within the left lung. (**c**) Coronal reformation of contrast-enhanced computed tomography at the level of the tracheal bifurcation demonstrates obstruction of the LMB and extensive infiltration of the mediastinum (*arrow*). Postobstructive pneumonitis is enhanced by contrast media administration while basal pleural effusion is of low density (*star*). (**d**) Virtual bronchoscopy confirms the complete obstruction of the origin of the LMB (*arrow*). (**e**) Coronal MIP shows the integrity of the left pulmonary artery and demonstrates the angiogram sign (*arrows*) within the postobstructive pneumonitis

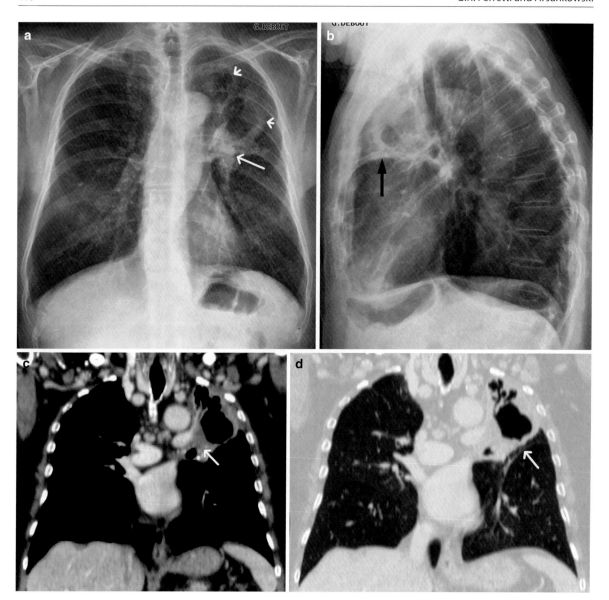

Fig. 17.4 Left upper lobe (LUL) postobstructive pneumonitis with distal necrosis due to a bacterial abscess in a 74-year-old man who has squamous cell carcinoma of the culmen. (**a**) Posteroanterior chest radiograph shows a dense, enlarged left hilum (*arrow*) associated with a heterogeneous consolidation of the LUL containing air bronchogram and thick-walled cavity (*arrowheads*). (**b**) Lateral chest radiograph demonstrates the location of the lesion within the culmen (*arrow*). (**c**) Contrast-enhanced computed tomography coronal reformation at the level of the LUL bronchus shows the obstruction of the LUL bronchus by a soft-density mass (*arrow*), a large irregular cavity of the culmen, and enlarged lymph nodes within the mediastinum. (**d**) Coronal reformation (lung windows) shows the thick wall of the cavity and air bronchogram. The convex upper bulge of the major fissure indicates LUL atelectasis (*arrow*)

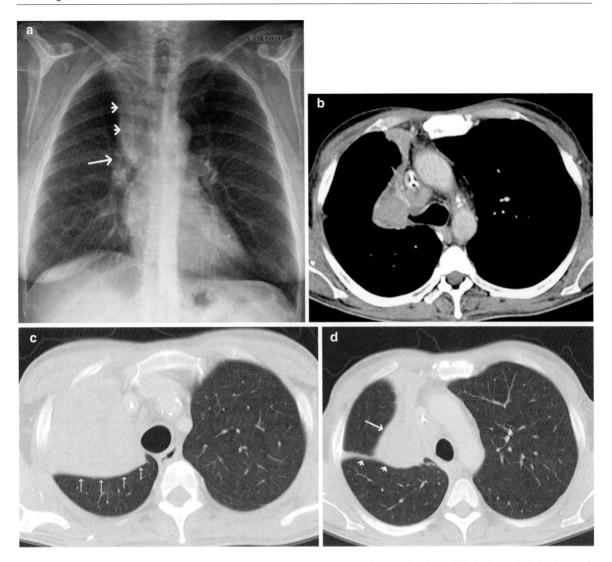

Fig. 17.5 S-sign of Golden in a 61-year-old woman with a right upper lobe (RUL) bronchus obstruction revealing squamous cell carcinoma. (**a**) Posteroanterior chest radiograph demonstrates atelectasis of the RUL (*arrowheads*) and focal convexity of the hilum (*arrow*). (**b**) Axial computed tomography (CT) at the level of the RUL bronchus shows a soft tissue density mass, 3 cm in diameter, obstructing the RUL bronchus. (**c**) Axial CT at the level of the upper thoracic trachea demonstrates an atelectatic RUL as a soft tissue density well limited posteriorly by the anteriorly displaced major fissure (*arrows*) and lying against the mediastinum. (**d**) Axial CT at the level of lower trachea shows the centrally located tumor and the atelectasis of the RUL. Note the medially displacement of the minor fissure (*arrow*) and the anterior displacement of the major fissure (*arrowheads*). The mediastinum is shifted to the right

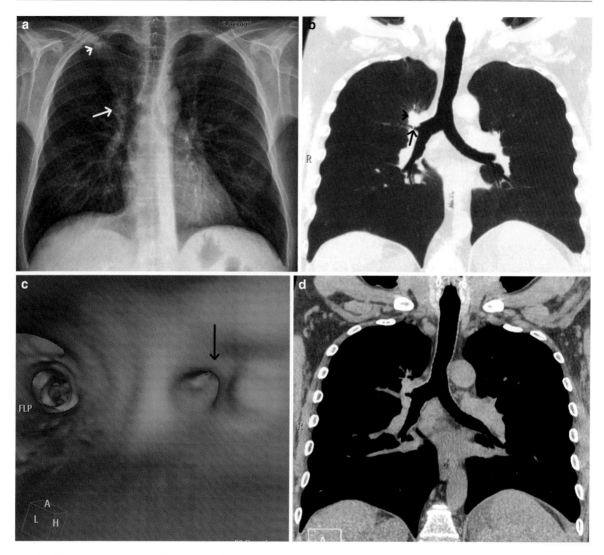

Fig. 17.6 Right upper lobe (RUL) carcinoma in a 73-year-old man with a history of RUL tuberculosis. (**a**) Posteroanterior chest radiograph demonstrates an elevation and enlargement of the right hilum compared with the left one (*arrow*). RUL subpleural opacity at the apex (*arrowhead*) and linear bands between the right hilum and the apex are also present. (**b**) Thin slab minimum intensity projection coronal reformation shows the irregu- lar narrowing of the RUL bronchus (*arrow*) and a spiculated mass above it obstructing the upper segmental bronchus (*arrow-head*). (**c**) Virtual bronchoscopy at the level of the RUL bron- chus reveals narrowing and irregularity (*arrow*) of the wall of the RUL bronchus. (**d**) Coronal reformation in mediastinal windows shows the tumor obstructing the bronchus

1999). These signs are usually associated with slow-growing, centrally located tumors such as carcinoids.

17.3.3.4 Bronchial Wall Thickening

When seen early, infiltration of peribronchial intersti- tial tissue by lung cancer can produce increased thickness of the bronchial wall or obscuration of the adjacent vessel (Fraser and Paré 1999). These signs have been described on the posteroanterior CXR for various bronchi, including the anterior segmental bron- chi of the right and left upper lobes, the superior seg- mental bronchus of the left lower lobe, and on the lateral CXR for the left main, lower lobe or intermediate bron- chus (Fig. 17.8). Thickening of the bronchial wall should be noticed on CT scans because it may represent the only sign of bronchogenic carcinoma in rare cases.

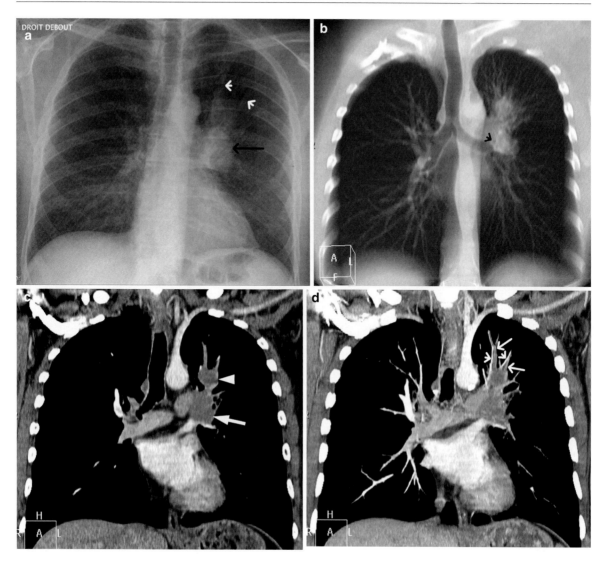

Fig. 17.7 Left enlarged hilum and bronchocele formation caused by centrally located adenocarcinoma with enlarged lymph nodes in a 52-year-old man with brain metastases. (**a**) Posteroanterior chest radiograph shows a dense enlarged left hilum (*arrow*) surmounted by a mass and finger-like opacities (*arrowheads*) extending into the culmen. (**b**) Coronal average reformation (35 mm thick) through the central airways demonstrates the obstruction of the culminal bronchus (*arrowhead*), the hilar and perihilar mass, and an increased number of tubular structures within the culmen distally to the hilar mass compared with the RUL. (**c**) Coronal reformation of contrast-enhanced computed tomography shows a well-limited mass within the left hilum (*arrow*) and a second well-defined mass above it (*arrowhead*). (**d**) Coronal thin slab maximum intensity projection shows the bronchoceles as enlarged bronchi filled with low-density material (*arrow*) and the satellite pulmonary arteries (*arrowheads*) within the left upper lobe

17.3.3.5 Mediastinal Involvement

In patients with significant mediastinal involvement, CXR shows lobulated, often asymmetrical widening of the mediastinum. It can be due to direct invasion from a contiguous tumor (Fig. 17.9) or the presence of enlarged lymphadenopathy (Fig. 17.10). All cell types of lung cancer may be associated with mediastinal involvement. However, bulky mediastinum is commonly seen in patients who have SCC, often in association with a hilar or perihilar mass. In these cases, encasement or invasion (Fig. 17.11) of mediastinal

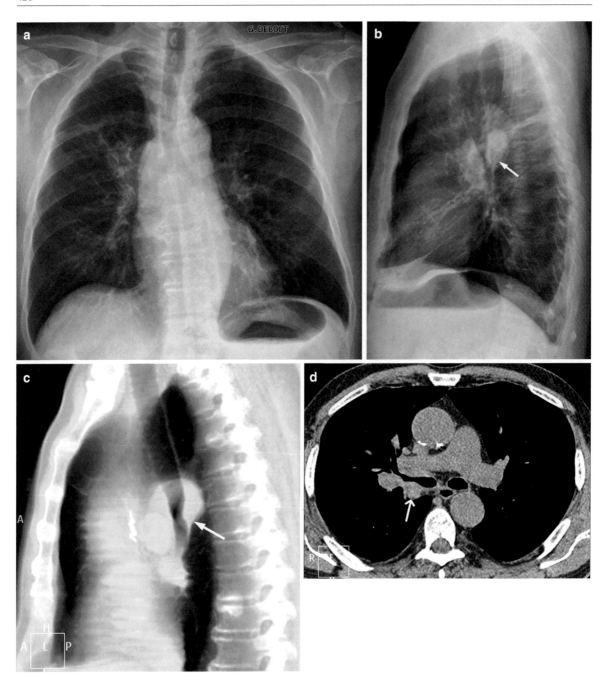

Fig. 17.8 Small cell carcinoma of the right hilum in a 56-year-old man. (**a**) Posteroanterior chest radiograph shows an enlarged and opaque right hilum. (**b**) Lateral chest radiograph demonstrates a thick and nodular intermediate bronchus line (*arrow*). (**c**) Sagittal average reformation confirms the thickening of the posterior wall of the intermediate bronchus (*arrow*). (**d**) Axial computed tomography shows the posterior wall thickening of the right intermediate bronchus (*arrow*)

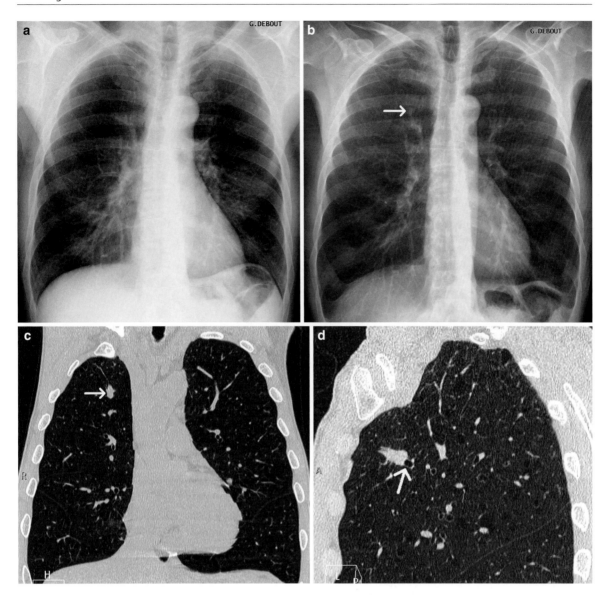

Fig. 17.9 Direct mediastinal extent of a small cell carcinoma. The patient received tracheal intubation because of acute respiratory distress. Pathological diagnosis was obtained by transthoracic needle biopsy because fiberoptic bronchoscopy did not provide adequate samples. (**a**) Anteroposterior chest radiograph taken in the intensive care unit reveals a large mass within the right upper lobe, shifting the mediastinum to the left. (**b**) Coronal average reformation (35 mm thick) demonstrates the obstruction of the right upper lobe (RUL) bronchus (*arrow*) and the mass of the RUL. (**c**) Coronal reformation without contrast enhancement shows a 12-cm soft tissue density mass involving the RUL and invading the right side of the mediastinum

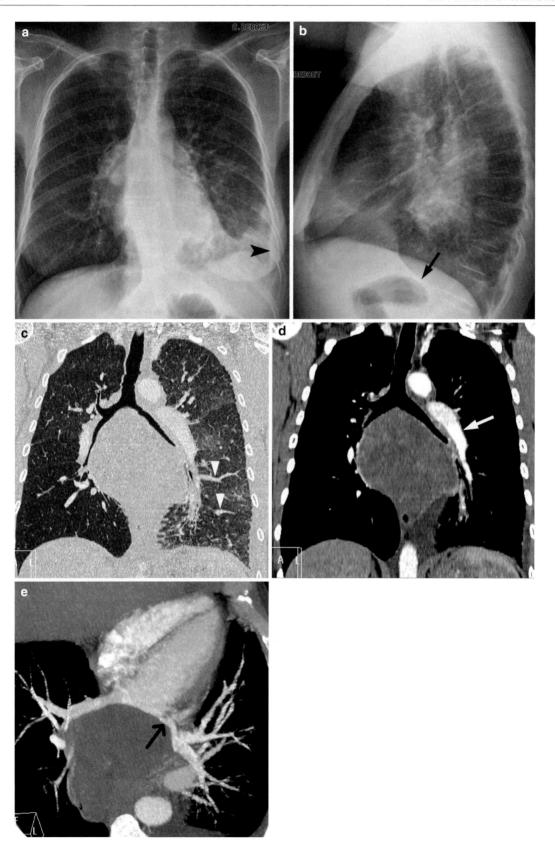

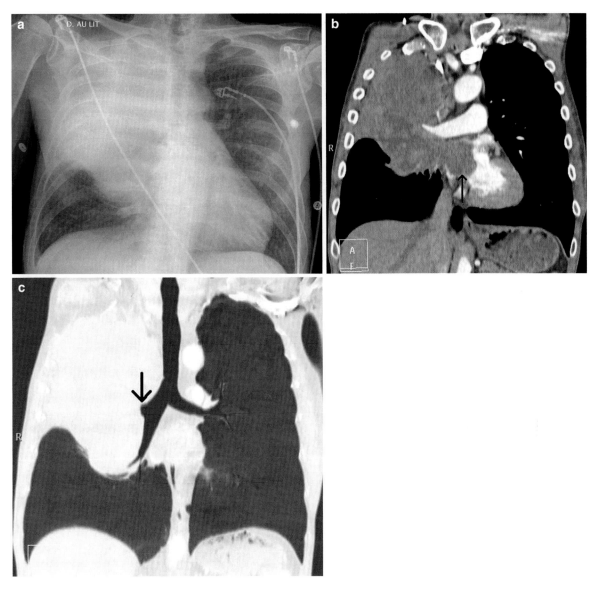

Fig. 17.11 A forty-seven-year-old man presented with acute thoracic pain. (**a**) Posteroanterior chest radiograph shows a large mass occupying the right upper lung and shifting the mediastinum to the left. (**b**) Coronal contrast-enhanced computed tomography scan shows direct extent of the tumor to the right atrium (*arrow*). (**c**) Coronal minimal intensity projection reconstruction at the level of the trachea shows the complete obstruction of the right upper lobe bronchus (*arrow*)

Fig. 17.10 Mediastinal lymph nodes in a 43-year-old woman with small cell carcinoma. (**a**) Posteroanterior chest radiograph reveals a large subcarinal mass elevating the main bronchi. Linear interstitial infiltration is visible in the left lower lung, along with pleural effusion (*arrowhead*). (**b**) Lateral chest radiograph demonstrates a lobulated mass within the subcarinal space, a left pleural effusion responsible for a silhouette sign with the left hemidiaphragm (*arrow*). (**c**) Coronal reformation (pulmonary window) shows the compression of the right and left central airways by the subcarinal mass. The left lower lobe veins (*arrowheads*) are enlarged compared with the right ones. (**d**) Coronal reformation shows the integrity of the left pulmonary artery (*arrow*). (**e**) Axial oblique maximum intensity projection reveals severe external compression of the left atrium and left pulmonary veins by the subcarinal mass. Compression of the left pulmonary veins (*arrow*) is supposed to be responsible for linear interstitial infiltration of the left lower lobe

structures and tracheobronchial compression are frequent (Pearlberg et al. 1988). In many cases, the primary tumor is not evident on the CXR.

Unilateral diaphragmatic paralysis resulting from tumoral extent to the phrenic nerve is a classic, although rare, presentation of lung cancer. CXR shows the elevation of one hemidiaphragm (Fig. 17.12), and in rare cases may not show any mediastinal abnormalities.

17.3.4 Peripheral Tumors

- The solitary nodule is a frequent incidental finding that may represent bronchogenic carcinoma.
- The larger the nodule, the more likely it is to be malignant.
- The most frequent malignant etiology of solitary nodules is adenocarcinoma.

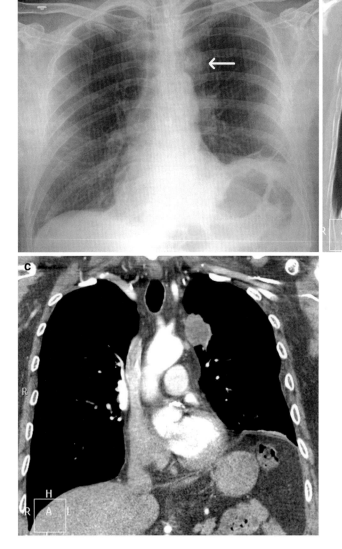

Fig. 17.12 Left diaphragmatic paralysis caused in a 63-year-old man complaining of dyspnea during recent exercise. Computed tomography (CT)-guided biopsy revealed mediastinal invasion from primary pulmonary squamous cell carcinoma. (**a**) Posteroanterior chest radiograph shows abnormal elevation of the left hemidiaphragm and a 3-cm mass projecting above the aortic arch (*arrow*).

(**b**) Coronal CT average reformation shows the integrity of the central airways, the mass abutting the left upper mediastinum (*arrow*), and the elevation of the left hemidiaphragm. (**c**) Coronal contrast-enhanced CT reformation shows the soft-density mass invading the mediastinal fat and a small lymph node in the left anterior mediastinum

- Precise morphologic analysis of pulmonary nodules requires volume high-resolution CT.
- Persistent or chronic air-space consolidation can be related to adenocarcinoma.
- Cavitation associated with a thick and irregular wall is highly suspicious of lung cancer.

They represent around 40% of bronchial carcinomas arising beyond the segmental bronchi. These tumors usually need to be more than 1 cm in diameter to be depicted on CXR, but larger lung cancers can be missed because of either intrinsic factors such as a low attenuation, as in nodular bronchioloalveolar carcinomas (BAC) or mixed adenocarcinoma, or either extrinsic factors such as an unfavorable anatomical location (i.e., within the apex, retrodiaphragmatic or retrocardiac location) (Sider 1990) (see Chap. 15).

Peripheral tumors are categorized as nodules (<3 cm in diameter) or masses (>3 cm in diameter). The larger the nodule, the more likely it is to be malignant; the majority of nodules larger than 2 cm are malignant. In rare cases, peripheral lung carcinoma appears as a chronic pulmonary consolidation or may mimic an apical cap.

17.3.4.1 Pulmonary Nodules and Masses

A great variety of benign or malignant conditions may result in a solitary pulmonary opacity. In clinical series in which solitary pulmonary lesions have been resected, about 40% were primary lung carcinomas, 10% were solitary metastases, and 50% were benign (McLoud and Swenson 1999). The role of the radiologist lies in attempting to approach noninvasively the origin of nodular opacities that are seen on CXR. Due to intrinsic limitations of CXR, radiographic signs are of greater value because they suggest with confidence the diagnosis of benignity rather than the diagnosis of malignancy. Therefore, nodules should be categorized into those with a formal benign pattern that deserve no further examination and those with an indeterminate pattern that require further exploration, with CT being the first imaging to be performed (Gould et al. 2007). This is mainly based on the examination of previous CXR to evaluate change in size over time and the assessment of morphologic details of the nodule. It is generally admitted that the stability in size of a pulmonary nodule for 2 years or longer is indicative of a benign etiology

(Yankelevitz and Henschke 1997). On the contrary, or in the absence of a previous radiograph, CT assessment is the next step in examination (Gould et al. 2007). Morphologic features that are of value include shape and margin, calcification, and doubling time.

Shape and Margin

Usually peripheral bronchial carcinomas appear as spherical or oval opacities (Fig. 17.13). Many signs have been described to separate malignant from benign pulmonary nodules. The analysis of the CXR is limited compared with the one provided by high resolution computed tomography High resolution computed tomography (high-resolution (HR) CT). Although the signs listed below are well demonstrated using HRCT, none of them is very specific for malignancy.

1. *Lobulation* (Fig. 17.14) is a common sign in bronchogenic carcinomas, indicating different growth rates of tumor populations within the tumor. This sign is, nevertheless, frequently demonstrated in hamartomas.
2. *Spiculations* (Fig. 17.14) are also frequent in lung carcinoma, sometimes creating a "corona radiata" around the tumor. Pathologic–radiologic correlations show that the strands extending into the surrounding lung can be either a result of direct tumor extension along interstitial planes or more usually a simple fibrotic reaction to the tumor. Approximately 90% of spiculated nodules are malignant (Zwirewich et al. 1991). It can also be demonstrated in benign conditions (subacute or chronic pneumonias, granulomas).
3. *The pleural tail sign* (Fig. 17.14) represents a linear band connecting the peripherally located tumor to the pleura (Hill 1982). They are seen predominantly in malignant nodules and represent fibrous strands or direct parenchymal invasion to the pleural surface.
4. Rarely, slow-growing bronchial carcinomas arise within the lumen of segmental or subsegmental bronchi, producing *bronchoceles* that appear on CXRs as V- or Y-shaped densities (Fraser and Paré 1999).

Calcifications

Calcifications are exceptionally visible within lung cancer opacities on CXRs and are frequently described

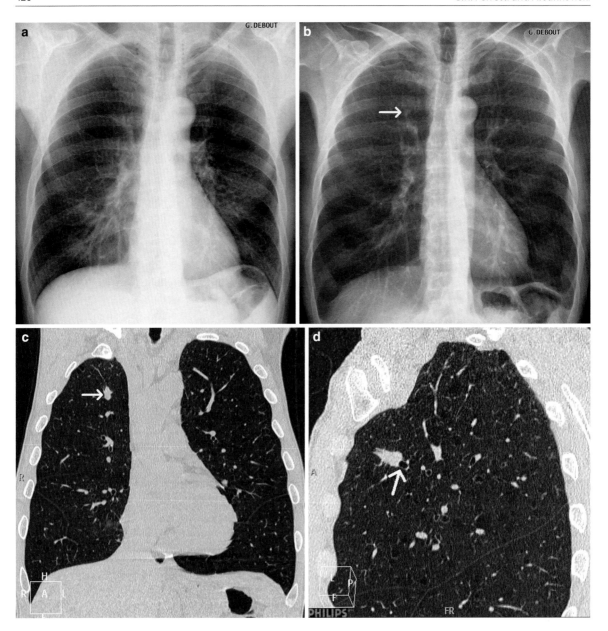

Fig. 17.13 Solitary pulmonary nodule (small cell carcinoma) in a 54-year-old smoker involved in the French Lung Cancer Screening Programm (DEPISCAN). (**a**) Posteroanterior chest radiograph at year 0 was unremarkable. (**b**) Posteroanterior chest radiograph at year 1 reveals a small pulmonary nodule, 10 mm in diameter, projecting between the fifth and sixth ribs (*arrow*). (**c**) Coronal computed tomography reformation demonstrates the small pulmonary nodule within the right upper lobe (*arrow*). (**d**) Sagittal reformation shows the endobronchial location of the tumor, obstructing the anterior segmental bronchus (*arrow*)

by pathologists. Because of a better contrast resolution, CT demonstrates such calcifications in about 6–10% of lung cancers (Heitzman 1977). Malignant calcifications are either large granulomatous calcifications engulfed by the growing tumor (usually eccentric in location) or dystrophic tumor calcifications (tiny, cloudlike, or punctate) (Fig. 17.15). They are different from benign calcifications, appearing as a central, laminated, or "popcorn" pattern (Mc Loud and Swenson 1999).

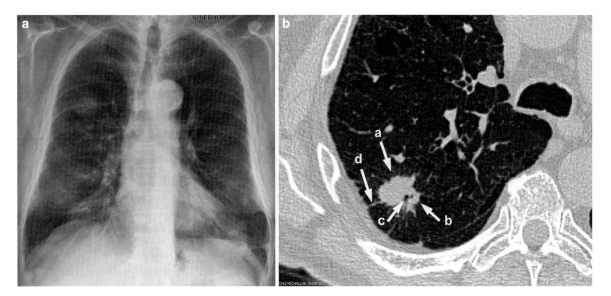

Fig. 17.14 Solitary pulmonary nodule in an asymptomatic 73-year-old smoker. (**a**) Posteroanterior chest radiograph reveals an oval, 2-cm, right-sided pulmonary nodule with regular margins. (**b**) Axial computed tomography shows morphologic criteria suggesting malignancy, such as spiculated margins (*arrow a*), lobulation (*arrow b*), cavitation (*arrow c*), and pleural tail sign (*arrow d*). Biopsy specimen showed adenocarcinoma

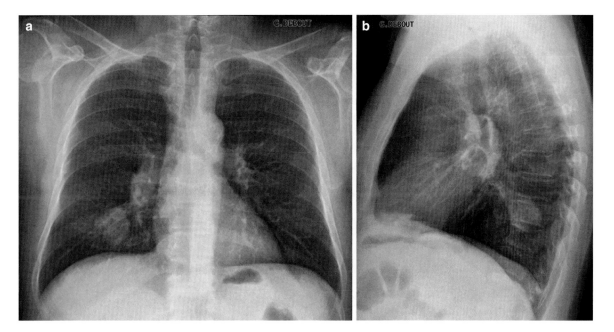

Fig. 17.15 Punctuate calcifications within a solitary mass (adenocarcinoma). (**a**) Posteroanterior chest radiograph shows a solitary pulmonary mass projecting in the right lung basis associated with dense and enlarged right hilum. (**b**) Lateral view shows the right lower lobe location of the mass. (**c**) Coronal computed tomography reformation (close up) without contrast administration shows that the mass has irregular, lobulated margins with punctuate calcifications. (**d**) Coronal reformation at the level of the trachea shows the presence of right hilar (*arrow*) and subcarinal (*arrowhead*) enlarged lymph nodes

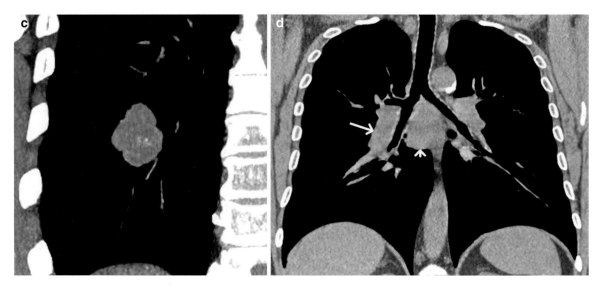

Fig. 17.15 (continued)

Cavitation

Cavitation secondary to necrosis and fistulization in a bronchus (Fig. 17.16) is seen in any type of tumor but most frequently in 10–20% of squamous cell carcinomas, particularly in large peripheral lesions (30%) (Patz 2000), and is more often demonstrated by CT. Liquefaction, air, or a mixture of both may be seen on CT and is better demonstrated after contrast media injection. Typically the walls of malignant cavities are thickened (>8 mm) and irregular. However, thin-walled cavities have also been reported in bronchogenic carcinomas. Cavitation can also be caused by an infection of the tumor; the diagnosis, however, is difficult for the pathologist.

Air Bronchogram and Bubble-Like Lucencies

Air bronchogram and bubble-like lucencies (pseudo-cavitation) are well demonstrated using HRCT and are frequently seen in BAC and adenocarcimomas. Due to their tiny size, these signs are not visible on CXR.

Pure or Mixed Nodular Ground Glass Opacification

Pure or mixed nodular ground glass opacification (GGO) representing BAC or adenocarcinoma is difficult to depict on CXR because of their low X-ray attenuation. However, HRCT's demonstration of GGO in a pulmonary tumor is associated with a better prognosis if a GGO component is more than 50%.

17.3.4.2 Chronic Air-Space Consolidation (Pneumonia-Like Appearances)

This is a rare presentation of lung carcinoma, mainly related to adenocarcinoma associated with a large BAC component. Radiographic presentation ranges from localized, hazy, unilateral air-space consolidation to diffuse, dense, bilateral consolidations (Lee et al. 1997). The lesion persists for weeks or months (Fig. 17.17), enlarging slowly or rarely cavitating. Air bronchogram can be seen on CXRs but are more frequently seen with CT. Contrast-enhanced CT also frequently displays an angiogram sign, which is not specific for a pneumonic type of adenocarcinoma and has been described in infectious pneumonitis, obstructive pneumonitis, lymphoma, pulmonary edema, and lipoid pneumonia. Differentiating BAC mimicking pneumonia and infectious pneumonia at the lung periphery is difficult when using CT (Kim et al. 2006). Transthoracic lung biopsy may be used to obtain histologic samples when fiberoptic bronchoscopy with bronchoalveolar lavage does not provide a diagnosis (Ferretti et al. 2008).

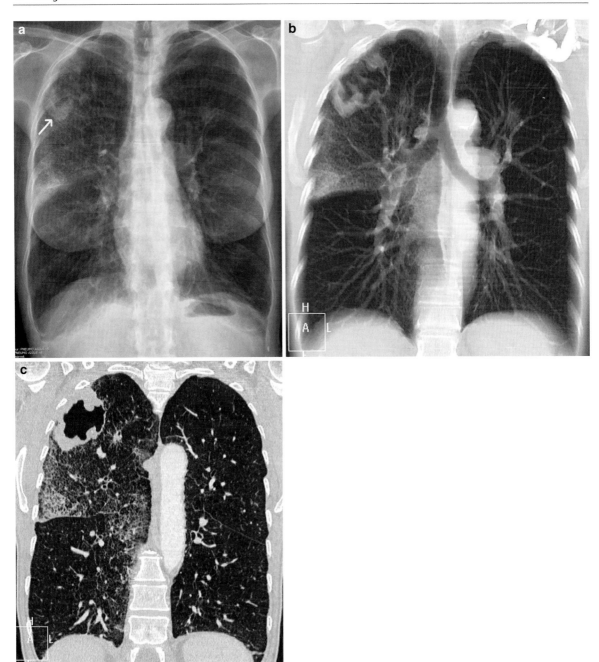

Fig. 17.16 Right upper lobe (RUL) mass (squamous cell carcinoma) with cavitation in 60-year-old woman who presented with hemoptysis. (**a**) Posteroanterior chest radiograph shows pulmonary overinflation, heterogenous pulmonary consolidation in the RUL containing a cavitated mass with a thickened wall (*arrow*). (**b**) Average thick slab coronal view confirms a cavitated mass within the RUL. (**c**) Coronal computed tomography reformation at the level of the descending aorta shows an irregular, thick-walled subpleural upper lobe mass and heterogeneous alveolar air-space consolidation within the RUL caused by hemorrhage

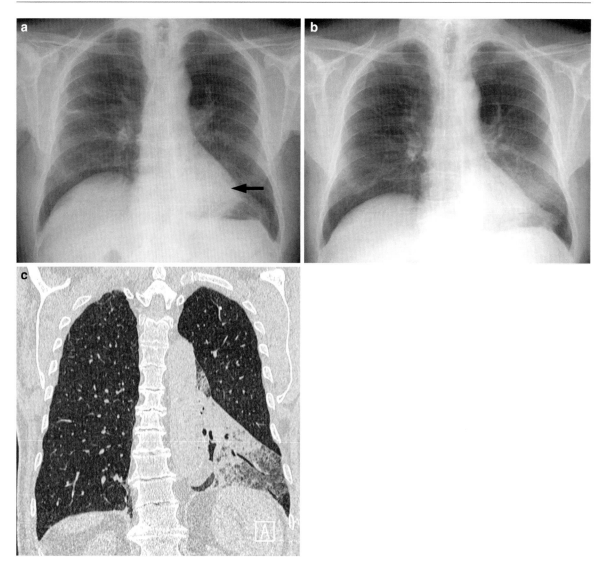

Fig. 17.17 Chronic pulmonary consolidation in a 65-year-old man caused by adenocarcinoma with a bronchioloalveolar component. (**a**) Posteroanterior chest radiograph (June 23, 2005) demonstrates pulmonary consolidation within the left lower lobe (LLL) (*arrow*). The patient was complaining of cough, fever, and expectoration. Suspected diagnosis was infectious pneu-

monitis. (**b**) Posteroanterior chest radiograph (September 15, 2005) shows enlargement of the LLL consolidation. (**c**) Coronal computed tomography (October 26, 2005) shows pulmonary consolidation and ground glass opacification of the LLL associated with slight volume loss of the LLL

17.3.4.3 Diffuse Interstitial Disease

It is quite uncommon that patients enter the disease with diffuse pulmonary interstitial infiltration. Lymphangitic carcinomatosis (Fig. 17.18) appears as localized or diffuse linear opacities often associated with hilar or mediastinal enlargement and pleural effusion. HRCT shows the lymphatic pattern of the disease

with interlobular septal thickening, sometimes nodular, thickened centrilobular dots, peribronchovascular thickening, and pleural effusion.

Multifocal BAC may appear as reticulonodular opacities simulating interstitial lung disease.

Chronic interstitial lung diseases, most often idiopathic pulmonary fibrosis, may be associated with an increased occurrence of lung cancer developing in the

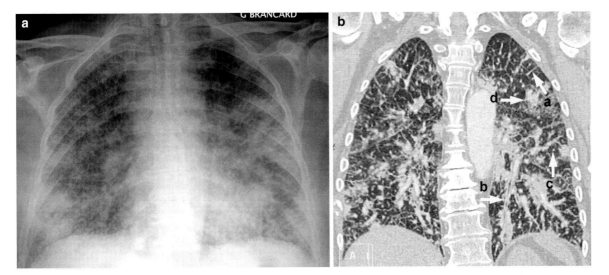

Fig. 17.18 A 52-year-old woman with progressively increasing dyspnea revealing diffuse lymphangitic carcinomatosis from pulmonary adenocarcinoma. (**a**) Posteroanterior chest radiograph shows diffuse linear and reticular pattern associated with areas of pulmonary consolidation. (**b**) Coronal high-resolution computed tomography demonstrates bilateral linear pattern with polygonal arcades (*arrow a*) due to thickening of the interlobular septa. Note thickened bronchoarterial bundles (*arrow b*), prominent centrilobular dots (*arrow c*), and focal air-space consolidations (*arrow d*)

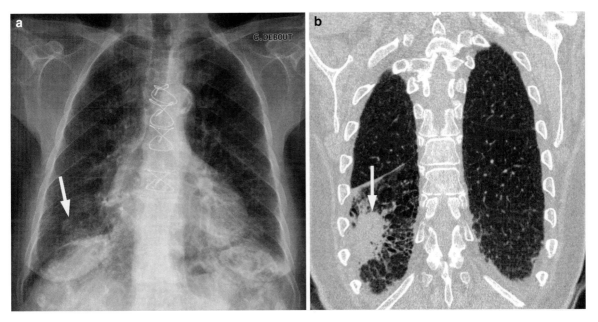

Fig. 17.19 Adenocarcinoma in an 80-year-old woman with usual interstitial pneumonia (UIP). (**a**) Posteroanterior chest radiograph shows a pulmonary mass (*arrow*) projecting on the right hemidiaphragm with a poorly defined border and bibasal pulmonary reticular infiltration. (**b**) Coronal computed tomography shows a mass 4.5 cm in diameter (*arrow*) within the right lower lobe and UIP pattern associating reticulation, and traction bronchiectasis with little honeycombing

lower part of the lungs, i.e., the area of fibrosis. Radiologic diagnosis of these cancers is often late because the infiltrative disease obscures the tumor (Fig. 17.19). Evaluation of sequential CXRs may help disclose the occurrence of a localized focal nodule. HRCT offers, however, a greater sensitivity and specificity than CXR.

17.3.5 Pleural Effusion and Pleural Thickening

- Pleural effusion may reveal bronchogenic carcinoma.

Pleural effusion occurs in about 10% of patients who have lung cancer. It is not always malignant and may be a serous or exudative effusion resulting from parenchymal infection or obstructive pneumonia.

The pleura can be involved by direct pleural invasion in the case of peripherally located lung cancer, or by hematogenous or lymphatic spread. When associated with a peripheral or central nodule or mass, obstructive pneumonitis or atelectasis, or hilar or mediastinal enlargement, it should raise the suspicion of lung cancer.

Pleural thickening (Fig. 17.20), either nodular or diffuse and encasing the lung with or without pleural effusion, is less frequently caused by lung carcinoma than by pleural metastases from extrathoracic malignancies, lymphoma, and pleural mesothelioma (Leung et al.1990). Pathological diagnosis is therefore required but can be difficult.

Spontaneous pneumothorax has been described as an inaugural presentation of lung cancer in rare cases.

17.3.6 Chest Wall Involvement

CXR has a low sensitivity and specificity for demonstrating chest wall involvement. Direct extension or metastatic spread to the ribs, sternum, or the vertebrae can be seen on CXR but is better depicted using CT (Pearlberg et al. 1987). Osteolytic lesions (Fig. 17.21) are much more frequent than osteoblastic ones.

17.3.7 Apical Tumors

- Apical tumors are rare (3%).
- The Pancoast syndrome is characterized by pain limited to the shoulder or radiating to the arm, Horner's syndrome, destruction of bone, and atrophy of hand muscles.
- CXR is less specific and sensitive than for CT showing an apical tumor.

A pulmonary apical tumor or Pancoast tumor develops in the superior sulcus of the lung and represents approximately 3% of primary NSCC (Bruzzi et al. 2008a). The Pancoast syndrome is associated with an apical lung cancer invading the costovertebral groove

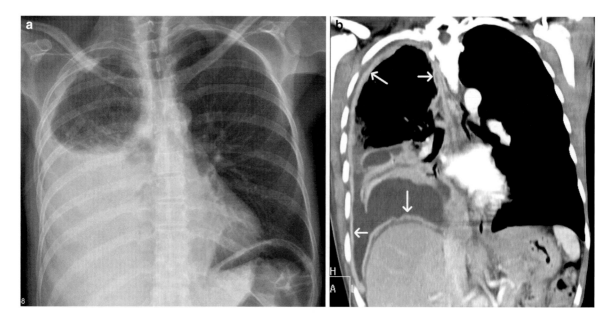

Fig. 17.20 A 47-year-old patient complained of dyspnea and right thoracic pain. Scans revealed a metastatic pleural effusion from bronchogenic adenocarcinoma. (**a**) Posteroanterior chest radiograph reveals a large right pleural effusion.

(**b**) Contrast-enhanced computed tomography in coronal view shows a large right pleural effusion, passive atelectasis of the right lower lobe, and circumferential contrast-enhanced pleural thickening (*arrows*)

in the posterior compartment of the superior sulcus, and symptoms include pain limited to the shoulder or radiating to the arm, Horner's syndrome, destruction of bone, and atrophy of hand muscles. CXR can show an apical cap more than 8 mm in thickness, convex inferiorly, an asymmetry in apical caps more than 5mm, an apical mass, and bone destruction of the first, second, or third ribs (Fig. 17.22) (Fraser and Paré

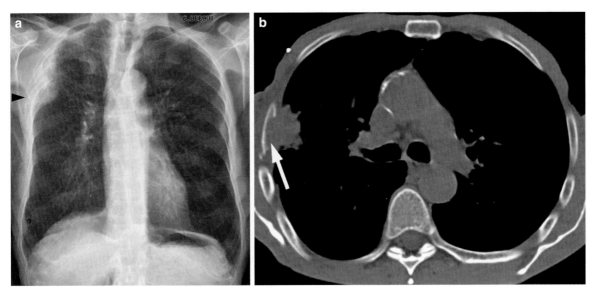

Fig. 17.21 Peripheral adenocarcinoma with chest wall invasion in an 82-year-old man with right upper anterior chest wall pain. (**a**) Posteroanterior chest radiograph shows a mass peripherally situated in the right upper lobe associated with destruction of the rib (*arrowhead*). (**b**) Axial computed tomography confirms the peripheral soft tissue density mass with destruction of the right lateral fourth rib (*arrow*)

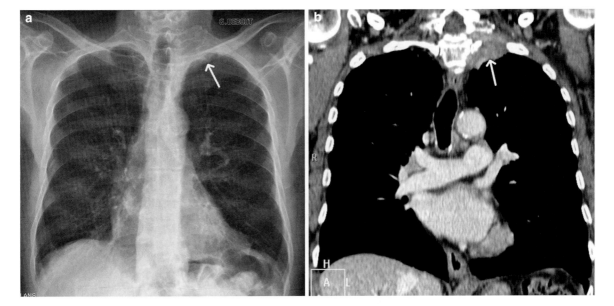

Fig. 17.22 Superior sulcus tumor (squamous cell carcinoma) in a 72-year-old man with a 2-month history of left shoulder pain. (**a**) Posteroanterior chest radiograph reveals a soft-tissue mass in the left lung apex with an inferior convex border (*arrow*). (**b**) Coronal computed tomography reformation depicts a soft-tissue mass within the superior sulcus (*arrow*). (**c**) Axial reformation (bone windows) shows focal destruction of the T2 vertebral body (*arrow*) and probable extension into the T2–T3 neurovertebral foramen (*arrowhead*). Note focal destruction of the first rib

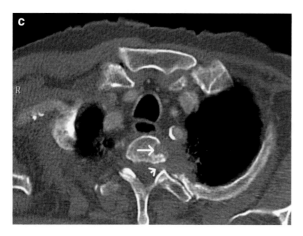

Fig. 17.22 (continued)

1999). CT is much more sensitive and specific than CXR, especially if isotropic multidetector coronal and sagittal reformations are performed (Chooi et al. 2005). CT is optimal for depicting bone erosion of the ribs and vertebral bodies and for the staging of intrathoracic disease (detection of enlarged lymph nodes and pulmonary metastases) (Bruzzi et al. 2008b). The subclavian artery, brachial plexus, vertebral bodies, and spinal canal should be assessed for tumor involvement. However, magnetic resonance imaging is superior to CT for evaluating tumor extension to the intervertebral neural foramina, the spinal cord, and the brachial plexus, primarily because of the higher contrast resolution and multiplanar capability available with magnetic resonance imaging (Bruzzi et al. 2008b).

17.4 Conclusion

CXR plays a pivotal role in the identification of lung cancer because it is commonly performed in patients who complain of respiratory symptoms and in asymptomatic persons. Correlations between CXR and CT images, particularly coronal and sagittal views, help radiologists to recognize and understand the radiographic presentation of bronchogenic carcinoma.

References

Bach PB, Jett JR, Pastorino U, Tockman MS, Swensen SJ, Begg CB (2007) Computed tomography screening and lung cancer outcomes. JAMA 297:953–961

Beckett WS (1993) Epidemiology and etiology of lung cancer. Clin Chest Med 14:1–15

Beckles MA, Spiro SG, Colice GL, Rudd RM (2003) Initial evaluation of the patient with lung cancer: symptoms, signs, laboratory tests, and paraneoplastic syndromes. Chest 123 (1 Suppl):97S–104S

Berg CD, Aberle DR, National Lung Screening Trial Executive Committee. (2007) CT screening for lung cancer. N Engl J Med 356:743–744

Brambilla E, Travis WD, Colby TV, Corrin B, Shimosato Y (2001) The new World Health Organization classification of lung tumours. Eur Respir J 18:1059–1068

Brogdon BG, Kelsey CA, Moseley RD Jr (1983) Factors affecting perception of pulmonary lesions. Radiol Clin North Am 21:633–654

Bruzzi JF, Komaki R, Walsh GL, Truong MT, Gladish GW, Munden RF, Erasmus JJ (2008a) Imaging of non-small cell lung cancer of the superior sulcus: part 1: anatomy, clinical manifestations, and management. Radiographics 28:551–560

Bruzzi JF, Komaki R, Walsh GL, Truong MT, Gladish GW, Munden RF, Erasmus JJ (2008b) Imaging of non-small cell lung cancer of the superior sulcus: part 2: initial staging and assessment of resectability and therapeutic response. Radiographics 28: 561–572

Byrd RB, Carr DT, Miller WE, Payne WS, Woolner LB (1969) Radiographic abnormalities in carcinoma of the lung as related to histological cell type. Thorax 24:573–575

Chen JJ, White CS (2008) Use of CAD to evaluate lung cancer on chest radiography. J Thorac Imaging 23:93–96

Chooi WK, Matthews S, Bull MJ, Morcos SK (2005) Multislice computed tomography in staging lung cancer: the role of multiplanar image reconstruction. J Comput Assist Tomogr 29:357–360

Ferretti GR, Jankowski A, Rodière M, Brichon PY, Brambilla C, Lantuejoul S (2008) CT-guided biopsy of nonresolving focal air space consolidation. J Thorac Imaging 23:7–12

Filderman AE, Shaw C, Matthay RA (1986) Lung cancer. Part I: Etiology, pathology, natural history, manifestations, and diagnostic techniques. Invest Radiol 21:80–90

Fraser RG, Paré JAP (1999) Diagnosis of diseases of the chest. W.B. Saunders, Philadelphia

Gould MK, Fletcher J, Iannettoni MD, Lynch WR, Midthun DE, Naidich DP, Ost DE (2007) Evaluation of patients with pulmonary nodules: when is it lung cancer?: ACCP evidence-based clinical practice guidelines (2nd edition). Chest 132:108S–130S

Hansell DM, Amstrong P, Lynch DA, Page McAdams H (2005) Imaging of diseases of the chest. Elsevier Mosby, Philadelphia

Heelan RT, Flehinger BJ, Melamed MR, Zaman MB, Perchick WB, Caravelli JF, Martini N (1984) Non-small-cell lung cancer: results of the New York screening program. Radiology 151:289–293

Heitzman ER (1977) Bronchogenic carcinoma: radiologic-pathologic correlations. Semin Roentgenol 12:165–173

Henschke CI, McCauley DI, Yankelevitz DF, Naidich DP, McGuinness G, Miettinen OS, Libby DM, Pasmantier MW, Koizumi J, Altorki NK, Smith JP (1999) Early Lung Cancer Action Project: overall design and findings from baseline screening. Lancet 354(9173):99–105

Hill CA (1982) "Tail" signs associated with pulmonary lesions: critical reappraisal. AJR Am J Roentgenol 139:311–316

Kim TH, Kim SJ, Ryu YH, Chung SY, Seo JS, Kim YJ, Choi BW, Lee SH, Cho SH (2006) Differential CT features of infectious pneumonia versus bronchioloalveolar carcinoma (BAC) mimicking pneumonia. Eur Radiol 16(8):1763–1768

Kubik A, Parkin DM, Khlat M, Erban J, Polak J, Adamec M (1990) Lack of benefit from semi-annual screening for cancer of the lung: follow-up report of a randomized controlled trial on a population of high-risk males in Czechoslovakia. Int J Cancer 45:26–33

Lee KS, Kim Y, Han J, Ko EJ, Park CK, Primack SL (1997) Bronchioloalveolar carcinoma: clinical, histopathologic, and radiologic findings. Radiographics 17:1345–1357

Leung AN, Müller NL, Miller RR (1990) CT in differential diagnosis of diffuse pleural disease. AJR Am J Roentgenol 154:487–492

Marcus PM, Bergstralh EJ, Fagerstrom RM, Williams DE, Fontana R, Taylor WF, Prorok PC (2000) Lung cancer mortality in the Mayo Lung Project: impact of extended follow-up. Natl Cancer Inst 92:1308–1316

McAdams HP, Samei E, Dobbins J, Tourassi GD, Ravin CE (2006) Recent advances in chest radiography. Radiology 241:663–683

McLoud T, Swenson SJ (1999) Lung carcinoma. Clin Chest Med 20:697–713

Muhm JR, Miller WE, Fontana RS, Sanderson DR, Uhlenhopp MA (1983) Lung cancer detected during a screening program using four-month chest radiographs. Radiology 148:609–615

Patz EF (2000) Imaging bronchogenic carcinoma. Chest 117:90–95

Pearlberg JL, Sandler MA, Beute GH et al (1987) Limitations of CT in evaluation of neoplasms involving chest wall. J Comput Assist Tomogr 11:290–293

Pearlberg JL, Sandler MA, Lewis JW Jr et al (1988) Small-cell bronchogenic carcinoma: CT evaluation. AJR Am J Roentgenol 150:265–268

Rosado-de-Christenson ML, Templeton PA, Moran CA (1994) Bronchogenic carcinoma: radiologic-pathologic correlation. Radiographics 14:429–446

Samei E, Flynn MJ, Peterson E, Eyler WR (2003) Subtle lung nodules: influence of local anatomic variations on detection. Radiology 228:76–84

Scagliotti G (2001) Symptoms, signs and staging of lung cancer. Eur Respir Mon 17:86–119

Sider L (1990) Radiographic manifestations of primary bronchogenic carcinoma. Radiol Clin North Am 28:583–597

Sone S, Sakai F, Takashima S, Honda T, Yamanda T, Kubo K, Fukasaku K, Maruyama Y, Li F, Hasegawa M, Ito A, Yang Z (1997) Factors affecting the radiologic appearance of peripheral bronchogenic carcinomas. J Thorac Imaging 12:159–172

Spiro SG, Gould MK, Colice GL (2007) Initial evaluation of the patient with lung cancer: symptoms, signs, laboratory tests, and paraneoplastic syndromes: ACCP evidenced-based clinical practice guidelines (2nd edition). Chest 132:149S–160S

Swensen SJ, Jett JR, Hartman TE, Midthun DE, Mandrekar SJ, Hillman SL, Sykes AM, Aughenbaugh GL, Bungum AO, Allen KL (2005) CT screening for lung cancer: five-year prospective experience. Radiology 235:259–265

Theros EG (1977) Varying manifestations of peripheral pulmonary neoplasms: a radiologic-pathologic correlative study. AJR Am J Roentgenol 128:893–914

Woodring JH (1988) Determining the cause of pulmonary atelectasis: a comparison of plain radiography and CT. AJR Am J Roentgenol 150:757–763

Yankelevitz D, Henschke CI (1997) Does 2-year stability imply pulmonary nodules are benign? AJR Am J Roentgenol 168:325–328

Zwirewich CV, Vedal S, Miller RR, Müller NL (1991) Solitary pulmonary nodule: high-resolution CT and radiologic-pathologic correlation. Radiology 179:469–476

Pulmonary Embolism and Pulmonary Hypertension

18

Kaushik Shahir, Lawrence Goodman, and Melissa Wein

Contents

Abstract

> Pulmonary thromboembolic disease spectrum is comprised of acute pulmonary embolism (PE), chronic PE, and pulmonary (arterial) hypertension. Approximately 8% of the untreated cases may result in death. Besides thrombus, fat, air, and amniotic fluid are also known to cause PE. Pulmonary hypertension is defined as a pulmonary systolic arterial pressure equal to or exceeding 25 mmHg or a mean pulmonary artery pressure greater than 18 mmHg during rest (normal level, 10 mmHg). Pulmonary venous hypertension is defined by a measurement of pulmonary venous pressure equal to or more than 18 mmHg. Pulmonary hypertension secondary to known cardiac, pulmonary, or hepatic disease is far more common than is primary pulmonary hypertension, which has no identifiable cause. This chapter will help correlate the plain radiographic features with computed tomography.

18.1 Pulmonary Embolism

Pulmonary thromboembolic disease spectrum is comprised of acute PE, chronic PE, and pulmonary (arterial) hypertension. Lower-extremity deep venous thrombosis is also considered to be a part of the same spectrum. PE is a common condition that, if undiagnosed, can prove fatal. Approximately 8% of untreated cases may result in death (Dalen and Albert 1975). Besides thrombus, fat, air, and amniotic fluid are also known to cause PE (Rossi et al. 2000).

K. Shahir (✉), L. Goodman, and M. Wein
Medical College of Wisconsin, 9200 West Wisconsin Avenue, Milwaukee, WI 53226-3596, USA
e-mail: kshahir@mcw.edu
e-mail: lgoodman@mcw.edu
e-mail: mwein@mcw.edu

E.E. Coche et al. (eds.), *Comparative Interpretation of CT and Standard Radiography of the Chest*, Medical Radiology, DOI: 10.1007/978-3-540-79942-9_18, © Springer-Verlag Berlin Heidelberg 2011

Various modalities have been utilized in the past for the diagnosis. These include chest radiography, pulmonary angiography, ventilation-perfusion (VQ) scan, computed tomography (CT) scan, magnetic resonance imaging, and ultrasound. Of these, CT and VQ scanning have been fairly accurate and feasible. Plain chest radiography is the least sensitive. This chapter will help correlate the plain radiographic features with CT.

18.1.1 Acute Pulmonary Embolism

18.1.1.1 Etiopathogenesis

The predisposing risk factors for PE are increasing age, hypercoagulable state, orthopedic surgery, malignancy, medical illness, instrumentation, pregnancy, and bed rest (Black et al. 1993). Clinical outcome of PE depends on the size of the embolus and pre-existing cardiopulmonary disease. Common clinical presentations are dyspnea, chest pain, cough, hemoptysis, and tachycardia. PE can also present as pulmonary edema, left ventricular failure, or cardiac arrest.

When the emboli lodge in a pulmonary artery, a sequence of events follows. Arterial hypoxia with cessation of blood flow to a portion of lung causes formation of an alveolar dead space. In the absence of adequate collateral pulmonary and bronchial circulation and initiation of fibrinolysis, a process of infarction sets in (Uhland and Goldberg 1964; Dalen et al. 1977).

18.1.1.2 Investigation

Nonimaging tests such as electrocardiogram, measurement of arterial pO_2, and D-dimers have low specificity for the diagnosis but help rule in, or rule out, other diagnoses. Imaging modalities include direct and indirect investigations (Egermayer et al. 1998; Ginsberg et al. 1998; Wells et al. 2001). The indirect modalities include chest radiography and radionuclide ventilation-perfusion imaging, whereas the direct modalities include CT, magnetic resonance imaging, and pulmonary angiography.

Chest radiography has low sensitivity (33%) and specificity (59%) for PE (Greenspan et al. 1982; Worsley et al. 1993). There are some radiographic abnormalities in 60% of patients who have PE. They can be divided into pulmonary-vascular, parenchymal,

and pleural abnormalities. Approximately 40% of cases with PE have a normal chest radiograph. The chest radiograph also serves to rule out other diagnoses that may simulate PE clinically, such as pneumonia, pneumothorax, large pleural effusion, pulmonary edema, or rib fractures. It also assists in interpretation of ventilation-perfusion scintigraphy.

18.1.1.3 Radiographic Features

Pulmonary Vascular Abnormalities

Westermark's sign consists of subtle peripheral parenchymal lucency, which can be either due to localized peripheral oligemia secondary to the blocked pulmonary artery or due to hypoxic vasoconstriction secondary to ventilation of a poorly perfused lung.

The enlargement of the central pulmonary arteries may be caused by the lodged embolus or an acute rise in pulmonary artery pressure (Fig. 18.1a, b, c).

The findings may only become apparent by comparison with prior radiographs. Figure 18.2b illustrates localized oligemia and dilation of the affected pulmonary artery as compared with a previous normal radiograph (Fig. 18.2a). CT angiography revealed acute central saddle pulmonary embolism (Fig. 18.2c). Pulmonary edema due to left ventricular failure after a PE may often be seen in patients who have underlying cardiopulmonary disease.

Acute PE on CT angiography is reliably diagnosed by the presence of an intraluminal filling defect surrounded to a variable degree by contrast. Depending on the vessel orientation, the doughnut sign and the railroad track sign are visible on cross-sectional and long axis images. Complete occlusion causes nonopacification of the distal vessel (Fig. 18.3) (Coche et al. 2004; Gotway 1999; Gulsun Akpinar and Goodman 2008; Patel and Kazerooni 2005).

Focal Parenchymal Opacities

Peripheral airspace opacification may represent parenchymal hemorrhage (Fig. 18.4) without infarction or true pulmonary infarction with ischemic necrosis (Fig. 18.5). Pulmonary hemorrhagic opacities tend to resolve rapidly compared with infarcts, which require weeks to months for resolution. Frequency of infarction is variable and ranges from 10% to 60%. Typically,

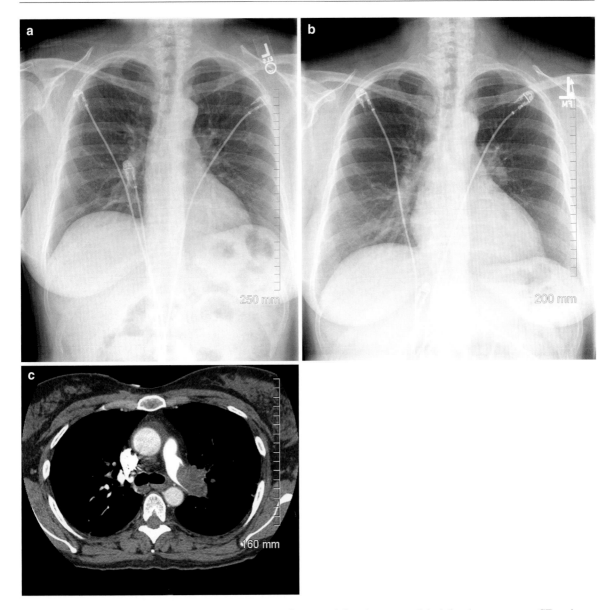

Fig. 18.1 Prior frontal chest radiograph reveals no abnormality in a 48-year-old female. Subsequent radiograph obtained during an episode of acute shortness of breath after knee surgery reveals a subtle enlargement of the left pulmonary artery. CT angiography demonstrates acute massive occlusive central PE

infarcts tend to be multiple or subpleural and have predilection for occurrence in lower lobes. They usually develop within 12–24 h of the onset of the symptoms. Infarcts are variable in size, poorly defined, and sometimes have a triangular shape. The infarct has been classically described as "Hampton's hump," which is characterized by a round subpleural opacity with medial convexity directed toward the hilum. The infarction usually progresses into a well-defined focal opacity over several days and then subsequently resolves completely or with mild residual scarring. Resolution of infarct is characterized by peripheral clearing similar to the melting of an ice cube, compared with the irregular patchy resolution of pneumonia (Woesner et al. 1971). Cavitation within an infarct is uncommon and occurs in infarcts larger than 4 cm. Typically, they are noninfected and occur within 2 weeks of development of the infarct.

Focal nonhemorrhagic/noninfarcted parenchymal opacities occur quite frequently in patients who have

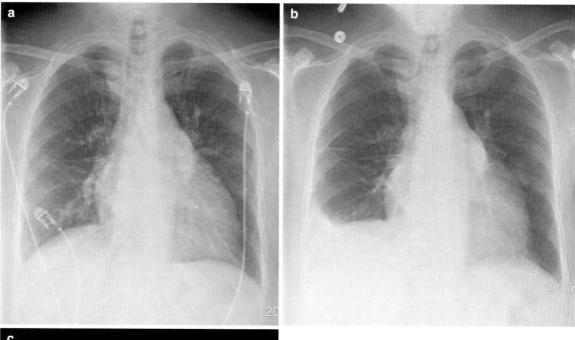

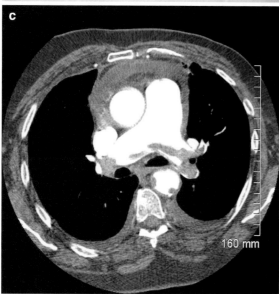

Fig. 18.2 A 65-year-old female with history of left breast cancer treated with mastectomy and radiation complained of acute onset right chest pain and shortness of breath. Frontal chest radiograph (**b**) compared with prior examination (**a**) demonstrates a new small right pleural effusion. In addition, careful observation reveals subtle reduced vascularity and increased translucency in upper lung fields. CT angiography (**c**) demonstrates central saddle embolism. Small bilateral pleural and pericardial effusions are also present

PE. These are mainly due to linear atelectasis secondary to hypoventilation, mucus plugging, and collapse secondary to depletion of surfactant. These are called Fleischner's lines. These are usually transient, but persistent opacities may develop into scars.

Pleural and Diaphragmatic Abnormalities

Pleural effusion is seen on chest radiographs in about half of patients who have PE and is often small and unilateral. Larger hemorrhagic effusions are seen in

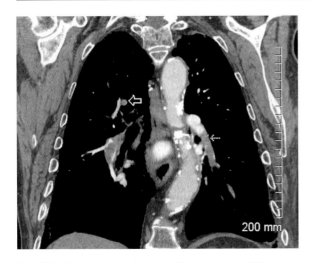

Fig. 18.3 Coronal reconstruction CT angio gram of the chest demonstrates acute occlusive central, lobar, and segmental PE. The orientation of the emboli simulates a doughnut (*black arrow*) and rail-road track (*dotted arrow*)

cases of infarction. The latter usually take longer to resolve. Elevation of the hemidiaphragm can be seen but is a nonspecific finding (Coche et al. 1998; Shah et al. 1999).

18.1.2 Chronic Pulmonary Thromboembolism

18.1.2.1 Etiopathogenesis

Repeated numerous small episodes or a few large thromboembolic events that fail to resolve completely are essentially the primary events that lead to chronic PE. Thromboemboli induce pulmonary arterial hypertension by occluding the vascular bed.

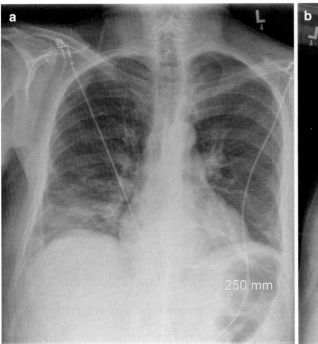
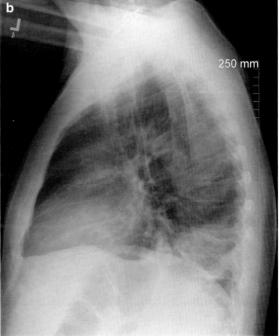

Fig. 18.4 A 68-year-old male with a history of sudden-onset shortness of breath and hemoptysis underwent an operation on his right hip 3 days before the onset of symptoms. Chest PA and lateral radiographs demonstrate a patchy opacity in the right lower lobe, mild cardiomegaly, and mildly enlarged central pulmonary arteries. Axial and sagittal CT angio gram images of the chest reveal right lower lobar, segmental occlusive PE, and patchy ground-glass opacities in the right lower lobe, consistent with hemorrhage. A small right pleural effusion is also seen. The parenchymal opacities resolved in 48 h after initiation of anticoagulation

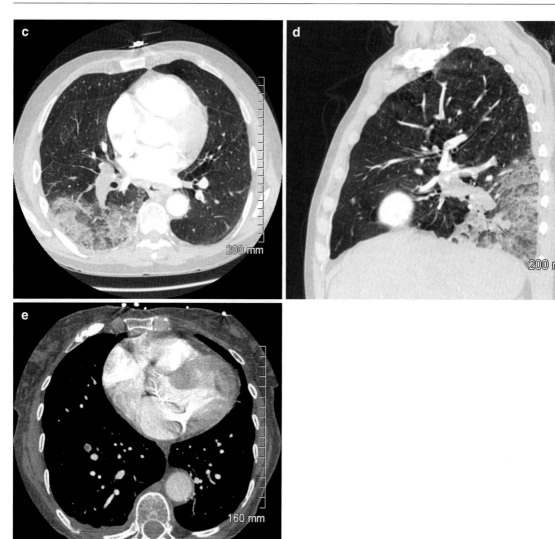

Fig. 18.4 (continued)

18.1.2.2 Radiographic Features

Plain radiographs typically demonstrate changes of pulmonary arterial hypertension characterized by large central pulmonary arteries with peripheral pruning. The features are described in Sect. 18.2.3. Pulmonary Arterial Hypertension on page 445. Small peripheral foci of consolidation from prior infarction may sometimes be seen.

CT also demonstrates classic changes of arterial hypertension (Fig. 18.6). Additionally, it reveals sequelae of thromboembolism, which include eccentric filling defects adjacent to the vessel wall. These represent organizing thrombi and are well demonstrated on multiformatted coronal and sagittal reconstruction images. Some of the partially recanalized thrombi are seen as linear web-like filling defects (Schwickert et al. 1994; Bergin et al. 1997; Roberts et al. 1997). Peripheral pruning on radiographs, on CT is seen as an abrupt reduction in arterial diameter. Areas of prior infarction are seen as peripheral subpleural opacities. Other commonly found features are large areas of mosaic attenuation due to perfusion defects in the lung parenchyma, similar to other causes of chronic pulmonary arterial hypertension.

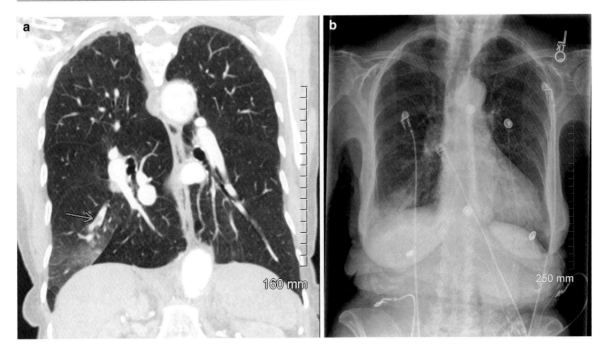

Fig. 18.5 A 75-year-old female who underwent recent abdominal surgery presented with acute onset of shortness of breath and hemoptysis. Coronal CT angio gram image reveals acute segmental PE in right lower lobe (*arrow*). Focal peripheral ground-glass opacity is seen in the subtended parenchyma. The opacity worsened during the next 48 h, with the development of peripheral consolidation on the chest radiograph consistent with development of an infarct

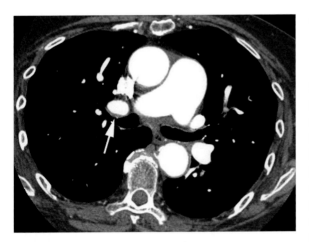

Fig. 18.6 A 53-year-old female with a history of recurrent PE on anticoagulation presented with dyspnea during exertion. CT angio gram of the chest depicts large central pulmonary arteries with peripheral pruning. The right pulmonary artery wall is thickened, consistent with chronic PE (*arrow*)

18.1.3 Nonthrombotic Pulmonary Embolism

This is a relatively rare group of abnormalities, which can have clinical implications. Nonthrombotic causes of embolism include tumor emboli and particulates such as talc, mercury, air, and fat. The clinical presentation depends on the specific embolic factor and can range from asymptomatic to marked respiratory failure. The radiographic manifestations are based on the etiopathogenesis. In the case of tumor embolism, one sees radiographic manifestations of pulmonary hypertension and thromboembolism. Nodularity may be visible along the vessels. Adenopathy and lymphangitis carcinomatosis may also be present. Air embolism can present acutely as frank pulmonary edema (Fig. 18.7) or can be asymptomatic. Air is quite often detected in

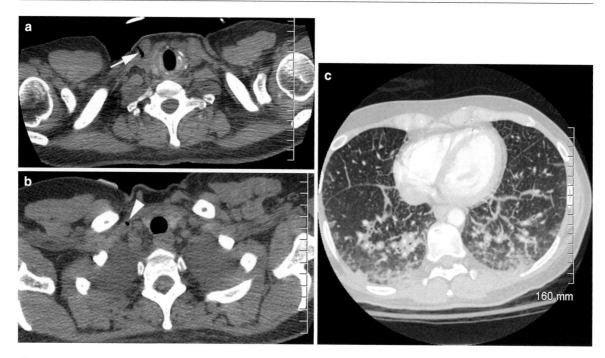

Fig. 18.7 A 34-year-old female with a history of sudden-onset shortness of breath after the removal of a large-bore jugular central catheter. (**a,b**) Initial noncontrast CT images revealed air pockets within the right internal jugular vein (*arrow*). (**c**) Contrast-enhanced CT revealed marked interlobular septal thickening and, peribronchial thickening consistent with acute pulmonary edema after air embolism. Radiographic findings reverted back to normal after conservative management

the central pulmonary arteries on a CT scan. The majority of these patients have a small amount of air injected and is asymptomatic. Fat embolism can present acutely as worsening shortness of breath with radiographic features consistent with increasing edema or acute respiratory distress syndrome (ARDS) in a case of trauma. This classically presents 2–3 days after major skeletal trauma. Very rarely, the fat as an embolus can be demonstrated using CT. Other particulate causes of embolism include mercury or cement from vertebroplasty, for which there are more radiographic features than clinical symptoms. Radiodense material is seen in the branching distribution of small pulmonary arteries on both X-ray and CT (Rossi et al. 2000).

Schistosomiasis is the most common parasitic embolization and is endemic in the Middle East, Africa, and South America. It is caused by migration of ova into the pulmonary circulation via porto-systemic collaterals (Shaw and Ghareeb 1938; Lapa et al. 2009). The most predominant cardiopulmonary changes that result from the infestation are pulmonary arterial hypertension and right heart failure. Chest radiography and CT demonstrate characteristic changes of pulmonary hypertension. Nodules representing parasitic granulomas are sometimes visualized.

18.2 Pulmonary Hypertension

Pulmonary hypertension is defined as a pulmonary systolic arterial pressure equal to or exceeding 25 mmHg or a mean pulmonary artery pressure greater than 18 mmHg during rest (normal level, 10 mmHg). Pulmonary venous hypertension (PVH) is defined as a measurement of pulmonary venous pressure greater than or equal to 18 mmHg. Pulmonary hypertension secondary to known cardiac, pulmonary, or hepatic disease is far more common than is primary pulmonary hypertension, which has no identifiable cause.

18.2.1 Pathophysiology

Elevated pressures are caused by increased vascular resistance, which in turn is caused by a decrease in the total number of small pulmonary arteries. The latter can be caused by intraluminal arterial occlusion, muscular contraction of small arteries, arterial wall thickening, and back pressure from PVH. It is a result of interplay between vasoconstrictors and dilators acting at the small arterial level (Remy-Jardin and Remy 1999).

18.2.2 Classification

Several models have been used to categorize various causes of pulmonary hypertension. Causes are best categorized into pre- and postcapillary pulmonary hypertension (Fraser et al. 1999; Frazier et al. 2000; Remy-Jardin and Remy 1999).

1. *Precapillary:* Changes mainly limited to pulmonary arterial circulation:

    (a) Primary pulmonary hypertension – idiopathic
    (b) Pulmonary hypertension associated with hepatic disease, HIV infection, drugs, and toxins
    (c) Congenital cardiovascular disease with Eisenmenger's physiology
    (d) Chronic thromboembolic disease
    (e) Nonthrombotic embolization – neoplastic, particulates and foreign material, and parasites (schistosomiasis)
    (f) Chronic alveolar hypoxia – chronic obstructive pulmonary disesase (COPD), interstitial lung disease, hypoventilation syndromes
    (g) Pulmonary capillary hemangiomatosis

2. *Postcapillary:* Changes within pulmonary venous circulation between the capillary bed and the left atrium:

    (a) Left-sided cardiovascular disease – mitral valve disease, cor triatriatum, cardiac tumor, chronic left heart failure
    (b) Extrinsic pulmonary venous compression
    (c) Pulmonary veno-occlusive disease (PVOD)
    (d) Mediastinal fibrosis

18.2.3 Pulmonary Arterial Hypertension

18.2.3.1 Radiographic Signs

Vascular signs

1. Dilatation of the central pulmonary arteries is commonly caused by increased vascular resistance. Based on CT criteria, a main pulmonary arterial diameter of more than 29 mm is strongly suggestive of arterial hypertension if it is associated with segmental artery to bronchus ratio of more than 1:1 in either of the lungs (Kuriyama et al. 1984; Tan and Goodman 1998). The individual left or right pulmonary arterial diameters of more than 18 mm are poor indicators of pulmonary

hypertension. The same can be assessed on the chest radiograph (Fig. 18.8 a, b). Right interlobar pulmonary artery dimension is measured at the hilar point on a frontal chest radiograph (Fig. 18.8). A measurement of more than 18 mm is considered abnormal.

2. In long-standing hypertension, the peripheral pulmonary arteries develop vasoconstriction, which is visualized as abrupt diminishing of peripheral vessels. This is termed "peripheral pruning" (Fig. 18.8 a, c) (Fleischner 1962).

3. Atherosclerotic calcification can be observed in the pulmonary arteries, usually in long-standing pulmonary arterial hypertension (Fig. 18.9).

Additionally, CT imaging may reveal bronchial arterial enlargement (more than 1.5 mm) and hypertrophy, especially in patients who have chronic thromboembolic disease (Remy-Jardin et al. 2005).

In chronic thromboembolic disease, CT angiography demonstrates eccentric filling defects along the vessel wall, which represents organizing thrombi.

Lung Parenchymal Signs

Pulmonary hypertension–induced peripheral vasoconstriction causes development of areas in the lung parenchyma with reduced vascularity and perfusion compared with ventilation. This is usually very subtle unless a large area is affected, and it can be seen as an area of translucency. This manifests as mosaic attenuation on CT (Fig. 18.10). The vessels in the region of decreased parenchymal attenuation are of smaller caliber compared with those within the normal or high attenuation parenchyma or smaller than the adjacent bronchi (Bergin et al. 1996; King et al. 1998; Griffin et al. 2007).

Other features include centrilobular ground-glass opacities representing foci of hemorrhage or cholesterol granulomas (Griffin et al. 2007; Nolan et al. 1999). Areas of subpleural consolidation may be seen in patients who have chronic thromboembolic diseases because of prior infarction. In cases of tumor embolization–induced pulmonary hypertension, CT may reveal vessels with a beaded appearance, which more peripherally at the centrilobular level would be seen in branching configuration resembling the tree-in-bud shape (Remy-Jardin and Remy 1999).

For other known causes of pulmonary arterial hypertension, radiographic and CT features would show

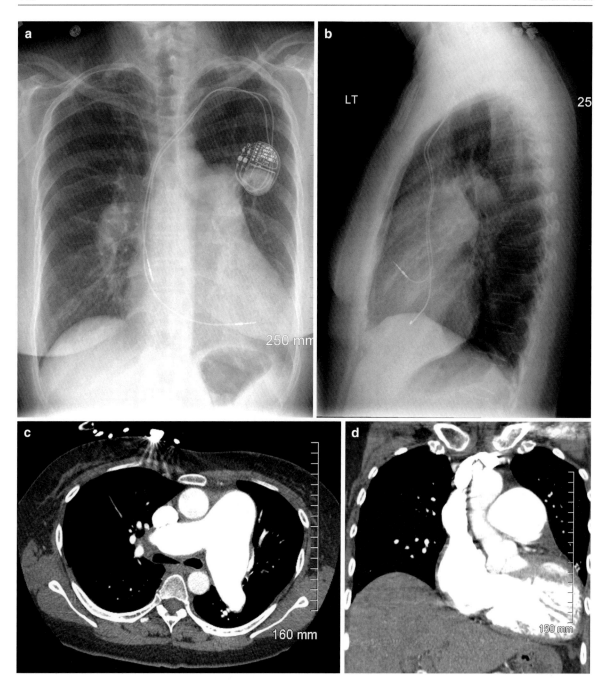

Fig. 18.8 Posteroanterior and lateral radiographs of the chest depict pulmonary hypertension in a case of Eisenmenger's syndrome in a 44-year-old female with an atrial septal defect. The right ventricular enlargement is seen encroaching on the retrosternal space. Large central pulmonary arteries and peripheral pruning are well demonstrated. Findings are well correlated with CT angio gram of the chest

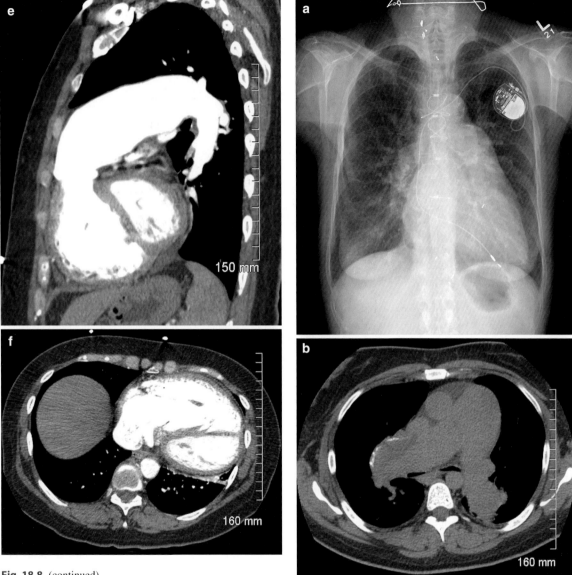

Fig. 18.8 (continued)

additional specific changes such as those seen in COPD or interstitial fibrosis. Pulmonary capillary hemangiomatosis and PVOD are rare diseases that show overlapping radiographic features of pulmonary arterial and venous hypertension with a normal pulmonary wedge capillary pressure (PWCP) (Lantuejoul et al. 2006; Resten et al. 2004). The degree of enlargement of the pulmonary arteries is often severe in patients who have long-standing untreated congenital heart diseases with a left-to-right shunt, such as ASD (atrial septal defect), VSD (ventricular septal defect) and PDA (patent ductus arteriosus). This is usually associated with marked right

Fig. 18.9 (**a**) Frontal chest radiograph demonstrates large pulmonary arteries with atherosclerotic calcification secondary to pulmonary hypertension. (**b**) Noncontrast axial CT image of the chest reveals large central pulmonary arteries and a thin rim of calcification along the anterior aspect of the right main pulmonary artery, consistent with long-standing pulmonary hypertension, which in this case was due to chronic PE. A subtle low-attenuation eccentric chronic embolus is seen anteriorly in the right pulmonary artery

ventricular dilatation. A decrease in right ventricular size suggests progression toward Eisenmenger's physiology with a rise in pulmonary arterial pressures and reversal of shunting (Griffin et al. 2007).

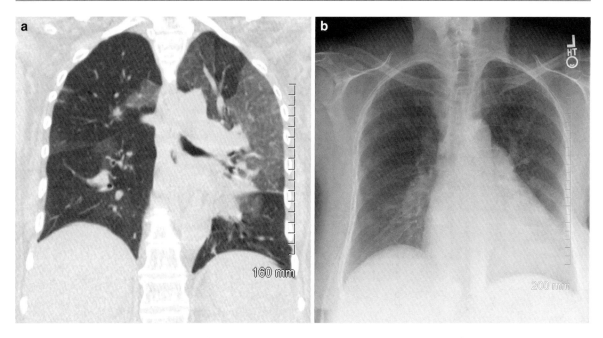

Fig. 18.10 (**a**) Coronal reconstruction CT image demonstrates large central pulmonary arteries and mosaic attenuation secondary to pulmonary hypertension. The low-density areas correspond to decreased attenuation. (**b**) Frontal chest radiograph shows moderate cardiomegaly and large pulmonary arteries in pulmonary hypertension. The vessels on the right are smaller than those on the left. There is a subtle discrepancy in lung translucency, which is seen as mosaic attenuation on CT because of reduced lung perfusion

Mediastinal and Cardiac Signs

Right-sided cardiac enlargement and hypertrophy develop as a result of pulmonary hypertension. This is seen as increased cardiac size on chest X-ray with upward deviation of the apex mainly due to right ventricular enlargement. Lateral radiograph reveals right ventricular enlargement encroaching on the retrosternal space (Fig. 18.8b and e).

CT scanning reveals additional features such as dilatation of the coronary sinus and inferior vena cava. Elevated right heart pressures may cause a reflux of contrast material into the inferior vena cava and hepatic veins, which is a sign of right heart failure. Other features of right atrial and ventricular enlargement are seen well with CT. An increase in right ventricular thickness and deviation of interventricular septum to the left are signs of severe pulmonary hypertension (Fig. 18.8f) (Yeh et al. 2004; Reid and Murchison 1998).

18.2.4 Pulmonary Venous Hypertension

18.2.4.1 Etiopathogenesis

PVH is another term for postcapillary pulmonary hypertension and is a result of increased resistance in the pulmonary veins. It is an important cause of secondary pulmonary arterial hypertension. The common causes are left ventricular failure, mitral valve disease, and aortic valve disease. Other causes include fibrosing mediastinitis and PVOD. With an increase in pulmonary venous pressure, sequential changes in pulmonary circulation occur, depending upon the degree of rise in pressures. This initially manifests as distension of upper lobe veins when compared with the lower lobe veins, which is known as "upper lobe venous diversion." With further rise in pressure, fluid begins to accumulate in the interstitium, which is known as interstitial pulmonary edema. Further rise in venous pressure leads to accumulation of fluid in alveolar air spaces, termed "alveolar edema." These changes are reversible. However, secondary pulmonary arterial hypertension ensues with long-standing venous hypertension. Edema may be due to noncardiogenic causes when the heart and vessel sizes are normal. Various causes include aspiration, ARDS, near-drowning, drugs, hepatorenal failure, and rapid lung expansion (Fraser et al. 1999; Frazier et al. 2000).

18.2.4.2 Radiographic Features

Plain radiographs have good sensitivity when demonstrating specific changes, depending on the degree of venous hypertension Simon et al. (1967). To a certain extent the changes can be correlated with PCWP. Normally, in an upright radiograph, the lower lobe veins have a slightly larger caliber compared with upper lobe veins because of gravity-dependent distribution. Upper lobe veins are distended when there is mild PCWP elevation. A further rise in PCWP (19–25 mmHg) leads to interstitial edema. Interstitial edema is characterized by thickening of the interlobular septa. These are called the Kerley lines. They are further divided into types A, B, and C. The term "Kerley C line" is no longer used. Kerley A lines are approximately 4 cm in length and are seen in the upper and middle-portions of the lung and radiate from the hila into the central portions of the lungs but do not reach the pleura. Kerley B lines are shorter (1 cm or less) interlobular septal lines (Fig. 18.11) found predominantly in the lower zones peripherally and parallel to each other but at right angles to the pleural surface. Other signs of interstitial fluid overload include perihilar haze, which is seen as an indistinct outline of the lower lobe and hilar vessels, and peribronchial cuffing (Fig. 18.12), which is apparent thickening of the bronchial walls as a result of fluid accumulation in the peribronchial interstitium. Airspace opacities appear when PCWP rises above 25 mmHg. This is suggestive of alveolar edema. This is accompanied by Kerley B lines, airspace nodules, bilateral symmetric consolidation in the middle and lower-lung zones, and pleural effusions. The common description of "perihilar bat-wing" pattern of airspace consolidation is seen most commonly

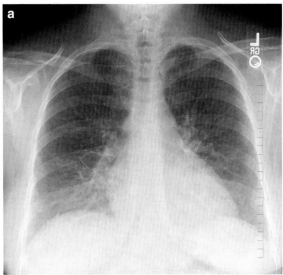

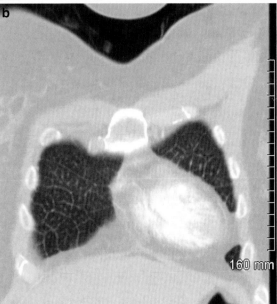

Fig. 18.11 Frontal chest radiograph reveals Kerley B lines (**a**), which correlate well with a coronal reconstruction CT image demonstrating interlobular septal thickening (**b**)

in left ventricular and renal failure (Fig. 18.13a), whereas alveolar edema localized to the right upper zone is seen with severe mitral regurgitation.

Signs of pulmonary arterial hypertension may develop in patients who have chronic PVH. Sometimes a fine nodular pattern from the deposition of

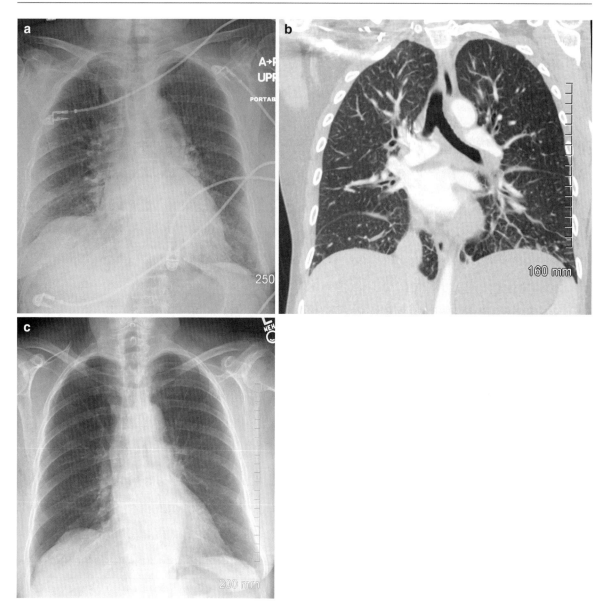

Fig. 18.12 Frontal chest radiograph (**a**) and coronal CT (**b**) demonstrate Kerley B lines, perihilar haziness, and peribronchial cuffing consistent with pulmonary edema. Findings reverted back to normal on subsequent radiograph (**c**)

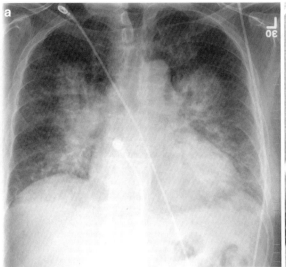
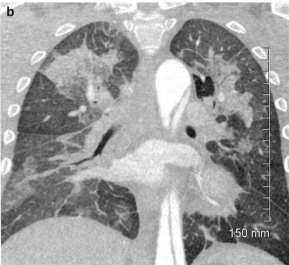

Fig. 18.13 (**a**) Frontal radiograph reveals a classic bat's wing distribution of pulmonary edema in a 40-year-old male with aortic dissection and acute left ventricular failure. (**b**) Coronal reconstruction CT angiography image reveals perihilar edema, septal lines, peribronchial cuffing, and an aortic dissection flap

hemosiderin may appear throughout both lungs and has been seen previously in patients with long-standing severe mitral stenosis. In very severe chronic PVH, pulmonary ossicles may form, measuring up to 1 cm in size (Fraser et al. 1999; Frazier et al. 2000).

CT is highly sensitive in the detection of PVH and edema. The findings include thickening of septal and bronchovascular structures. Patchy perihilar ground-glass opacities may be seen in cases of mild parenchymal edema. Alveolar edema may initially be recognized as peribronchovascular airspace nodules progressing to dense airspace consolidation (Fig. 18.13b).

References

Bergin CJ, Rios G, King MA et al (1996) Accuracy of high-resolution CT in identifying chronic pulmonary thromboembolic disease. AJR Am J Roentgenol 166:1371–1377

Bergin CJ, Sirlin CB, Hauschildt JP et al (1997) Chronic thromboembolism: diagnosis with helical CT and MR imaging with angiographic and surgical correlation. Radiology 204: 695–702

Black MD, French GJ, Rasuli P, Bouchard AC (1993) Upper extremity deep venous thrombosis. Underdiagnosed and potentially lethal. Chest 103:1887–1890

Coche EE, Müller NL, Kim KI, Wiggs BR, Mayo JR (1998) Acute pulmonary embolism: ancillary findings at spiral CT. Radiology 207:753–758

Coche E, Verschuren F, Hainaut P, Goncette L (2004) Pulmonary embolism findings on chest radiographs and multislice spiral CT. Eur Radiol 14:1241–1248

Dalen JE, Alpert JS (1975) Natural history of pulmonary embolism. Prog Cardiovasc Dis 17:259–270

Dalen JE, Haffajee CI, Alpert JS III et al (1977) Pulmonary embolism, pulmonary hemorrhage and pulmonary infarction. N Engl J Med 296:1431–1435

Egermayer P, Town GI, Turner JG et al (1998) Usefulness of D-dimer, blood gas, and respiratory rate measurements for excluding pulmonary embolism. Thorax 53:830–834

Fleischner FG (1962) Pulmonary embolism. Clin Radiol 13: 169–182

Fraser RS, Muller NL, Colman N, Pare PD (1999) Diagnosis of diseases of the chest. W.B. Saunders, Philadelphia, pp 1897–1945

Frazier AA, Galvin JR, Franks TJ, Rosado-de-Christenson ML (2000) Pulmonary vasculature: hypertension and infarction. Radiographics 20:491–524

Ginsberg JS, Wells PS, Kearon C et al (1998) Sensitivity and specificity of a rapid whole-blood assay for D-dimer in the diagnosis of pulmonary embolism. Ann Intern Med 129: 1006–1011

Gotway MB, Edinburgh KJ, Feldstein VA et al (1999) Imaging evaluation of suspected acute pulmonary embolism. Curr Probl Diagn Radiol 28:129–184

Greenspan RH, Ravin CE, Polansky SM, McLoud TC (1982) Accuracy of the chest radiograph in diagnosis of pulmonary embolism. Invest Radiol 17:539–543

Griffin N, Allen D, Wort J et al (2007) Eisenmenger syndrome and idiopathic pulmonary arterial hypertension: do parenchymal lung changes reflect aetiology? Clin Radiol 62: 587–595

Gulsun Akpinar M, Goodman LR (2008) Imaging of pulmonary thromboembolism. Clin Chest 29(1):107–116

King MA, Ysrael M, Bergin CJ (1998) Chronic thromboembolic pulmonary hypertension: CT findings. AJR Am J Roentgenol 170:955–960

Kuriyama K, Gamsu G, Stern RG et al (1984) CT-determined pulmonary artery diameters in predicting pulmonary hypertension. Invest Radiol 19:16–22

Lantuejoul S, Sheppard MN, Corrin B et al (2006) Pulmonary veno-occlusive disease and pulmonary capillary hemangiomatosis: a clinicopathologic study of 35 cases. Am J Surg Pathol 30:850–857

Lapa M, Dias B, Jardim C et al (2009) Cardiopulmonary manifestations of hepatosplenic schistosomiasis. Circulation 119: 1518–1523

Nolan RL, Mcadams HP, Sporn TA et al (1999) Pulmonary cholesterol granulomas in patients with pulmonary artery hypertension: chest radiographic and CT findings. AJR Am J Roentgenol 172:1317–1319

Patel S, Kazerooni EA (2005) Helical CT for the evaluation of acute pulmonary embolism. AJR Am J Roentgenol 185: 135–149

Reid JH, Murchison JT (1998) Acute right ventricular dilatation: a new helical CT sign of massive pulmonary embolism. Clin Radiol 53:694–698

Remy-Jardin M, Remy J (1999) Spiral CT angiography of the pulmonary circulation. Radiology 212:615–636

Remy-Jardin M, Duhamel A, Deken V et al (2005) Systemic collateral supply in patients with chronic thromboembolic and primary pulmonary hypertension: assessment with multi-detector row helical CT angiography. Radiology 235: 274–281

Resten A, Maitre S, Humbert M et al (2004) Pulmonary hypertension: CT of the chest in pulmonary venoocclusive disease. AJR Am J Roentgenol 183:65–70

Roberts HC, Kauczor HU, Schweden F, Thelen M (1997) Spiral CT of pulmonary hypertension and chronic thromboembolism. J Thorac Imaging 12:118–127

Rossi SE, Goodman PC, Franquet T (2000) Nonthrombotic pulmonary emboli. AJR Am J Roentgenol 174:1499–1508

Schwickert HC, Schweden F, Schild HH et al (1994) Pulmonary arteries and lung parenchyma in chronic pulmonary embolism: preoperative and postoperative CT findings. Radiology 191:351–357

Shah AA, Davis SD, Gamsu G et al (1999) Parenchymal and pleural findings in patients with and patients without acute pulmonary embolism detected at spiral CT. Radiology 211: 147–153

Shaw AF, Ghareeb A (1938) The pathogenesis of pulmonary schistosomiasis in Egypt with special reference to Ayerza's disease. J Pathol Bacteriol 46:401–424

Simon M, Sasahara AA, Cannilla JE (1967) The radiology of pulmonary hypertension. Semin Roentgenol 2:368–388

Tan RT, Goodman LR (1998) Utility of CT scan evaluation for predicting pulmonary hypertension in patients with parenchymal lung disease. Chest 113:1250–1256

Uhland H, Goldberg LM (1964) Pulmonary embolism: a commonly missed clinical entity. Dis Chest 45:533–536

Wells PS, Anderson DR, Rodger M et al (2001) Excluding pulmonary embolism at the bedside without diagnostic imaging: management of patients with suspected pulmonary embolism presenting to the emergency department by using a simple clinical model and D-dimer. Ann Intern Med 135:98–107

Woesner ME, Sanders I, White GW (1971) The melting sign in resolving transient pulmonary infarction. Am J Roentgenol 111:782–790

Worsley DF, Alavi A, Aronchick JM et al (1993) Chest radiographic findings in patients with acute pulmonary embolism: observations from the PIOPED Study. Radiology 189:133–136

Yeh BM, Kurzman FE et al (2004) Clinical relevance of retrograde inferior vena cava or hepatic vein opacification during contrast-enhanced CT. AJR Am J Roentgenol 183:1227–1232

Chest Trauma

Monique Brink and Helena M. Dekker

19

Contents

Abstract

> Chest injury is an important contributor to mortality and deserves rapid diagnosis. Although conventional radiography (CR) is not as accurate for chest injuries as multidetector computed tomography (MDCT), CR remains an important initial diagnostic tool in trauma care.

> Signs of chest injuries are, however, often subtle and difficult to identify during CR of supine anteroposterior trauma. This chapter reviews subtle CR findings that suggest relevant chest injuries by correlating these CR signs with the appearance of injuries on coronal reformatted MDCT. Attention will be paid to the following diagnoses: aortic injury, diaphragmatic injury, tracheobronchial tree injury, pulmonary contusion, pneumothorax, hemothorax, rib fractures, and scapulothoracic dissociation.

19.1 Introduction

Chest injury is an important contributor to mortality in trauma patients (Trupka 1997; Stiell 1999); therefore, rapid and accurate diagnosis of chest injuries is imperative to direct definitive therapy. Conventional chest radiography (CR) classically has been used as the sole diagnostic tool in the primary evaluation of trauma patients, but is now increasingly being replaced by computed tomography (CT) (Rieger 2002; Broder 2006; Wurmb 2007).

It is especially multidetector computed tomography (MDCT) that has a high diagnostic accuracy for

M. Brink (✉) and H.M. Dekker
Department of Radiology, Radboud University Nijmegen
Medical Centre, Geert Grooteplein 10, PO Box 9101,
6500 HB Nijmegen, The Netherlands
e-mail: m.brink@rad.umcn.nl; h.dekker@rad.umcn.nl

predominantly pulmonary and vascular injuries (Rowan 2002; Abboud 2003; Mirvis 1998; Parker 2001; Chen 2004) and seems to improve diagnostic thinking and to influence the patient's treatment (Trupka 1997; Guerrero-Lopez 2000; Salim 2006a; Omert 2001). However, the negative side effects of CT cannot be neglected. Firstly, the risk of potential harmful effects of ionizing radiation exposure associated with CT is substantial, especially because the trauma population is young and therefore sensitive to those harmful effects. Secondly, CT might cause a delay in the diagnosis and treatment because transportation and positioning of the often obtunded patient dictate the time that is available for CT scanning examinations. Thirdly, CT is relatively expensive.

Although CR has increasingly been reported as a less accurate imaging tool when used for blunt trauma patients (Rowan 2002; Lopes 2006; Scaglione 2006; Wisbach 2007), this is nonetheless a quick method that uses a far smaller radiation dose. Effective radiation dose of CR is approximately 0.05 mSv, whereas effective dose is 5 mSv in chest CT (Mettler 2008; Brenner 2008). Furthermore, CR can be quickly used as an adjunct in the primary survey for abnormalities that require rapid treatment, such as tube malposition, large pneumothoraces, or massive intrathoracic bleeding (American College of Surgeons Committee on Trauma 2004). Finally, CR remains the primary screening method for trauma patients in many European institutions when deciding whether CT is warranted: subtle CR signs might predict the presence of more, relevant chest injuries that can be accurately visualized during CT.

It is therefore imperative for radiologists to recognize these signs on CR to establish the need for CT. The purpose of this pictorial chapter is to evaluate subtle CR signs of relevant injuries and to correlate these with the appearance of these injuries on CT. The relevant injuries evaluated in this chapter include aortic injury, diaphragmatic injury, tracheobronchial tree injury, pulmonary contusion, pneumothorax, hemothorax, rib fractures, and scapulothoracic dissociation.

19.2 Chest Radiographs and MDCT

At our institution, we obtain CR scans of the chest in the trauma room within several minutes after arrival. These radiographs consist of at least one supine view of the chest in anterior–posterior direction. The majority of patients undergo CR while they are still positioned on a spine board.

MDCT is executed in the room adjacent to the trauma bay. We position the patient with the arms raised above the acromioclavicular region and use automated tube current modulation for optimal image quality at the lowest radiation dose possible (Brink 2008a). The chest MDCT is often obtained as a part of a thoracoabdominal scanning examination from the acromioclavicular joint to the lesser trochanter at a tube potential of 120 kV, with a reference value of effective tube current time product of 200 mAs and a small collimation size of 1.5 mm or less. For optimal imaging of soft tissue trauma and arterial injuries, we preferably inject 100–150 mL of iodinated contrast medium (at an iodine concentration of 300–350 mg/mL, depending on the patient's habitus) according to the following split-bolus protocol: two thirds of the contrast medium is injected at a rate of 3 mL/s, followed by a saline chaser bolus. Thereafter, the remaining one-third of the contrast medium is injected at a rate of 4 mL/s, followed by a saline chaser bolus. The patient is scanned with a delay of 60 s. For optimal imaging of the aortic arch, we use bolus tracking software and a contrast agent at a concentration of 350 mg/mL, which is administered at 4–5 mL/s followed by a saline chaser.

For reconstruction, lung, soft tissue, and bone kernels are used, and sagittal and coronal multiplanar reformatted (MPR) images are obtained.

19.2.1 Aortic Injury

Traumatic aortic injury is considered to be caused by a mechanism of severe acceleration–deceleration. It occurs in 1–2% of blunt trauma patients who have suffered from a significant mechanism of trauma and who reach the hospital alive (Fabian 1998; Dyer 2000). Patients have a low survival rate if this injury is not detected and treated at an early stage (Parmley 1958).

Several radiographic signs have been described for aortic injury. These signs are based on the fact that aortic rupture causes a local or more generalized mediastinal hematoma. A mediastinal hematoma can be reflected by mediastinal widening on CR, which has classically been described as a distance of more than 8 cm from the right border to the left border of the mediastinum at the level of the aortic knob (Marsh 1976). Although a widened mediastinum has been reported to be 100% sensitive for aortic injury in several studies (Grieser 2001; Wong 2004; Mengozzi 2000; Haramati 1996), this sign has also been reported to be negative in some cases (Demetriades 1998; Ho 2002; Cook 2001). In addition, mediastinal widening is not specific for aortic injury: firstly, because patients are scanned positioned on top of a spine board with long mediastinum-to-film distances that result in a broad mediastinal projection. For this reason, a new upper limit of up to 9.7 cm has been proposed (Gleeson 2001). Secondly, patient compliance to breathing instructions often fails in trauma patients (Costantino 2006). Thirdly, a widened mediastinum may also be present secondary to venous hemorrhage (Sandor 1967), thoracic vertebral fractures (Fig. 19.10) (Sandor 1967), spinal ligamentous injuries (Costantino 2006), first rib fractures (Sandor 1967), clavicular or sternal fractures (Demetriades 1998), or a fatty mediastinum (Wicky 2000).

Other findings that might reflect aortic injury are loss of sharpness of the aortic contour (Fig. 19.1) (Cook 2001; Ungar 2006; Mengozzi 2000), opacification of the aortopulmonary window (Fig. 19.1) (Cook 2001; Ungar 2006), rightward deviation of the nasogastric tube within the esophagus (Ungar 2006; Cook 2001), rightward deviation of the trachea (Ungar 2006; Cook 2001), downward displacement of the left mainstem bronchus (Cook 2001; Mengozzi 2000; Ungar 2006),

widening of the right paratracheal stripe (>5 mm) (Woodring 1990; Ungar 2006), left apical capping (Ungar 2006; Cook 2001), which reflects a migrated mediastinal hematoma into the extrapleural space over the apex of the left lung (Simeone 1975), a displaced left or right paraspinous line (Gibbs 2007; Cook 2001; Ungar 2006), and a displaced vena cava superior (Ungar 2006). Finally, signs of hemothorax, pneumothorax and pulmonary contusion at conventional radiography are associated with a higher incidence of aortic injury (Ungar 2006; Kirkham 2007).

None of these above signs occur in all patients with aortic injuries, and none of the signs are 100% specific for this injury. Hence, several authors have suggested that to rule out aortic injury at CR it is necessary to consider a combination of all signs and the radiologist's overall impression of the mediastinal contour (Ho 2002; Sriussadaporn 2000; Erpenbach 1995). However, predicting the presence of aortic injury via CR remains a challenge in daily practice (Fig. 19.2).

19.2.2 Diaphragmatic Injury

Although the incidence of diaphragmatic injury is high in penetrating trauma (occurring in 10–24% of patients

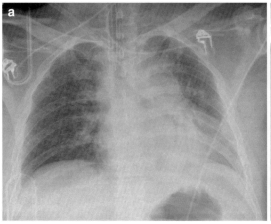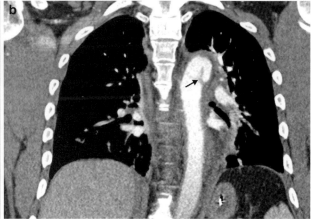

Fig. 19.1 A 37-year-old man was involved in a high-energy car accident and was intubated at the scene of the accident. During primary survey at the emergency department this patient had sufficient respiration and was normotensive, but he had a tachycardia of 109 beats per minute and lacerations across the abdomen. (**a**) The initial chest radiograph showed a widened mediastinum, with an abnormal aortic contour and an opacified aortopulmonary win-

dow. In addition, this chest radiograph showed atelectasis of the left lower lung. (**b**) Coronal reconstructions of the chest multidetector computed tomography (MDCT) demonstrated a hematoma around the aortic arch and an aortic rupture (*arrow*). In addition, MDCT demonstrated pulmonary contusion, atelectasis, rib fractures, and a pneumothorax (not shown). This patient was treated with an endovascular aortic stent

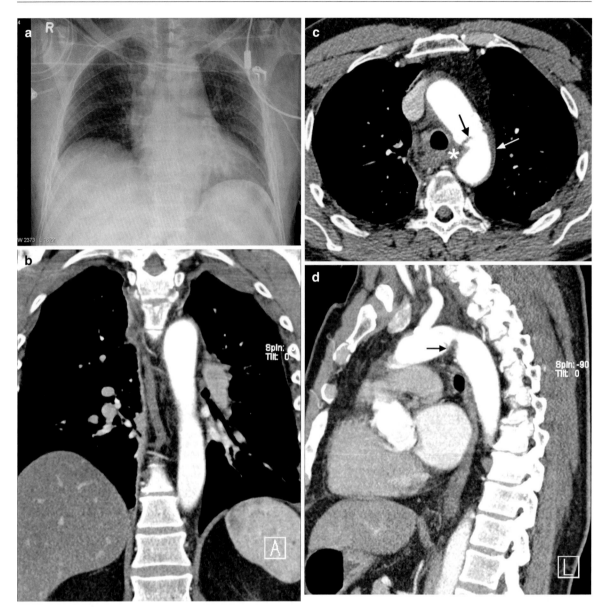

Fig. 19.2 A 56-year-old man entered the trauma room after a high-energy car collision, during which another occupant died. This patient had no respiratory problems and was hemodynamically stable. (**a**) During initial resuscitation and before multidetector computed tomography (MDCT), the supine anteroposterior chest radiograph showed elevation of the right diaphragm, rightward deviation of the trachea, a widened paratracheal stripe, and a widened mediastinum. However, because there was a sharply marked aortic contour, aortic injury was not suspected during the initial interpretation of this chest radiograph. (**b**) Although coronal reconstructions of MDCT with intravenous contrast did not show remarkable mediastinal widening, (**c**) transversal imaging showed a small periaortic hematoma in the central mediastinum (*asterisk*), partial thickening of the aortic wall (*white arrow*), and (**c, d**) an aortic transection with an intimal flap (*black arrows*) of the aortic arch. This patient was treated with an endovascular aortic stent

who have a penetrating injury to the left lower chest [Murray 1998; Mirvis 2003]), this injury is found in only 0.8% of blunt trauma patients (Costantino 2006). If diaphragmatic injury is present in blunt trauma patients, the left dome of the diaphragm is most frequently injured. Diaphragmatic injury has a substantial impact on patient mortality and morbidity if left untreated (Reber 1998).

Injury to the diaphragm is difficult to diagnose with CR unless typical findings are present. CR findings with a high positive predictive value include asymmetric elevation of the diaphragm (sensitivity: 50% in blunt trauma patients) (Shackleton 1998) and herniation of the nasogastric tube or of bowel gas into the thoracic cavity (sensitivity: 44–60%) (Guth 1995; Shackleton 1998) (Fig. 19.3). The latter can appear as the collar sign: a waist-like constriction of the gas containing viscera at the level of the diaphragmatic tear (Mirvis 2003).

It should be noted that herniation of abdominal contents especially occurs in spontaneously breathing patients; this sign is often absent in patients who receive mechanical ventilation that causes a positive intrathoracic pressure (Shapiro 1996; van Vugt and Schoots 1989). Diaphragmatic injury might also be accompanied by a mediastinal shift away from the injured site (Shapiro 1996). In addition, less specific, but still suggestive, findings of diaphragmatic injury are pleural effusion or plate-like atelectasis above an indistinct diaphragm

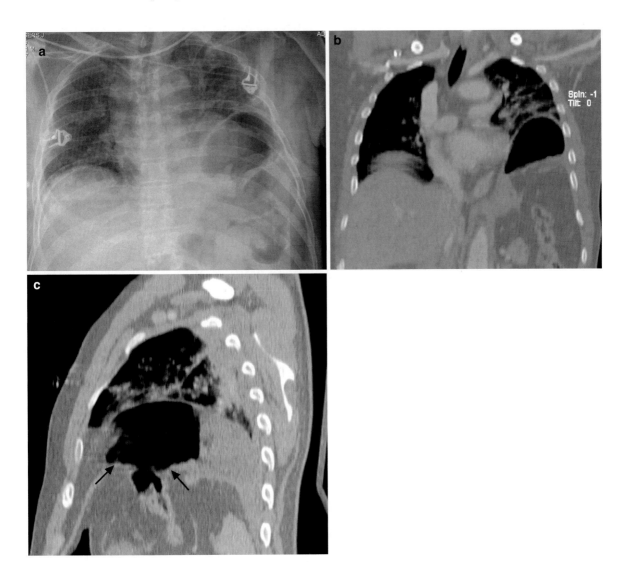

Fig. 19.3 A 56-year-old man was involved in a car accident. During clinical evaluation, this patient had a normal breathing frequency. However, oxygen saturation was 88% and no respiratory sounds could be heard across the left hemithorax. (**a**) Chest radiography showed a pulmonary contusion, rib fractures, a tracheal shift, and signs of a diaphragmatic injury: asymmetric elevation of the left hemidiaphragm and herniation of abdominal contents (bowel gas) into the thoracic cavity. (**b, c**) Coronal and sagittal reconstructions of multidetector computed tomography verified these findings and demonstrated a diaphragmatic rupture (*arrows*). This diaphragmatic defect was confirmed and primarily closed during a laparotomy

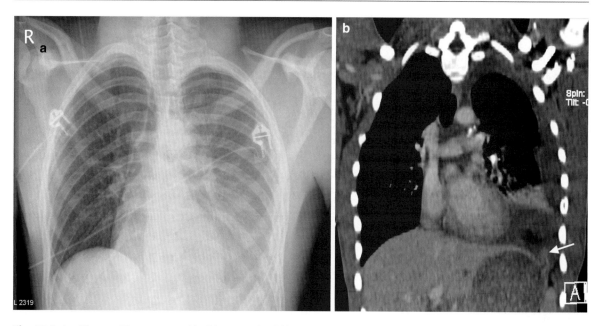

Fig. 19.4 An 18-year-old man was stabbed between the fifth and sixth ribs in the left hemithorax. On arrival at the emergency department the airway was not occluded. Oxygen saturation and breathing sounds were normal. However, the patient had a high breathing frequency of 30 breaths per minute. (**a**) Chest radiography showed a hemopneumothorax above an indistinctly delineated diaphragm. (**b**) Multidetector computed tomography demonstrated a hemopneumothorax with the stomach herniating through a defect (*arrow*) in the diaphragm. A laparotomy was subsequently performed. This procedure confirmed the presence of injury to the left hemidiaphragm and a laceration of the stomach wall. Both injuries could be successfully repaired

(Costantino 2006; Guth 1995; Shapiro 1996) (Fig. 19.4) and, in case of gunshot injuries, an unexplained hemothorax (sensitivity: 33%) or a missile near the diaphragm (sensitivity: 36%) (Shackleton 1998).

19.2.3 Tracheobronchial Injury

Injury to the trachea or bronchi occurs in only 0.4–1.5% of blunt trauma patients (Brink 2008b; Mirvis 2003) but can be a direct threat to airway continuity (Cassada 2000) and oxygenation.

CR might indicate tracheobronchial injury by showing subcutaneous emphysema (sensitivity: 75% [Ayed 2004] (Fig 19.5); pneumomediastinum (Fig. 19.5) (i.e., free air surrounding mediastinal arteries and veins, trachea, and esophagus, which is indicated by the thymic sail sign, "ring around the artery" sign, tubular artery sign, double bronchial wall sign, continuous diaphragm sign, extrapleural sign [Zylak 2000], and the elevation of the aortic-pulmonary stripe) (sensitivity: 67% [Ayed 2004]); or a pneumothorax (sensitivity: 67% [Ayed 2004]) that typically persists despite chest tube drainage (Wicky 2000) (Fig. 19.5). More specific, though rarely encountered signs are malposition of the endotracheal tube (overdistension or oblique or extraluminal position of the endotracheal balloon cuff) (Scaglione 2006), distortion of the normal tracheal configuration (Scaglione 2006), intramural gas in the proximal airways (Costantino 2006), or the fallen lung sign. The latter comprises a posterolateral position of a collapsed lung at the distal end of the tracheobronchial injury (Wintermark 2001).

19.2.4 Pulmonary Contusion

Pulmonary contusion is considered to contribute to morbidity and mortality in trauma patients in a substantial way. Depending on the injury severity of the patient population, pulmonary contusion is estimated to occur in 7–75% of blunt trauma patients (Mirvis 2003; Salim 2006b; Blostein 1997). Pulmonary contusion is constituted of disruption of the alveolar capillary membrane, secondary hemorrhage, and parenchymal oedema. On

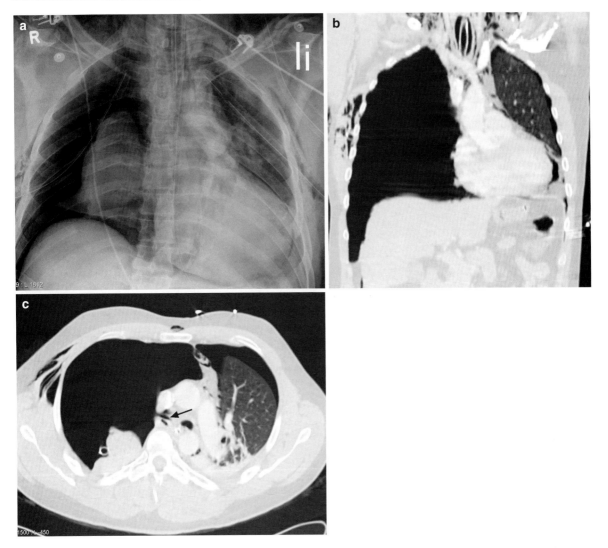

Fig. 19.5 A 35-year-old man was crushed between two heavy vans. This patient's airway was secured with orotracheal intubation, and two chest tubes were placed while the patient was still at the scene of the accident. On arrival at the trauma bay, this patient had respiratory distress with reduced breathing sounds across the right hemithorax, an oxygen saturation of 75%, and a massive air leak from the right chest tube. (**a**) Chest radiography showed mediastinal and subcutaneous emphysema, bilateral persistent pneumothoraces with a mediastinal shift to the left side atelectasis, and signs of pulmonary contusion. (**b**) Multidetector computed tomography confirmed these findings and (**c**) demonstrated a subtotal rupture of the right main bronchus (*arrow*). After selective intubation of the left main bronchus to ensure optimal oxygenation of the left lung, the rupture was repaired by primary closure of the defect after a lateral thoracotomy. The patient fully recovered

CR this shows as irregular focal or multifocal areas of either discrete or confluent ground glass opacities or consolidation, not confined to anatomic limits of the segments and lobes (Fig. 19.6) (Trupka 1997; Wagner 1989). The sensitivity of CR for pulmonary contusion ranges from 27% to 83% (Soldati 2006; Blostein 1997) depending on the severity of the contusion (Figs. 19.6 and 19.7). Pulmonary contusion may be accompanied with pulmonary lacerations or traumatic pneumatoceles in severe cases (Mirvis 2003). These are blood- or air-filled cavities resulting from disruption of the alveolar spaces (Mirvis 2003). Although these lesions are frequently encountered on CT, they are seldom diagnosed with CR (Wagner 1989).

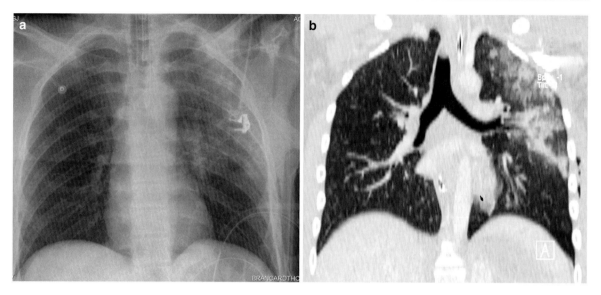

Fig. 19.6 A 16-year-old car occupant was involved in a collision in which the driver died. This patient had orotracheal intubation and received a chest drain in the prehospital setting. On arrival at the emergency department, oxygen saturation was low (76%) with a normal breathing frequency. The patient's hemodynamic status was normal. (**a**) Chest radiography showed subcutaneous emphysema and a large, ill-defined dense area of the left upper lung. (**b**) Multidetector computed tomography (MDCT) demonstrated subcutaneous emphysema and pulmonary contusion: irregular opacities in the area of the left superior lobe. In addition, MDCT demonstrated a pneumothorax and rib fractures of the left hemithorax (not shown)

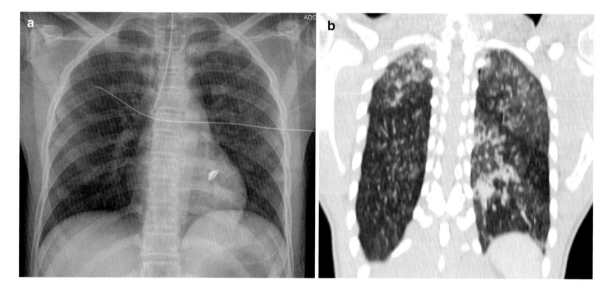

Fig. 19.7 An 18-year-old male driver of a motor-assisted bicycle was involved in a collision with a car. This patient was treated with orotracheal intubation because of a depressed level of consciousness. During physical examination oxygen saturation was 94% and breathing sounds were minimal across both hemithoraces. (**a**) Chest radiography showed selective intubation of the right main bronchus, but there was no suspicion of pulmonary contusion during the initial interpretation of this CR. (**b, c**) However, multidetector computed tomography demonstrated a small ventral pneumothorax and multiple opacities in the dorsal region of both lungs, suggestive of pulmonary contusion. In retrospect, this pulmonary contusion could already have been identified with CR, which showed a subtle decrease in translucency in the left hemithorax

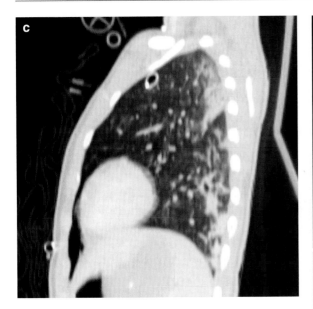

Fig. 19.7 (continued)

19.2.5 Pneumothorax

Although a pneumothorax is encountered in 20–50% of blunt trauma patients (Lamb 2007; Blostein 1997), CR of a patient in a supine position is not very sensitive for pneumothoraces, especially if these lesions have a minimal to moderate size (sensitivity ranges from 24% to 64% [Haramati 1996; Sampson 2006]) (Figs. 19.8 and 19.9). Most patients with pneumothoraces that were missed on CR do not require chest tube insertion (Brasel 1999; Ball 2005). However, it has been suggested that patients who receive ventilatory support have a higher chance of progression of missed pneumothoraces and might therefore benefit from chest tube drainage (Ball 2005).

Signs suggestive of pneumothoraces on CR done with the patient in the supine position include the following: a relatively hyperlucent hemithorax, visualization of the visceral pleura separated from the chest wall with loss of lateral lung markings (Mirvis 2003; Trupka 1997), subcutaneous emphysema (Ball 2005) (Fig. 19.5), demonstration of a deep sulcus sign (Ball 2006; Rhea 1979) (Fig. 19.8), a crisp outline of the mediastinal border or hemidiaphragm (Ball 2006), and a double diaphragm sign that is created by the outlines of the ventral and dorsal portions of the pneumothorax at the anterior and posterior aspects of the hemidiaphragm (Zinck 2000).

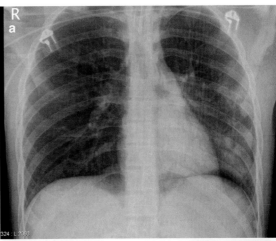

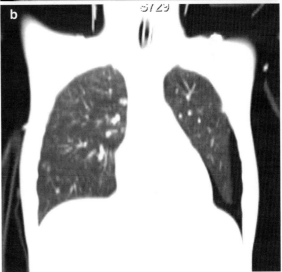

Fig. 19.8 A 19-year-old man who fell from a height of 10 m had orotracheal intubation because of neurological deterioration during the prehospital phase. The primary survey and further physical examination did not reveal any abnormalities. (**a**) Chest radiography demonstrated areas of pulmonary contusion of the left lung and a left, deep, abnormally lucent costophrenic sulcus, suggestive of a pneumothorax. (**b**) This along with other trauma-related abnormalities were verified with multidetector computed tomography. The patient was treated with a chest drain

19.2.6 Hemothorax

Hemothorax is present in 6–11% of blunt trauma patients (Brink 2008b; Traub 2007), but occurs more frequently in patients who have suffered penetrating injury to the chest. Massive arterial hemothoraces may induce ventilation-perfusion mismatch and hypotension. They

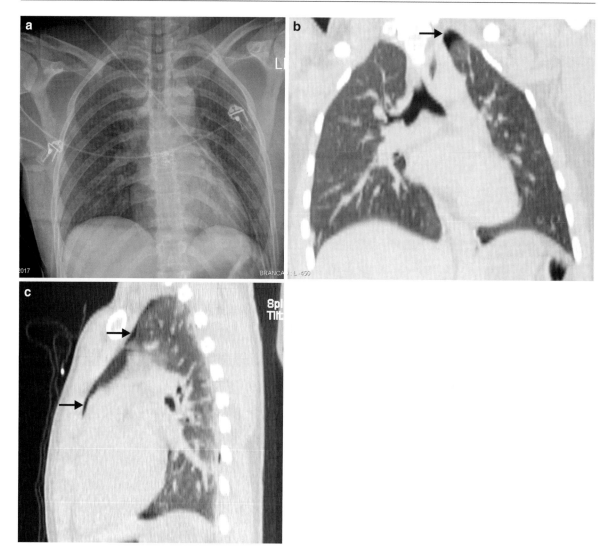

Fig. 19.9 A 24-year-old woman fell from a horse. This patient had no respiratory or hemodynamic abnormalities on arrival at the hospital but had tenderness to palpation of the left hemithorax. (**a**) Chest radiography did not demonstrate any traumatic abnor- mality. (**b, c**) However, multidetector computed tomography revealed several rib fractures of the left hemithorax (not shown) and small pneumothoraces (*arrows*). This patient did not receive chest tube drainage

therefore require adequate diagnosis and immediate drainage or surgical intervention.

Signs of a hemothorax on CR of the supine patient are an increased opacity of the hemithorax, blunting of the costophrenic angles, or an apical pleural cap (Raasch 1982) (Fig. 19.10). However, CR fails to detect a large proportion of patients with hemothoraces; sensitivity ranges from 12% to 44% (Massarutti 2004; Kalavrouziotis 1997) (Fig. 19.11).

19.2.7 Rib Fractures

Rib fractures (incidence of 14–31% among blunt trauma patients [Salim 2006b; Brink 2008b]) are not in them- selves life-threatening injuries; however, their presence has prognostic implications. They are associated with potentially life-threatening chest injuries (Rosado de Christenson 2005; Ungar 2006; Simon 1998), especially if a flail chest (defined as at least two fractures within

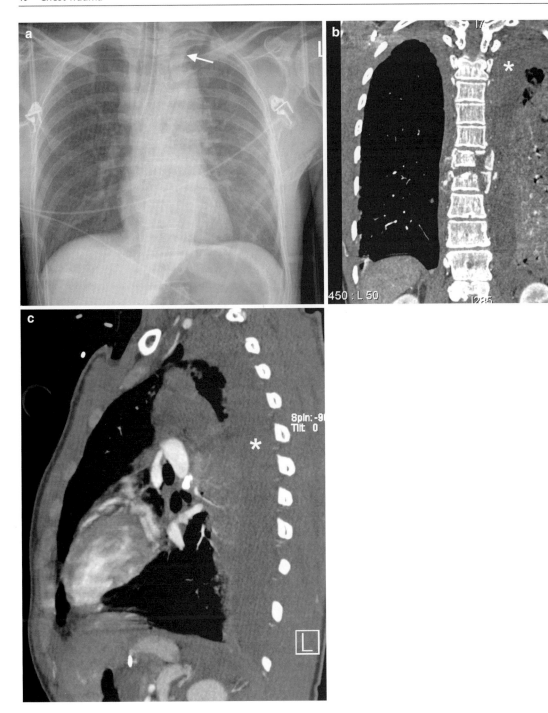

Fig. 19.10 A 32-year-old patient who fell from a height and who was intubated at the scene of the accident because of a depressed level of consciousness had neurological signs of instable spinal injury. On arrival at the hospital the patient's respiratory status was good. However, there was a short episode of hypotension with a systolic blood pressure of 63 mmHg and a heart rate of 80 beats per minute. (**a**) Chest radiography demonstrated selective intubation of the right main bronchus, a left crescent-shaped apical cap (*arrow*), an abnormal and widened mediastinal contour, and abnormal configuration of the thoracic spine, especially at the level of the eighth thoracic vertebra. (**b**) Coronal and (**c**) sagittal multidetector computed tomography reconstructions showed two fractured thoracic spinal corpora, dorsal atelectasis, and pleural effusion with a mean density of 36 Hounsfield units, suggesting a dorsal hemothorax (*asterisks*), which was treated with a chest drain

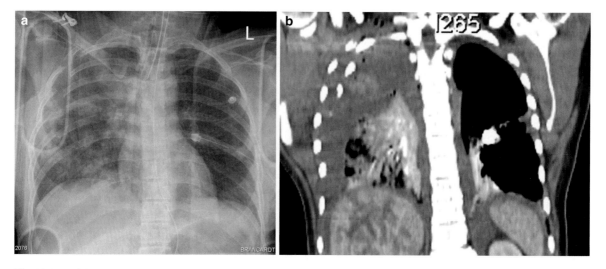

Fig. 19.11 A 34-year-old woman who fell from a height showed a right-sided flail chest during physical examination. She received ventilatory support and a chest tube in the left hemithorax because of clinical suspicion of a pneumothorax. Oxygen saturation was, thereafter, normal. The patient had a tachycardia of 109 bpm at a systolic blood pressure of 120 mmHg. (**a**) Chest radiography demonstrated several rib fractures at the right side and a relatively dense right hemithorax that initially was considered to reflect a pulmonary contusion. (**b**) However, multidetector computed tomography also revealed, among other things, a severe hepatic injury, pleural effusion with a Hounsfield unit density of 40, suggestive of a severe hemothorax. She first underwent chest drain positioning in the right hemithorax, and, eventually, a thoracotomy. She did not survive

one rib in three or more consecutive ribs) is present (Borman 2006) (Fig. 19.11).

CR is specific but not sensitive in the detection of rib fractures; CR demonstrates rib fractures in only 60–87% of patients with this injury (Exadaktylos 2001; Brink 2008b) (Figs. 19.6 and 19.9). The suspicion for rib fractures should be raised if one or more associated injuries are seen on CR. These injuries include pneumothorax, hemothorax, and pulmonary contusions.

(Wicky 2000). The degree of displacement can be quantified by comparing the distance between the medial border of the scapula and the spinous process of the third vertebra or the distance between the sternal notch and the medial margins of the coracoid process or the glenoid fossa. In addition, associated injuries that can indicate scapulothoracic dislocation are acromioclavicular separation, a displaced clavicular fracture, or sternoclavicular separation (Ebraheim 1988; Brucker 2005) (Fig. 19.12).

19.2.8 Scapulothoracic Dissociation

This injury is very rare and often is associated with injury to the brachial plexus and the thoracic inlet veins and arteries. It is therefore important to recognize this injury on CR to indicate the need for further diagnostic workup to evaluate damage of the vessels and nerves (Ebraheim 1988).

The presence of scapulothoracic dissociation is reflected by lateral displacement of the medial border of the scapula on CR (specificity: 80%; sensitivity: 60%)

19.3 Conclusion

CR of the supine trauma patient is difficult to interpret and not as sensitive as CT for relevant traumatic injuries. However, besides the fact that CR can quickly confirm the clinical diagnosis of abnormalities that need rapid treatment, CR also serves as an initial screening to direct the need for further imaging. For this, special attention should be paid to subtle signs on CR that indicate relevant injuries that can only be accurately diagnosed with CT.

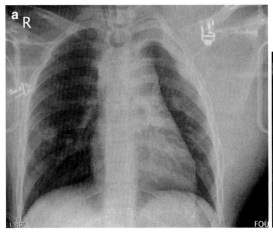
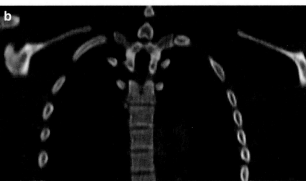

Fig. 19.12 A 16-year-old man whose scooter collided with a tractor showed massive soft tissue swelling of the shoulder. (**a**) Among a widened mediastinum, a left apical cap, opacification of the aortopulmonary window, and pulmonary contusion, chest radiography and (**b**) multidetector computed tomography demonstrated signs of severe scapulothoracic dissociation: sternoclavicular separation, lateral displacement of the scapula, and enlargement of (*1*) the distance between the medial border of the scapula and the spinous process of the third vertebra and (*2*) the distance between the sternal notch and the medial margins of the coracoid process and the glenoid fossa. This patient had severe injuries of the brachial plexus and subclavian artery and vein. These lesions were all treated surgically

References

Abboud PA, Kendall J (2003) Emergency department ultrasound for hemothorax after blunt traumatic injury. J Emerg Med 25:181–184

American College of Surgeons Committee on Trauma (2004) Thoracic trauma. In: Advanced Trauma Life Support for Doctors. 7th American College of Surgeons Committee on Trauma, Chicago, pp 103–124

Ayed AK, Al-Shawaf E (2004) Diagnosis and treatment of traumatic intrathoracic major bronchial disruption. Injury 35: 494–499

Ball CG, Kirkpatrick AW, Laupland KB, Fox DI, Nicolaou S, Anderson IB, Hameed SM, Kortbeek JB, Mulloy RR, Litvinchuk S, Boulanger BR (2005) Incidence, risk factors, and outcomes for occult pneumothoraces in victims of major trauma. J Trauma 59:917–924

Ball CG, Kirkpatrick AW, Fox DL, Laupland KB, Louis LJ, Andrews GD, Dunlop MP, Kortbeek JB, Nicolaou S (2006) Are occult pneumothoraces truly occult or simply missed? J Trauma 60:294–298

Blostein PA, Hodgman CG (1997) Computed tomography of the chest in blunt thoracic trauma: results of a prospective study. J Trauma 43:13–18

Borman JB, Aharonson-Daniel L, Savitsky B, Peleg K (2006) Unilateral flail chest is seldom a lethal injury. Emerg Med J 23:903–905

Brasel KJ, Stafford RE, Weigelt JA, Tenquist JE, Borgstrom DC (1999) Treatment of occult pneumothoraces from blunt trauma. J Trauma 46:987–991

Brenner D, Huda W (2008) Effective dose: a useful concept in diagnostic radiology. Radiat Prot Dosimetry 128:503–508

Brink M, de Lange, Oostveen LJ, Dekker HM, Kool DR, Deunk J, Edwards MJR, van Kuijk C, Kamman RL, Blickman JG (2008a) Arm raising at exposure-controlled multidetector trauma CT of thoracoabdominal region: Higher image quality, lower radiation dose. Radiology 249:661–670

Brink M, Deunk J, Dekker HM, Kool DR, Edwards MJR, van Vugt AB, Blickman JG (2008b) Added value of routine chest MDCT after blunt trauma: evaluation of additional findings and impact on patient management. AJR Am J Roentgenol 190:1591–1598

Broder J, Warshauer DM (2006) Increasing utilization of computed tomography in the adult emergency department, 2000–2005. Emerg Radiol 13:25–30

Brucker PU, Gruen GS, Kaufmann RA (2005) Scapulothoracic dissociation: evaluation and management. Injury 36:1147–1155

Cassada DC, Munyikwa MP, Moniz MP, Dieter RA Jr, Schuchmann GF, Enderson BL (2000) Acute injuries of the trachea and major bronchi: importance of early diagnosis. Ann Thorac Surg 69:1563–1567

Chen MY, Miller PR, McLaughlin CA, Kortesis BG, Kavanagh PV, Dyer RB (2004) The trend of using computed tomography in the detection of acute thoracic aortic and branch vessel injury after blunt thoracic trauma: single-center experience over 13 years. J Trauma 56:783–785

Cook AD, Klein JS, Rogers FB, Osler TM, Shackford SR (2001) Chest radiographs of limited utility in the diagnosis of blunt traumatic aortic laceration. J Trauma 50:843–847

Costantino M, Gosselin MV, Primack SL (2006) The ABC's of thoracic trauma imaging. Semin Roentgenol 41:209–225

Rosado de Christenson, M L D S e (2005) ACR Appropriateness Criteria: Rib fractures.

Demetriades D, Gomez H, Velmahos GC et al (1998) Routine helical computed tomographic evaluation of the mediastinum in high-risk blunt trauma patients. Arch Surg 133:1084–1088

Dyer DS, Moore EE, Ilke DN et al (2000) Thoracic aortic injury: how predictive is mechanism and is chest computed tomography a reliable screening tool? A prospective study of 1, 561 patients. J Trauma 48:673–682

Ebraheim NA, An HS, Jackson WT, Pearlstein SR, Burgess A, Tscherne H, Hass N, Kellam J, Wipperman BU (1988) Scapulothoracic dissociation. J Bone Joint Surg Am 70: 428–432

Erpenbach S, Gerlach A, Arlart IP (1995) Rational diagnosis of traumatic aortic rupture. Bildgebung 62:24–30

Exadaktylos AK, Sclabas G, Schmid SW, Schaller B, Zimmermann H (2001) Do we really need routine computed tomographic scanning in the primary evaluation of blunt chest trauma in patients with "normal" chest radiograph? J Trauma 51:1173–1176

Fabian TC, Davis KA, Gavant ML, Croce MA, Melton SM, Patton JH Jr, Haan CK, Weiman DS, Pate JW (1998) Prospective study of blunt aortic injury: helical CT is diagnostic and antihypertensive therapy reduces rupture. Ann Surg 227:666–676

Gibbs JM, Chandrasekhar CA, Ferguson EC, Oldham SA (2007) Lines and stripes: where did they go?–From conventional radiography to CT. Radiographics 27:33–48

Gleeson CE, Spedding RL, Harding LA, Caplan M (2001) The mediastinum – is it wide? Emerg Med J 18:183–185

Grieser T, Buhne KH, Hauser H, Bohndorf K (2001) Significance of findings of chest X-rays and thoracic CT routinely performed at the emergency unit: 102 patients with multiple trauma. A prospective study. Rofo 173:44–51

Guerrero-Lopez F, Vazquez-Mata G, cazar-Romero PP, Fernandez-Mondejar E, guayo-Hoyos E, Linde-Valverde CM (2000) Evaluation of the utility of computed tomography in the initial assessment of the critical care patient with chest trauma. Crit Care Med 28:1370–1375

Guth AA, Pachter HL, Kim U (1995) Pitfalls in the diagnosis of blunt diaphragmatic injury. Am J Surg 170:5–9

Haramati LB, Hochsztein JG, Marciano N, Nathanson N (1996) Evaluation of the role of chest computed tomography in the management of trauma patients. Emerg Radiol 3:225–230

Ho RT, Blackmore CC, Bloch RD et al (2002) Can we rely on mediastinal widening on chest radiography to identify subjects with aortic injury? Emerg Radiol 9:183–187

Kalavrouziotis G, Athanassiadi K, Exarchos N (1997) Emergent axial computed tomography in the diagnosis and management of blunt thoracic trauma. Eur J Cardiothorac Surg 12:158–159

Kirkham JR, Blackmore CC (2007) Screening for aortic injury with chest radiography and clinical factors. Emerg Radiol 14:211–217

Lamb AD, Qadan M, Gray AJ (2007) Detection of occult pneumothoraces in the significantly injured adult with blunt trauma. Eur J Emerg Med 14:65–67

Lopes JA, Frankel HL, Bokhari SJ, Bank M, Tandon M, Rabinovici R (2006) The trauma bay chest radiograph in stable blunt-trauma patients: do we really need it? Am Surg 72:31–34

Marsh DG, Sturm JT (1976) Traumatic aortic rupture: roentgenographic indications for angiography. Ann Thorac Surg 21:337–340

Massarutti D, Berlot G, Saltarini M, Trillo G, D'Orlando L, Pessina F, Modesto A, Meduri S, Da RT, Carchietti E (2004) Abdominal ultrasonography and chest radiography are of limited value in the emergency room diagnostic work-up of severe trauma patients with hypotension on the scene of accident. Radiol Med (Torino) 108:218–224

Mengozzi E, Burzi M, Miceli M, Lipparini M, Sartoni GS (2000) Application of spiral computerized tomography in the study of traumatic lesions of the thoracic aorta. Radiol Med (Torino) 100:139–144

Mettler FA Jr, Huda W, Yoshizumi TT, Mahesh M (2008) Effective doses in radiology and diagnostic nuclear medicine: a catalog. Radiology 248:254–263

Mirvis SE, Shanmuganathan K (2003) Diagnostic imaging of thoracic trauma. In: Ross A (ed) Imaging in thoracic trauma and critical care, 2nd edn. Saunders, Philadelphia, pp 297–368

Mirvis SE, Shanmuganathan K, Buell J, Rodriguez A (1998) Use of spiral computed tomography for the assessment of blunt trauma patients with potential aortic injury. J Trauma 45:922–930

Murray JA, Demetriades D, Asensio JA, Cornwell EE III, Velmahos GC, Belzberg H, Berne TV (1998) Occult injuries to the diaphragm: prospective evaluation of laparoscopy in penetrating injuries to the left lower chest. J Am Coll Surg 187:626–630

Omert L, Yeaney WW, Protech J (2001) Efficacy of thoracic computerized tomography in blunt chest trauma. Am Surg 67:660–664

Parker MS, Matheson TL, Rao AV, Sherbourne CD, Jordan KG, Landay MJ, Miller GL, Summa JA (2001) Making the transition: the role of helical CT in the evaluation of potentially acute thoracic aortic injuries. AJR Am J Roentgenol 176:1267–1272

Parmley LF, Mattingly TW, Manion WC, Jahnke EJ (1958) Nonpenetrating traumatic injury of the aorta. Circulation 17:1086–1101

Raasch BN, Carsky EW, Lane EJ, ÓCallaghan JP, Heitzman ER (1982) Pleural effusion: explanation of some typical appearances. AJR Am J Roentgenol 139:899–904

Reber PU, Schmied B, Seiler CA, Baer HU, Patel AG, Buchler MW (1998) Missed diaphragmatic injuries and their long-term sequelae. J Trauma 44:183–188

Rhea JT, vanSonnenberg E, McLoud TC (1979) Basilar pneumothorax in the supine adult. Radiology 133:593–595

Rieger M, Sparr H, Esterhammer R, Fink C, Bale R, Czermak B, Jaschke W (2002) Modern CT diagnosis of acute thoracic and abdominal trauma. Anaesthesist 51:835–842

Rowan KR, Kirkpatrick AW, Liu D, Forkheim KE, Mayo JR, Nicolaou S (2002) Traumatic pneumothorax detection with thoracic US: correlation with chest radiography and CT–initial experience. Radiology 225:210–214

Salim A, Sangthong B, Martin M, Brown C, Plurad D, Demetriades D (2006) Whole body imaging in blunt multisystem trauma patients without obvious signs of injury: results of a prospective study. Arch Surg 141:468–473

Sampson MA, Colquhoun KB, Hennessy NL (2006) Computed tomography whole body imaging in multi-trauma: 7 years experience. Clin Radiol 61:365–369

Sandor F (1967) Incidence and significance of traumatic mediastinal haematoma. Thorax 22:43–62

Scaglione M, Romano S, Pinto A, Sparano A, Scialpi M, Rotondo A (2006) Acute tracheobronchial injuries: Impact of imaging on diagnosis and management implications. Eur J Radiol 59:336–343

Shackleton KL, Stewart ET, Taylor AJ (1998) Traumatic diaphragmatic injuries: spectrum of radiographic findings. Radiographics 18:49–59

Shapiro MJ, Heiberg E, Durham RM, Luchtefeld W, Mazuski JE (1996) The unreliability of CT scans and initial chest radiographs in evaluating blunt trauma induced diaphragmatic rupture. Clin Radiol 51:27–30

Simeone JF, Minagi H, Putman CE (1975) Traumatic disruption of the thoracic aorta: Significance of the left extrapleural cap. Radiology 117:265–268

Simon BJ, Chu Q, Emhoff TA, Fiallo VM, Lee KF (1998) Delayed hemothorax after blunt thoracic trauma: an uncommon entity with significant morbidity. J Trauma 45:673–676

Soldati G, Testa A, Silva FR, Carbone L, Portale G, Silveri NG (2006) Chest ultrasonography in lung contusion. Chest 130:533–538

Sriussadaporn S, Luengtaviboon K, Benjacholamas V, Singhatanadige S (2000) Significance of a widened mediastinum in blunt chest trauma patients. J Med Assoc Thai 83:1296–1301

Stiell IG, Wells GA (1999) Methodologic standards for the development of clinical decision rules in emergency medicine. Ann Emerg Med 33:437–447

Traub M, Stevenson M, McEvoy S et al (2007) The use of chest computed tomography versus chest X-ray in patients with major blunt trauma. Injury 38:43–47

Trupka A, Waydhas C, Hallfeldt KK, Nast-Kolb D, Pfeifer KJ, Schweiberer L (1997) Value of thoracic computed tomography in the first assessment of severely injured patients with blunt chest trauma: results of a prospective study. J Trauma 43:405–411

Ungar TC, Wolf SJ, Haukoos JS, Dyer DS, Moore EE (2006) Derivation of a clinical decision rule to exclude thoracic aortic imaging in patients with blunt chest trauma after motor vehicle collisions. J Trauma 61:1150–1155

van Vugt AB, Schoots FJ (1989) Acute diaphragmatic rupture due to blunt trauma: a retrospective analysis. J Trauma 29:683–686

Wagner RB, Jamieson PM (1989) Pulmonary contusion. Evaluation and classification by computed tomography. Surg Clin North Am 69:31–40

Wicky S, Wintermark M, Schnyder P, Capasso P, Denys A (2000) Imaging of blunt chest trauma. Eur Radiol 10:1524–1538

Wintermark M, Schnyder P, Wicky S (2001) Blunt traumatic rupture of a mainstem bronchus: spiral CT demonstration of the "fallen lung" sign. Eur Radiol 11:409–411

Wisbach GG, Sise MJ, Sack DI, Swanson SM, Sundquist SM, Paci GM, Kingdon KM, Kaminski SS (2007) What is the role of chest X-ray in the initial assessment of stable trauma patients? J Trauma 62:74–78

Wong YC, Ng CJ, Wang LJ, Hsu KH, Chen CJ (2004) Left mediastinal width and mediastinal width ratio are better radiographic criteria than general mediastinal width for predicting blunt aortic injury. J Trauma 57:88–94

Woodring JH (1990) The normal mediastinum in blunt traumatic rupture of the thoracic aorta and brachiocephalic arteries. J Emerg Med 8:467–476

Wurmb TE, Fruhwald P, Hopfner W, Roewer N, Brederlau J (2007) Whole-body multislice computed tomography as the primary and sole diagnostic tool in patients with blunt trauma: searching for its appropriate indication. Am J Emerg Med 25:1057–1062

Zinck SE, Primack SL (2000) Radiographic and CT findings in blunt chest trauma. J Thorac Imaging 15:87–96

Zylak CM, Standen JR, Barnes GR, Zylak CJ (2000) Pneumomediastinum revisited. Radiographics 20:1043–1057

Index